Scott-Brown's
DISEASES OF THE EAR,
NOSE AND THROAT

VOLUME 4

Scott-Brown's

DISEASES OF THE

Edited by

JOHN BALLANTYNE
F.R.C.S., D.L.O.

Consultant Ear, Nose and Throat Surgeon,
Royal Free Hospital, London

and

JOHN GROVES
M.B., B.S., F.R.C.S.

Consultant Ear, Nose and Throat Surgeon,
Royal Free Hospital, London

Titles of other volumes:
VOLUME 1: BASIC SCIENCES
VOLUME 2: THE EAR
VOLUME 3: THE NOSE

EAR, NOSE AND THROAT

THIRD EDITION

VOLUME 4
THE THROAT

PHILADELPHIA
J. B. LIPPINCOTT COMPANY

First published by Butterworth & Co. (Publishers) Ltd.

Distributed in the United States of America by
J. B. Lippincott Company, East Washington Square
Philadelphia, Pa. 19105

First Edition 1952
Second Edition 1965
Reprinted 1967
Reprinted 1968
Third Edition 1971

Suggested U.D.C. Number: 616·21

ISBN 0 407 14987 2   Individual copies
ISBN 0 407 14983 X   Set of 4 volumes

Printed and bound in Great Britain by
R. J. Acford Ltd., Industrial Estate, Chichester, Sussex.

CONTENTS

		PAGE
LIST OF CONTRIBUTORS		vii
LIST OF COLOUR PLATES		ix
INTRODUCTION TO THE THIRD EDITION		xi
INTRODUCTION TO THE SECOND EDITION		xiii
INTRODUCTION TO THE FIRST EDITION		xv

PART I

DISEASES OF THE MOUTH, PHARYNX AND OESOPHAGUS

CHAPTER

1. METHODS OF EXAMINATION OF THE MOUTH AND PHARYNX — 3
   A. Bowen-Davies

2. DISEASES OF THE MOUTH — 17
   David Downton

3. DISEASES OF THE SALIVARY GLANDS — 37
   Douglas Ranger

4. PHARYNGITIS—ACUTE AND CHRONIC — 67
   A. Bowen-Davies

5. PHARYNGEAL LESIONS ASSOCIATED WITH GENERAL DISEASES — 87
   A. Bowen-Davies

6. DISEASES OF THE TONSILS AND ADENOIDS (EXCLUDING NEOPLASMS) — 103
   S. Mawson

7. TUMOURS OF THE PHARYNX — 147
   R. S. Lewis

8. HYPOPHARYNGEAL DIVERTICULUM (PHARYNGEAL POUCH) — 197
   John Ballantyne

9. OESOPHAGEAL CONDITIONS IN THE PRACTICE OF EAR, NOSE AND THROAT SURGERY — 207
   E. H. Miles Foxen and John Groves

CONTENTS

PART II

DISEASES OF THE LARYNX AND TRACHEOBRONCHIAL TREE

10. METHODS OF EXAMINING THE LARYNX AND TRACHEOBRONCHIAL TREE 249
    R. S. Lewis

11. CONGENITAL DISEASES OF THE LARYNX   –   –   –   –   – 281
    R. Pracy

12. TRAUMA AND STENOSIS OF THE LARYNX   –   –   –   –   – 301
    Douglas Ranger

13. ACUTE LARYNGITIS –   –   –   –   –   –   –   – 311
    Maxwell Ellis

14. CHRONIC LARYNGITIS   –   –   –   –   –   –   – 333
    Maxwell Ellis

15. TUMOURS OF THE LARYNX   –   –   –   –   –   – 375
    Henry Shaw

16. CERVICAL NODE DISSECTION   –   –   –   –   – 459
    Maxwell Ellis

17. SKIN GRAFTING   –   –   –   –   –   –   – 473
    R. L. G. Dawson

18. PRINCIPLES OF RADIOTHERAPY AND CHEMOTHERAPY IN MALIGNANT
    DISEASE OF THE HEAD AND NECK   –   –   –   –   – 489
    D. F. N. Harrison

19. INTUBATION OF THE LARYNX, LARYNGOTOMY AND TRACHEOSTOMY – 505
    Douglas Ranger

20. NEUROLOGICAL AFFECTIONS OF THE LARYNX   –   –   – 525
    John Ballantyne

21. OCCUPATIONAL DISORDERS OF THE LARYNX   –   –   – 541
    John Ballantyne

22. DISORDERS OF SPEECH   –   –   –   –   –   –   – 559
    C. H. Edwards

23. LOWER RESPIRATORY CONDITIONS IN THE PRACTICE OF EAR, NOSE
    AND THROAT SURGERY   –   –   –   –   –   –   – 583
    E. H. Miles Foxen

CONTRIBUTORS TO THIS VOLUME

JOHN BALLANTYNE, F.R.C.S., D.L.O.
Consultant Ear, Nose and Throat Surgeon, Royal Free Hospital, London

A. BOWEN-DAVIES, M.B., B.Ch., F.R.C.S.
Consultant Surgeon, Ear, Nose and Throat Department, The London Hospital

R. L. G. DAWSON, M.B., B.S., F.R.C.S.
Consultant Plastic Surgeon, Royal Free Hospital, London, Mount Vernon Centre for Plastic Surgery, Northwood, and Royal National Orthopaedic Hospital, London

DAVID DOWNTON, F.D.S.R.C.S.
Senior Consultant Oral Surgeon, Royal Free Hospital, London

C. H. EDWARDS, F.R.C.P.
Consultant Physician, Department of Nervous Diseases, St. Mary's Hospital, London; Consultant Neurologist to the Royal National Throat, Nose and Ear Hospital, London; Lecturer in Neurology, Institute of Laryngology and Otology, London; Consultant Neurologist, King Edward VII Hospital, Windsor, Canadian Red Cross Memorial Hospital, Taplow, and Maidenhead Hospital

MAXWELL ELLIS, M.D., M.S., F.R.C.S.
Dean of the Institute of Laryngology and Otology; Surgeon, Royal National Throat, Nose and Ear Hospital, London; Ear, Nose and Throat Surgeon, Central Middlesex Hospital, London

E. H. MILES FOXEN, F.R.C.S., D.L.O.
Consultant Surgeon, Ear, Nose and Throat Department, Westminster Hospital and Westminster Teaching Group of Hospitals, London; Consultant Ear, Nose and Throat Surgeon, Chelsea Hospital for Women and Queen Charlotte's Maternity Hospital, London

JOHN GROVES, M.B., B.S., F.R.C.S.
Consultant Ear, Nose and Throat Surgeon, Royal Free Hospital, London

D. F. N. HARRISON, M.D., M.S., F.R.C.S.
Professor of Laryngology and Otology, Institute of Laryngology and Otology, London; Surgeon, Royal National Throat, Nose and Ear Hospital, London

CONTRIBUTORS TO THIS VOLUME

R. S. LEWIS, M.A., M.B., B.Ch., F.R.C.S.

> Consultant Surgeon, Ear, Nose and Throat Department, King's College Hospital, London; Ear, Nose and Throat Surgeon, Mount Vernon Hospital, Northwood

S. MAWSON, F.R.C.S., D.L.O.

> Consultant Surgeon, Ear, Nose, and Throat Department, King's College Hospital and Belgrave Hospital for Children, London; Consultant Ear, Nose and Throat Surgeon, Queen Mary's Hospital, Roehampton

R. PRACY, M.B., B.S., F.R.C.S.

> Director of the Department of Otorhinolaryngology, University of Liverpool; Consultant Ear, Nose and Throat Surgeon, United Liverpool Hospitals and Alder Hey Children's Hospital

DOUGLAS RANGER, M.B., B.S., F.R.C.S.

> Consultant Senior Surgeon, Ear, Nose and Throat Department, The Middlesex Hospital, London; Ear, Nose and Throat Surgeon, Mount Vernon Hospital, Northwood; Ear, Nose and Throat Surgeon, St. Andrew's Hospital, London

HENRY SHAW, V.R.D., M.A., F.R.C.S.

> Director of the Head and Neck Unit, Royal Marsden Hospital; Consultant Ear, Nose and Throat Surgeon to the Royal National Throat, Nose and Ear Hospital, London, Royal Marsden Hospital, London, and Northwood and Pinner Memorial Hospital

COLOUR PLATES IN THIS VOLUME

FACING PAGE

I   Diphtheria of the fauces   –   –   –   –   –   –   –   –   112

II Acute laryngitis –   –   –   –   –   –   –   –   –   320

III Radio-necrosis and perichondritis with abscess formation   –   –   321

IV (a) Massive tuberculous infiltration of the epiglottis and ventricular
      bands   –   –   –   –   –   –   –   –   –   –   –   336
     (b) Healed tuberculosis with massive fibrosis
     (c) Lupus showing the fibrosis of healing over the arytenoids and ary-
      epiglottic folds
     (d) Syphilis. A gummatous involvement of the whole of the left side
      of the larynx

V (a) Chronic localized hyperplastic laryngitis –   –   –   –   –   337
   (b) Interarytenoid pachydermia

VI (a) Intubation granulomas on the vocal processes of the arytenoids   384
    (b) Fibroma growing from the edge of the right vocal cord
    (c) Retention cyst of the left vallecula
    (d) Pedunculated papilloma growing from the anterior commissure
    (e) Single papilloma of right vocal cord on quiet respiration
    (f) Effect of phonation on papilloma shown in (e)

VII (a) Multiple papillomas in the larynx   –   –   –   –   –   384
    (b) Bilateral vocal nodules in the typical position
    (c) Multiple congenital telangiectases in the larynx (Osler–Rendu
     disease)
    (d) Large angioma of the right ventricular band and aryepiglottic fold
    (e) Chondroma growing from the right arytenoid
    (f) Retention cyst of left laryngeal ventricle projecting into the larynx
    between the left vocal cord and ventricular band

VIII (a) Stage 1 carcinoma limited to the membranous right vocal cord.
     Irradiation is the treatment of choice   –   –   –   –   385
    (b) Carcinoma involving the anterior commissure and anterior thirds
    of both vocal cords (Stage 2). Irradiation preferable to partial
    laryngectomy
    (c)Stage 3 glottic carcinoma involving the anterior third of the left cord,
    the anterior commissure, the base of the epiglottis and the whole
    length of the right vocal cord to include the arytenoid. Some reduced
    mobility of the right cord. Total laryngectomy would be the treat-
    ment of choice

COLOUR PLATES IN THIS VOLUME

FACING PAGE

(*d*) Early (Stage 1) carcinoma of left aryepiglottic fold. Treatment by 385
    irradiation or partial laryngectomy

(*e*) Stage 2 carcinoma of right ventricle involving the middle third of
    the right vocal cord. Treatment by irradiation or total laryngectomy

(*f*) Subglottic (Stage 1) carcinoma beneath mobile right vocal cord.
    No posterior extension. Irradiation is the treatment of choice

(*g*) Extensive epiglottic carcinoma (Stage 2). Treatment by total
    laryngectomy

(*h*) Massive carcinoma involving whole fixed right hemilarynx with
    subglottic extension and two mobile palpable homolateral neck nodes
    (Stage 3). Treatment by total laryngectomy with right radical
    block dissection in continuity

IX   The use of Disulphine Blue as a tracer dye –   –   –   –   – 496

X   (*a*) Non-infective laryngitis   –   –   –   –   –   –   – 552
   (*b*) Submucosal haemorrhages of the vocal cords
   (*c*) Singers' nodules
   (*d*) Contact ulcer

INTRODUCTION TO THE THIRD EDITION

A radical new departure is made in the presentation of this work in four separately available volumes. This has been done for two main reasons. First, there is a real need, we feel, to recognize the diverse requirements of different readers—the newcomer to the specialty who needs a compact presentation of the special anatomy, physiology and radiology (for preparation for the D.L.O. Part I and Primary F.R.C.S. examinations), and the specialist who is more interested in, say, the ear than in the throat. Secondly, advances are more numerous and more rapid in some sub-divisions of the specialty than in others so that it will be advantageous in the future to revise one volume at a time. The reduction in bulk of the individual volumes results, we hope, in easier handling and more pleasant reading.

A consequence of this change in format and policy is that page and chapter cross-references between different volumes cannot be given, nor is it practicable any longer to compile the symptom index featured in the last edition. To offset the former disadvantage some overlapping of subject material has been deliberately introduced wherever it was felt that too frequent referral to another volume would otherwise be necessary. Each volume has its own Table of Contents and Index, the latter compiled on the basis of noun-entries only.

The text throughout has been comprehensively revised. As a matter of general editorial policy, for this and for any subsequent editions which may appear under our direction, we have invited contributions only from those of our colleagues who are still actively engaged in hospital, university or college practice; and it has been our pleasure to welcome several new contributors. By including several new chapters, we have been able to remedy some of the omissions from earlier editions (for example, "Congenital Diseases of the Larynx"), and also to give due emphasis to such topics as "Acoustic Trauma" and "Acoustic Neuroma", each of which now demands a separate chapter. The weights and liquid measures of all drugs, as well as the measures of distance, are all given in the metric system.

We are grateful to all the authors for submitting their work on schedule so that the production can be uniformly up-to-date. We warmly appreciate the efforts and enthusiasm of the Publisher's Editorial Staff, and the kind help we have received from colleagues, artists, and many friends too numerous to be named. It has been a tremendous encouragement to have the continuing interest of Mr. W. G. Scott-Brown, C.V.O., M.D., F.R.C.S., who has read and contributed substantially to the editing of a large part of this edition. We wish to thank him for the honour of his invitation to join in the Editorship of this standard textbook, which was established solely by him in the First Edition of 1952. Although he has now handed over completely the pleasant duties of joint Editorship to us and our successors, it remains his book and it retains his name.

London, 1971
JOHN BALLANTYNE
JOHN GROVES

xi

INTRODUCTION TO THE SECOND EDITION

The objects set out in the Introduction to the First Edition have been the guiding principles in the present work. In order to make this new edition authoritative and contemporary in outlook, I asked two of my colleagues to join me as co-editors and I have been most fortunate in having the help and inspiration of John Ballantyne and John Groves. We have together re-cast the main sections, subsections and chapters and have given more emphasis to those departments of the specialty which have undergone the greatest changes. We have also made great efforts to have all contributions written and despatched to the printer within one year of starting the project, in order that all the articles shall be finished at the same time and be up to date when published. This object has been achieved thanks to the co-operation of our contributors.

It will be seen that the sections on physiology have been extended and improved and the chapters on the ear have been considerably altered and enlarged to include the many fresh ideas and techniques associated with both infective and non-infective ear conditions. The sections on endoscopy have been re-arranged to make the subject as practical as possible for our specialty. It is hoped that the necessary curtailment has not given rise to any major omissions. Neoplasms of the larynx and pharynx have been separated and new chapters on voice and speech have been introduced.

The index has been completely revised, and an innovation in a textbook of this size is an additional index—a symptom index—which is complete for the whole work at the end of each volume. It is hoped that this may be particularly useful to candidates for higher examinations and to general practitioners looking for causes of particular symptoms.

It is a pleasure to acknowledge the generous help which has been given by all the contributors, a number of them new to this book, and to artists and friends, for their kindly and stimulating interest. It is not possible here to record individual acknowledgments, but a special word of thanks must be made to the Editorial Staff of the Publishers.

London, 1965   W. G. SCOTT-BROWN

INTRODUCTION TO THE FIRST EDITION

This work has been compiled with the object of presenting a textbook on Diseases of the Ear, Nose and Throat which would include most of the subject matter required by students and post-graduates with sufficient detail for those taking the higher specialized qualifications. It should also be a suitable reference book for general practice.

To achieve this it was decided to ask a number of teachers, examiners and other well-recognized authorities in the specialty to contribute articles on this general plan while leaving them free to put forward their own views of the particular subject in their own way. This has in some cases meant the presentation of individual preferences, classifications or theories, but as far as possible these have been integrated with the more usual views to give a balanced appreciation of the subject. It is hoped that this individuality of articles will give a more stimulating approach to the subject in spite of some overlapping of subject matter and differences of opinion.

Each section is prefaced by its anatomy and physiology as an essential basis to the understanding of the subject, and also to include in a concise manner the material necessary for the examinee. Methods of examination on the other hand have been cut to a minimum as they can only be learnt by the practical examination of patients. After considerable deliberation it was decided to include a chapter on plastic surgery of the nose and ear which should set out what can be done rather than entering into details of technique which are largely the province of the Plastic Surgeon.

My thanks are due in the first place to all the contributors who have lightened the editorial burden: they have all been most co-operative and have given freely of their time, knowledge and, in many cases, helpful criticism. Acknowledgment is made in the text for opinions and illustrations used.

I must particularly thank the Publisher's team, all of whom have been not only helpful but also encouraging during the many unavoidable delays and difficulties in the production of a new work.

London, 1952

W. G. SCOTT-BROWN

PART I
DISEASES OF THE MOUTH, PHARYNX AND OESOPHAGUS

METHODS OF EXAMINATION OF THE MOUTH AND PHARYNX

A. BOWEN-DAVIES

INTRODUCTION

Lighting is provided by a concave forehead mirror with a focal length of 23·6 cm. (9 in.) and a hole 2 cm. ($\frac{3}{4}$ in.) in diameter at the centre through which the surgeon looks and by means of which light is reflected from a bullseye lamp. Thus, any part that can be seen is brilliantly illuminated. The diameter of the mirror is 9 cm. ($3\frac{1}{2}$ in.), so the vision of the other eye is not obscured and binocular vision is retained.

The bullseye lamp is suspended from a bracket on the wall, or attached to a stand with a heavy base. It is movable from side to side and backwards and forwards so that it may be placed in the proper position, just behind the patient's left ear and 30 cm. (12 in.) to the left of it. This protects the patient from the considerable heat of the lamp and ensures that the beam does not fall directly on the eyes of the examiner, which are protected by the head mirror. An advantage of this form of lighting is that both hands are free to carry out the examination. Movement of the examiner's head is very much restricted however, as the mirror must be kept in the beam of light. The patient must be moved to bring the part under examination into the appropriate position.

An alternative source of lighting is a headlight. This has a low voltage bulb and a lens by which the beam may be focused. It is worn on the head with the light as close to the bridge of the nose as possible (the lamp becomes very hot) so that the beam of light coincides as nearly as possible with the line of vision. Illumination by this means is not as perfect as that provided by a head mirror, but the movement of the surgeon's head is not restricted, which is an advantage when operating under general anaesthesia. It is also convenient when visiting patients at home, when it may be run off a dry battery. Whatever form of lighting is used, illumination is greatly improved if the room is darkened.

EXAMINATION OF THE MOUTH

First, examine the lips and note whether the mouth is closed during quiet respiration. Prominent upper incisor teeth, usually associated with a short upper lip, may be a familial characteristic which naturally predisposes to mouth breathing, while the habit of sucking the thumb may aggravate the situation. Nasal or postnasal obstruction of the airway necessitates mouth breathing, which may persist as a habit after the obstruction has been relieved unless corrected by breathing exercises. Chronic mouth breathing causes hypertrophy of the gum in the region of the upper incisor teeth.

In cases of illness with a high temperature, the lips become dry and cracked. Chapped lips are common in cold weather and may cause a fissure in the middle of the lower lip, which bleeds easily and may lead to a permanent scar. Angular stomatitis may be associated with anaemia, as in the case of the Paterson–Brown Kelly, or Plummer Vinson, syndrome. The upper lip is one of the commoner sites for an extragenital chancre of primary syphilis. Owing to the lack of secondary infection, it may remain quite a small lesion and be mistaken for a boil. It is associated with considerable "rubbery" enlargement of the submandibular and cervical glands, which are distinct from the hard, fixed glands associated with an epithelioma which usually occurs on the lower lip. Herpes catarrhalis affects the upper lip and is associated with the common cold. It appears as a group of blisters which become dry and cracked, with considerable discomfort and a tendency to bleed. Hare-lip is a cleft in the upper lip due to an incomplete fusion of one maxillary process with the globular process, and a fissure is present between the philtrum and the lateral part of the upper lip. It is frequently associated with a cleft palate. Congenital haemangioma may affect the lower lip and cause considerable deformity.

The mouth is a delicate part of the body and the co-operation of the patient is essential if a satisfactory examination is to be achieved. A rapport between the surgeon and the patient should have been established whilst the history was being taken, bearing in mind that many are apprehensive of the result of a consultation. In the case of children, it is important that they should be asked questions to make them feel that they are participating in the procedure. Difficulty in carrying out the examination may arise because some people are hypersensitive in the mouth and throat to such an extent that they retch when they open their mouths and experience difficulty in cleaning their teeth. In such subjects, only a limited view of the mouth and pharynx is possible, and a complete examination can only be carried out under general anaesthesia. Others find it difficult to relax, often owing to nervousness, but with a little patience their co-operation can usually be obtained. If the gag reflex is rather brisk, the examination may be facilitated by the use of a local anaesthetic spray, such as 10 per cent cocaine. Some neurotic individuals are very insensitive in the mouth and pharynx, and submit to examination without any difficulty. Children rarely cause difficulty; if they are treated as adults they will behave like them. Should a child prove fractious, it may have to be restrained. The child is placed on the nurse's right thigh and her legs are crossed over the child's so that it cannot kick. With her left hand she presses the child's arms to its chest, while the other hand is placed on the child's forehead so that its head may be held against her chest. An infant is easily restrained by wrapping it in a blanket, with the arms included.

The normally co-operative patient is instructed to open his mouth and take regular breaths, which should enable him to become perfectly relaxed. The left hand is rested on the patient's head. This places him in the correct position, and the synergistic impulses between the examiner's two hands enable him to estimate the pressure which he is exerting with his right hand, with which the spatula is introduced at the angle of the mouth. This manoeuvre permits inspection of the buccal mucosa, the opening of the parotid duct, the teeth and gums, the tongue and the palate. Furthermore, introducing the spatula in this manner gives the patient confidence that it will not be pushed down his throat.

The buccal mucosa is moist and pink. In cases of pulmonary tuberculosis it is strikingly pale, as it is in those suffering from anaemia. If there is stomatitis, the mucosa is grossly congested and it may become dry, with a varying amount of debris adherent to it; this is common when the mouth has been subjected to a full course of radiotherapy. Thrush, due to infection with *Candida albicans*, was commonly seen in children, but adults taking oral antibiotics may also become infected. It covers considerable areas of the mucosa with milky white patches which are easily removed; examination of a smear taken from the lesion confirms the diagnosis. Koplik spots are white lesions, the size of a pinhead, surrounded by an area of erythema, and are diagnostic of measles before the morbilliform rash appears. Leucoplakia may affect the cheeks or the "milky streaks" of lichen planus may be seen. Bullae due to pemphigus or erythema multiforme must be distinguished from pemphigoid. A carcinomatous ulcer has characteristic hard everted edges with a slough in the base, and the regional lymph nodes may be enlarged and hard, and fixed to surrounding structures. In the secondary stage of syphilis, there is a generalized upper respiratory infection, and the patient may complain of "a nasty cold". The buccal mucosa is congested and "snail track ulcers" may affect the cheeks and palate. There is a symmetrical rash on the body and limbs, which also affects the forehead when it is called the "corona veneris". There is a generalized lymph node involvement, and examination of a smear from an ulcer under dark-ground illumination reveals the *Treponema pallidum*. In Addison's disease, the mucosa is pigmented.

The mouth of the parotid duct is a slit in the mucosa opposite the second upper molar tooth. If there is an infection of the gland, as in epidemic parotitis (mumps), the orifice of the duct becomes red and congested, whilst in suppurative parotitis pus may be seen coming from it as well. This is often a terminal event in a cachectic patient who has been suffering for a long time from a fatal disease. Rarely calculus may be present at the opening of the parotid duct. Aphthous ulcers frequently occur on the inner aspect of the lips, and a common site for them is in the gingivolabial fold where they will be overlooked unless a deliberate search is made for them.

If examination under general anaesthesia is necessary, access to the palate, pharynx and nasopharynx may be obtained by placing the patient in the position employed in tonsillectomy and inserting a Boyle Davis gag. An adenoid curette or a catheter passed up one nostril and brought out through the mouth retracts the soft palate, and a small laryngeal mirror may be used to examine the nasopharynx. Finer detail can be observed with the operating microscope. Yankauer's speculum permits direct inspection. Much can be learned by palpation and if the adenoids are large they may be removed. If the tongue is to be examined, a Mason or Doyen gag should be used to open the mouth.

EXAMINATION OF THE TEETH

The teeth and gums merit close attention. A child has 20 deciduous teeth, two incisors, one canine, and two molars on each side of the upper and lower jaws. Eruption of the deciduous teeth begins at six to nine months of age, the first to appear being the lower central incisors, and is completed by the eruption of the second molars at the age of 20–24 months, but there is considerable variation. The first permanent tooth is the first molar which erupts behind the deciduous molars, which are later replaced by the permanent premolars. It erupts at the age of six years, and is followed by the incisors. The dentition is completed by the eruption of the second molars at the age of 12 or 13 years, with the exception of the third molars, the "wisdom teeth", which erupt between the age of 18 and 25 years. In fact, the wisdom teeth may never erupt and instead become impacted. As a result of this a certain amount of pain may arise and this is quite often referred to the ear, causing the patient to consult an otologist. If no local cause for the pain is evident, and particularly if it is said to be in the vicinity of the ear rather than in the ear itself, the teeth must always come under suspicion; similar symptoms may be due to a carious lower molar. When the teeth and gums are heavily infected the tonsils and pharynx may become inflamed and painful. This is due to the normal response of the lymphoid tissue to a constant stream of infected material passing over it and does not indicate that it is the site of chronic infection.

Much can be learned by an inspection of the individual permanent teeth. Ridges on the incisors may indicate a period of malnutrition during childhood, or a severe illness at some time. Congenital syphilis may cause Hutchinson teeth; the permanent incisors are affected. The biting edge is notched and becomes semilunar, whilst the tooth is deformed and becomes peg-shaped. There may be stigmata of the disease elsewhere, saddle shaped deformity of the bridge of the nose, interstitial keratitis and perceptive deafness.

The bite should be inspected to see that the teeth have a normal articulation or that dentures fit properly. The upper dental arch is somewhat larger than the lower so that the upper incisors overlap the lower when the jaw is closed. The molars of the upper and lower jaws come into exact apposition when the jaw is closed however, and anything interfering with this arrangement, such as the loss of molar teeth or ill fitting dentures, may throw the temporomandibular joints out of alignment. This may cause pain in the ear or, by pressure on the chorda tympani, a disturbance of the sense of taste; it may also interfere with the function of the eustachian tube (Costen's syndrome).

The roots of the upper molars, and particularly the premolars, are in close relationship with the maxillary sinus, and an apical abscess may give rise to acute maxillary sinusitis, which is usually associated with a very foul nasal catarrh. Sometimes the root of a premolar projects into the maxillary sinus, possibly as a result of necrosis of the thin bone separating them, so that when the tooth is extracted an oro-antral fistula is formed.

Dental sepsis is the commonest cause of swelling of the tissues of the face, sometimes erroneously thought to be due to acute maxillary sinusitis. This never causes swelling of the face unless it is complicated by osteomyelitis of the maxilla, a rare condition sometimes affecting infants.

Gingivitis, whilst usually due to local infection, may be a manifestation of some serious general illness. In acute leukaemia the gums may become hypertrophied to such an extent that the teeth may be almost completely enveloped; gums in the edentulous are unaffected. Scurvy gives rise to spontaneous haemorrhage from the gums which become infected so that the teeth are loosened and may fall out.

The commonest cause of gingivitis is lack of dental hygiene. The teeth should be scaled at regular intervals to remove tartar and they should be brushed regularly, ideally after every meal, to remove food particles. When the gums are infected they become spongy and tend to bleed easily. They may harbour Vincent's organisms, which may affect other parts of the mouth and throat. The tendency to bleed may only be noticed when the teeth are brushed, but some people appear to suck their gums whilst sleeping and complain of coughing up a little blood in the morning, whilst it is a well known trick of malingerers to feign haemoptysis. In all such cases it is wise to have a radiograph of the chest to exclude infection there. A blue line on the gum, about 1 mm. from its free margin, indicates poisoning by a heavy metal, such as lead.

EXAMINATION OF THE TONGUE AND FLOOR OF THE MOUTH

The patient is instructed to protrude his tongue as far as possible and it is noted whether it is straight or deviated. If the hypoglossal nerve is paralysed, the tongue will deviate towards the affected side and there is hemi-atrophy. Inability to protrude the tongue may be due to tongue-tie or to a neoplasm infiltrating the muscles.

The dorsum of the tongue is dried with a tongue cloth, which facilitates inspection of the papillae. The patchwork markings of geographical tongue are immediately evident. The markings tend to migrate, making an ever changing pattern; it is of no significance. A smooth clean tongue devoid of papillae is suggestive of some form of anaemia, often associated with the Paterson–Brown Kelly syndrome, and there may be angular stomatitis as well. In the case of pernicious anaemia, the tongue is red and beefy in contrast to the pallor of the buccal mucosa. In scarlet fever the tongue is at first coated with a yellow fur through which the inflamed papillae project, "strawberry and cream tongue"; later, the fur disappears and the grossly inflamed organ is described as "raspberry tongue". "Black hairy tongue" is caused by the appearance of long pigmented filaments of keratin on the dorsum of the tongue. It may cause a certain amount of discomfort but is of no significance, tending to clear up spontaneously. Aphthous ulcers may affect any part of the tongue; they are small ulcers with clean bases and heal spontaneously. They are extremely painful and cause much distress since they tend to come in crops over a period of weeks.

A carcinoma of the tongue may affect any part, and may appear as a lump pushing up the mucous membrane. In this case the movement of the tongue may be severely restricted and it may not be protruded. It may also appear in a patch of leucoplakia on the surface of the tongue, but sooner or later breaks down to form a typical malignant ulcer with hard everted edges and involvement of the cervical lymph nodes. In either case, palpation reveals it as a hard lesion which should lead to a biopsy to establish the diagnosis. Chronic superficial glossitis affects the dorsum of the tongue, and appears as a considerable area of leucoplakia. There are deep fissures on the tongue which may become malignant, and the patient should be under constant supervision so that a timely biopsy can lead to early diagnosis of carcinoma. It is said to be due to smoking, sepsis, syphilis or spirits, and surprisingly its incidence is markedly on the decline.

The tip of the tongue is now grasped with a tongue cloth and moved from side to side so that the edges may be examined. In the case of macroglossia, the edges are scalloped by indentations made by the teeth. The edge of the tongue is a common site for aphthous ulcers or a carcinoma. A dental ulcer lies opposite a jagged tooth, and the cause of the condition may be suggested by the patient. The tooth should receive immediate attention and if the ulcer is not healed within ten days it should be regarded as a carcinoma.

Towards the base of the tongue the vallate papillae may be seen. They are a row of large papillae formed in the shape of a V with its apex at the foramen caecum. A tumour here may be an ectopic thyroid gland, or a cyst may form in connection with the thyroglossal duct. Behind the vallate papillae lies the pharyngeal portion of the tongue. The lymphoid deposits are large, and there may be large blood vessels as well. If a patient has cause to look at his tongue and protrudes it far enough to bring this part into view, he may well become alarmed fearing that he has a neoplasm. This collection of lymphoid tissue is known as the lingual tonsil. It is usually separated from the palatine tonsil by a sulcus, but sometimes there is no clear line of demarcation. The lingual tonsils may become acutely infected, especially when the palatine tonsils have been removed, but they do not have crypts.

The patient is now told to put the tip of his tongue on his hard palate and the under surface is examined. The frenum can be seen in the midline running down a variable distance behind the tip, to the floor of the mouth. In some cases the frenum extends almost to the tip of the tongue, severely limiting its movement; a condition called "tongue-tie". It can be divided if necessary, but it rarely causes much trouble unless the patient requires indirect laryngoscopy. Abrasions of the frenum are sometimes seen in children suffering from whooping cough, for the tongue is strongly protruded with each cough and the frenum impinges on the lower incisor teeth.

In the floor of the mouth, the submandibular ducts are seen under the mucosa with their orifices on each side of the attachment of the frenum. They may be distended by calculi, or a calculus may present at one orifice. Calculi are easily palpated in the duct, and swelling of the submandibular salivary gland is readily identified by bimanual palpation with one finger on the floor of the mouth and the tips of the fingers of the other hand on the skin of the submandibular triangle of the neck. An enlarged submandibular lymph node cannot be felt in this way because it does not lie in the floor of the mouth. Ludwig's angina may complicate dental infection, but it may arise spontaneously. There is cellulitis of the floor of the mouth, extending to the tissues beneath the chin, causing a hard brawny swelling. There may be respiratory embarrassment, and it is a potentially dangerous condition.

The rest of the mouth is now palpated with the forefinger; bimanual palpation can be applied to the cheeks. Any tumour or ulcer is felt, to determine whether it is hard or soft, mobile or fixed. If the patient takes deep breaths, it is possible to palpate the tonsils without causing distress. It may also be thought advisable to express the contents of the tonsillar crypts to see whether they contain pus, cheesy collections of debris and food particles, or a tonsillolith. It is wise to defer these manoeuvres until the examination of the mouth and pharynx has been completed in case retching is induced, making further instrumentation difficult.

In certain cases it is necessary to test the sense of taste. The taste buds of the anterior two-thirds of the tongue are supplied by the chorda tympani, and those on the posterior one-third by the glossopharyngeal nerve. They are capable of appreciating only four basic sensations—sweet, acid, salt and bitter. Sweet and salt are most appreciated at the tip of the tongue, acid along the side, and bitter on the posterior part. Sugar, salt, vinegar and quinine are suitable substances for the test. The major part of the sense of taste is, of course, connected with the sense of smell, and it may be of importance from the medico-legal aspect in establishing the veracity of a man who claims that he has lost his senses of smell and taste as a result of a head injury, but admits that the basic sense of taste is retained.

In electrogustometry a device is used by which a measured current can be applied to either side of the tongue to determine the threshold at which an acid taste is produced. As a quantitative test, the technique can be used in assessment of chorda tympani and facial nerve function.

EXAMINATION OF THE OROPHARYNX AND PALATE

When both sides of the mouth have been examined the spatula is placed on the dorsum of the tongue and depressed to bring the fauces, the palatine tonsils, the soft palate and the oropharynx into view. The spatula should not encroach on the posterior one-third of the tongue, innervated by the glossopharyngeal nerve, which induces a gag reflex; this is resented by the patient. If the patient is properly relaxed little pressure is required, but if there is some resistance a firm and gradually increasing pressure may be exerted. Should it be necessary to change the position of the spatula, it should be lifted off the tongue and replaced in the desired position.

The hard palate forms the roof of the mouth and the floor of the nose while the alveolus lies in the base of the maxillary sinus. The soft palate is a muscular curtain which is attached to the posterior margin of the hard palate, from which it extends backwards to the level of the anterior pillar of the fauces with which it is in continuity. In the centre of its free margin there is an appendage of variable length, the uvula. The palate is freely mobile and by its elevation together with contraction of the pharyngeal muscles the nose is completely shut off from the oropharynx. This mobility is very important and may be restricted by scarring due to operations for the removal of tonsils and adenoids, a severe attack of scarlet fever, or more chronic disease, such as lupus, gummatous ulceration or malignant infiltration; it may also be affected by acute infection, such as quinsy.

Paralysis of the palate may be due to bulbar poliomyelitis or diphtheria, in which case it always recovers, or some other disease of the central nervous system, such as multiple sclerosis or pseudobulbar palsy, of which it is usually only one manifestation. Unilateral paralysis is demonstrated by making the patient say "Ah", when the palate is pulled towards the sound side with a "curtain movement". If both sides are paralysed it may be necessary to make the patient gag to demonstrate it, and paralysis of the pharynx may be noted at the same time. When immobility of the palate is bilateral, there may be serious disability owing to rhinolalia aperta, and drink and food may be regurgitated through the nose, particularly if the pharynx is involved as well; this may necessitate a tracheostomy and tube feeding. When movement of the palate is restricted by local scarring, a degree of disability is experienced, for it is by the free movement of the palate that secretions in the nasopharynx are aided in their passage into the oropharynx.

Cleft palate is represented in its least severe form by a bifid uvula, but the soft palate and the hard palate may be involved and it may be associated with a hare-lip. These cases require the services of a plastic surgeon.

On the soft palate there may be a herpetic eruption sometimes associated with geniculate herpes, the Ramsey Hunt syndrome. Herpangina, due to infection with a

9

Coxsackie A virus, causes lesions resembling aphthous ulcers but rather larger and usually affecting the free margin of the palate. Other parts affected are the pillars of the fauces, the pharyngeal wall and the roof of the mouth. The hard palate is brought into view by tilting the patient's head backwards. A high arch to the palate is associated with a crowded dentition, causing prominence of the upper incisor teeth and a short upper lip predisposing to mouth breathing, as evidenced by the hypertrophy of the gum in that region. An orthodontist can do much to remedy the condition, which is usually hereditary.

Aphthous ulcers may affect any part of the mouth, but ulcers on the palate are commonly due to syphylitic or tuberculous infection. Secondary syphilis causes snail track ulcers associated with mucous patches; a gumma forms an ulcer with punched out edges and a slough in the base. It erodes bone and may cause a perforation of the hard palate; it is relatively painless. Tuberculous ulcers are shallow, with rolled edges, and are extremely painful. Lupus usually affects the soft palate; in some areas there is activity with the formation of "apple jelly" nodules, whilst other parts heal with gross scarring causing considerable deformity.

Papilloma is a fairly common tumour on the soft palate, frequently pedunculated and arising near the uvula. Angioma is uncommon unless it is part of a generalized angiomatosis. Torus palatinus is a bony outgrowth in the midline of the hard palate; it is of no consequence unless it interferes with the fitting of a denture, when it should be removed.

A fibrolipoma usually occurs in the soft palate; it has a lobulated outline which is easily discernible on palpation. Mixed salivary tumours affect either the hard or soft palate; they are not malignant but they are locally invasive and may ulcerate and cause perforation of the palate.

An epithelioma breaks down to form a typical ulcer with hard everted edges and a dirty base; either the soft or hard palate may be involved, and perforation occurs. The cervical lymph nodes may be enlarged, hard, and fixed to surrounding structures. A reticulum celled sarcoma or fibrosarcoma may also be encountered. Malignant tumours in the nose may cause depression of the soft palate and even ulcerate through it, causing a perforation. A carcinoma of the maxillary sinus may push the molar or premolar teeth down into the mouth; they become loosened and may fall out.

Wounds of the palate may be due to gunshot, sometimes self inflicted. In children, they may be the result of a fall with something like a pencil in the mouth.

The fauces and palatine tonsils are now examined, with the posterior wall of the oropharynx. The anterior pillar of the fauces is formed by the palatoglossus muscle, and the posterior pillar by the palatopharyngeus muscle. The mucous membrane is pink, like that of the palate. Injection of the vessels is suggestive of infection in the tonsils. The tonsils are paired organs which have a remarkable degree of symmetry. Their surfaces are smooth and their size is very variable and of no consequence unless they attain such proportions as to interfere with the functions of the alimentary and respiratory tracts, a condition rarely seen today but not uncommon in the early part of the century when nutrition and hygiene among the less fortunate left much to be desired. The best guide to their condition is provided by the history, but there are certain characteristics which suggest that they are the site of chronic infection.

Chronic infection is suspected when the tonsil has been partly destroyed by successive infections with the haemolytic streptococcus. This leads to scarring of the surface, and the tonsil becomes "buried" behind the anterior pillar of the fauces. It is confirmed when the vessels round the mouth of the crypts are injected and pus can be expressed from them. Enlargement of the tonsillar lymph node supports the diagnosis. Asymmetry of the tonsils suggests that one of them is undergoing a pathological process, possibly neoplastic, lymphosarcoma in children. In adult life there is a progressive atrophy of the tonsils.

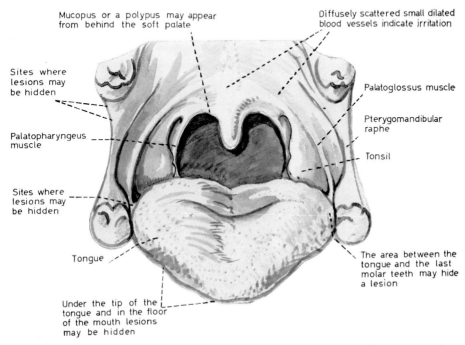

FIG. 1.—The pharynx from the front, showing areas of special interest on clinical examination.

Acute infection in the throat may affect the tonsils and the pharynx. Acute follicular tonsillitis is characterized by white spots overlying the mouths of the crypts, while acute parenchymatous tonsillitis causes acute congestion of the tonsil with some oedema. The membrane of acute diphtheria is firmly adherent to the tonsil, and attempts to remove it lead to bleeding; it may also extend over the adjacent palate. This is a potentially lethal disease and it is essential that a throat swab should be taken in every acute throat infection to exclude it from the diagnosis. Angina of glandular fever resembles it, but this can be diagnosed by means of a blood count or Paul Bunnell reaction. Vincent's infection causes considerable destruction of the tonsil, and the membrane appears to be inlaid rather than laid on the surface; the organisms can be identified by examination of a smear taken from the lesion. Peritonsillar abscess (quinsy) causes the anterior pillar of the fauces in the region of the upper pole to bulge and the tonsil is displaced medially. It must be distinguished from a parapharyngeal abscess, when the whole lateral wall of the pharynx is displaced. Trismus, inability to open the mouth except to a limited extent owing to reflex spasm of the masseter muscle, may make examination and treatment of the patient difficult. Trismus may also be the first manifestation of tetanus.

Acute infection of the pharynx may cause it to become congested and the lymphoid tissue to become oedematous. A stream of mucopus trickling down the pharynx may be due to an acute nasal infection, while hypertrophy of the lateral bands of lymphoid tissue situated between the lateral and posterior walls of the pharynx is suggestive of chronic nasal or sinus infection. Acute retropharyngeal abscess occurs in children as a complication of acute infection of the throat or acute otitis media, or it may arise spontaneously. It is due to suppuration in the retropharyngeal lymph nodes which lie to either side of the midline. It presents as a swelling in the pharynx and may cause difficulty in swallowing and breathing. In infants it is not always easily seen, but can be palpated with the finger. This condition cannot arise in adults, for the retropharyngeal lymph nodes atrophy in early childhood. A midline retropharyngeal abscess may, however, complicate tuberculous infection of the cervical vertebrae, presenting as a bulging of the posterior pharyngeal wall.

Atrophic pharyngitis is often associated with atrophic rhinitis, frequently due to congenital syphilis with "snuffles" and destruction of the ethmoid cells; there is an excessive airway which causes the mucosa to become dry, with destruction of the mucous glands, which aggravates the situation. The process may extend as far as the larynx and trachea. In the pharynx the mucosa is atrophic and thin, so that the pharynx appears large and the outline of the cervical vertebrae may be clearly seen. The diminution of mucous secretion leads to the formation of crusts, with secondary infection and foetor oris.

Keratosis may affect the tonsils, pharynx and tongue, and may even extend to the larynx. There are white keratin processes firmly adherent to the mucosa, which may be mistaken for the follicles of acute tonsillitis. It causes unnecessary alarm, for it is a benign condition which may disappear spontaneously.

Retention cysts in the tonsil appear as yellow smooth tumours and may cause some alarm to the patient; they are easily evacuated after the throat has been sprayed with a local anaesthetic. A papilloma may arise from the surface of the tonsil, but otherwise it is rarely affected by simple tumours.

Ulceration of the tonsil is commonly due to an epithelioma. It breaks down to form an ulcer with hard everted edges and a slough in the base. The cervical lymph nodes are hard and fixed, and often the reason for the patient seeking advice. Lymphosarcoma may occur at any age and cause a swelling of the tonsil, but it rarely ulcerates. The cervical nodes may be enlarged but are not very hard. Syphilis may cause ulceration of the tonsil. A primary chancre is not unknown, and in the secondary stage there may be ulcers and mucous patches on the surface. A gumma causes considerable destruction of the tonsil, with a punched out ulcer with clean edges and a slough in the base.

EXAMINATION OF THE NASOPHARYNX

Examination of the nasopharynx is carried out with the aid of a postnasal mirror. It is warmed by holding it with the glass in the flame of a methylated spirit lamp until it is sufficiently warm to prevent condensation from the patient's breath. The temperature of the mirror is checked by applying it to the hand, and if the patient appears to be apprehensive he may be reassured by placing it on his cheek. The tongue is depressed with a spatula and the patient told to relax and breathe quietly when the soft palate should fall away from the posterior pharyngeal wall to expose the nasopharynx. The mirror is inserted below and behind the free margin of the soft palate. If the uvula is long, it is advisable to insert the mirror on either side of it. The shaft of the instrument may be steadied against the angle of the mouth, but the mirror must not touch the base of the tongue or the posterior pharyngeal wall, which causes retching so that no view can be obtained. The largest mirror which the patient can accommodate should be used, for not only the extent of the view but the brilliance of the illumination depends upon the size of the mirror.

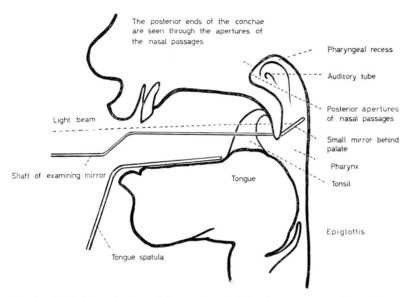

Fig. 2.—Clinical examination of the nasal part of the pharynx; areas of importance on clinical examination.

It is unfortunate that this examination can rarely be carried out in children. It can give valuable information about the adenoids, but few children are able to co-operate sufficiently and the smallness of the part militates against it. On no account should the adenoids be palpated in a conscious child. It is far better to examine the child under a general anaesthetic, when the adenoids may be removed if it is considered necessary. The first landmark is the posterior end of the nasal septum, which is always in the midline. This is followed up to the vault of the nasopharynx when the adenoids, if present, are brought into view. By turning the mirror slightly to each side both posterior nares may be inspected. The posterior ends of the inferior turbinates can always be seen and usually the posterior ends of the middle turbinates as well. A trickle of pus from the middle meatus is suggestive of infection in the maxillary, ethmoid or frontal sinuses, whereas if it is seen high up in the vault of the nasopharynx the sphenoid is suspect. This emphasizes the importance of this examination in assessing the state of the nose. Nasal secretions are propelled backwards into the nasopharynx by the cilia of the nasal mucosa, so anything abnormal is first seen here. It is only when the secretions are so profuse that the nose can scarcely contain them that they are seen on anterior rhinoscopy.

If the nose is full of polypi they may be seen protruding from the posterior nares whilst an antrochoanal polypus, arising in the maxillary sinus and entering the nose through the ostium, is directed backwards to appear in the posterior nares. It may give rise to characteristic symptoms, in that it acts as a ball valve so that inspiration through the affected nostril may be possible, but obstruction to expiration is complete when the polypus is blown into the posterior nares. By turning the mirror a little further to each side, the eustachian cushions are brought into view and conditions such as neoplasms, which may obstruct the tubes, may be seen.

A carcinoma is the commonest tumour in the nasopharynx and is seen as an ulcerating mass, either in the roof or on the lateral wall where it may involve the eustachian cushion and cause deafness and earache. There is obstruction to the airways, and there may be an offensive blood-stained nasal catarrh. The upper deep cervical lymph nodes are commonly involved and may be hard and fixed to surrounding structures. A sarcoma presents a similar appearance. A plasmocytoma is a rare tumour resembling a carcinoma, but it does not normally give rise to metastases. A lymphoepithelioma differs from other tumours in that the primary growth is very small and may only give the impression that one lateral wall of the nasopharynx is slightly more prominent than the other. There is sometimes involvement of the eustachian tube, but the feature of the condition is the gross enlargement of the upper deep cervical lymph nodes; they are not as hard as those involved by carcinoma. A fibro-angioma appears in the roof of the nasopharynx, commonly in youths in their early teens. It is not malignant but may cause a good deal of damage by invasion of neighbouring structures, such as the orbit. A chondroma or myxochondroma may arise in connection with the eustachian cushion, and a hamartoma sometimes occurs in this region.

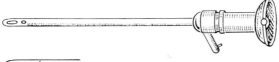

FIG. 3.—An electric nasopharyngoscope.

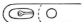

The nasopharyngoscope is an instrument similar to a cystoscope with an eyepiece and a light and prism, and a side window at its distal end. The direction in which the window is pointing is indicated by a small knob on the eyepiece. It is introduced along the floor of the nose which has first been sprayed with a local anaesthetic. Deformities of the septum, particularly septal spurs, may prevent introduction of the instrument. It gives a limited field of view and is not used very much in this country, but is used as a routine in the United States of America.

EXAMINATION OF THE LARYNGOPHARYNX

The tip of the protruded tongue is now grasped with a tongue cloth and pulled forward, but not so far as to damage the frenum with the lower incisor teeth.

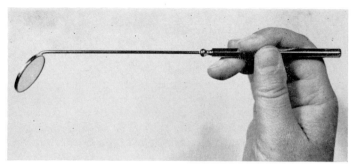

FIG. 4.—Holding the mirror for examination of the lower pharynx.

The patient is made to flex his cervical spine and extend the atlanto-occipital joint so as to bring the mouth and pharynx as nearly as possible into alignment. A laryngeal mirror, previously warmed by holding the glass over a methylated-spirit lamp, is introduced into the mouth and applied to the soft palate with firm pressure until it is in contact with the posterior pharyngeal wall. It is essential that firm pressure be exerted; light pressure serves only to tickle the palate and

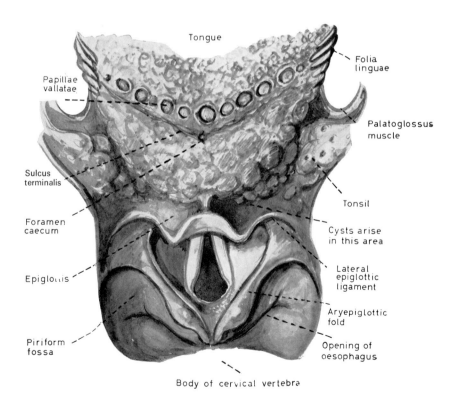

FIG. 5.—The lower pharynx seen in the examining mirror. Areas of importance in clinical examination.

cause the patient to gag. The mirror is adjusted so that the back of the tongue may be inspected as far as the base of the epiglottis. The space in front of the anterior aspect of the epiglottis is called the vallecula, and is sometimes the site of a carcinoma. The base of the tongue and the adjacent pharyngeal walls are carefully examined for any sign of tumour or ulceration. By making the patient say "E" the aryepiglottic folds are drawn medially and the pyriform fossae are brought into view. They may be ulcerated by carcinoma or Behçet's disease. A postcricoid carcinoma cannot be seen unless it is very advanced, when an ulcerating mass may be seen behind the larynx. A useful sign in this condition is the loss of crepitus, normally elicited by moving the larynx from side to side across the cervical spine, owing to the mass interposed between the structures. The neck should now be palpated for evidence of enlargement of the cervical lymph nodes.

RADIOLOGICAL EXAMINATION

Radiological examination of every part of the mouth and pharynx can provide essential diagnostic information. The normal radiographic appearances are described in Vol. 1.

REFERENCES

Costen, J. B. (1937). *Miss. Doct.*, **15**, 33.
Keogh, C. A. (1957). *Ann. Otol., etc. St. Louis*, **66**, 416.

DISEASES OF THE MOUTH

DAVID DOWNTON

ORAL HYGIENE

On examining the mouth, note must first of all be taken of the general state of hygiene. Chronic oral sepsis, if severe, can easily mask other pathology. Even in edentulous mouths ill-fitting and uncleaned dentures can produce chronic irritation.

In cases of neglected oral hygiene, food debris collects around the teeth, and there are heavy deposits of salivary calculus. Irregular teeth, partial dentures, and carious teeth help to make this condition worse, and in the long run gingivitis with periodontal disease will ensue.

Mouth breathing can cause gingivitis by preventing the normal flow of saliva over the gingivae, which become dry and cracked—secondary infection then follows. With mouth-breathing, even if nasal obstruction is cured, the habit may persist.

During eruption of deciduous teeth the oral mucosa is particularly prone to inflammatory processes, and particular attention should be paid to oral hygiene at this time. Eruption of the permanent teeth usually occurs without complication apart from the third molar, or wisdom tooth. In particular the mandibular wisdom tooth is not infrequently impacted, or there is insufficient space for its normal eruption. A gum flap, therefore, presents over part of the tooth and this can lead to severe acute infection, which may proceed to a cellulitis of the face or neck.

One should also bear in mind when examining a mouth, that even when it appears to be well cared for a tooth with a large filling may have an apical infection which can result in abscess formation. Apical abscesses usually point into the oral cavity, but may occasionally point extra-orally (Fig. 6). It should not be forgotten that due to the proximity of the apices of upper molars and premolars to the floor of the antrum abscesses on these teeth may point therein and present a picture of maxillary sinusitis.

Pain referred to the ear or face might be due to dental causes especially with impacted lower wisdom teeth.

In the normal healthy mouth many organisms are found, but when chronic oral sepsis is present their numbers are increased enormously.

With severe oral sepsis infection can spread along the normal anatomical pathways which are connected with the mouth, and when the gingivae and periodontal membrane are involved organisms can enter the systemic circulation.

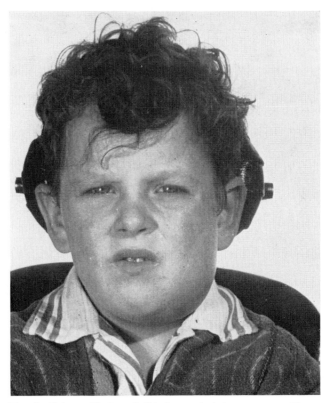

FIG. 6.—Submandibular cellulitis from apical abscess on mandibular deciduous molar.

CONGENITAL AND DEVELOPMENTAL ANOMALIES

Fordyce spots

These present as small elevated yellowish spots on the buccal mucosa. They are due to sebacous glands and are more apparent in adult life, being present in about 60 per cent of the population.

Malformations of the tongue

Bifid tongue is rare and due to failure of the lateral tubercles of the mandibular arch to coalesce during development.

Macroglossia is uncommon, and usually is seen in association with cretinism, mongolism and acromegaly. A lymphangioma of the tongue can also produce severe enlargement.

The treatment is to remove a wedge-shaped portion of the tongue, but when a lymphangioma (Fig. 7) is the cause radiotherapy should be considered.

Microglossia is a smallness or complete absence of the tongue.

Ankyloglossia is tongue-tie, due to maldevelopment of the fraenum, or of the anterior two-thirds of the tongue. If severe enough to cause difficulty in articulation, the tongue-tie should be freed surgically before the patient learns to speak.

Median rhomboid "glossitis" presents as a smooth oval reddish patch in the midline of the dorsum of the tongue anterior to the circumvallate papillae. It is due to the persistence of the tuberculum impar on the tongue's surface.

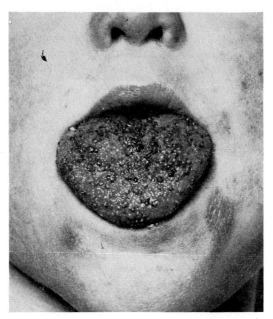

Fig. 7.—Lymphangioma of the tongue.

Furrowed tongue is a congenital fissuring of the dorsum of the tongue and no treatment is indicated unless soreness is produced by particles of food debris collecting and stagnating in the fissures. In such cases regular hygiene of the tongue should be applied.

Accessory thyroid tissue may present as a lingual thyroid at the back of the tongue as a purplish red swelling, or may be found deeply placed along the line of the original thyroglossal tract. Thyroglossal cysts appear anywhere in this midline tract between the supersternal notch and the foramen caecum of the tongue.

The treatment of the cysts is by removal. Lingual thyroid should be removed only if it causes bleeding, or is so large as to endanger the airway, and it must first be determined whether the gland itself is present and functioning.

Geographical tongue (*erythema migrans linguae*) (Fig. 8) presents as reddish patches surrounded by yellow elevated borders. It occurs on the dorsum of the tongue and frequently several patches may develop and coalesce. The characteristic feature of this condition is that the configuration changes from time to time. The filiform papillae have disappeared from the red areas, but at the borders they have become more prolific producing the typical appearance. The condition may start in childhood and continue throughout life, or it may remit spontaneously.

The aetiology is unknown and it rarely gives rise to symptoms.

19

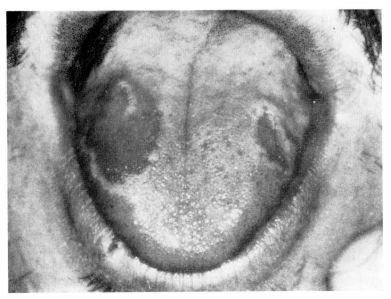

FIG. 8.—Geographical tongue.

Hairy tongue (Fig. 9) presents on the dorsum of the tongue as a profusion of fine "hairs" usually black or brown in colour. These hairs are produced by an overgrowth of the filiform papillae and can be as much as 1·25 cm. in length. The discoloration is possibly due to chromogenic bacteria, tobacco smoking or medicaments.

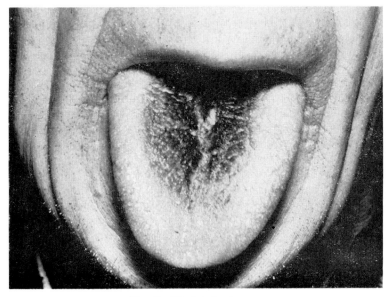

FIG. 9.—Black hairy tongue.

The aetiology is not understood but it has been noticed to follow the local application of antibiotics or oxidizing antiseptics especially if they have been used for some time.

The treatment is the removal of the filaments by gentle scraping and the patient is then instructed to brush the tongue twice a day with a soft brush using a weak solution of bicarbonate of soda.

STOMATITIS

Stomatitis can be produced by local or systemic diseases. Clinical diagnosis is frequently possible, but in some cases this is extremely difficult and one may have to resort to haematological, serological, bacteriological and biopsy investigations.

Traumatic injuries to the gingivae and oral mucosa can be caused by very stiff bristles on a tooth brush, or by fish bones becoming detached and embedded in the mucosa. Cheek-biting, ill-fitting dentures and jagged teeth also play their part. These lesions may vary somewhat in appearance but usually the cause can easily be ascertained and when the aetiological factor is removed in the normal healthy individual, healing occurs rapidly.

Thermal injuries from hot foods, or *chemical injuries* following the use of medicaments, may present varied lesions but the history will frequently give the diagnosis. Healing may take from several days to several weeks according to the severity of the damage.

Tobacco smoking may well have an effect on the mucosa, varying from an inflamed patch to one of excessively keratinized epithelium possibly leading to leucoplakia. The treatment will depend on the severity of the lesion. In early cases one should attempt to prevent the patient continuing the habit, but when leuco-plakia is present, the treatment may well be surgical (*see* "Leucoplakia", p. 27).

Radiotherapy produces an inflammatory reaction in the skin and mucosa. The tongue frequently becomes smooth, with atrophy of the papillae. Dryness of the oral mucosa is apparent when the salivary glands have been affected. The dryness of the mouth is extremely unpleasant and may make the wearing of dentures very difficult or even impossible. The mucosa frequently cracks and ulcerates. At this stage the topical use of an antibiotic with hydrocortisone may be helpful. The patient must be instructed in strict oral hygiene. The coating of the lips and mucosa with a lubricant, such as liquid paraffin, may prove beneficial especially when applied last thing at night.

Avitaminosis

Deficiency of the vitamin B₂ complex

In severe deficiencies of riboflavin and nicotinic acid pellagra is the end result. This condition is rarely found in civilized countries, although milder degrees of the deficiency can be found among old people who live alone and neglect their diet. The milder degrees of the deficiency have a less severe clinical picture than pellagra, the lips become red, swollen, painful and cracked, especially at the angles of the mouth. There is a painful glossitis, the tongue becoming inflamed and fissured.

Deficiency of vitamin C

Deficiency of vitamin C produces scurvy. This is uncommon today in civilized countries, but it may occur in elderly people living alone. When the teeth are present the gingivae become hyperaemic and swollen, and haemorrhagic when ulceration occurs.

Oral manifestations of diseases of the blood

Anaemias

Occasionally the oral lesions of the anaemias are the first sign to appear, as extreme pallor of the lips and oral mucosa and glossitis. The tongue is red and sore and in the typical Hunter's glossitis, which may well be the first sign of pernicious anaemia, it is also smooth.

Polycythaemia

In this condition there is a bluish-red discoloration of the oral mucosa, and glossitis and/or cheilitis may be present in varying degrees.

Infectious mononucleosis (glandular fever)

The cause of this disease is a virus. There is a considerable increase in the total number of white cells and a relatively great increase in the number of large mononuclear cells.

Frequently there are no oral lesions but the uvula may be swollen and oedematous, and an inflammatory reaction in the buccopharangeal mucosa together with sore throat may occur. In about 20 per cent of all cases there are petechial spots on the palate.

The submandibular and cervical lymph nodes are enlarged but are part of the general symptoms and usually occur without any oral signs being present.

Besides the increase in the white cell count, the Paul Bunnell test usually becomes positive five days after the onset of symptoms.

There is no specific treatment for this condition.

Agranulocytosis

This is caused by sensitivity to drugs containing the benzene ring especially amidopyrine, the sulphonamides and more recently the cytotoxic agents. There is a marked reduction in the neutrophil polymorphs.

Agranulocytosis is a severe disorder and frequently fatal. There is a sore throat of sudden onset and ulceration of the tongue, buccal mucosa and pharynx occurs, together with false membrane formation. Pyrexia is high and the patient is extremely ill. Diagnosis is confirmed by a typical blood picture. The treatment should consist of the withdrawal of any causal drug, while antibiotics, steroids and vitamin B_{12} therapy are instituted, with blood transfusion as required.

The leukaemias

Acute lymphatic leukaemia is the commonest form, and occurs chiefly in children. The first signs may well be enlargement of, and bleeding from the gingival margin, rapidly worsening with severe ulceration ensuing. Leucocytosis may be in the region of 100,000 cells/mm.³ and immature cells are always present in relatively large numbers.

In the chronic leukaemias, the oral lesions are not nearly as well marked and in many cases do not appear at all.

The diagnosis is always made from the blood picture.

Stomatitis associated with specific micro-organisms

Acute coccal stomatitis presents as an acute gingivitis which is often super-imposed upon a pre-existing chronic inflammatory condition of the gingivae. The gingival margins are inflamed and may be painful and ulcerated. A false membrane appearing greyish-white may form on the gingivae, and when detached it leaves a raw bleeding area. In severe cases the patient may have a pyrexia and a local adenitis. The condition may sometimes be mistaken for Vincent's infection, but lacks the typical halitosis associated with this disease. Diagnosis can be confirmed and clarified by smear examination.

The treatment is strict attention to oral hygiene, and systemic antibiotic therapy may be necessary in severe cases.

Acute ulcerative stomatitis (Vincent's). It has been suggested that a virus may be the actual exciting cause for this condition with the true Vincent's organisms being secondary invaders. However, these organisms are always present in the fully developed clinical condition. Vincent's stomatitis showed a marked increase during the two world wars and in World War I was so prevalent in the trenches that it was called "trench mouth". These facts lead one to think that it is more likely to appear when there is a low general resistance to infection together with a deficiency of certain vitamins and when the oral hygiene of the individual has been neglected.

A marked foetor is present and the ulceration commences on the gingival margins, usually between the teeth, spreading and coalescing to involve the rest of the gingivae. The soft palate, tonsils, and faucial pillars can also be affected (Vincent's angina).

The condition is painful and a lymphadenitis is usually present. In severe cases the pyrexia and malaise may be well marked.

In severe cases systemic antibiotic therapy may be necessary. Daily treatment by a dental surgeon is initially essential, all calculus being removed from the teeth and the oral hygiene restored. The local application of 10 vol/vol hydrogen peroxide followed by gentle atomizing or rinsing is of value. Chromic acid may be used as a 5 per cent solution in conjunction with the hydrogen peroxide.

After the acute phase has passed, the teeth and gingivae must be treated, otherwise a chronic Vincent's infection will remain with a tendency to acute exacerbations.

Tuberculosis in the oral cavity. A primary lesion in the mouth is extremely rare but it may be seen as a single painful ulcer in the gingivae, tongue or buccal mucosa. Biopsy will give the diagnosis.

Syphilis may present in the mouth in any of its stages. *Primary chancre* may occur on the tongue or lips. *Secondary syphilis* occurs on the oral mucosa and palate as snail track ulcers while mucous patches may also appear on the tongue. *Gumma* may occur in the tertiary stage of the disease usually on the palate or tongue, in the midline.

Fungal infections of the mouth

Monilia (thrush) is the commonest and is due to *Candida albicans*. The lesions occur on the oral mucosa and tongue. It is more frequently found in infants or debilitated adults. The lesions appear as white or greyish papules which frequently coalesce to form a membrane which is surrounded by a slight erythema. The membrane can be removed leaving a raw area.

Nystatin used locally in tablet form is curative in many cases and the local application of a 2 per cent solution of gentian violet may be helpful with infants. Good nursing is important. Angular cheilitis is not infrequently described as one of the lesions produced by monilia, but in the vast majority of these cases the causal agent is faulty dentures which do not support the soft tissues sufficiently, and drooping at the angles of the mouth occurs. This results in cracking of the skin and mucosa in this region and monilia are secondary invaders. It is, therefore, essential to exclude faulty dentures prior to any other treatment.

Actinomycosis, blastomycosis and *histoplasmosis* also occur within the oral cavity, but are extremely rare.

Scarlet fever and dipthheria also have their own oral lesions but can be diagnosed from the general signs and symptoms of the patient.

Stomatitis associated with virus diseases

Many well known virus diseases such as measles and chicken-pox have oral lesions, but there are several that may have oral lesions alone.

Catarrhal stomatitis

This usually arises in conjunction with coryza, pharyngeal infection or one of the exanthemata.

Cultures from affected surfaces may yield growths of *Neisseria catarrhalis*, *Diplococcus pneumoniae* and various streptococci. The oral cavity shows similar signs of inflammation to those found in the pharynx. Lack of oral hygiene is always a contributory factor.

Herpes

Herpes simplex.—In this condition, small vesicles appear which break down to form shallow painful ulcers. The margins of the ulcers are hyperaemic and they may be found in any part of the oral mucosa. One of the diagnostic points is that they are commonly seen in the hard palate, especially round the palatal gingivae when teeth are present.

Recurrent herpetic stomatitis.—This may appear in an herpetic subject following quite mild trauma by a toothbrush or the injection of a local anaesthetic. The lesions are similar to those found in herpes simplex.

Recurrent herpes labialis.—A well known lesion frequently referred to as a "cold sore". The initial symptom is a burning feeling in the lip, followed by vesicle formation which finally breaks down to form a crust. This separates after several days leaving an erythematous area which disappears a few days later. The lesion occurs on the skin at its junction with the oral mucosa.

For typical herpetic stomatitis a mouthwash of 2 per cent aureomycin can be used. This in no way treats the herpes, but it deals with the secondary infection and removes a considerable amount of discomfort.

Herpes zoster.—Whereas in herpes simplex the causal agent is the herpes simplex virus, in zoster it is thought the causal agent is the virus responsible for chicken-pox. The oral lesions which occur in herpes zoster are clinically indistinguishable from those of herpes simplex.

Coxsackie virus infections

These include herpangina, hand-foot-and-mouth disease and acute nodular meningitis. These infections have oral lesions similar to those found on the fauces and oropharynx.

Allergic stomatitis

This often occurs as part of a generalized allergic reaction to certain foodstuffs.

Chemical or contact allergy

Lipstick is a well known cause of cheilitis and glossitis, and reaction in the buccal mucosa might follow the use of certain antiseptics in mouthwashes or toothpastes. Aspirin, iodine and acriflavin are some examples of drugs that may produce such a reaction.

Dental materials especially acrylic resins used in dentures are very rarely the cause of an allergic reaction.

Stomatitis due to metals and drugs

Metals

Mercury and bismuth.—Stomatitis may occur when these metals are used medicinally and is not uncommon in workers handling them. The gingivae become red and swollen and if left untreated the periodontal membrane and alveolar bone become involved. A black or purplish line appears around the gingival margin due to the fact that the soluble salts circulating in the blood come into contact with hydrogen sulphide formed during the decomposition of debris around the teeth. The insoluble sulphide of the metal is then deposited in the gingivae. If untreated the condition is progressive and may lead to necrosis of the jaws and involvement of the salivary glands.

Lead.—The lesions are similar to those produced by bismuth and may occur in painters, lead metal workers and small children.

Gold.—Still occasionally used for the treatment of certain arthritic conditions and may produce a gingivitis.

Drugs

Epanutin.—Used in treatment of epilepsy may produce a considerable gingival hyperplasia which in some cases covers the teeth. Inflammation is not a primary effect of the drug but where present has arisen from other sources. The drug should be stopped if possible and a gingivectomy may be necessary. If the drug is continued after a gingivectomy is performed the condition will recur.

Antidepressants.—Certain of these drugs produce oral symptoms, usually associated with a dry mouth which may be severe.

Stomatitis and oral lesions of obscure aetiology

Recurrent ulcerative (aphthous) stomatitis

This is a common condition which can occur in varying degrees of severity. There is no definite known cause. Viruses, psychogenic and endocrine disturbances, and the anaemias have all been said to play a part, but more recent work indicates the condition is probably the result of an auto-immune reaction.

Small vesicles are the earliest sign to appear but may not be noticed. Ulceration soon occurs leaving an ulcer which varies in size from that of a pinhead to soon occurs leaving an ulcer which varies in size from that of a pinhead to one 2–3 cm. There may be a single lesion or several occurring in all parts of the oral cavity. The ulcers have a sloughing base and a marked area of hyperaemia around the edge. They are usually extremely painful and may last for several days. Healing is usually complete in 14 days although occasionally they have been known to last for some weeks. In patients suffering from this condition mild trauma may bring on an ulcer.

Every effort should be made to discover in these patients if there is any underlying general condition such as nutritional deficiency or anaemia. Small isolated lesions may require no more treatment than reassurance. In more severe cases hydrocortisone lozenges have been used with reported success. Strict attention to oral hygiene is important and in the isolated lesion the single application of a caustic such as phenol or silver nitrate shortens the duration and removes the pain.

Behçet's syndrome

The cause of this disease is not known. The ulceration that occurs in the mouth is of the aphthous type and there are also ulceration of the external genitalia and lesions on the eyes. Neurological manifestations may appear after a delay of two to five years and resemble an encephalitis or an acute lesion of the brain stem. Blindness may result from the ocular lesions.

The treatment is non-specific but steroids have been tried and are perhaps the drugs of choice at present.

Reiter's Syndrome

This disease which typically produces arthritis, urinary tract infection and ocular lesions occasionally produces oral lesions which are similar to aphthous ulceration.

Gangrenous stomatitis (cancrum oris)

This is a severe and rare disease the cause of which is obscure, but bacteriologically the micro-organisms found are similar to those in Vincent's stomatitis. Severe malnutrition is the real predisposing cause, the condition being found more commonly in the underdeveloped and starving countries.

Stomatitis is usually the first sign of this disease with ulceration rapidly occurring, followed by gangrene. This causes the destruction of whole areas of the cheeks with involvement of maxilla and mandible. Foetor is intense and the patient extremely ill.

The use of systemic penicillin has revolutionized the treatment of this condition, but the affected areas should be cleaned with 5 per cent solution of sodium bicarbonate and attention to oral hygiene is of first importance. An increasing number of these patients now survive and plastic surgery frequently is necessary for the repair of the defects produced.

Pemphigus

Pemphigus is a rare condition and may occur in acute or chronic form. It is characterized by the formation of bullous lesions on the skin and oral mucosa. Its origin is not known.

Several types of pemphigus have been described and classification of these has been attempted.

Pemphigus vulgaris is the more common form and is characterized by the formation of large flaccid bullae which rupture easily leaving a denuded area which tends to increase in size by progressive detachment of the epidermis. Extensive oral lesions are not infrequently the first sign of the disease. In the days before cortisone therapy the lesions often failed to heal and death resulted within several months. Slight friction of the mucosa produces separation of the superficial from the deep layers of the epithelium (Nikolsky's sign) which means that the wearing of dentures and even normal oral hygiene is impossible. There are variations of pemphigus vulgaris but the signs and symptoms described are similar in them all.

Benign mucous membrane pemphigoid

In this condition there is formation of bullae in the mucosa similar to those found in pemphigus vulgaris, and the eyes may also be involved. The condition runs a chronic benign course but severe scarring may result and if the eyes are involved blindness might follow. The diagnosis and the differentiation between pemphigoid and pemphigus vulgaris rests on the biopsy of the bullae.

The steroid drugs have revolutionized the treatment and prognosis of all forms of pemphigus and pemphigoid, but very large doses may be necessary to bring the condition under control.

Lichen planus

Lichen planus is an inflammatory condition of the skin and mucous membranes. The aetiology is not known. On the skin it presents as pinkish patches which are irritable, and there may be lesions on the oral mucosa. It must be noted that skin and oral mucosa lesions may appear separately or together.

In the mouth the condition may be symptomless, but it presents as glistening white papules which form varied patterns. Sometimes they may be plaque-like or arranged in lines giving a lace-like appearance. Hyperkeratosis may be present in varying degrees. Although the patient may in some cases be unaware of the condition, there are occasions when the lesions erode and ulcerate giving rise to severe pain. The wearing of dentures may then become very difficult.

This condition must always be differentiated from leucoplakia and a biopsy is generally necessary. Even histologically the distinction may not be easy.

The only treatment required in many cases is reassurance but oral hygiene is important especially if ulceration occurs. Certain authorities advocate the systemic use of cortisone. Occasionally spontaneous remissions occur.

Leucoplakia (Fig. 10)

This is a clinical term meaning literally a *white patch*. There are many diseases in which white patches appear in the mouth. They may appear in scleroderma, they may be seen with a white spongy naevus, and monilia can also give this appearance.

Biopsy or excision biopsy is usually necessary and the term leucoplakia is now generally reserved for those cases where no other diagnosis can be made.

A simple hyperkeratosis can be associated with local irritation and if when the irritation is removed the mucosa returns to normal, this should not be regarded as true leucoplakia. If, however, hyperkeratosis becomes irreversible it should be regarded in that light. Chronic irritation whether from a tooth, smoking, strong alcohol or spiced foods, is undoubtedly of some aetiological significance.

This condition should be regarded as pre-cancerous and where possible excision should be carried out.

There may be no symptoms in the early stages when the appearance is usually that of several raised, rather hard plaques which may coalesce. On the dorsum of the tongue there may be isolated white patches and on the cheeks there may be several whitish bands which can give the appearance of lichen planus. In the severe case the normal mucosa may disappear completely. Pain follows when these plaques crack and ulcerate.

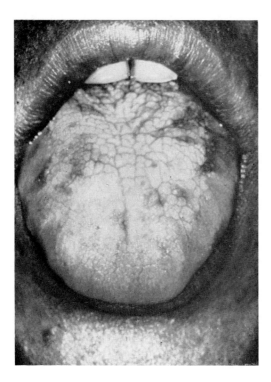

FIG. 10.—Leucoplakia of the tongue.

When the leucoplakia appears on a very inflamed area (erythroplakia) it must be regarded as very far advanced, with malignant change already having occurred.

The treatment is to remove any source of chronic irritation, excise the lesion completely if possible, and observe at regular intervals post-operatively.

DISORDERS OF THE TEMPOROMANDIBULAR JOINT

Costen was the first to draw attention to dysfunction of this joint as a cause of earache. Clicking noises from the joint are not always significant. They may be produced voluntarily without pain or restriction of movement, and they may also disappear spontaneously. The condition can, however, present as clicking of the jaw with restricted movement, with or without pain. There may be a complaint of earache or facial pain not associated necessarily with clicking. The pain in the ear is due to a referred otalgia whilst that in the face is frequently due to spasm of the associated muscles. Conductive deafness which is usually slight may result from dysfunction of the eustachian tube. Loss of mobility or stiffness in mandibular movement especially on wakening is also a common symptom.

The onset of symptoms may be associated with a blow, yawning, or following dental treatment, although frequently there is no such history. The main cause is malocclusion. The condition is more common in young women.

Radiography is usually negative unless osteoarthritic changes have occurred.

In the treatment and management of these patients exercises can be of value where the patient has produced "a bite of convenience". The patient can frequently be shown how to relax the muscles of mastication to open the jaw without deviation and to masticate on both sides. If the occlusion is definitely deranged a bite plate should be made in the first instance to restore the occlusion and in some cases where bruxism occurs and might well be the main aetiological factor the plate can be worn at night only. The correction of the occlusion should aim at restoration of the vertical dimension, replacement of missing teeth, and correction of dentures if already worn. The aim should be to allow free sliding movements of the mandible in mastication so that there is minimal cuspal interference. In cases of sudden onset such as following acute trauma intra-articular hydrocortisone injection is of value, but thereafter the joint must be rested for a minimum of 14 days. If malocclusion is present this must be treated after the rest period. The operations of condylectomy or condylotomy may become necessary in those cases which do not respond to treatment, but are usually only advisable if osteoarthritic changes have occurred.

CYSTS OF THE MOUTH

Developmental cysts

Medial group

These cysts are situated in the line of fusion of the two maxillae and are usually symptomless unless they become infected. They are frequently found on routine dental radiographs. The nasopalatine cyst, also in the midline, arises from tissue in the incisive canal or cell rests in the incisive papillae and presents usually in the palate or occasionally in the floor of the nose.

Lateral group

The lateral group of developmental cysts occur in the line of fusion of the maxillary and premaxillary elements of the palate and may cause separation of the canine and lateral incisor teeth.

Cysts of dental origin

These are derived from the epithelium that has been associated with the development of the tooth concerned.

The primordial cyst arises from the epithelium of the enamel organ before the formation of the dental tissues. The most common site is in the third molar region of the mandible and that tooth will of course be absent.

Cysts of eruption occur over a tooth that has not yet erupted and arise from the epithelial remains of the dental lamina. They are found in young people and may occur over deciduous or permanent teeth. They appear as small bluish fluctuant swellings and usually an elliptical incision is sufficient for the cyst to be removed and the underlying tooth to erupt.

The dentigerous cyst (Fig. 11) arises from the follicle around an unerupted tooth, the tooth projecting into the cyst cavity.

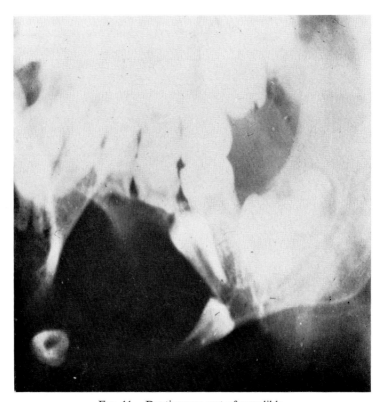

FIG. 11.—Dentigerous cyst of mandible.

The dental cyst arises from epithelial remains in the periodontal membrane and is the most common cyst to occur in the jaws. Chronically infected dead teeth or roots produce a granulomatous reaction at the apex. This granuloma contains epithelium which proliferates initially to produce the cyst lining. It is, therefore, common to find a dead tooth or root in conjunction with a cyst. Occasionally teeth or roots might have been removed and the cyst left behind (residual cyst).

Most of these cysts are symptomless unless they become infected. Many are found on routine radiographs, or it might be noticed that a tooth is missing, or the patient may simply complain of a swelling of the jaw. Fluctuation does not occur until the cyst has perforated the outer or inner alveolar plate.

In the maxilla a dental cyst arising from a premolar or molar tooth might easily invade the antrum and in some cases completely fill it.

Retention cysts

These are not uncommonly found in the oral cavity, palate and buccal mucosa. They are due to occlusion of the mucous glands present there. In the floor of the mouth such a retention cyst can progress to a very large size lifting the oral mucosa and base of the tongue (Ranula).

X-ray examination is essential for diagnosis of cysts in the hard tissue and the important point is that they show, as a rule, a very clear outline. When there is a multilocular radiolucent area in the jaws or the outline is not clear a differential diagnosis must be made from metastases or endosteal tumours. It must be remembered that the brown tumour of hyperparathyroidism is sometimes the first sign of this disease and the jaws are not an uncommon site for its appearance.

ODONTOMES

Several different types of odontome are described and they should be regarded as developmental anomalies. They arise from epithelial and mesenchymal parts of the tooth germ and consist of a number of tooth-like structures surrounded by a capsule or a cyst, whilst others are merely calcified masses.

Clinically one or two normal teeth are missing and frequently a hard swelling is noticed at this site. They rarely give rise to pain unless infection occurs.

Radiographic examination is necessary and the treatment is by surgical removal.

TUMOURS OF THE JAWS AND ORAL CAVITY

The most common tumour-like lesions that appear in the oral cavity arising from soft tissues are probably due to an inflammatory reaction. They are fibrous epulis, the giant-celled epulis and the fibro-epithelial polyp. Although not true tumours they are usually treated as such.

The great majority of tumours that occur in various parts of the body may also occur in the oral cavity and therefore there are many types to be considered. Always the most important consideration is whether the lesion is benign or malignant. It must be remembered that the mouth may be invaded by tumours arising from the nose, pharynx and other related structures in the neck. Furthermore the mandible or maxilla may be the site of a metastasis.

Benign epithelial tumours

Papilloma is not uncommon and may present as a pedunculated or sessile tumour in any part of the oral cavity. Its treatment is by excision.

Adenoma occurs rarely in the mouth but the most common site is in the palate. It is frequently one of the varieties of the so-called mixed salivary tumour. This can be a most unpleasant tumour and whilst not invariably malignant has the tendency to become so. It should be removed completely and even then close follow-up is essential for a long time.

Benign connective tissue tumours

Fibroma

Fibroma is not an uncommon tumour in the mouth and may be found in any site, not infrequently on the buccal mucosa when it may become painful if ulcerated by the teeth. It can be pedunculated or sessile and should be removed completely.

Fibrous epulis

"Epulis" means *on the gums*, and therefore any lump on the gum may be referred to as an epulis with the descriptive adjective immediately before it. Fibrous epulis is pedunculated and attached to the gum, and is usually situated between two teeth. The colour is similar to that of the normal gum although if inflamed it might appear much redder. The size can vary from 0·5 cm. to 3 cm., or more, in diameter and it may occur at any age. This epulis probably arises initially through an inflammatory response to irritation and on histological examination it is sometimes noticed that there has been an abscess formation and then the epulis may be referred to as a granuloma pyogenicum.

The treatment is by complete surgical excision, extraction of the associated teeth being unnecessary in the first instance.

Giant-celled epulis (Fig. 12)

This is occasionally referred to as a peripheral osteoclastoma or even a myeloid epulis but it is almost certainly not a true osteoclastoma. It consists of multi-nucleated giant cells in a fibrous matrix and in appearance it is much more purple

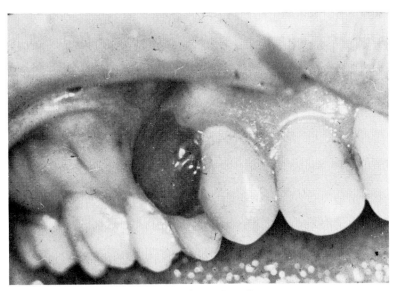

FIG. 12.—Giant cell epulis.

in colour than the fibrous epulis, and bleeds easily. Histologically two types are sometimes described; the first type, where many spindle cells can be seen in which multinucleated giant cells are embedded, and the second, the vascular type, where the connective tissue matrix is much looser in structure, many giant cells are present and the vascularity is increased. The treatment is by complete excision. There is a tendency to recurrence and in such cases the adjacent teeth must be extracted.

With these giant-celled lesions it is always advisable to have the serum electrolytes estimated with a view to eliminating the possibility of hyperparathyroidism.

Pregnancy tumour

This is not a true tumour, but is included as an "epulis". During pregnancy there is a period of disturbance in the endocrine secretions and subacute gingivitis may occur. This may appear as a generalized gingival inflammation with hypertrophy, but occasionally it may be localized on the gingivae between one or two teeth producing a tumour, which clinically is an epulis. Histologically it is very vascular.

Lipoma

This tumour may be found in the floor of the mouth, lips or tongue, and should be excised.

Muscle tumours

Muscle tumours may be found in the tongue and oral cavity but they, like the myxomata, are only rarely found in this situation.

Haemangiomatous formations

Scattered telangiectiases, and cavernous and capillary haemangiomata, may be found in the oral cavity, as indeed may some of the rarer tumours that are found in other parts of the body.

Osteoma

True compact or cancellous osteoma may be found in either jaw, but not commonly. A more frequent bony abnormality which is sometimes given the name of an osteoma may appear in the hard palate, the so-called *torus palatinus*, or on the lingual side of the mandible in the premolar region, the so-called *torus mandibularis*. These latter are usually bilateral.

Torus palatinus (Fig. 13)

This is not a true tumour, but is an overgrowth or exostosis in the midline of the hard palate. It is bony hard and is usually bilateral involving both the maxillary processes though they may not be equally affected. The shape and size vary from a small and flat elevation to a larger mass, and the surface may be fissured or smooth.

In slight cases no treatment is necessary but if very large and causing discomfort or interfering with a denture then this overgrowth should be removed.

Torus mandibularis

The cause is not known but these bony protuberances can be extremely large on the lingual side of the mandible. If they make the fitting of a denture impossible they should be removed.

33

Benign reparative giant-celled granuloma

It is more commonly found in females and may affect either jaw. Microscopically many giant cells are seen in a fibrous matrix and are evenly distributed, the tumour grows slowly and deformity is caused by size. Egg-shell crackling may be present when a considerable amount of bone has been resorbed. Radiographs show a soap bubble trabeculation within a partial or complete boundary wall, but without erosion of other parts of the jaw. The treatment is by radical excision. In the past this granuloma has been frequently referred to as an osteoclastoma. The latter is a rare tumour in the jaws and when it does occur its behaviour is similar to osteoclastoma in any other situation.

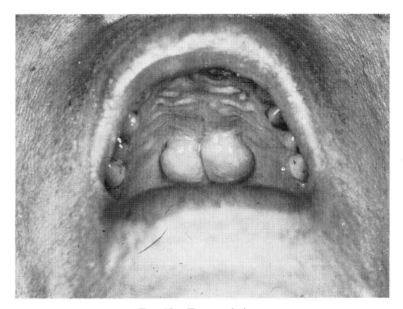

Fig. 13.—Torus palatinus.

Plasmacytoma

This may occur anywhere in the mouth but occasionally presents as an epulis; hence the importance of sending such tumours that are excised for histological examination. The plasmacytoma tends to recur and multiple myelomatosis may follow.

Ameloblastomas

These are sometimes classified as odontomes. They have been known previously as adamantinomata, or multilocular cysts. The tumour however does not contain enamel, it is not necessarily multiloculated and may not even be cystic. It may arise from any part of the epithelium responsible for tooth formation.

The tumour increases in size slowly and invades the bone which may become completely resorbed and it will progress, unless treated, to a large mass. It may be monocystic or polycystic. This is why even apparently simple dental cysts should be sent for histological examination. Some of these tumours may remain solid

34

and microscopically there are masses of cells arranged in palisaded groups separated by connective tissue. In many instances they appear histologically rather like a basal cell carcinoma. It is in this solid mass of cells that cystic degeneration may occur.

Clinically these tumours occur more commonly in young adults and the mandible is more frequently affected than the maxilla. In the first instance they appear as slow expansion of the jaw but when the bone has been destroyed the tumour feels firm or fluctuant according to its type. The teeth in the region of the lesion become loosened and occasionally their roots resorb. In very large tumours which perforate the oral cavity, ulceration occurs.

The radiographic appearance is that of a multilocular cyst or occasionally even a radicular or dentigerous cyst.

These tumours must be regarded as locally malignant and radical excision is therefore necessary. In very large lesions resection of considerable parts of the mandible may be necessary, followed by bone grafting. If the lesion is small it is sometimes possible to leave the lower border of the jaw as sufficient tissue can be removed from around the tumour.

Malignant epithelial tumours

By far the most frequent carcinoma is the squamous cell carcinoma but occasionally adenocarcinoma or the mixed salivary type of tumour may occur in the palate, floor of the mouth and buccal mucosa, arising from the mucous glands and occasionally from aberrant salivary tissue.

Carcinoma of the anterior two-thirds of tongue

This is more frequent in men than women and occurs mainly in middle and old age. It varies in type from a highly keratinized to an anaplastic tumour.

Hyperkeratosis may be a precursor. It is certain that chronic irritation plays a part and syphilis may also be a contributory factor.

In the initial stages it may vary clinically. It may appear as a small warty growth or papilloma. Ulceration may occur in leucoplakia, the base of the ulcer being indurated and sloughing with an everted edge.

Pain is common in the later stages, foetor is frequently marked and the tongue becomes fixed on the side of the lesion.

Lymph node metastases are common and if the lesion is at the tip of the tongue the submental nodes are usually the first to be involved.

Any doubtful lesion should be subjected to a biopsy (excision if possible) and one should remember that cytological examination can be useful in this area.

Cancer of the tongue may be treated by excision or radiotherapy or a combination of these methods. With the advances in radiotherapeutic equipment and techniques this is becoming the method of choice, in preference to mutilating surgery. The cytotoxic drugs have also been used in these cases and in the advanced case where metastases into the cervical lymph nodes have occurred a block dissection of the neck and hemiresection of the mandible may be necessary. Some authorities advocate so-called "prophylactic" neck dissection. Oral hygiene is of the utmost importance.

Carcinoma of the buccal mucosa and floor of the mouth (Fig. 14)

This presents similar clinical features to carcinoma of the tongue. Primary growth may occur in any part of the mouth especially in the region of the opening of the submandibular ducts. The oral mucosa may also be affected by spread from carcinoma of the tongue or alveolus. The principles of diagnosis and management are similar to those outlined above for carcinoma of the tongue.

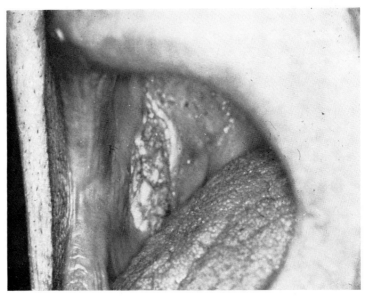

Fig. 14.—Carcinoma in leucoplakia of buccal mucosa.

Carcinoma of the lip

This has a more favourable prognosis than the other oral lesions. Surgical excision with plastic reconstruction is giving way to radiotherapy, especially in the more advanced cases. Lymph node metastases require block dissection.

Melanoma

Pigmented tumours both benign and malignant may occur on the lips and within the oral cavity. They are extremely rare and the majority of malignant melanomata reported have occurred in the maxilla. It must be remembered that melanine spots may occur rather like freckles on the lips in cases of intestinal polyposis and melanin deposits are not uncommon in the oral cavity in certain races. Addison's disease not infrequently causes melanin deposits on the gingivae and a differential diagnosis must be made before treatment is planned.

Malignant connective tissue tumours

Sarcoma of the tongue and jaws is very rare and frequently fatal. Various types such as fibrosarcoma, lymphosarcoma, osteogenic sarcoma and the reticulum celled sarcoma have all been reported. Radical excision followed by irradiation is necessary, but even in the early stages the chances of recovery are very small.

FOR FURTHER READING

Farmer, E. D., and Lawton, F. E. (Eds.) (1966). *Stones' Oral and Dental Diseases* (5th ed.) Edinburgh; Livingstone.

3

DISEASES OF THE SALIVARY GLANDS

DOUGLAS RANGER

It is customary to divide the salivary glands into two main groups—the major and the minor. The sublingual glands are commonly grouped in the major category together with the parotid and submandibular but they more closely resemble and are more easily considered with the other minor glands which are scattered widely throughout the pharyngeal and oral mucosa including the lips.

Although they will not be considered here it is worth noting that similar glands with comparable secretions are found in the nose, sinuses, postnasal space, larynx, trachea and bronchi. The lacrimal gland is of the same general type and may (rarely) be the site of tumours identical with those arising in the salivary glands.

SURGICAL ANATOMY

Parotid glands

The parotid glands are the largest of the salivary glands and in the adult each gland weighs on average 20–25 g. Patey and Ranger have shown that in 25 subjects in whom the gland was removed *post-mortem* the weight of the gland varied from 11 g. to 30 g. and that the lower weights were found in subjects who were elderly or emaciated.

The gland is enclosed in and adherent to a well-defined fibrous capsule derived ftom the deep cervical fascia. A particularly thickened part of this fascia forms the stylomandibular ligament which supports the gland antero-inferiorly and separates it from the submandibular gland.

The parotid gland forms a somewhat irregular mass roughly triangular on hotizontal section with its base externally and its apex projecting into the space between the mandible in front and the mastoid process and sternomastoid muscle behind. These structures groove the anteromedial and posteromedial surfaces. Upwards the gland extends forwards over the masseter muscle. It is from this part of the gland that the parotid duct, about 5 cm. long, emerges to curve around the anterior border of the masseter muscle and open into the mouth opposite the second upper molar tooth. The direction of the duct is indicated by a line drawn from the tragus to the midpoint of the upper lip.

The deep aspect of the parotid gland is related to the upper portion of the posterior belly of the digastric muscle and to the styloid process, stylohyoid and stylomandibular ligaments and the stylohyoid, styloglossus and stylopharyngeus muscles. These structures separate the gland from the carotid sheath and related nerves and more anteriorly from the parapharyngeal space. As a result of this relationship a small proportion of tumours arising in the deep portion of the parotid gland may present as a swelling of the faucial region and soft palate.

A number of structures traverse the parotid gland or are closely applied to it and have relationships of considerable surgical significance. They will be considered in the order of their depth from the surface.

The great auricular nerve arises from the second and third cervical nerves and curves around the posterior border of the sternomastoid muscle near its centre, pierces the deep fascia and ascends across that muscle running with the external jugular vein deep to the platysma muscle. It reaches the postero-inferior portion of the parotid gland and then runs upwards on the capsule or in the most superficial part of the gland before dividing into an anterior branch which supplies the skin over the angle of the jaw and a posterior branch which supplies sensation to the lobe of the ear.

The facial nerve traverses the gland in a postero-anterior direction deep to the great auricular nerve and immediately superficial to the veins. After emerging from the stylomastoid foramen, about 7 mm. deep to the tympanomastoid suture, the facial nerve runs forwards 4–5 mm. below the bony external auditory meatus to enter the posterior surface of the parotid gland accompanied by a branch of the stylomastoid artery which runs just below it. Within the substance of the gland 1–2 cm. from its point of entry the nerve nearly always divides into two main divisions, temporofacial and cervicofacial and these soon divide into a number of terminal branches which spread out to supply the muscles of facial expression including the buccinator. These branches emerge from the gland on its deep surface near its anterior margin and cross the surface of the masseter muscle to their destinations. There are usually a number of filamentous communications between adjacent branches and it is therefore often possible to sacrifice, if necessary, some main branches without a paralysis developing. They are inconstant and cannot be assumed to be present between any branches. However the uppermost branch, to the frontalis, and the lowermost, the cervical branch, only exceptionally have connections with adjacent branches and as a result damage to these branches nearly always leads to paralysis. Occasionally there are two cervical branches—a smaller superficial one and a larger deep branch.

The plane of the facial nerve divides the gland artificially into superficial and deep portions. There is no anatomical separation of the two parts into separate lobes but the gland can be divided surgically in the plane of the nerve and as a result it is possible to resect the whole parotid gland while preserving the facial nerve intact.

Immediately deep to the facial nerve lies a plexus of veins draining into the posterior facial vein running from above downwards in the same plane. This vein originates by the union of the superficial temporal and maxillary veins and at the lower part of the parotid it divides into an anterior division which joins the anterior facial vein to form the common facial vein, and a posterior division which becomes the external jugular vein after being joined by the posterior auricular vein. Very occasionally the posterior facial vein runs between the lower branches of the facial nerve lying immediately superficial, instead of deep, to the lowest one or two branches of the nerve.

Just above the posterior belly of the digastric muscle the external carotid artery enters the deep aspect of the parotid gland and at this point is separated from the veins by a moderate amount of gland tissue. As the artery travels upwards it becomes more and more superficial until at the upper pole the arteries and veins lie together. In the parotid gland the external carotid artery divides into the maxillary and superficial temporal arteries.

The auriculotemporal nerve arising from the mandibular division of the trigeminal nerve passes backwards on the surface of the tensor palati muscle deep to the lateral pterygoid muscle and then between the neck of the mandible and sphenomandibular ligament just above the maxillary artery. The nerve then turns laterally to the deep aspect of the upper part of the parotid gland behind the neck of the mandible. Passing around the upper pole of the parotid gland the auriculotemporal nerve emerges just behind the superficial temporal vessels at the condyle of the mandible. It then runs upwards with the vessels to cross the zygomatic arch before dividing into superficial temporal branches.

It is the auriculotemporal nerve which is generally considered to carry the parasympathetic secretomotor fibres to the parotid gland. Reaching the glossopharyngeal nerve from the inferior salivary nucleus the fibres run in the lesser superficial petrosal nerve to emerge from the skull through the foramen ovale (or the foramen innominatum) and relay in the otic ganglion before joining the auriculotemporal nerve. However clinical observations in patients after intracranial division of the glossopharyngeal nerve and in other patients with gustatory sweating suggest the possibility that secretomotor fibres to the parotid gland may also be supplied through the chorda tympani nerve, and Diamant considers that there is this dual parasympathetic supply. The sympathetic supply to the parotid glands is derived from the plexus around the external carotid artery after relay in the superior cervical ganglion.

The relative importance of the parasympathetic and sympathetic nerves in producing secretion of saliva is not known with certainty. In the past it has been customary to regard the parasympathetic nerves as having the dominant secretomotor role and the sympathetic as supplying the blood vessels and possibly also the myoepithelial cells in the ducts. However, studies by Eneroth, Hokfelt and Norberg (1969) using catecholamine fluorescence, choline esterase staining and electron microscopy suggest that the human parotid and submandibular glands are supplied by fairly equal numbers of sympathetic and parasympathetic nerves and that both sets of fibres innervate parenchymal cells. It has not yet been established to what extent sympathetic activity can produce a secretion of saliva but some clinical observations are certainly in keeping with the suggestion that the sympathetic nerves to the salivary glands have at least some secretomotor activity.

The parotid gland contains a considerable amount of lymphoid tissue. Some of this is aggregated into discrete lymph nodes under the capsule or within the substance of the gland while in other areas masses of lymphocytes surround acini and ducts without having any nodal pattern.

Submandibular glands

The submandibular glands lie beneath the floor of the mouth on each side deep to the body of the mandible and extending below it in the submandibular triangle. Like the parotid the submandibular gland also has a well defined capsule derived from the deep cervical fascia but in contrast it is not normally adherent to it and it is possible to excise the submandibular gland by intracapsular dissection unless inflammatory or other conditions have rendered it abnormally adherent.

The larger part of the submandibular gland lies superficial to the mylohyoid muscle extending as far forwards as the anterior belly of the digastric muscle covered by skin, platysma and fascia in the lower part and also by the mandible and medial pterygoid muscle in the upper part. Around the posterior border of the mylohyoid muscle the superficial portion of the gland becomes continuous with the deep portion lying on the hyoglossus and styloglossus muscles and extending forwards deep to the mylohyoid muscle.

The lingual and hypoglossal nerves cross the hyoglossus deep to the gland—the lingual above and the hypoglossal below. The submandibular duct emerges from the deep part of the gland between the lingual and hypoglossal nerves and runs forwards and upwards to open into the mouth just to the side of the frenum of the tongue. The lingual nerve first descends across the lateral side of the duct and then curves upwards and forwards medial to it. The duct thus passes upwards, inwards and forwards through a loop in the nerve.

The facial artery usually enters the postero-inferior part of the deep lobe of the gland and after traversing the gland at a variable depth emerges from the upper surface to cross the body of the mandible just in front of the origin of the masseter muscle where it is readily located. Anatomically the facial artery is merely embedded in the gland and sometimes its groove is so shallow that the artery is readily separated from the surface of the gland and can be preserved without difficulty during excision of the submandibular gland. The artery is accompanied by veins lying superficially to it.

Just deep to the mandible the artery and veins are crossed superficially by the cervical branch of the facial nerve which can be found at the junction of the planes of the lower border of the mandible and the facial artery by reflecting the platysma upwards. As the submandibular gland can be excised, for non-neoplastic conditions, by intracapsular dissection the nerve can best be safeguarded by opening the capsule well below the mandible.

The parasympathetic nerve supply to the submandibular gland travels from the superior salivary nucleus in the nervus intermedius, and then in the chorda tympani to join the lingual nerve. The fibres leave the lingual nerve to relay in the submandibular ganglion lying on the hyoglossus muscle just below the lingual nerve at the upper portion of the deep lobe of the gland. Just as it has been postulated that the parotid has a double parasympathetic nerve supply there is also the possibility of a dual supply to the submandibular gland from the tympanic branch of the glossopharyngeal nerve and lesser superficial petrosal nerve as well as from the chorda tympani. The sympathetic nerve supply is derived from the carotid plexus along fibres accompanying the facial artery.

Some lymph nodes lie within the capsule of the submandibular gland but lymphoid tissue is not normally found scattered in the substance of the gland itself.

Both the parotid and submandibular glands are compound racemose glands with a single duct dividing into multiple branches arranged into lobes and lobules and ending terminally in alveoli enclosed in a basement membrane continuous with that of the duct. Almost all the alveolar cells of the parotid produce a serous secretion but there are usually a few cells in the alveoli which secrete mucus and there are nearly always a number of mucus-secreting goblet cells opening into the ducts. The submandibular gland contains a roughly equal proportion of mucous and serous alveolar cells.

Minor salivary glands

The minor salivary glands are widely scattered throughout the oral and pharyngeal mucosa. Although separate groups are described according to their anatomical situation there is little to be gained by detailed description. The sub-lingual glands lying just to the side of the lingual frenum, are the largest of the minor glands and open into the floor of the mouth and into the submandibular duct through several small ducts. The palatal glands are the most numerous and there are some 400 glands distributed over the hard and soft palates and the uvula (Fig. 15). Their distribution is often readily assessed by the beads of secretion to be seen on the palate after the administration of drugs with cholinergic activity used during the course of anaesthesia.

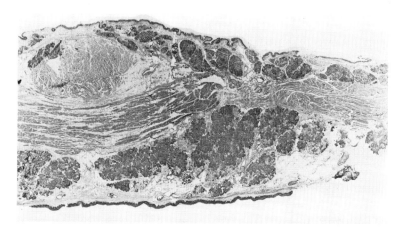

FIG. 15.—Transverse section of palate showing numerous mucous glands on both upper and lower aspects.

The secretions of the minor salivary glands may be serous or mucous but the term "mucous gland" is commonly used to designate the minor salivary and other glands of similar type whatever may be the type of secretion.

GENERAL CLINICAL CONSIDERATIONS

The salivary glands have such a large reserve capacity for producing saliva to aid chewing and swallowing that diminution of secretion is not noticeable unless it is severe as occurs in widespread interference with salivary secretory activity. It is not uncommon for patients to have both submandibular glands removed and some patients may have both parotids excised but such a loss does not produce any noticeable disability as far as the secretion of saliva is concerned. However, patients do have great difficulty with mastication when there is extensive interference with the activity of the salivary glands as may occur in association with the irradiation of malignant neoplasms in the region of the mouth and pharynx or in certain disorders of the glands constituting the sicca syndrome.

Dryness of the mouth in itself does not act as a stimulus to secretion of saliva as is well shown in patients with nasal obstruction who are forced to breathe through the mouth.

Total salivary secretion can be determined only in patients with a complete pharyngeal fistula but it is possible to measure the secretion of each parotid gland separately by fitting a suction cup over the orifice of the duct (Fig. 16).

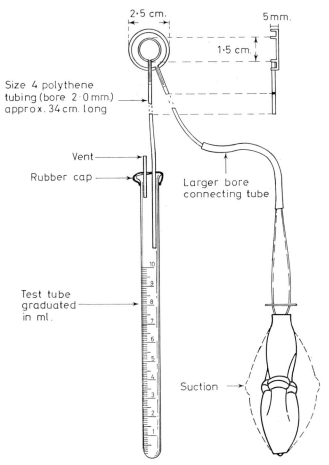

FIG. 16.—Apparatus for collection of saliva from the parotid duct. The metal cup is held in position around the opening of the duct by means of the suction applied to the rim.

Such a procedure does not seem to act as a stimulus to secretion as occurs with the introduction of a catheter into the duct and accordingly some other stimulus must be employed in order to obtain measurable amounts of saliva. Physiological stimulation of the taste buds by standardized solutions applied to the tongue and palate have not proved satisfactory in practice because they do not produce a uniform response in normal subjects. More reliable and consistent results are obtained by the intravenous injection of pilocarpine (in a dosage of 5 mg. for adults) as advocated by Curry and Patey (1964) and this is a more convenient method than the technique of slow intravenous infusion of methacoline used by Diamant (1960), and by Enfors (1962).

In most patients palpation does not give any clear indication of the size or outline of the parotid gland because it has much the same consistency as the surrounding tissues. However, in some people the parotid is distinguishable and appears enlarged without there being any other indication of abnormality. Some of these patients whose glands have been explored have been found on biopsy to have merely a generalized increase of interlobular fat.

The submandibular gland is often palpable externally and can usually be felt easily on bimanual palpation with one finger in the mouth and the fingers of the other hand under the mandible. In some patients the submandibular gland lies unduly low in the neck and can be readily seen and felt below the mandible.

The minor salivary glands are not normally distinguishable through the intact mucosa of the mouth or pharynx but are often encountered in operations on these regions and should not be confused with aggregations of lymphoid tissue.

RETENTION CYSTS

Obstruction of the parotid duct usually leads to suppression of the secretion from the serous alveoli and a tendency to recurrent infection. However, secretion of mucus is not inhibited in the same way and obstruction of the submandibular duct leads to swelling of the gland when secretion of saliva is stimulated by eating. Because the gland is enclosed in a firm fascial capsule this swelling produces a considerable increase in pressure and this is accompanied by pain.

Similar obstruction of the opening of a minor salivary gland usually leads to the development of a thin walled cyst which is painless because there is no firm capsule surrounding it and the overlying mucosa stretches easily. The condition presents as a smooth painless swelling covered by thin mucosa and the cystic nature of the swelling is usually obvious on inspection and palpation.

Such cysts may occur in any part of the mouth or pharynx. When they occur on the lips they are readily noticed by the patient and his relatives and when they occur on the buccal surface of the cheek they tend to interfere with the closure of the teeth. In those situations therefore they are unlikely to become very large before advice is sought. However, when they occur in the floor of the mouth they may enlarge to a considerable size before causing any discomfort or disability and for that reason have tended to be given a separate name—*ranula*. In some instances the cyst wall is so thin that it ruptures and the contents extravasate into the tissues as was shown by Bhaskar, Bolden and Weinmann (1956). This explains the extent of some of these ranulae and the difficulty of their complete eradication in some instances. When the extravasation has extended widely through the tissue planes the term sometimes applied to the condition is "burrowing ranula".

Treatment of retention cysts generally presents no problems. Excision can be carried out immediately outside the cyst wall, which usually separates easily from the surrounding tissues unless there has been previous infection. In the floor of the mouth care must be taken to avoid damage to the lingual nerve and submandibular duct. In patients with burrowing ranulae the essential aspect of the operation is to remove the gland from which the mucoid secretion is arising by adequate excision of the mucosa forming the wall.

SALIVARY FISTULAE

Parotid fistulae occasionally occur from the cut surface of the gland when it is damaged in accidental injuries or surgical incisions. Thus fistulae may (rarely) develop in the postauricular region after mastoidectomy or on the cheek after drainage of an abscess or other operation or injury there. In spite of the large area of cut surface of the parotid which is left exposed after partial parotidectomy it is very rare for a fistula to develop. Provided the parotid duct is normal and provided there is no neoplasm such glandular fistulae present no special problems. If they persist after the rest of the incision has healed they can be dealt with simply by ligating and excising the fistulous track a short distance from the surface and suturing the skin without drainage.

Injuries to the parotid duct, on the other hand, are more difficult to deal with. The first principle of treatment is to try to establish free drainage into the mouth. In any recent injury if there is reason to suppose that the parotid duct might have been injured because of the position of the wound then the duct should be identified and examined. If it is found to be divided or injured the cut ends should be identified and a fine polyethylene catheter inserted as far as possible into the posterior part of the duct after being passed through the natural opening of the duct and along the remaining anterior portion. If the two cut ends can then be approximated without tension this is done, but if not the catheter is left to bridge the gap. The catheter is sutured to the buccal mucosa and left in position for three weeks before being removed. If the natural opening of the parotid duct is involved in the injury then the catheter is brought into the mouth through a stab wound at an appropriate point.

If a salivary fistula has developed on the cheek from a previous injury then a similar method is employed and is usually successful. Even if the duct cannot be identified because of scar tissue but there is a cavity containing saliva associated with the fistula then drainage of this cavity into the mouth with a catheter may well succeed in establishing adequate drainage into the mouth and healing of the fistula. Morel and Firestein (1963) report such a result in a patient explored six weeks after a knife wound and at follow-up 15 months later there was free flow of saliva through the surgically-created buccal opening. Such methods are much simpler and probably more effective than attempts to construct a new portion of duct from oral mucosa.

Abolition of salivary secretion by radiotherapy is a procedure which has been used in patients with parotid fistulae but a full tumour dose may be necessary and even this cannot be guaranteed to prove effective. Such dosage has considerable disadvantages and if all attempts at repairing the fistula should fail conservative parotidectomy with preservation of the facial nerve can be carried out with less hazard than with radiotherapy.

Submandibular salivary fistulae are uncommon and when they do occur they are not difficult to control because of the comparative simplicity of excising the submandibular gland.

SALIVARY CALCULI

Calculi sometimes form in the salivary glands. Over 90 per cent occur in association with the submandibular gland and only rarely are they found in the sublingual gland. The calculi consist of an organic matrix similar to that found in urinary calculi but with somewhat less tendency to form concentric laminations (Harrill, King and Boyce, 1959). The main inorganic constituent is calcium in the form of calcium phosphate but there are usually also traces of magnesium. These inorganic constituents account for the almost invariable opacity of salivary calculi on x-ray examination but small calculi in the parotid gland may be obscured by overlying bony shadows. In both the submandibular and parotid regions intra-oral films may show calculi which would otherwise be missed.

Calculi in the submandibular gland are usually larger than in the parotid and are less likely to be multiple. The calculi may be situated anywhere in the course of the ducts. Sometimes the calculus ulcerates through the duct wall and is extruded into the mouth or into an abscess cavity in the tissues surrounding the duct. In either case the obstruction will be relieved at least temporarily although a stricture may form subsequently at the site of ulceration. The symptoms produced by the presence of salivary calculi will depend on the site and degree of obstruction, on the effect of the obstruction on salivary secretion and on whether or not there is infection present. Glands which secrete mucus are capable of functioning against considerable resistance and mucoceles may develop in many parts of the body when drainage of mucous glands is obstructed in the absence of any infection. On the other hand serous glands cease to function early in the presence of obstruction.

Because there are large numbers of mucus-secreting alveoli in the submandibular gland, secretions continue to be produced even if the duct is completely occluded and as a result the usual symptom produced by a calculus in the submandibular duct is recurrent swelling of the gland in association with meals. Infection may occur but is not common. On the other hand calculi in the parotid duct lead to a greatly diminished secretion of saliva from the gland and infection is much more likely to develop. As a result of this the common effect produced by parotid calculi is the occurrence of repeated attacks of acute parotitis.

The treatment of salivary calculi will depend on the symptoms produced and these will be largely determined by the site. In the parotid gland the problem is usually one of recurrent infections and is more conveniently dealt with under that heading in the next section.

In the submandibular gland the common symptom is recurrent swelling and pain in the submandibular region on eating. Stimulation of salivary activity by lemon juice or a sweet containing fruit juice usually produces a demonstrable enlargement of the submandibular gland. A calculus may be felt on bimanual palpation of the duct and gland. Calculi in the submandibular gland or duct are almost invariably opaque to x-rays and are revealed on plain x-rays provided intra-oral views are taken. If the calculus is situated in the duct itself it is usually a simple matter to remove it by an incision through the oral mucosa and a substantial proportion of patients treated in this way have no further trouble. If the calculus recurs, or if it is situated in the gland itself so that it cannot be removed via the duct, then excision of the submandibular gland is required.

INFECTIONS

Non-suppurative infections of the salivary glands may occur in mumps and there is usually little difficulty in diagnosis except when the condition is unilateral or involves only the submandibular glands without the parotids being affected. A blood count shows no leucocytosis and in any cases of doubt estimations of anti-body titres provide conclusive diagnostic evidence. Occasionally non-suppurative infection may occur in the course of glandular fever.

As with other systems in the body bacterial infection is more common in the presence of obstruction. In the salivary glands this may be caused by the presence of a foreign body in the form of a calculus or by a stricture of the duct. The obstruction may block the main duct in which case the whole gland is involved, or one of the minor ducts when the process will be confined to only a lobe or a lobule of the gland. Reduced salivary secretion such as occurs in dehydrated states and in some pathological conditions of the glands may also be a factor in the aetiology. Infection itself is liable to reduce salivary secretion by damaging or destroying acinar cells and may also lead to strictures of the ducts. Both of these processes increase the likelihood of further infection developing later. Oral sepsis increases the chances of infection spreading along the ducts but glands which are secreting normally and are not obstructed are remarkably resistant to even gross infections in the mouth.

Acute bacterial infection of the salivary glands is normally not difficult to diagnose. The condition follows the general course of such infections elsewhere in the body and is characterized by the rapid development of pain and tenderness in the gland with a variable but usually slight degree of systemic effects and there are usually inflammatory changes evident in the opening of the duct. There is usually a purulent exudate which discharges from the duct spontaneously or in response to pressure. The common organism is a streptococcus but sometimes mixed flora are responsible. If the condition is untreated a tense abscess may develop and this will tend to rupture. In the case of the parotid gland rupture may occur into the external auditory meatus. In the submandibular gland rupture into the floor of the mouth is most likely. However, most of these infections respond rapidly to antibiotics and abscess formation is unusual in any patient so treated. Swabs should be taken from the pus expressed from the duct but while the result of this is awaited ampicillin is probably the antibiotic of choice.

Although a single attack of acute infection may occur in a previously normal gland chronic and recurrent infections of the salivary glands are nearly always associated with obstruction or with diseases in which there is reduced salivary secretion. In the submandibular gland the problem of chronic or recurrent infection is not a difficult one because the offending gland can be removed easily and safely. It is in the parotid gland where operation carries the risk, however slight, of a permanent facial paralysis that recurrent infections present difficulties in management.

As has been mentioned already acute attacks of bacterial parotitis usually respond to antibiotics and some will settle even without them, often with a sudden gush of purulent mucoid material from the duct into the mouth. Initial attacks are often diagnosed as mumps and second attacks may also be so regarded in spite of the fact that such an event must be exceptionally rare if it occurs at all.

The investigation of a patient who has had recurrent attacks of parotitis involves plain x-rays of the region including intra-oral films. Parotid calculi are often very small and there are other shadows in the area which may obscure the calculi. Contrast radiography to outline the duct system with an opaque material is a valuable diagnostic measure but must be done with care. Thackray (1955) has shown that duct walls which have been damaged by inflammatory changes are liable to rupture easily under pressure and that saccular or globular opacities seen on the x-rays after injection of an opaque material into the duct represent extravasated material in the substance of the gland. The appearance of fusiform sialectasis seen in some films indicates a true dilatation of the ducts with the epithelial lining remaining intact while the appearance of sialectasis in any form indicates the presence of chronic infection of the gland, Thackray provided pathological evidence that extravasation produces a marked fibrous reaction and this may prevent resolution of the existing infection as well as predisposing to further infection and rendering surgical excision more difficult with the possible consequence of damage to the facial nerve during operation. Once a duct has ruptured injection of any more material tends to increase the extravasation and is of no further value in outlining the duct system. In an experimental study Ian Ranger (1957) showed that in 20 parotid glands and 20 submandibular glands removed *post mortem* from adults a complete duct pattern was seen in all cases when 0·5 ml. of neo-hydriol was injected and that the injection of further material tended to obscure the duct pattern by acinar filling and by duct rupture in the case of the parotid gland. Pattinson (1969) has advised that initial injection of the parotid duct should be limited to 0·5 ml. in adults or 0·25 ml. in children and further injection made only if required after inspection of the original films. In the submandibular gland amounts of 1·5 ml. may be used.

Estimation of the secretory activity of the parotid gland is indicated in those patients with recurrent or chronic infection who show no evidence of duct obstruction on sialography. Using the technique described by Curry and Patey already mentioned, normal patients secrete from 3 ml. to 13 ml. in the five minutes after injection of 5 mg. pilocarpine intravenously. Although the absolute values vary to this extent there is usually a close correlation between the two sides in the absence of any disease and therefore any appreciable difference between them is significant even though both values may be within the normal range.

The treatment of an acute bacterial parotitis has already been considered. The management of patients who have recurrent or chronic parotitis will depend on the result of the investigations just mentioned.

If x-rays show a single calculus in the main parotid duct then dilatation of the orifice of the duct may result in passage of the stone. Incision of the duct through the mouth or through an incision in the cheek to remove the calculus are often not the simple operations they might seem in that there is nearly always considerable surrounding fibrosis and the procedure is likely to be followed by stricture formation.

If there is a stricture of the main duct intermittent dilatation with bougies may succeed. Insertion of a small polyethylene catheter if possible and suture to the buccal aspect of the cheek to retain it in position for a period of three weeks (based on experience of injuries to the duct) is a technique of value in some patients but even after the passage of bougies it is not always possible to insert a catheter.

If investigations do not show any obstruction in the ducts and if secretion is within normal limits then there is a good chance that the attacks will subside. Any oral sepsis is dealt with and steps taken to ensure that the patient does not become dehydrated at any time.

If x-rays show multiple calculi or obstruction of the ducts which is not amenable to treatment or if treatment of the obstruction fails, or if there is greatly diminished secretion, then the likely course of events is that attacks of parotitis will recur with increasing frequency as each attack produces further damage and predisposes to further infections. In this situation parotidectomy may be the only means of ensuring a cure but other methods mentioned below may be successful and are worth trying if otherwise parotidectomy would be advocated.

Intra-oral ligation of the parotid duct as described by Laage-Helman (1955) and by Diamant (1958) may be successful in a large proportion of patients. Diamant found that six out of his seven patients were cured by the procedure, combined with pre-operative radiotherapy, and Maynard has reported 73 per cent successful results in a series followed up for one year. Although Diamant advised pre-operative radiotherapy the possible disadvantages of this, especially in young people, are such that some workers would regard it as unjustifiable. An alternative method of temporarily reducing parotid secretion in the immediate post-operative period is to perform a tympanotomy and divide the tympanic branch of the glossopharyngeal nerve on the promontory of the middle ear and possibly also the chorda tympani. These intratympanic procedures in themselves do not seem adequate to cure recurrent parotitis but seem to reduce parotid secretion temporarily and appear to be a reasonable and less damaging alternative to radiotherapy as an adjunct to ligation of the parotid duct. The problem about ligation of the duct arises from the fact that the mucous elements in the gland may continue to secrete and as a result the condition may be made worse and parotidectomy become essential. Accordingly the treatment can be carried out only on patients who have accepted this risk and in centres which are prepared to undertake parotidectomy for this condition if it is needed.

The indications for parotidectomy, because of recurrent parotitis, will depend on the frequency and severity of the attacks and the acceptance by the patient of the risk of a facial paralysis. This risk must be very slight with surgeons who have considerable experience of parotid surgery and although Patey (1965a) reported that temporary functional facial paralysis is commoner after operations for parotitis than for tumours all his patients had recovered full facial movements.

Specific infections of the salivary glands are uncommon. Tuberculosis may occur in the gland substance but is more likely to develop in a lymph node within the capsule. In the parotid the condition presents as a parotid "tumour" and there are no particular features to distinguish it from a true neoplasm. In the submandibular gland the condition is even more uncommon and again is more likely to be diagnosed as a tumour than an infection. In either gland excision is usually undertaken before the diagnosis is apparent. In a patient recently treated by the author the histological and cultural findings provided conclusive evidence of tuberculosis even though a pre-operative Mantoux test was negative.

Sarcoidosis occasionally involves the parotid glands and rarely the submandibular glands. Unlike tuberculosis, it generally produces a diffuse enlargement of the gland and is usually bilateral. The condition is part of a generalized disease and occurs in about 5 per cent of patients with sarcoidosis. In the great majority of patients, a radiograph of the chest shows either hilar lymphadenopathy or pulmonary infiltration or both. The Kveim test is positive in about 80 per cent of the patients and there is usually enlargement of peripheral lymph nodes, commonly including the epitrochlear nodes. In about one-third of patients with parotid sarcoidosis, there is an associated uveitis and ophthalmic examination is necessary whenever sarcoidosis of the salivary glands is suspected. Peripheral neuritis, especially of the cranial nerves, is not uncommon and when the facial nerve is involved it is natural to associate it directly with the parotid enlargement. However, Pennell (1951) and later Hook (1954) showed that facial paralysis occurs no more commonly in sarcoidosis with parotid involvement than in sarcoidosis generally and concluded that pressure from the enlarged parotid gland is not the cause of the paralysis. This view has been supported by others having considerable experience of sarcoidosis, such as Greenberg, Anderson, Sharpstone and James.

In most patients with sarcoidosis of the salivary glands, the presenting symptom is usually a swelling of the glands and some patients also notice some dryness of the mouth. In a few patients, ocular symptoms occur first. The activity of the process varies considerably and in a proportion of patients, there is a persistent low-grade fever—the "febris uveoparotidea subchronica" described by Heerfordt in his classical description of the syndrome. In about half the patients, the salivary glands return to normal within six months. In the others, resolution may take up to three years. Corticosteroids reduce the size of the glands in the more acute conditions, but seem to have little influence on the overall course of the disease and are usually not indicated.

Actinomycosis is very uncommon in this country now and syphilis rarely involves the salivary glands.

OTHER CONDITIONS

Enlargement of the parotid glands, usually bilateral, as a result of increase of the intraglandular fat has already been mentioned. It is of no cosequence and requires no treatment but may cause confusion in diagnosis. Sialography and secretion are normal. Differential diagnosis includes hypertrophy of the masseter muscles but this is unlikely to cause difficulty provided it is thought of.

Enlargement of the parotid occasionally occurs in patients receiving treatment with thiouracil. Barbero and Sibinga (1962) reported that 92 per cent of patients with mucoviscidosis had significant enlargement of the submandibular glands but the parotids seem to escape.

In a few patients the lymphoid tissue in the parotid or submandibular glands is involved in a reticulosis and sometimes this can be difficult to distinguish clinically and histologically from a sialoadenitis when it is the presenting symptom and when there is no evidence of other lymphoid tissue being involved.

Enlargement of the parotids and sometimes the submandibular glands with diminished secretion also occurs in an ill-understood group of conditions which, for this reason, are described under various names. In 1888 at a meeting in Konigsberg, Mikulicz described a patient with swelling of the lacrimal, submandibular and parotid glands and this was reported in 1892. Since then the term "Mikulicz Disease" or "Mikulicz Syndrome" has been used as an eponymous title and other names such as Gougerot and Sjogren have been added by some people. More recently the term "sicca syndrome" has been used as a descriptive title to emphasize one of the main features of the disorder.

Histological evidence shows that the gland is infiltrated by lymphocytes and plasma cells leading to fibrosis. Patey and Thackray (1955) also reported atrophy of acinar cells with squamous epithelial proliferation of the ducts and multiple minute calculi. Sialography shows a picture of punctate sialectasis and Jones reported that 50 per cent of patients had a significantly raised γ-globulin. Some patients have other diseases such as rheumatoid arthritis or dermatomyositis and in some antinuclear factors have been demonstrated in the blood suggesting an auto-immune process. In a few patients the changes in lymphoid elements in the gland have made it difficult to distinguish the condition from an adenolymphoma.

49

Whatever the aetiology of the condition, or group of conditions, the clinical features which present problems are the liability to recurrent infection, the enlargement of the gland suggesting a diagnosis of neoplasm and last, but often the most important to the patient, the associated xerostomia. If the lacrimal glands are also involved there will be diminished tear formation and a tendency to kerato-conjunctivitis. The problem of infection has been referred to already and neoplasia will be considered in the next section. Symptomatic relief of xerostomia is never satisfactory but patients sometimes obtain some relief from glycerin.

NEOPLASMS

Although tumours arising from the lymphoid or supporting connective tissues may occur in the salivary glands they are rare, as also are secondary malignant neoplasms, and most of the tumours found in the salivary glands arise from the specialized epithelial cells of the ducts or acini. They form only 2–3 per cent of all tumours but are of particular significance because of the special features which they exhibit and the consequent difficulty in classification and terminology. Rewell (1963) has aptly remarked that "in this field terminology has proliferated madly enough to be termed 'malignant'".

Although salivary tumours of almost any type may occur in any of the glands there is considerable variation in the frequency with which different types of tumour occur in individual glands and in the proportional distribution of benign and malignant tumours, not only between the major and minor glands but also between different groups of minor glands. Approximately 80 per cent of the tumours are situated in the parotid gland, 10 per cent in the submandibular gland and 10 per cent in the minor salivary glands. This distribution does not correspond with the relative weights of the glandular tissue and among the minor glands the frequency in different sites is not related to the number of glands in a particular area.

Classification

No system of classification so far devised has received universal acceptance but with the increasing frequency of excision of salivary tumours in the last 20 years and the greater opportunity for correlating the histological findings with the subsequent history of the patients, certain general principles have emerged. In particular it has now been recognized that local recurrence of tumour in these situations is not necessarily, or usually, a feature to be equated with frank malignancy. Also benign tumours may occasionally undergo malignant change which is not only manifested by the clinical behaviour of the tumour but also by demonstrable changes which have occurred in the histological appearance.

The distribution of the main types of tumours is shown for the different sites in Table I, which has been compiled from the comprehensive detailed figures given by Bardevill, Luna and Healey; Eneroth; Eneroth, Hjertman and Moberger; Farr; Foote and Frazell; Harrison; Naunton Morgan and Mackenzie; Patey (1965b); Patey, Thackray and Keeling; Ranger, Thackray and Lucas; Thackray (1961).

The main types of salivary tumour will now be considered in more detail and then their management will be discussed in relation to the site of origin.

TABLE I

DISTRIBUTION OF MAIN TYPES OF TUMOUR OCCURRING IN DIFFERENT SALIVARY GLANDS EXPRESSED AS AN APPROXIMATE PERCENTAGE OF THE TOTAL

Type of tumour	Parotid gland	Sub-mandibular gland	Lip and cheek	Palate	Floor of mouth and tongue	Peri-tonsillar area	Total
Pleomorphic adenoma	61	4	1	2·7		1	69·7
Muco-epidermoid tumour	3·5	1		0·7			5·2
Adenoid cystic carcinoma	1·5	1·5	0·4	1·2	1·3	0·2	6·1
Other types of carcinoma	11	2·5	0·1	0·4			14
Miscellaneous	5						5
Total	82	9	1·5	5	1·3	1·2	100

Note: This table refers to only those glands which can properly be classed as "salivary" glands, major or minor, and does not include similar tumours found in the nose, sinuses, larynx, trachea, bronchi etc.

Pleomorphic adenoma

For many years these tumours have been referred to as "mixed" tumours on account of their histological appearance. They are the commonest of all the salivary tumours and occur more than twice as frequently as all the other types combined. The tumours are essentially benign but may recur locally if removal is incomplete and a small proportion (less than 5 per cent) undergo malignant change, sometimes after a very long interval. Patey, Thackray and Keeling report such a change in a woman whose history went back 46 years.

These tumours occur most commonly in young adults, the majority developing before the age of 40. Males and females are almost equally affected. The parotid gland is by far the commonest site and nearly 90 per cent of all salivary pleomorphic adenomas occur in that gland.

Macroscopically the tumour is firm and usually lobulated with a well-defined capsule surrounding it. However, histologically it can be seen that portions of tumour frequently extend through the capsule. In single sections these outgrowths may appear to be detached from the main tumour (Fig. 17) but as has been demonstrated by Patey and Thackray (1953), serial sections show that there is always a projection through the capsule although the strand may be quite slender. As any tumour may have several such outgrowths, the strands of which are easily torn across if the tumour is enucleated, recurrences are usually multicentric in type and serial sections of recurrent neoplasms show no connecting strands between the different recurrent tumours which are growing apparently as one mass.

A pleomorphic adenoma has a slowly progressive rate of growth and if left untreated may come to weigh as much as 2 or 3 kg. Recurrences tend to grow steadily at the same rate.

Microscopically the tumour consists of epithelial cells in a hyaline stroma having a chondroid appearance and it was this that led to the original description of "mixed" tumour. However, it is now generally regarded that the stroma is a secretion but there is still considerable difference of opinion about its exact origin and significance. The amount of matrix present varies considerably from one tumour to another and even in different areas of the same tumour.

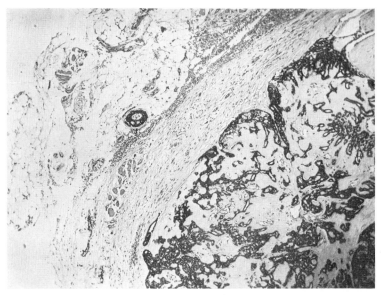

FIG. 17.—Pleomorphic adenoma with a well-defined capsule and an extension of neoplasm outside the capsule. In this single section the nodule appears to be separate from the main mass of tumour but serial sections showed that the two were connected by a fine strand penetrating the capsule. (× 35, reduced to three-quarters on reproduction.) (*From Ranger, Thackray and Lucas* (1956), *reproduced by courtesy of the Editor of* British Journal of Cancer.)

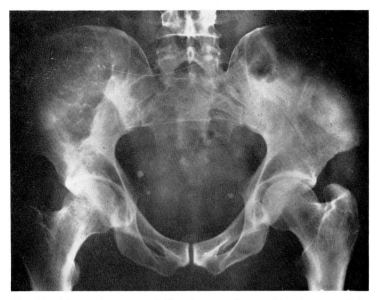

FIG. 18.—Metastatic tumour of ilium from a pleomorphic adenoma of the parotid. The metastasis, from which a biopsy was taken in 1942, showed the histological features of a typical pleomorphic adenoma identical in appearance with a parotid tumour removed in 1919.

Rarely, metastases in distant parts of the body have had histological appearances identical with the original pleomorphic adenoma removed many years previously. Fig. 18 shows the x-ray appearances of such a tumour in the ilium. A biopsy taken from it in 1942 showed a typical pleomorphic adenoma indistinguishable from the sections of a tumour removed from the patient's parotid gland in 1919.

Muco-epidermoid tumours

Muco-epidermoid tumours form about 5 per cent of parotid tumours and are also occasionally found in the submandibular gland and in the palate but are very rare elsewhere. When these tumours were first clearly described by Stewart, Foote and Becker (1945) and later by Linell (1948) they were considered to include both benign and malignant varieties. However, it is now generally accepted that none can be regarded as truly benign although the degree of malignancy is variable.

Histologically these tumours contain varying proportions of epidermoid cells, mucus-secreting cells and intermediate cells and as a result the cut surface of the tumour may appear to be a solid mass or collection of mucous cysts.

Although some of these tumours may be of high grade malignancy the prognosis is generally better than with other types of malignant salivary tumours. There is evidence that at least some of these tumours are radio-sensitive.

Adenoid cystic carcinoma

These tumours are frequently referred to by other names such as cylindroma or basalioma. These terms serve to describe two of the characteristic features of the pathology but fail to include the predominant concept of malignancy and therefore fail to distinguish them adequately from "mixed" tumours with a cylindromatous appearance. For this reason the term "adenoid cystic carcinoma" has come to be used increasingly throughout the literature on salivary tumours.

In the parotid gland adenoid cystic carcinomas form only a small proportion of the total tumours (less than 2 per cent) but in the palate they form a much higher proportion (about 30 per cent) and in the tongue and floor of mouth virtually all the salivary gland tumours are of this type.

These tumours are invasive and often infiltrate along tissue planes, particularly in perineural and perivascular spaces. Although malignant, their rate of growth is usually slow and it may be several years before they reach appreciable size or recur after removal. They are liable to metastasize widely, especially after local recurrences have developed but the metastases usually also grow slowly and patients with metastases may continue to live for several years in a generally fit state.

Histologically the tumours are characterized by the occurrence of masses of cells around cystic or alveolar spaces in a scanty connective tissue stroma but in some instances the cells occur in solid sheets without any cystic spaces.

Acinic cell tumours

These are malignant tumours with a distinctive histological appearance of masses of uniform acinic cells with a well marked cell membrane and small deeply staining nucleus. The cells are usually arranged in solid masses but sometimes exhibit a microcystic or papillary cystic form. They occur predominantly in women and almost entirely in the parotid gland. A small proportion of the tumours are painful.

The acinic cell tumours are malignant but appear to have a better prognosis than the other malignant neoplasms.

Other carcinomas

In addition to the muco-epidermoid tumours, acinic cell tumours and adenoid cystic carcinomas which have been described already, other malignant tumours are found in the salivary glands. The commonest of these is the spheroidal cell carcinoma without any recognizable glandular elements and with masses of undifferentiated rounded cells. Some of these tumours arise *de novo* but from 30–40 per cent develop in glands which have previously been the site of a pleomorphic adenoma. The next most common type is the adenocarcinoma and in approximately 50 per cent of these there is also evidence of a pre-existing pleomorphic adenoma. Histologically these tumours have obvious tubule formation of frankly malignant type but without the special features found in the adenoid cystic tumours. About 50 per cent of spindle cell carcinomas arise in pleomorphic adenomas and occasionally they have been found in association with adenoid cystic carcinoma. They are characterized by masses of spindle-shaped cells without any glandular structure. Squamous cell carcinomas with varying degrees of keratinization are sometimes found in the parotid and may occur in the minor salivary glands as well but in those sites it is impossible to distinguish them from squamous cell carcinomas arising from the mucosa of the area.

Secondary tumours

Occasionally secondary tumours may be found in the parotid gland and even more rarely in the submandibular gland, although of course either may be secondarily involved by direct extension of malignant neoplasms occurring in the neighbourhood.

Melanomata of the face and scalp may give rise to a metastatic lymph node in the parotid without the primary lesion being obvious and the patients may be regarded as having a primary parotid tumour. Blood-borne metastases have also occurred from carcinoma in such distant sites as bronchus, breast, kidney, stomach, pancreas etc.

Miscellaneous tumours

Occasionally other tumours not already discussed may occur in the salivary glands, especially in the parotid. These may arise from epithelial or lymphoid structures or from connective tissue.

Adenolymphoma

These are completely benign encapsulated tumours which form about 7 per cent of all the tumours in the parotid gland and are sometimes referred to as "Wartins" tumours. They may be multiple and bilateral and are predominantly found in males of middle age. Histologically they contain both lymphoid and epithelial elements, the latter usually being arranged in a papillary manner in cystic cavities. Although, because of their tendency to multiple origin, apparent recurrences may develop, they are not malignant and are not sensitive to irradiation.

Oncocytoma

These are uncommon benign tumours which account for only about 0·5 per cent of all parotid tumours. They arise from the oncocytes which are found in the parotid glands of adults, but seldom before the age of 50. Histologically the tumours are composed of uniform masses of eosinophilic granular oncocytes with a deeply staining peripheral nucleus.

Retention cysts and branchial cysts

These have been referred to already on p. 43 but are mentioned again here as often they are indistinguishable from neoplasms until the gland is explored.

Connective tissue tumours

Tumours which arise in connective tissue may occasionally occur in the salivary glands. Neurofibroma is probably the least uncommon and other tumours which have been found include fibroma, lipoma, haemangioma and lymphangioma. Haemangiomas and lymphangiomas are softer in consistency than other tumours and usually appear to be more diffuse. Sometimes a diagnosis of cavernous haemangioma can be confirmed by the appearance of multiple calcified thrombi on x-ray which differ from parotid calculi in that they have no tendency to produce recurrent parotitis.

THE MANAGEMENT OF SALIVARY TUMOURS

Although the behaviour of any salivary neoplasm is largely determined by its pathological type, the diagnosis and treatment will depend on its site of origin and its relationship to adjacent anatomical structures as well as its histological classification. In view of this it is convenient to discuss the management of tumours according to the gland which is affected.

Parotid tumours

In the parotid gland more than three-quarters of the neoplasms are benign and in addition some inflammatory lesions present as painless tumours indistinguishable from neoplastic conditions. The frequency of various types of parotid tumour is shown in Table II.

TABLE II

Parotid tumours	Percentage incidence
Pleomorphic adenoma	65
Adenolymphoma	5
Oncocytoma	0·5
Benign cysts and connective tissue tumours (neurinoma, lipoma, haemangioma, lymphangioma)	6·5
Acinic cell tumours	1·5
Muco-epidermoid tumours	5
Adenoid cystic carcinoma	5·5
Other carcinomas and sarcomas (including metastases)	11

Only very few parotid tumours, e.g. haemangiomas, have any special features which enable a pathological diagnosis to be made pre-operatively on clinical and radiographic evidence. Most tumours present as painless swellings without any particular distinguishing features. Although evidence of involvement of the facial nerve is an indication of malignancy the majority of malignant tumours are not associated with any facial weakness when the patient is first seen.

Biopsy of parotid tumours leads to spillage of cells and may well lead to the development of tumour in the scar. Fig. 19 shows a typical example. Because of this it is inadvisable to perform a preliminary biopsy of any parotid tumour and biopsy at the time of operation is indicated only in particularly difficult cases. Cytological examination of material obtained by aspiration biopsy is a method which is used in some centres but the results are unlikely to provide a certain answer on which treatment can be soundly based. Eneroth, Franzen and Zajicek (1966) were able to confirm the presence of a tumour in 92 per cent of cases, but this degree of probability is no greater than that resulting from simple clinical examination. More particularly, in only about 50 per cent of cases could the question of malignancy be correctly evaluated. Few people can have had such extensive experience as these workers and in less skilled hands the figures would be even less favourable.

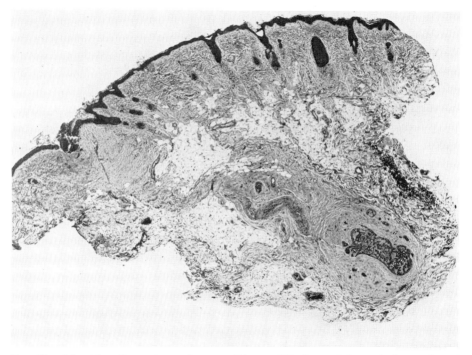

FIG. 19.—Adenoid cystic carcinoma in a parotid scar. Histology of the excised scar showed active viable adenoid cystic carcinoma after a radical course of radiotherapy administered before total radical parotidectomy with excision of the scar. (*Photomicrograph by Mr. D. Bishop, Ferens Institute of Otolaryngology, from a slide provided by Professor A. C. Thackray, Bland Sutton Institute of Pathology.*)

Surgical exploration remains the most certain way of determining the correct diagnosis of any swelling in the parotid gland and of assessing the most appropriate form of management. The passage of the facial nerve through the parotid gland dominates the anatomical features and the exact relationship of the tumour to the nerve can be determined precisely only at operation. As a result of the types of operation which have been developed over the years by Redon (1965) and others the plane of the facial nerve can be defined with exactitude and the superfacial portion or the subfacial portion of the gland can be removed with any contained tumour. If the pathological nature of the condition allows it the superfacial and subfacial portions can both be excised with preservation of the facial nerve. Clinical experience and pathological studies have shown that in a large number of tumours enucleation from within any capsule which is present is liable to leave residual small nodules of tumour which lead to multicentric recurrences although the rate of growth of many tumours is such that this may not be obvious for some years. When there is no connective tissue capsule and the tumour is contained merely within a surrounding area of compressed normal gland tissue then clearly any attempt at enucleation in this plane must be surgically unsound.

The common tumours of the parotid gland are not radio-sensitive and radio-therapy is not an alternative to surgical excision although some people regard it as an adjuvant to be used in conjunction with enucleation of the tumour. Excision of the tumour with a surrounding area of normal parotid gland is preferred by most surgeons and Morrison (1966) has described the indications for radiotherapy in the management of pleomorphic adenomas of the parotid as being confined to those cases in which the capsule of the tumour ruptures at operation or, exceptionally, the tumour is large and for some reason is inoperable.

A small proportion of patients with parotid tumours arising in the deep lobe of the gland present with a mass in the parapharyngeal space. These will be considered in more detail later under the heading of peritonsillar tumours but, in general, the principles of management are the same as with other parotid tumours although some modification of technique may be required at operation.

For the reasons given above the management of patients with parotid tumours consists essentially of surgical exploration of the parotid gland; identification of the facial nerve and determination of its exact relationship to the tumour; an assessment of the pathological nature of the tumour and the degree of any infiltration which may be present followed by a resection of an appropriate amount of the gland except in a few patients in whom the growth appears to be inoperable. In those few patients with extensively infiltrating malignant tumours in whom resection is impossible the best management will be by radiotherapy. In others, if histological evaluation after excision shows that the tumour is a mucoepidermoid or adenoid cystic carcinoma or some other form of malignancy then post-operative radiotherapy is indicated.

Operative technique

The operation starts with a vertical incision in front of the ear, in a pre-auricular skin crease, extended in a wide S-shaped curve below the ear and then prolonged forwards in an upper cervical skin crease to the level of the tip of the greater cornu of the hyoid bone. The incision is extended through superficial and deep fascia exposing the sternomastoid muscle with the external jugular vein and great auricular nerve crossing it obliquely. These are preserved at this stage and the deep fascia dissected off the muscle to its anterior edge, dividing in the process any posterior fibres of the platysma which are in the way. The muscle is cleared posteriorly as far back as the mastoid process and the greater auricular nerve is now exposed with the posterior fibres running to the lobe of the ear. These fibres can usually be preserved intact unless there is a tumour situated in the posterior part of the gland.

Unless there is a very large tumour posteriorly, dissection then proceeds in the interval between the anterior border of the base of the mastoid process and the mandible by division of the fascia extending from the parotid to be firmly attached to the cartilage of the external auditory meatus. The upper part of the sternomastoid muscle is retracted backwards and the stylohyoid muscle and posterior belly of the digastric exposed and identified. The main trunk of the facial nerve is then located by blunt dissection after it has emerged from the stylomastoid foramen and is running forwards in the angle between the external auditory meatus and the digastric muscle to enter the posterior surface of the parotid. A small artery accompanies the nerve, usually lying just below it and if this can be preserved it probably reduces the risk of a temporary facial paralysis.

Once the nerve has been identified it can be followed forwards into the gland where it soon divides into its main upper and lower divisions. At this point an assessment is made of the site of the tumour in relation to the nerve and of any infiltration which may be present. In most instances the tumour will be entirely superficial to the plane of the facial nerve and in that case the treatment of choice is a resection of the superficial portion of the gland with preservation of the nerve. If the tumour lies deep to the nerve then the deep portion of the gland should be removed; to allow this, in some instances the superficial portion need only be reflected upwards with the nerve, but in other patients adequate access to the deep lobe may be obtained only after resecting the superficial part of the gland.

If there is evidence that the tumour is malignant and is infiltrating the nerve then the nerve will have to be sacrificed in whole or in part, together with any other structures in the neighbourhood, such as the masseter muscle, which may also be involved. In such patients operation should be followed by post-operative radiotherapy.

The post-operative complication most feared after parotidectomy is, of course, facial paralysis but with the development of the technique of precise identification of the nerve any permanent paralysis can be avoided except when it is necessary to deliberately sacrifice the nerve.

The most frequent post-operative complication is gustatory sweating—sweating of the side of the face on eating—shown by Glaister and his colleagues (1958) to be the result of divided parasympathetic secretomotor fibres coming to activate sweat glands in the area. Although this seems to be the explanation of the phenomenon treatment by intratympanic division of the parasympathetic nerves has not always been effective in curing the condition in those few patients in whom the condition is a considerable disability. Patey (1968) has referred to one such patient treated in conjunction with the author. Fortunately in most patients the complication amounts to only a minor nuisance.

Salivary fistula after parotidectomy is rare and has been referred to already under "Salivary Fistulae", p. 44. It usually presents no difficulty in management.

Submandibular tumours

In the submandibular gland most swellings are associated with an obstruction of the duct, usually by a calculus, and neoplasms are uncommon. Of the neoplasms a significant proportion are malignant. Among 187 primary tumours of the submandibular gland Eneroth, Hjertman and Moberger (1967) found that one-third were malignant and this figure is lower than that in many other series. As is seen in Table I the composite figures obtained from many different series show that more than one-half of the submandibular neoplasms are malignant.

In the management of submandibular tumours the first essential is to suspect the condition. In patients with a swelling of the gland the majority will have a history of recurrent swelling with meals and clinical or radiological evidence of a calculus in the gland or the duct. If both of these features are not present then a neoplastic condition must be suspected as a possibility.

As in the parotid gland treatment consists essentially of excision but in this case there are no important anatomical structures to interfere with complete removal of the gland. If subsequent histological examination of the gland shows that the tumour is malignant then post-operative radiotherapy is indicated.

Operative technique

The operation of excision of the submandibular gland starts with an incision in the upper skin crease of the neck extending from a point opposite the angle of the jaw almost to the midline of the neck. In excision of the gland for inflammatory conditions and to deal with the problems of calculi the fascial capsule of the gland can be opened immediately and all subsequent dissection carried out in that plane to avoid the risk of damage to the mandibular branch of the facial nerve supplying the muscles of the lower lip at the corner of the mouth; the facial artery and veins can also be ligated and divided close to the gland and, on the deep surface of the gland, the lingual nerve above and hypoglossal nerve below can be identified lying on the hyoglossus muscle and are preserved carefully while the duct is divided as it runs forwards and inwards in the loop of the lingual nerve. However, in suspected neoplasms, as in the parotid gland, at an early stage of the operation there must be a careful assessment of the nature of the lesion and the degree of any infiltration of surrounding structures. In view of the fact that adenoid cystic carcinomas are known readily to involve and spread in perineural and perivascular spaces it is desirable, if the condition appears to be malignant, to ligate the vessels well away from the gland and it may be necessary also to sacrifice the lingual and hypoglossal nerves and parts of the mylohyoid, digastric and hyoglossus muscles depending on the size and site of the tumour and the degree of any infiltration which is found.

Minor salivary glands

In the *lip* it is almost exclusively the upper lip which is likely to be the site of salivary tumours (Fig. 20) and here, as in the cheek, the tumour is unlikely to be malignant. The differentiation from a retention cyst is usually easy on palpation and because of their situation such tumours are easily excised with a surrounding area of soft tissue. If the histology of the resected tissue shows that the tumour is malignant then post-operative radiotherapy should be given to the area but such an event is a rarity.

In the *palate* the tumours are often neglected and may become large before the patient seeks medical advice. A typical palatal salivary tumour is shown in Fig. 21 while an unusually large one is shown on a lateral x-ray film in Fig. 22. In approximately half the patients the tumour is malignant, commonly an adenoid cystic carcinoma, and the bone of the palate may be involved without there being any evidence of this until the bone is removed and examined histologically (Fig. 23). If such tumours are not adequately removed they extend upwards and eventually may invade the middle cranial fossa (Fig. 24).

Because of their situation in relation to bone, salivary tumours arising in the area of the hard palate are most easily removed by simple enucleation off the bone and

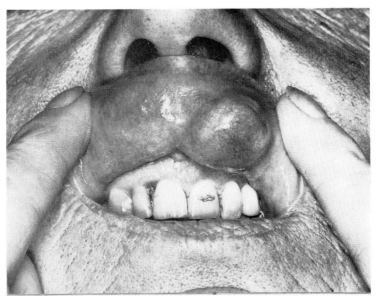

FIG. 20.—Typical pleomorphic adenoma of the upper lip.

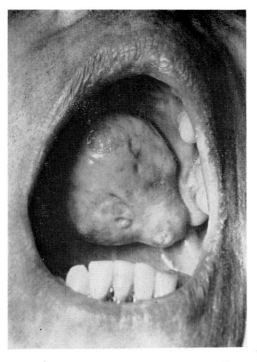

FIG. 21.—Typical pleomorphic adenoma of the hard palate. (*From
Ranger, Thackray and Lucas* (1956),
*reproduced by courtesy of the Editor
of* British Journal of Cancer.)

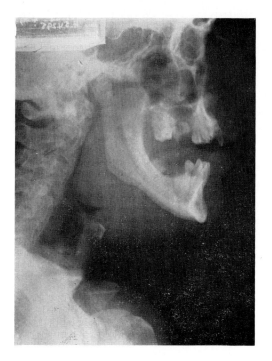

FIG. 22.—Lateral radiograph showing the extent of a very large pleomorphic adenoma arising in the palate. The patient was aged 30 and the tumour had first been noticed at the age of 19. (*From Ranger, Thackray and Lucas* (1956), *reproduced by courtesy of the Editor of* British Journal of Cancer.)

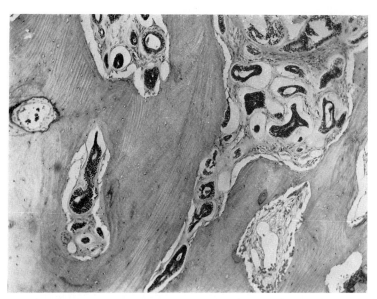

FIG. 23.—Adenoid cystic carcinoma in the hard palate. There is extensive spread of tumour throughout the Haversian system without any destruction of bone and therefore without any clinical, radiological or operative evidence of involvement of bone. (× 70, reduced to three-quarters on reproduction.) (From *Ranger, Thackray and Lucus* (1956), *reproduced by courtesy of the Editor of British Journal of Cancer.*)

61

undoubtedly this fact has contributed largely to the high recurrence rate of even pleomorphic adenomas in this situation as stressed by Ranger, Thackray and Lucas (1956). As has been mentioned already enucleation of almost any salivary tumour is liable to leave behind residual neoplastic areas and in addition statistics show that in the palate approximately half the tumours are malignant. For these

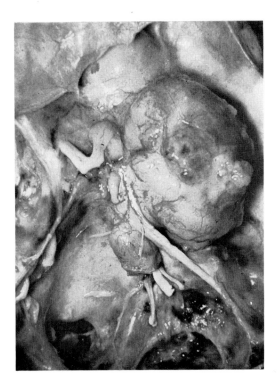

FIG. 24.—Adenoid cystic carcinoma invading the middle cranial fossa. The patient presented with a tumour of the palate which had been present for four years. Treatment was by excision followed by radio-therapy. Multiple pulmonary meta-stases developed six years later and death occurred from the intracranial extension after a further two years.

reasons it is considered that the treatment of choice for palatal tumours is to remove the tumour by excising the area of palate to which it is attached and this applies whether the tumour is situated in the hard or soft palate. The resulting defect can be closed by an obturator and the defect to be covered in this way will be smaller than any deficiency resulting from attempts to treat multicentric recurrences. Furthermore, operation for eradication of recurrence is unlikely to be successful.

In the *floor of the mouth* and tongue salivary tumours are almost invariably malignant and are clinically similar to squamous cell carcinomas invading that area of the mouth. Also in this area surgical excision of malignant tumours may require extensive resection of tissues including possibly the mandible. For these reasons this is one situation in which it is considered that the management of salivary tumours is governed by the fact that they are not clearly distinguishable from other malignant tumours occurring in the same area and as a result biopsy will be the initial requirement. In the light of the histological evidence the decision will rest between primary excision and primary radiotherapy.

In the *peritonsillar region,* in striking contrast with the floor of the mouth, most salivary tumours are of the pleomorphic adenoma type and in the author's experience, the majority of them arise from the deep portion of the parotid gland. Occasionally tumours develop in a peritonsillar mucous gland and these appear localized to the soft palate and fauces. Tumours arising in the deep portion of the parotid are likely to be larger and may present with a tumour visible externally as well as in the peritonsillar area (Fig. 25).

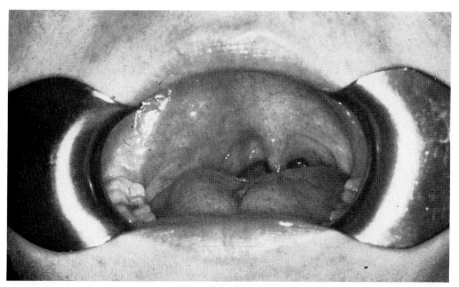

FIG. 25.—Pleomorphic adenoma of the deep lobe of the parotid presenting in the soft palate and peritonsillar region. There was also an obvious swelling externally in the parotid area.

While it may be possible to excise a tumour arising from a peritonsillar mucous gland by an incision through the pharyngeal mucosa, those arising in the deep lobe of the parotid can be excised safely only by an external approach and removal of the whole of the deep lobe after defining the plane of the facial nerve with exactitude. The author has found that in some instances the facial nerve has run within a few millimetres of the external aspect of the tumour.

Preliminary biopsy of a tumour bulging into the pharynx, although a technically simple procedure, is inadvisable. Once a biopsy has been taken in this way tumour cells are spilled into the tissues and the scar becomes adherent to the tumour. As a result excision of this area of mucosa is necessary and makes the excisive procedure more hazardous when an external operation is required. In any event if it is not possible to remove the tumour via a pharyngeal incision then an external operation will be required whether the biopsy shows that the tumour is a pleomorphic adenoma or, much more uncommonly, a parapharyngeal neurofibroma or some other tumour. If it is considered possible to excise the tumour through a pharyngeal approach then a preliminary biopsy is not needed.

The removal of a tumour of the deep lobe of the parotid presenting in the parapharyngeal region follows the same lines as has already been described in the account of parotidectomy but there are added difficulties because of the large mass lying deeply in the space between the styloid process and the mandible. Division of the stylomandibular ligament and fracturing of the styloid process as advocated by Patey and Thackray (1957) improves the access but in some large tumours even this is inadequate and considerable help can be obtained by division of the mandible with retraction of the ramus forwards and upwards (Fig. 26). Cook and Ranger (1969) reported that in six patients such a procedure made removal very much easier and had no troublesome post-operative sequelae. The loss of lip sensation gradually improved and in most patients returned to normal.

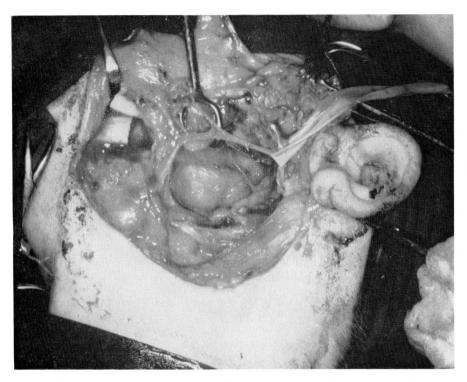

FIG. 26.—Exposure of the deep parotid area. The body of the mandible has been divided in the region of the second premolar tooth and a retractor placed around the angle of the mandible retracts the ramus forwards, upwards and outwards. The facial nerve is retracted with thin latex. (*From Cook and Ranger* (1969), *reproduced by courtesy of the Editor of* Journal of Laryngology and Otology.)

They advocated repairing the mandible with a small Vitallium (chrome cobalt) Venables fracture plate to allow immediate mobilization (Fig. 27). Berdal and Hall (1970) in the six patients in whom they found it necessary to divide the mandible fixed the bone afterwards with stainless steel wire and found satisfactory healing per primam.

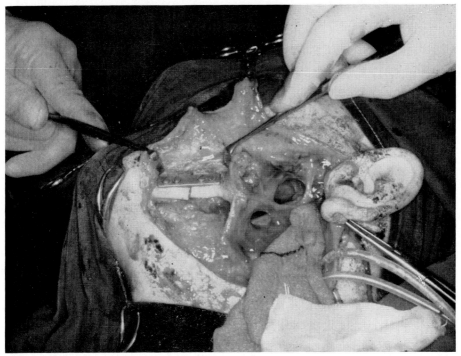

Fig. 27.—Method of fixation of the divided mandible by means of a Vitallium Venables fracture plate. (*From Cook and Ranger* (1969), *reproduced by courtesy of the Editor of* Journal of Laryngology and Otology.)

REFERENCES

Barbero, G. J., and Sibinga, M. S. (1962). *Paediatrics*, **29**, 788.
Bardwil, J. M., Luna, M. A., and Healey, J. E. Jnr. (1967). *Cancer of the Head and Neck* (Ed. by W. S. Maccomb and G. H. Fletcher). Baltimore; Williams and Wilkins.
Berdal, P., and Hall, J. G. (1970). *Acta otolaryng. Stockh.* Suppl., 263, p. 164.
Bhaskar, S. N., Bolden, T. E., and Weinmann, J. P. (1956). *J. dent. Res.*, **35**, 852.
Cook, H. P., and Ranger, D. (1969). *J. Laryng.*, **83**, 863.
Curry, R. C., and Patey, D. H. (1964). *Brit. J. Surg.*, **51**, 891.
Diamant, H. (1958). *Acta otolaryng. Stockh.*, **49**, 375.
— (1960). *Proc. R. Soc. Med.*, **53**, 461.
— and Wiberg, A. (1965). *Acta otolaryng. Stockh.*, **60**, 255.
Eneroth, C-M. (1964). *Acta otolaryng. Stockh.* Suppl., 191.
— Franzen, S., and Zajicek, J. (1966). *Acta otolaryng. Stockh.* Suppl., 224, p. 168.
— Hjertman, L., and Moberger, G. (1967). *Acta otolaryng. Stockh.*, **64**, 514.
— Hokfelt, T., and Norberg, K-A. (1969). *Acta otolaryng. Stockh.*, **68**, 369.
Enfors, Bo. (1962). *Acta otolaryng. Stockh.* Suppl., 172.
Farr, H. W. (1967). In *Proceedings of the International Workshop on Cancer of the Head and Neck* (Ed. by J. Conley). Washington; Butterworths.
Foote, F. W., and Frazell, E. L. (1954). "Tumours of the Major Salivary Glands". In *Atlas of Tumour Pathology* (Sect. IV; Fasc. II). Washington, D.C.; Armed Forces Institute of Pathology.
Glaister, D. H., Hearnshaw, J. R., Heffron, P. F., and Peck, A. W. (1958). *Brit. med. J.*, **2**, 942.
Goujerot, H. (1926). *Bull. Med. Paris*, **40**, 360.
Greenberg, G., Anderson, R., Sharpstone, P., and James, D. G. (1964). *Brit. med. J.*, **2**, 861.
Harrill, J. A., King, J. S. Jnr., and Boyce, W. H. (1959). *Laryngoscope*, **69**, 481.
Harrison, K. (1956). *Ann. R. Coll. Surg. Engl.*, **18**, 99.
Heerfordt, C. F. (1909). *Albrecht v. Graefes Arch. Ophthal.*, **70**, 254.
Höök, O. (1954). *Arch. Neurol. Psychiat., Chicago*, **71**, 554.

65

Jones, B. R. (1958). *Lancet*, **2**, 773.
Laage-Hellman, J. E. (1955). *Svenska Lak-Tidn.*, **52**, 3150.
Linell, F. (1948). *Acta path. microbiol. scand.*, **25**, 801.
Maynard, J. D. (1965). *Brit. J. Surg.*, **52**, 784.
Mikulicz, J. Von (1892). *Beitr-z. Chir., Festschrift.*, 610.
Morel, A. S., and Firestein, A. (1963). *Arch. Surg.*, **87**, 623.
Morrison, R. (1966). *Proc. R. Soc. Med.*, **59**, 429.
Naunton Morgan, M., and MacKenzie, D. H. (1968). *Brit. J. Surg.*, **55**, 284.
Patey, D. H. (1965a). *Ann. R. Coll. Surg. Engl.*, **36**, 26.
— (1965b). In *Clinical Surgery* (Vol. 9). *Head and Neck* (Ed. by Charles Rob and Rodney Smith). London; Butterworths.
— (1968). *J. Laryng.*, **82**, 853.
— and Ranger, I. (1957). *Brit. J. Surg.*, **45**, 250.
— and Thackray, A. C. (1953). *Ann. Rep. Brit. Emp. Cancer Campgn.*, **31**, 74.
— — (1955). *Brit. J. Surg.*, **43**, 43.
— — (1957). *Brit. J. Surg.*, **44**, 352.
— — and Keeling, D. H. (1965). *Brit. J. Cancer*, **19**, 712.
Pattinson, J. N. (1969). In *Operative Surgery* (Vol. 6). *Head and Neck and Lymph Nodes* (Ed. by Charles Rob, Rodney Smith and Maurice Ewing). London; Butterworths.
Pennell, W. H. (1951). *Arch. Neurol. Psychiat.*, *Chicago*, **66**, 728.
Ranger, D., Thackray, A. C., and Lucas, R. B. (1956). *Brit. J. Cancer*, **10**, 1.
Ranger, I. (1957). *Brit. J. Surg.*, **44**, 415.
Redon, H. (1965). *Chirurgie des Glandes Salivaires*. Paris; Masson.
Rewell, R. E. (1963). *Pathology of the Upper Respiratory Tract*. Edinburgh; Livingstone.
Sjogren, H. (1933). *Acta Ophthal.* Suppl., 2.
Stewart, F. W., Foote, F. W., and Becker, W. F. (1945). *Ann. Surg.*, **122**, 820.
Thackray, A. C. (1955). *Arch. Middx Hosp.*, **5**, 151.
— (1961). *Clin. Radiol.*, **12**, 241.

4

PHARYNGITIS—ACUTE AND CHRONIC

A. BOWEN-DAVIES

CORYZA

The signs and symptoms of the common cold are fully dealt with elsewhere. There is usually a degree of pharyngitis, which causes the sensation of roughness in the throat or burning behind the nose. There is some injection of the pharynx, but the pharyngeal condition is not severe and is soon overshadowed by the nasal condition which is characteristic of the disease.

ACUTE PHARYNGITIS

Aetiology

Acute pharyngitis is usually due to infection with haemolytic streptococci, but virus infections are responsible for a number of cases. The tonsils are usually involved and may indeed bear the brunt of the infection, when the condition is more accurately described as acute tonsillitis.

Symptoms

The disease may be trivial, with a slight sore throat lasting for a few days, a little malaise and a mild degree of pyrexia. In this form the disease often occurs in epidemics. In severe cases there is intense sore throat with marked toxaemia, high temperature and headache. The patient looks ill and is suffering considerably, as is evident when he attempts to swallow his saliva; he may refuse to do so, holding his head on one side to allow the accumulation to dribble from the corner of his mouth. When the palate is oedematous there may be an irritating cough caused by the elongated uvula touching the back of the tongue, and fluids may regurgitate through the nose.

Signs

In mild cases the pharynx may be uniformly injected, or redness may be confined to the pillars of the fauces. The regional lymph nodes may be enlarged and tender. In severe cases the pharynx is grossly injected, particularly in the region of the lateral bands. The surface of the mucosa is oedematous and is covered with mucus; there is often oedema of the palate and uvula. The pharyngeal lymph nodules stand out and may be covered with sloughs, and the lingual tonsils may be similarly affected. The tonsils are injected and there may be follicles or exudate on their surface, or a quinsy may have formed.

67

Examination of the throat may be difficult owing to trismus. The breath is foul and the mouth is full of saliva and mucus; the teeth are caked with debris. Breathing is difficult and is accompanied by much bubbling of mucus in the throat. There is high temperature and a rapid and perhaps irregular pulse rate.

Diagnosis

In mild infections diagnosis presents no difficulties, but when exudate is present diphtheria must be excluded. Culture of a throat swab establishes the diagnosis, but treatment must rely on clinical judgment. In diphtheria the degree of toxaemia is usually out of proportion to the rise in temperature, but the pulse rate is unduly raised. Although there is exudate on the tonsils, the inflammatory reaction of the pharynx is not, as a rule, so marked as it is in the case of streptococcal infection. The exudate is firmly adherent and may extend to the soft palate: its removal leaves a bleeding area. Diphtheria antitoxin and penicillin should be given without delay. In all cases of sore throat a swab must be taken before antibiotic therapy is started.

Complications

The patient may be desperately ill with toxaemia, and some die in a few hours from toxic myocarditis, or oedema may spread to the glottis, leading to fatal respiratory obstruction. Infection may spread to the neck and floor of the mouth, causing Ludwig's angina, or a cervical abscess may arise. In severe cases streptococci may be grown from a blood culture.

Treatment

The patient should be confined to bed and given abundant fluids by mouth, per rectum, subcutaneously or by intravenous injection if necessary, in order to minimize the effect of toxaemia. Frequent hot gargles of saline solution or potassium chlorate and phenol are soothing, and aspirin, 650 mg. four-hourly, relieves pain and helps to reduce the temperature. Potassium chlorate lozenges, or glycerin and blackcurrant lozenges, may give relief. Systemic antibiotics and chemotherapy may be given, should the severity of the case warrant their use, whilst a small fresh blood transfusion may be advisable in grave cases. Difficulty in breathing may be relieved by steam inhalations, but should respiratory obstruction appear imminent, a tracheostomy set should be available at the bedside.

Ludwig's angina

Aetiology

Ludwig's angina is the name given to cellulitis of the floor of the mouth and of the neck. It is usually due to infection with a haemolytic streptococcus and may be regarded as a serious complication of acute pharyngitis or sepsis in the mouth.

Symptoms

The patient is in great distress because movement of the tongue causes excruciating pain, and for this reason he may have deprived himself of food and drink and thus have delayed his recovery. There is difficulty in breathing, and talking may be almost impossible. The saliva is not swallowed and may run freely from the mouth, since salivation is increased.

Signs

The striking feature of the disease is the hard brawny swelling which fills the space between the chin and neck, and which is found on bimanual palpation to occupy the floor of the mouth; it may also extend to the neck. Fluctuation is not obtained, because pus, when present, is at a considerable distance from the surface. The patient is gravely ill with severe toxaemia and there is respiratory distress, with great danger of oedema of the glottis leading to sudden death.

Treatment

Full doses of antibiotics and chemotherapy are indicated as the first line of treatment in view of the nature of the infecting organism. This has revolutionized the treatment of the disease, and it is rare for active surgery to be necessary in the acute stage.

If the condition is not responding to treatment, it may be necessary to consider incision and drainage owing to the dangerous complexities of mediastinitis and oedema of the glottis.

Halothane is the anaesthetic of choice; intravenous anaesthesia is contra-indicated.

The incision is made in the midline of the neck, because pus is likely to form in the thyroglossal remnant, and because the risk of damage to important structures is eliminated; Hilton's method is employed.

Acute cervical adenitis

When acute cervical adenitis complicates acute pharyngitis the group of glands which includes the "tonsillar gland", just below and behind the angle of the jaw, is involved. Sometimes the primary lesion is on the skin, commonly on the scalp when the head is infested, or in the external auditory meatus. In this case, the upper cervical group of nodes is most affected, and there may be pre-auricular and post-auricular adenitis as well. As a rule, when the primary lesion has subsided, the nodes resolve, although they remain palpable for an indefinite period. Occasionally, lymph node involvement forms the major part of the disease and the primary lesion may have healed before the patient seeks advice.

Sometimes children are referred for treatment because of repeated attacks of "glands". A history of sore throat is denied, but although no definite primary lesion can be found during an attack, the portal of entry is presumably in the pharynx, for it is the nodes draining this area that are involved. The child is ill, refusing his food and disturbing the household at night; the temperature is raised and vomiting may be troublesome. There may be considerable discomfort from glandular enlargement, or there may be a little pain with tenderness on palpation. The attack usually lasts for a few days, but sometimes a subacute condition runs a more prolonged course.

Treatment

The child should be confined to bed and a liberal fluid diet should be given. Hot fomentations or kaolin poultices are applied to the affected area, under a large pad of wool secured with a crêpe bandage, which may with advantage be brought round the forehead to limit movement of the neck and to secure rest to the part. Sedatives may be necessary to ensure sleep, and the severity of the condition may justify the use of antibiotics and chemotherapy. When the attacks are repeated at frequent intervals, the condition of the tonsils and adenoids is suspect and their removal during a quiescent period must be considered.

Acute cervical abscess

In the event of adenitis proceeding to suppuration, with the formation of an acute cervical abscess, surgical intervention is necessary. An incision is made over the area of softening or fluctuation; it must not be brought within 1·25 cm. of the angle of the jaw, however, lest the cervical branch of the facial nerve be injured. Hilton's method is used, and after the wound has been adequately extended with sinus forceps or with a finger, a rubber glove drain should be inserted.

PARAPHARYNGEAL ABSCESS

The rare condition of parapharyngeal abscess may complicate tonsillitis or pharyngitis, but more commonly occurs after tonsillectomy or injury to the pharyngeal wall. If there is perforation of the pharyngeal wall, surgical emphysema in the neck may arise. It is a serious condition, because infection may spread rapidly along the tissue planes to the mediastinum.

There is constitutional disturbance with high temperature, intense dysphagia and respiratory obstruction. The neck is swollen; the pharynx is oedematous, and oedema may have spread to the arytenoids. The lateral pharyngeal wall is displaced medially, but this displacement may not easily be recognized because of difficulty in carrying out examination of the throat owing to trismus, and a mistaken diagnosis of quinsy may be made.

Treatment

Antibiotics and chemotherapy may control the infection, but incision of the abscess may be necessary. The abscess should be incised either through the pharynx or through the neck, according to the direction in which the infection has spread. Precautions must be taken to deal with respiratory obstruction, should it arise.

THE INFECTIOUS FEVERS

It would be out of place to give a full account of the specific fevers here but, as many of them exhibit lesions in the mouth or pharynx, they must be considered in the differential diagnosis of acute infection in this region.

Diphtheria

Aetiology

Diphtheria is caused by *Corynebacterium diphtheriae*, a thin beaded Gram-positive bacillus containing metachromatic granules demonstrable by special staining techniques. Although growing mainly on the tonsils it produces its most serious effect by wide diffusion of diphtheria toxin, which can cause myocarditis or neuritis.

Pathology

The lesion is usually confined to the pharynx, but may occur in the nose, larynx or elsewhere. The tonsils are commonly affected, and there is superficial ulceration, with the formation of a false membrane, which may spread to the soft palate and the uvula. The exudate is grey-white, firmly adherent, and appears to have been laid on the surface rather than inlaid, as in the case of Vincent's infection; its removal leaves a bleeding area. There is relatively little reaction in the surrounding parts, although, in severe cases, there may be oedema of the palate and uvula.

The disease is usually spread by exposure of susceptible subjects to those suffering from the disease or incubating it, but individuals may carry infection and infect others without showing any evidence of disease themselves. These "carriers" may have had the disease, but some have never shown any clinical signs of it. Many suspected carriers are harbouring organisms which prove, on biological examination, to be avirulent, and others respond to treatment with penicillin.

Symptoms

Children are commonly affected, and the disease starts with general malaise, headache, vomiting and sore throat. There is not a marked degree of pyrexia, but the pulse rate is unduly raised. The breath is foul, with a sweetish odour, which is regarded as an important diagnostic feature. The regional lymph nodes are enlarged and tender, and may be grossly affected as in the classical "bull neck". In cases in which the nose is involved, constitutional symptoms are not severe and bleeding from the nose, with purulent nasal discharge, often unilateral, is frequently associated with impetigo of the upper lip. In laryngeal cases, respiratory obstruction is the presenting feature, and life is very often threatened.

Complications

Complications may arise from the spread of infection, causing respiratory obstruction or pneumonia, and also from the action of the toxin, which has an affinity for neuromuscular junctions and the myocardium; for this reason early diagnosis and treatment are of the greatest importance.

Diagnosis

The condition must be differentiated from acute streptococcal infection, Vincent's infection, and other forms of acute ulceration in the pharynx. In nasal cases, the presence of a foreign body may be suspected.

The organism can be identified by culture, but many hours must elapse before the diagnosis can be established by this means, so one must rely on clinical acumen if the treatment is not to be delayed; examination of direct smears and other rapid bacteriological methods are unreliable. When in doubt, it is better to treat a suspected case as one of diphtheria and to administer adequate doses of antitoxin until the diagnosis is established by bacteriological examination.

Treatment

Prophylactic.—Much can be done to prevent the disease by active immunization. Susceptibility can be determined by the Schick test, and if this is positive, immunization can be induced by graduated doses of toxoid. An attack of the disease usually confers immunity, but if antitoxin has been given early in the disease, permanent immunity may not be acquired, so a history of a previous attack does not necessarily exclude the possibility of a further infection.

Passive immunity can be produced by prophylactic injection of 16,000 units of antitoxin, and it is justifiable to do this in the case of one who has been seriously ill and has been inadvertently exposed to infection. In the case of healthy individuals exposed to infection, it is better to keep them under close observation than to induce passive immunity, because a carrier state may be produced in this way.

Curative.—The most important measure is the administration of adequate doses of antitoxin intramuscularly, or intravenously if necessary. The initial dose should never be less than 16,000 units, and as much as 72,000 units intravenously may be indicated. The patient must be kept absolutely at rest, and complications must be dealt with as necessary. Antibiotics are indicated, and a throat swab must be taken before they are administered. The importance of this was illustrated in a recent epidemic of diphtheria among children attending the same school. They were treated as cases of acute streptoccal tonsillitis, and the nature of the infection was only suspected when one of them died of myocarditis. Since they all had been treated with penicillin, it was impossible to confirm the diagnosis by taking throat swabs. However, a routine swabbing of the pupils unaffected by the disease revealed a number of carriers of *Corynebacterium diphtheriae*. Another disturbing revelation was that a number of those affected by the disease had previously received active immunization with toxoid.

Scarlet fever
Aetiology
Scarlet fever is caused by the spread of toxin from a streptococcal infection of the pharynx and tonsils. The incubation period is from two to seven days.

Clinical picture
The onset is sudden, with a rise of temperature, malaise and shivering; headache is a feature, and vomiting may be pronounced. The throat is sore and the regional lymph nodes are enlarged and tender. In the early stage the pharynx may be red, or there may be a yellow slough on the tonsils; this can be easily wiped from them. The tongue undergoes characteristic changes, being first covered with a yellow fur through which the papillae project, "strawberry-and-cream tongue", becoming later "strawberry tongue" or "raspberry tongue" as the fur disappears. Within two days of the onset of the disease an erythematous rash appears on the trunk and limbs, but rarely on the face, which is flushed save for an area of circumoral pallor.

Complications
Fortunately the disease runs a relatively mild course at the present time, but in the past the mortality rate was high. Acute otitis media, sinusitis, nephritis and pneumonia are frequent complications, and many who have recovered from the disease become carriers. The patient must be bacteriologically free from infection before he is released from isolation, and surgical measures may be necessary for the throat, ear or sinuses in order to eliminate the infection. Antibiotics are given in all but the mildest cases.

Measles
Aetiology
Measles is caused by a virus infection and occurs in epidemics; the incubation period is 10–12 days. It is a serious disease, particularly in the young, because of the possible development of pneumonia, which may be viral or bacterial.

Symptoms

The prodromal stage lasts for three or four days, when the symptoms are those of severe coryza with conjunctivitis, nasal catarrh, diarrhoea and vomiting. Laryngitis (measles croup) may be pronounced and may lead to a mistaken diagnosis of laryngeal diphtheria unless the nature of the disease is recognized.

Signs

Diagnosis may be made at this stage by inspection of the buccal mucosa; this is injected and, scattered over its surface particularly in the region of the molars, are small white spots (Koplik's spots) about the size of a pinhead, surrounded by an area of erythema. After four or five days the typical morbilliform rash appears and Koplik's spots fade.

Complications

Acute otitis media, mastoiditis or pneumonia may complicate the condition, but since the introduction of antibiotics and chemotherapy they may be largely prevented by prophylactic treatment. In ill-nourished children infection can lead to gangrene of the mouth (cancrum oris) or of the vulva (noma vulvae), but such cases are rarely seen now.

Chicken-pox

Aetiology

Chicken-pox is due to a virus infection and the incubation period is 14–21 days.

Symptoms and signs

There is a short prodromal period with a feeling of general malaise, followed by the eruption of macules or maculopapules. They are centripetal in distribution, which serves to differentiate them from the lesions of smallpox. The eruption takes place over a period of two or three days, so that fresh lesions are appearing while the older ones become superficial vesicles or pustules. The scab separates with, in some cases, ulceration, which may give rise to pock marks. The lesions may affect the buccal mucosa early in the disease and may be confused with the vesicles of herpes. The conjunctivae are also affected, but only with superficial lesions which leave no permanent effects unless secondary infection occurs.

Relation to herpes zoster.—There is no doubt that the virus responsible for chicken-pox is also responsible for herpes zoster. Many cases of herpes zoster have been recorded amongst those in contact with chicken-pox, and we have heard of a colleague and his house surgeon who both developed chicken-pox within three weeks of examining a case of geniculate herpes.

CHRONIC PHARYNGITIS

Primary aetiological factors

Pharyngitis may be due to a primary infection in the pharyngeal tissues but such cases are rare, and more commonly the pharynx becomes infected as a result of disease in other parts of the upper respiratory tract or other systems.

Secondary aetiological factors

Rhinitis and sinusitis

In some cases, inspection of the oropharynx reveals mucopus festooned over the posterior pharyngeal wall, and it is evident that a quantity of infected material is passing from the nose into the pharynx. In other cases, examination with a post-nasal mirror shows a thin stream of mucopus coming from the posterior end of the middle meatus and tracking down the lateral pharyngeal wall. It may be temporarily halted at the level of the soft palate, but evidence of its passage below this is seen in the hypertrophied and inflamed lymphoid tissue down the lateral columns of the pharynx.

Since mucus is normally passed backwards from the nose into the nasopharynx, infection in the nose or paranasal sinuses may not lead to any nasal symptoms and, indeed, many patients deny excessive use of the handkerchief, even when there is clear evidence of postnasal catarrh. Unless a careful examination of the naso-pharynx is made, therefore, the cause of the pharyngeal condition may be overlooked. Even if the nose and nasopharynx appear healthy, infection in the paranasal sinuses cannot be definitely excluded, and all methods of examination may be necessary to establish the correct diagnosis.

The mouth

Teeth.—A number of patients consult laryngologists for conditions which are greatly aggravated by dental sepsis, even if not directly attributable to it. One has only to observe the improvement in the state of carcinomatous ulcer in the pharynx after dental sepsis has been corrected to realize the importance of this source of infection. Chronic pharyngitis is common where dental sepsis prevails, and tonsillitis and laryngitis may also occur.

Tonsils.—Chronic infection in the tonsils naturally exerts an unfavourable effect on the condition of the pharynx, and if the primary focus of infection lies here, tonsillectomy should benefit the patient. If the focus of infection is elsewhere, however, the tonsils may be merely the site of secondary infection and their removal cannot improve the pharyngeal condition.

Mouth-breathing

When the air is breathed in through the mouth, it is not subjected to the humidification, warming and cleansing which normally take place during its passage over the nasal mucosa. Consequently, the pharynx becomes dry and is subjected to an abnormal degree of infection. The cause of mouth breathing may be:

Nasopharyngeal.—The most common cause of mouth-breathing in the young is obstruction due to excessive adenoid tissue. In older subjects, tumours of the nasopharynx or antrochoanal polypi are found.

Nasal.—Nasal obstruction may be due to maldevelopment, congenital atresia of the posterior choanae, or to structural defects, e.g. deflection in the nasal septum or large turbinates. Inflammatory conditions, such as acute or chronic rhinitis, may cause thickening of the nasal mucosa, as also may allergic states. Nasal polypi or, more rarely, tumours may cause complete obstruction, or the nasal airway may be narrowed by scarring after acute infections, syphilis, lupus or leprosy.

Dental.—Protruding teeth prevent the lips coming into apposition, and consequently there is a tendency for mouth-breathing to occur. This prevents the normal development of the alveolus and palate, with aggravation of the dental condition.

Habitual.—Some people breathe through their mouths habitually, even though their nasal airways are free. This is particularly the case in those in whom an organic nasal obstruction has been relieved. It is important, after the removal of adenoids, to ensure that nasal respiration is established and breathing exercises may be necessary.

Faulty voice production

The pharynx plays an important part in the production of the voice, because not only does it regulate the flow of air through the nose during speech, but by contraction of its muscles it regulates the size of the lumen of the pharynx to effect a change in resonance. Excessive use of the voice, particularly should voice production be faulty, predisposes to chronic pharyngitis.

External conditions

Living in industrial areas, where the atmosphere is laden with smoke and other waste products of industry, undoubtedly predisposes to chronic pharyngitis, and in the past many people in the course of their duties were exposed without adequate protection from harmful gases. Although much has been done to purify the atmosphere and to provide protection against irritant fumes, some subjects appear to be unduly sensitive to such agents and consequently develop pharyngitis when others would suffer no inconvenience.

Smoking is a common cause of pharyngitis, and few heavy smokers do not show some evidence of it.

Digestive disorders

Since the pharynx is part of the alimentary tract, pharyngitis may be a manifestation of disorders of digestion. In addition, dyspeptics may refer to the pharynx symptoms due to gastritis, water-brash or eructations after aerophagy.

Those who indulge excessively in alcohol, especially spirits, usually suffer from some degree of pharyngitis, and the habitual use of condiments and highly spiced foods is an aggravating factor.

Pulmonary conditions

In cases of chronic bronchitis and bronchiectasis, heavily infected sputum is constantly passing into the pharynx and exerting an adverse influence there.

General conditions

It is important to consider the general condition of the patient, lest one's attention be concentrated on what amounts to no more than an insignificant complication of a grave disease.

Symptoms

The symptoms experienced by people who suffer from chronic pharyngitis vary considerably and seem to bear little relationship to the pathological changes in the pharynx. Thus a man who indulges freely in alcohol and tobacco may have a pharynx which would be expected to cause acute discomfort and yet he is free from symptoms, whereas an introspective individual may complain bitterly of pharyngeal symptoms when his pharynx may well be regarded as normal. The most constant symptom is discomfort in the throat, which may amount to actual pain, especially early in the morning; or there may be the sensation of a foreign body in the throat. There is undue irritability, and spasms of coughing and retching may be induced by factors which would leave most undisturbed.

Once the dryness and discomfort experienced on waking, often due to mouth-breathing during sleep, have passed off, the throat is more comfortable until later in the day, when the symptoms return owing to the strain of talking and exposure to irritating agents. Indeed, in some cases the only complaint is that of "tiredness of the voice" while the patient is conscious of the undue effort required in speaking; this, of course, is an aggravating factor.

The voice may lose its quality and singers become uncertain in getting the note, or the voice may crack with the production of a sound akin to "falsetto". For this the blame may be wrongly laid upon the larynx.

Owing to the constant discomfort in the throat, there is a tendency to cough or to clear the throat, or to interrupt speech in order to swallow.

Signs

Chronic catarrhal pharyngitis

In chronic catarrhal pharyngitis there is congestion of the pharynx with engorgement of the vessels, which may be seen coursing across the posterior pharyngeal wall. The pillars of the fauces may appear somewhat thickened. There is increased secretion of mucus, and the walls of the pharynx may be covered with frothy fluid.

The condition may persist for some time, or it may pass gradually into one of the other forms of chronic pharyngitis.

Chronic hypertrophic pharyngitis

In this form of the disease there is considerable hypertrophy of the pharyngeal mucosa. The tonsils and adenoids may be similarly affected, but hypertrophic pharyngitis may arise after these organs have been removed. The whole of the pharyngeal wall may be involved, or hypertrophy may be limited to the lateral bands of lymphoid tissue. This hypertrophy may also extend to the muscular coat in this region, and the masses may attain proportions which lead to their being mistaken for faucial tonsils, when these have been removed.

At first there is excessive secretion of mucus, but later the mucous glands may become obstructed by hypertrophied lymph nodules and there may be a little sticky secretion on the pharyngeal wall; this causes the patient to make repeated attempts to swallow and so further aggravates the disease. The pharynx is engorged and large vessels may be seen running over its surface. The palate is injected, and the uvula may be elongated and may appear almost oedematous, or it may be short and thickened. The pharyngeal wall may appear granular because of hypertrophy of the lymph nodules, which may coalesce to form large masses. Granulations may form round the openings of the mucous glands and obstruct them, causing them to become distended and adding to the general thickening of the pharyngeal wall. This form of pharyngitis is often seen in those who use their voices excessively, particularly when voice production is faulty; hence the name "clergyman's throat".

76

Treatment

Rest is the most important factor in treating chronic pharyngitis, and much can be done to secure rest by explaining exactly the cause of the symptoms to the patient. He must be told that it is detrimental to swallow repeatedly in order to remove the "crumb" or "lump in the throat" because, in fact, none is there; he must be forbidden to clear his throat, hawk, or perform any of the pharyngeal contortions which he has devised; his cough must be suppressed. He must rest his voice, and in the case of a patient whose calling demands the use of his voice, a long holiday is advisable; a course of instruction in voice production will do much to help.

Assistance can be given by prescribing applications to reduce the discomfort in the throat. Gargles of hot saline solution, Glycothymoline brand solution, or potassium chlorate and phenol should be used on rising, or a steam inhalation of compound tincture of benzoin or of menthol may be preferred. Mandl's paint may be applied with a camel-hair brush, and lozenges of potassium chlorate, formalin, or glycerin and blackcurrant may be sucked during the day. Temporary relief may be obtained by the use of a spray containing the following:

Tinct. Ferr. Perchlor.	4 ml.
Stovaine	300 mg.
Menthol	300 mg.
Sp. Vin. Rect.	12 ml.
Glycer.	12 ml.
Aqua	30 ml.

The nasal cavities may be used as a reservoir for pharyngeal applications, since any substance placed there is slowly passed into the pharynx, and the use of a bland oil containing white soft paraffin (one part) and liquid paraffin (three parts), warmed before use, can give relief for considerable periods. A potent linctus, such as linctus codeine, should be given in doses sufficient to suppress the cough, especially at night.

In cases in which hypertrophy is marked, the lymphoid tissue may be cauterized with 10 per cent silver nitrate used sparingly on a probe, or with the electric cautery, but it is doubtful whether symptoms are relieved by this, and the procedure may serve only to fix the patient's attention more firmly on his throat.

In the case of secondary pharyngitis, the primary cause must receive appropriate treatment. The nose and sinuses must be restored to health, and the teeth and tonsils must receive attention. The patient's diet and habits must be regulated, and he should be removed from unsuitable surroundings, at least for a reasonable period. The pharynx must receive treatment as well, however, because once the pharyngitis has become established, it may persist after the cause has been removed, owing to the faulty habits the patient has developed.

CHRONIC ATROPHIC PHARYNGITIS

Aetiology

Chronic atrophic pharyngitis is usually associated with atrophic rhinitis, and perhaps with laryngitis as well. It may be of a secondary nature, but most often is regarded as a direct extension of disease from the nose. In its milder form, sometimes known as pharyngitis sicca, it may follow granular pharyngitis, or conditions which lead to mouth-breathing. It is sometimes associated with diabetes mellitus or gout, or with some other constitutional disorder.

Symptoms

The symptoms are similar to those in other forms of chronic pharyngitis, but dryness of the throat is very marked and may cause great discomfort. The patient may find relief in taking sips of water. Talking aggravates the condition, and the presence of crusts may cause constant hawking and coughing.

Signs

There is atrophy of the pharyngeal mucosa and of the mucous glands in particular, so that the pharynx assumes a dry parchment-like appearance. The surface appears glazed and becomes wrinkled when the muscles contract. Absence of mucus leads to the formation of crusts, which favour secondary infection; this causes foetor oris. The lumen of the pharynx appears large and, owing to the thinning of the walls, the outline of the cervical spine is clearly visible.

Treatment

Causes for the condition must be sought in the nose or elsewhere and must be appropriately treated. This form of pharyngitis also calls for special forms of local treatment to prevent the formation of crusts, or to remove them when they have been formed. Alkaline lotions should be sprayed on to the pharynx as often as the severity of the case demands, but not less than three times a day. Ten per cent glucose in glycerin as a nasal application improves the condition of the nose, and also trickles into the pharynx; or an oily preparation may be indicated. Crusts must be removed, and this is facilitated by the use of an oily application, or by hydrogen peroxide; it is important to prevent the formation of crusts, however, because, in their removal, the surface epithelium is damaged and infection perpetuated. Potassium iodide administered in 325 mg. doses promotes secretion of mucus and may give relief, but it should be prescribed only for short periods. "Airbron" spray effectively loosens crusts and assists in their removal.

The regime advised for chronic pharyngitis should be followed.

SYPHILIS

Syphilitic lesions in the pharynx may occur at any stage of the disease, but it is in the secondary stage, when spirochaetes are most widely distributed throughout the body, that manifestations are most regularly seen.

Primary syphilis

Probably the most common site for an extragenital chancre is the lip or the mouth. The lesion may be mistaken for a boil on the lip, or impetigo, but the characteristic rubbery feel of the enlarged regional lymph nodes should suggest its nature and lead to further investigation. The lesion presents the typical features of a primary chancre, with the "cartilaginous" base and ulceration with a dirty slough, but it may remain small owing to the relative absence of secondary infection.

In other cases, the chancre may be situated on the tonsil, or cheek, when it may be mistaken for a carcinoma or Vincent's infection. In the early stages, the Wassermann reaction may be negative, but examination under dark ground illumination of a smear taken from the lesion reveals *Treponema pallidum*. Experience is necessary to discriminate between it and the spirochaetes which normally inhabit the mouth.

Secondary syphilis

In the secondary stage of the disease, which usually arises in 6–8 weeks, the spirochaetes are widely distributed throughout the body, and the mucous surfaces are particularly affected. There is some degree of sore throat, which may cause acute discomfort, or merely the symptoms associated with a bad cold. When the disease is florid, there may be a rash symmetrically distributed over the body, and of a colour likened to that of raw ham; when the forehead is involved, it is called corona veneris. There is associated anaemia, the hair tends to fall out, and there is a general enlargement of the lymph nodes. The pharynx is uniformly injected, and on the fauces and palate there are mucous patches and snail track ulcers symmetrically placed, with the characteristic lymphadenitis of syphilis. The disease is now in its most infective state and an early diagnosis is important; the Wassermann reaction is probably positive, and the spirochaetes can be seen in smears taken from the mucous patches and ulcers.

Tertiary syphilis

By now the invasive stage of the disease has been overcome, but localized activity continues and the manifestations may occur almost coincidently with the secondary stage, or many years after. The typical lesion is a gumma, which is formed as a result of chronic infection of the tissues, with endarteritis of the arterioles and necrosis in the area of their distribution. Secondary infection leads to the formation of a punched-out ulcer with a wash-leather slough at the base. Bone is commonly involved, thus there may be perforation of the hard palate, but the soft tissues may be affected and ulceration of the tonsil and pharynx is often seen. Since the nerve endings are destroyed early in the disease, there is little pain, and ulceration of the palate and fauces may have progressed to a remarkable extent before the patient seeks advice. The regional lymph nodes become affected owing to secondary infection.

Congenital syphilis

In congenital syphilis the pharynx may be involved in gummatous infiltration owing to infection acquired *in utero*. The lesions resemble those seen in tertiary syphilis but progress more slowly, with considerable scarring in consequence. There may be perforation of the palate.

The permanent teeth, particularly the upper central incisors, may be affected and show the well-known deformity described by Hutchinson. The cutting edges are eroded and tend to become semilunar, while the whole tooth is malformed and shaped like a peg.

Differential diagnosis

The ulcer may be confused with that due to tuberculous infection but, in this condition there is a shallow ulcer with undermined edges; there is much pain and there is evidence of pulmonary involvement; nevertheless large terminal pharyngeal tuberculous ulcers may be painless.

In the case of epithelioma, the ulcer is hard with everted edges, and the regional lymph nodes, if involved, are hard and may be attached to surrounding tissues. Vincent's ulceration may resemble either secondary or tertiary syphilis, but pain is more severe, and direct examination of the exudate, and the Wassermann reaction, should establish the diagnosis.

Treatment

Local relief can be obtained by the administration of potassium iodide, and this may serve as a useful therapeutic test in doubtful cases, but the case should be referred to a venereologist for treatment and observation. Early treatment is important to arrest the progress of the ulceration, which may rapidly cause a perforation of the palate or other permanent scarring.

TUBERCULOSIS

Tuberculosis is seen in the pharynx in three forms, acute miliary tuberculosis, chronic tuberculous ulceration and lupus vulgaris.

Acute miliary tuberculosis

This manifestation of the disease is associated with spread of tubercle bacilli to the blood stream. There is an eruption of tubercles on the fauces, soft palate, base of the tongue or buccal mucosa. There is some discomfort at this stage, but when the tubercles break down to form ulcers, there is acute pain and dysphagia. There is a tendency to bleed and to excessive salivation; mucus adheres to the ulcerated area. There is considerable constitutional disturbance, with high temperature, and the general condition of the patient deteriorates rapidly.

Chronic ulcerating tuberculosis

Chronic ulcerating tuberculosis is always associated with advanced pulmonary tuberculosis, and the sputum is laden with tubercle bacilli. There is ulceration in the pharynx and on the tongue, where the ulcers are usually situated at the tip. The ulcers are shallow, with undermined edges and relatively clean bases; their progress is indolent. The nerve endings are intact, so there is much pain with all the symptoms associated with acute dysphagia.

Treatment

There is great improvement in tuberculous ulceration of the upper respiratory tract when treatment of the pulmonary lesion is instituted. There may be little change in the appearance of the lesions for a few weeks, but pain is rapidly relieved and the lesions eventually heal. If there are bacilli in the sputum, a culture should be made and sensitivity tests carried out. Initially, treatment should be instituted with the daily administration of streptomycin 1 g., isoniazid 300 mg. and para-aminosalicylic acid 10–12 g. daily.

Streptomycin is a toxic drug and may cause degeneration of the labyrinth, with perceptive deafness and vertigo; the onset of these symptoms should lead, therefore, to the immediate withdrawal of the drug. It should not be used unless the renal function is normal. Similarly, if sensitivity tests show the organism to be resistant to any of the drugs, their administration should be stopped. Treatment with streptomycin should cease after three months, but treatment with other drugs should continue for at least 18 months. If the organisms are resistant to the three drugs, ethionamide, cyclosim, pyrazinamide or biomycin provide alternative means of treatment. Dihydrostreptomycin is more ototoxic than streptomycin and should never be used.

Lupus vulgaris

Pathology

Lupus vulgaris is essentially a cutaneous manifestation of tuberculosis, and perhaps the most benign. The favourite site in the upper respiratory tract is the anterior end of the nasal septum and the inferior turbinate, whence the disease may spread to the face or the pharynx.

In the pharynx, the soft palate and fauces may be affected, but rarely the tonsils. There is often associated disease in the nose, larynx or, infrequently, the chest; occasionally, however, the pharyngeal lesion is the sole manifestation of the disease.

There is an eruption of "apple jelly nodules" which soon become grey and appear more solid; microscopically they resemble tubercles. The mucosa becomes hard and loses its mobility; the nodules break down and the surface of the mucosa is destroyed, with exposure of a granular area which hardly amounts to ulceration. Both sides of the soft palate may be involved, but perforation does not occur. In the rare cases in which the hard palate is affected, bone may be exposed but is not involved in the disease process. The disease runs a very chronic course, with a tendency to heal in parts while activity continues elsewhere; consequently there is considerable scarring and the palate becomes shrunken, the mucosa assumes the appearance of orange peel, and the uvula may be reduced to a little knob.

Symptoms

In the early stages, or when the disease resumes activity, there is a burning sensation and a slight degree of sore throat. Later, the quality of the voice may change owing to a fixation of the palate, and there may be some dysphagia, but it is only in very advanced cases that regurgitation of fluids through the nose occurs.

Diagnosis

The lesion may be confused with syphilis; in this case, however, the disease runs a much more rapid course with greater destruction of tissue, and the Wassermann reaction is positive. A diagnosis of lupus vulgaris may be confirmed by biopsy.

Treatment

As with other tuberculous infection the most efficacious mode of treatment is by the administration of streptomycin, isoniazid and para-aminosalicylic acid. Streptomycin should be administered by subcutaneous injection, 1 g. twice weekly for three months. Treatment with isoniazid, 300 mg. daily and para-aminosalicylic acid 10–12 g. daily, should be continued for 18 months.

81

The patient should be kept under observation for many years, however, owing to the remittent nature of the disease. Nothing can be done to prevent the gross scarring which is a feature of the disease.

KERATOSIS PHARYNGEUS

Keratosis pharyngeus is a condition of unknown origin, and one which may cause much needless distress because the appearance of the throat suggests some serious lesion, whereas, in fact, the disease runs a singularly benign course, tending to undergo spontaneous resolution in a matter of months. Symptoms are negligible, amounting to no more than slight discomfort, but the patient may be prompted to examine his throat. The lesions appear in the throat as grey-white or yellow horny outgrowths; they are in fact formed by hypertrophy and keratinization of the epithelium. They are firmly adherent and can only be removed with difficulty. The tonsillar crypts are most frequently involved, but the lesion may be scattered over the pharynx, and the lingual tonsils seldom escape. The lesions may extend to the hypopharynx, and the larynx may be implicated. Swabs taken from the lesions show a variety of organisms and fungi, but there is no evidence that they are in any way responsible for the condition. The disease has been likened to black hairy tongue, since in this case the "hairs" consist of keratinized epithelium.

When the lesions are plentiful, diagnosis should present no difficulty, but when they are confined to the faucial tonsils they may be mistaken for the follicles of acute follicular tonsillitis; there is, however, no acute pharyngitis or constitutional disturbance. They may be mistaken for collections of debris in the tonsillar crypts, but these are cheesy and yellow and may be expressed with a spatula.

The disease does not require treatment, but the patient may be assured that no harm will result even should the lesions persist, while it is likely that they will disappear spontaneously in the course of time. The application of 40 per cent urea in saline may hasten the resolution of the condition.

STENOSIS OF THE PHARYNX

Aetiology

Stenosis of the pharynx is due to scar tissue. This may follow acute infections, such as scarlet fever or gangrenous tonsillitis. Chronic disease, notably syphilis or lupus vulgaris, may be followed by extensive scarring, with narrowing of the pharynx or fixation of the palate. Operative measures for neoplastic disease, or removal of tonsils and adenoids, may also cause a narrowing of the pharynx. Other cases are due to wounds, or the swallowing of corrosives.

Symptoms and signs

Usually the upper parts of the oropharynx and nasopharynx are involved, with resulting obstruction to nasal respiration. The voice may be altered so that the patient speaks with rhinolalia clausa. Examination of the pharynx immediately reveals the state of affairs, with gross scarring of the palate and pharynx.

Treatment

Treatment is unnecessary except in the most severe cases. Dilatation with bougies may be successful, but if there is no relief, surgical intervention is necessary.

Division of adhesions and mobilization of the palate is doomed to failure unless a Thiersch graft is inserted to prevent further scarring. The graft, which should be taken from a hairless area of the body, should be held in position for a week or two by a stent mould, and a similarly shaped obturator should be prepared for insertion after the mould has been removed. This obturator must be worn for 6–12 weeks to prevent the contraction of scar tissue that will otherwise take place.

The results of these operations are often unsatisfactory but it is nearly always possible to give some nasopharyngeal opening that allows nasal breathing. Operation should be reserved for severe stenosis.

VIRUS INFECTIONS
Clinical manifestations of infection

Many viruses cause well-recognized clinical diseases, such as mumps or measles, but others cause more varied clinical manifestations.

Enterovirus infection

Acute anterior poliomyelitis.

Coxsackie virus infection

Isolated in Coxsackie, New York State.
(1) Aseptic meningitis and paralysis simulating acute anterior poliomyelitis.
(2) Bornholm disease.
(3) Herpangina.
(4) Neonatal carditis.
(5) Acute upper respiratory infection resembling the common cold.

Enterocytopathogenic human orphan virus (ECHO)

(1) Aseptic meningitis and paralysis.
(2) Epidemic febrile disease sometimes accompanied by meningitis. It is often accompanied by a maculopapular rash.
(3) Acute respiratory disease resembling the common cold.
(4) Gastro-enteritis.

Viruses affecting the respiratory tract. Myxoviruses—influenza

Type A and its variants are responsible for most epidemics. It tends to undergo frequent antigenic variation. The pandemic in 1918 was probably caused by a mutant of type A, and since then localized epidemics occurred in 1932 and 1934. In 1946 another strain gave rise to an epidemic and it was classed as A.1. In 1957 this was superseded by the A.2 strain, which caused the "Asian 'flu' " epidemic, and in 1969 yet another variant of A.2, the Hong Kong strain, caused widespread epidemics.

Adenovirus infections. DNA virus

(*a*) Types 1, 2 and 5 infect the tonsils and adenoids of children, seldom produce ill-effects and tend to lie latent. It is unknown whether they play a part in hyperplasia.
(*b*) Types 3, 4, 7, 7a and 14 cause epidemics of febrile pharyngitis and other acute respiratory diseases, including primary atypical pneumonia syndrome.

(c) These viruses also have an affinity for the conjunctiva (pharyngoconjunctival fever).

(d) Type 8. Epidemic keratoconjunctivitis.

(e) Adenovirus when swallowed may give rise to acute mesenteric adenitis. Bowel hyperplasia may result in intussusception.

The common cold. Rhinovirus infection

A number of serotypes have been isolated. They are distantly related to the ECHO virus. The common cold may also be simulated by infections due to para-influenzal viruses, ECHO viruses, the Coe virus, respiratory syncitial viruses and the REO (respiratory enteric orphan, an enterovirus) viruses.

Manifestations of virus infection of the pharynx

Although virus infection of the pharynx does not usually assume a characteristic clinical picture, some cases have been described in which the clinical manifestations are typical of certain virus diseases.

Herpangina

Zahorsky described this condition in 1924 and although, of course, he had no idea what was the cause of the condition, he recognized that it was not due to bacterial infection nor was it typical of herpes. Since that time several epidemics have been reported and Coxsackie A virus has been identified.

There are minute vesicles, about the size of a millet seed or a pea, situated on the anterior pillars of the fauces or along the free margin of the soft palate. These vesicles are occasionally seen on the posterior part of the buccal mucous membrane or on the roof of the mouth, but more frequently on the tonsils or pharyngeal mucous membrane. The vesicle begins as a small papule which undergoes vesiculation in 24 hours. The vesicle ruptures and leaves a punched-out ulcer. The ulcer often becomes covered with a thin exudate and its edges are undermined. The ulcer heals leaving a slight depression.

Pharyngoconjunctival fever

Many cases of pharyngoconjunctival fever have been described. It usually occurs in epidemics, and young adults are normally affected. It is usually due to infection with adenovirus types 3, 4 and 7.

The clinical features of the disease are acute pharyngitis, acute conjunctivitis and pyrexia, which may be severe and last for up to a week. The pyrexia resolves by lysis. There is a considerable pharyngitis, with large lymphoid follicles and mucopus in the nasopharynx. In the eye, inflammation is more marked in the palpebral than the sclerotic conjunctiva and one eye is more severely affected than the other. When the injection fades the sclerotic conjunctiva clears first and the palpebral conjunctiva may remain injected for a further two weeks. There is usually a raised white cell count in the blood of up to 10,000/mm³. Bacterial complications are mild but include bronchitis, pneumonia and acute otitis media.

Acute lymphonodular pharyngitis

Acute lymphonodular pharyngitis is similar to herpangina but is distinguished from it because the lesions in the pharynx do not ulcerate. There is a sore throat and the temperature may be raised to 38°–41°C. There is mild headache and malaise. The disease runs a course of 10–14 days. Each lesion is raised and discrete, white or yellow in colour. It is solid and not vesiculated, and surrounded by a zone of erythema. The lesions are frequently seen on the uvula, the anterior pillars of the fauces, and the posterior pharyngeal wall. If a biopsy is performed, there is little bleeding and the lesions fade. Cropping is not observed.

Attempts to produce an effective chemotherapeutic agent to combat an established infection have yielded disappointing results. Idoxuridine inhibits replication of certain DNA viruses, particularly those responsible for corneal herpetic ulcers. Many other forms of chemotherapy have been produced, but they are ineffectual because the infecting virus has usually undergone an antigenic variation before their influence can be exerted. Gamma globulin, which may be obtained from the blood of those convalescent from an infection or unselected donors, confers some protection on those who are not infected, but has no influence on the course of the disease once it is established.

REFERENCES AND BIBLIOGRAPHY

Duxbury, A. E. (1960). *Med. J. Aust.*, **47**, 413.
Heath, R. B. (1969). *Brit. J. hosp. Med.*, **11**, 1807.
Ormerod, F. C. (1939). *Tuberculosis of the Upper Respiratory Tract*. London; John Bale.
Schroeder, R. (1936). *J. Laryng.*, **51**, 631.
Stark, J. (1969). *Brit. J. hosp. Med.*, **11**, 1791.
Steigman, A. J. (1962). *J. Paediat.*, **17**, 97.
Swinburne, G. (1940). *J. Laryng.*, **55**, 237.
Walters, J. B., and Israel, M. S. (1963). *General Pathology*. London; Churchill.
Zahorsky, J. (1924). *Arch. Paediat.*, **41**, 181.

5

PHARYNGEAL LESIONS ASSOCIATED WITH GENERAL DISEASES

A. BOWEN-DAVIES

ALTERATION IN THE BLOOD PICTURE

Anaemia

In all cases of anaemia there is a reduction in the haemoglobin content of the blood. There are many types of anaemia and in many cases their aetiology is unknown. They are divided into normoblastic and megaloblastic anaemias, according to the development of the red cells in the bone marrow. We may recognize normocytic, macrocytic and hyperchromic, and microcytic and hypochromic anaemia.

Normocytic anaemia—Normocytic anaemia is found after acute haemorrhage when the blood volume has been replaced; it is a feature in aplastic anaemia and some forms of haemolytic anaemia.

Microcytic anaemia—This accompanies chronic haemorrhage from any cause, including the nose, haemorrhoids or peptic ulcer.

Symptoms and signs

The symptoms and signs common to all the anaemias are due to a reduction in the capacity of the blood to ensure oxygenation of the tissues. The patient complains of lassitude, breathlessness, pallor, palpitations and fainting attacks. His mucous membranes are pale, and if heart failure develops he will have oedema of the ankles.

Treatment

Treatment of the associated conditions may suffice to restore the blood to its normal condition. The hypochromic anaemias respond to iron therapy, in most cases by mouth but, if absorption is deficient, by intramuscular or intravenous injection. Pernicious anaemia responds to vitamin B_{12}, but megaloblastic anaemia resulting from idiopathic steatorrhoea, coeliac disease, and sprue responds better to treatment with folic acid. Megaloblastic anaemia may be associated with iron deficiency anaemia, when both vitamin B_{12} and iron should be administered.

Pernicious anaemia

Pernicious anaemia occurs usually in middle age. The patient is pale, with a lemon tint, and symptoms appear insidiously. They are those associated with other forms of anaemia, breathlessness and weakness, but gastro-intestinal symptoms may be marked; the mouth becomes sore, particularly the tongue, and there may be vomiting with diarrhoea or constipation. Subacute combined degeneration in the spinal cord gives rise to neurological disturbances associated with posterior and lateral column dysfunction.

Examination of the blood shows reduced haemoglobin content; the number of red corpuscles is reduced, but the cells tend to be larger than normal. Anisocytosis is marked and poikilocytosis occurs. There may be nucleated red cells, normoblasts or megaloblasts in the circulation, and punctate basophilia and polychromasia are seen.

The condition is usually associated with absence of hydrochloric acid in the gastric secretions. The spleen may be palpable.

Mucous membrane

The appearance of the mucous membrane forms a guide to the haemoglobin content of the blood, and whilst it is customary to examine the conjunctiva the mucous membrane of the mouth yields the same information. In cases of severe haemorrhage or of anaemia from other causes, there is uniform pallor of the buccal and faucial mucosa.

The tongue

In pernicious anaemia the tongue does not participate in the general pallor of the mucous membrane but becomes swollen, red and beefy, and there may be considerable pain. There is a tendency to fissure, particularly at the tip, and there may be loss of the papillae; this may be more easily demonstrated after the tongue has been dried with a cloth.

In the Paterson–Brown Kelly, or Plummer Vinson, syndrome there is glossitis with loss of papillae, so that the tongue appears glazed. This is associated with dysphagia, microcytic anaemia and achlorhydria; there may be sores at the angles of the mouth, and koilonychia. Middle-aged women are mostly affected.

Dysphagia is localized to the upper end of the oesophagus, but examination may reveal nothing abnormal. In other cases, a web may have formed across the upper end of the oesophagus or, in severe cases, there may be hypopharyngitis or oesophagitis.

A number of patients subsequently develop a carcinoma of the pharynx or oesophagus.

Haemorrhagic states

Haemorrhage into the tissues can occur when there is a vascular abnormality as in scurvy, or a disorder of coagulation as in haemophilia. In purpura there is a tendency to bleed from mucous surfaces, the mouth, nose or into the bowel and into the skin where petechial rashes or ecchymoses occur. The condition may occur in septicaemia, but there is also a group of cases in which the manifestations are associated with a deficiency of blood platelets in the circulating blood, thrombocytopenic purpura. This commonly occurs in children and recovers spontaneously, or as a result of treatment with steroids. In resistant cases, splenectomy may have to be considered. This gives excellent results but, owing to the haemorrhagic state of the patient, the operation is not devoid of risk.

Agranulocytic angina

Aetiology

Agranulocytic angina may arise spontaneously or in the course of an acute infection, but the majority of cases are caused by toxic substances administered therapeutically. The worst offenders were those containing coal tar derivatives and administered as analgesics, Pyramidon in particular, but since the introduction of chemotherapy, the sulphonamides or chemotherapy for malignant diseases have been responsible for the majority of cases. Cases have been seen after the administration of thiouracil.

Haematology

There is a marked leucopenia affecting the granulocytes, so that there is a relative lymphocytosis. The deficiency of granulocytes is thought to be due to a failure on the part of the granulopoietic tissues rather than to excessive destruction of the cells. The total white count may be reduced to less than a thousand cells per mm³., with the result that the general resistance of the patient is grossly impaired.

Signs

There is a sudden deterioration in the general condition of the patient, which may have been preceded for a few days by a rise in temperature. Very soon loss of resistance is shown in the sites where organisms are generally present, the mouth, the vagina and the region round the anus.

In the mouth there is ulceration on the gums, cheeks, fauces and tonsils. At first the lesions are small indolent ulcers, with ragged edges and clean bases, and with little inflammatory reaction around. Later, ulceration becomes much more extensive, and a form of gangrenous tonsillitis may occur.

Diagnosis

The condition must be distinguished from acute leukaemia, glandular fever, syphilis and tuberculosis. In the case of acute leukaemia, there is generalized glandular involvement and the spleen may be palpable. Glandular fever may resemble the condition closely, particularly when the glandular enlargement is confined to the cervical group of glands. In syphilis and tuberculosis, the ulceration progresses less rapidly, and in the former the Wassermann reaction is positive. Estimation of the number of white cells in the blood shows a marked granulopenia, which is typical of the condition.

Treatment

Whilst excessive use of the responsible drugs may cause the condition, many individuals appear to be unduly sensitive to the toxin and succumb after small doses. Much can be done to prevent the condition becoming serious by frequent examination of the blood during treatment with any of the responsible agents; this is particularly desirable should there be a sudden rise of temperature.

Once the condition has become established, it is important to recognize its nature, lest the dose of the offending substance be increased to combat secondary infection. The drug must be immediately withheld and vitamin B_{12} administered. In grave cases a fresh blood transfusion may help the patient to overcome a critical situation. The hygiene of the mouth is important, and frequent mouthwashes should help to keep it clean. Nystatin lozenges prevent infection with Candida albicans. Antibiotics may help to control the infection. Application of caustics or any operative intervention is strictly contra-indicated, owing to the absence of local tissue reaction.

Leukaemia

Leukaemia is a disease in which there is characteristically an increase in the number of white cells circulating in the blood stream. In some cases, however, there is no increase in the total white count, but the ratio of lymphocytes to granulocytes is disturbed. In either case, many immature forms of white cells are seen and it is on their presence that the diagnosis should be made. There is often an associated anaemia, with an increase in the number of erythroblasts in the blood.

The cause of the disease is unknown, and either the lymphopoietic tissue or granulopoietic tissue may be affected; accordingly, myelogenous and lymphatic leukaemia are recognized. It has been noted that the disease may develop an aleukaemic phase, but even when the number of white cells is greatly increased, resistance to infection is impaired and secondary infection is common. As is usual in such cases, the mouth and pharynx are involved at an early stage, and in the acute form of the disease the condition of the mouth may be the presenting feature.

The disease occurs in acute and chronic forms. Acute leukaemia occurs in children and young adults, and is nearly always of the lymphatic type; chronic leukaemia is more often seen in middle age and is usually of the myelogenous variety.

Acute leukaemia

Acute leukaemia is a fulminating disease affecting children and young adults. The onset is sudden; there is rapid deterioration of the general condition of the patient, with ulceration of the mouth and pharynx, and a mistaken diagnosis of some acute infection may be made. Haemorrhage from the ulcerating areas in the mouth, or from the nose, may be profuse, and internal haemorrhage may occur. There is generalized enlargement of the lymph glands, and the spleen is usually palpable but not grossly enlarged. In the mouth, the lymphatic tissue becomes hypertrophied, and secondary infection quickly follows. The gums become spongy and bleed readily, and the tonsils become ulcerated; gangrene often supervenes. The temperature may be high. The condition must be distinguished from acute streptococcal tonsillitis, diphtheria, infectious mononucleosis (glandular fever), Vincent's angina, or agranulocytosis.

In the early stages, the total number of white cells in the blood may not be increased or may even be diminished. Examination of a blood smear, however, shows the presence of large numbers of immature cells. Later, the total white count is raised considerably, 200,000 cells/mm³. being found in some cases. The increase is due to the great preponderance of lymphocytes.

Blood transfusion and deep x-ray therapy applied to the affected glands give temporary relief, while the use of cytotoxic drugs has produced some encouraging results. Nevertheless, the disease is always fatal. The mouth should receive constant attention to make the patient as comfortable as possible.

Chronic myelogenous leukaemia

Gross enlargement of the spleen is the feature of this disease, and it is often the discovery of an abdominal tumour that brings the patient under observation. There is a general loss of well-being, and there may be haemorrhage from the mucous surfaces or into an organ. The number of white cells in the blood is greatly increased owing to an abundance of granular cells, and a total cell count of 500,000 cells mm$_3$. is frequent; there are many immature cells and it is on the number in which they are present, rather than on the total number of cells, that the prognosis should be assessed.

Although the outcome of the disease is always fatal, its course may run for several months or even years. There are often remissions for quite long periods, and the number of cells in the blood can usually be controlled by the application of deep radiotherapy to the spleen and long bones.

Chronic lymphatic leukaemia

The onset is insidious, and advice is sought because of generalized painless enlargement of the lymph glands and loss of well-being. The spleen may be palpable, but is not greatly enlarged. The tonsils and lymphoid tissue in the pharynx may show signs of hypertrophy, and the gums may become hypertrophied to such an extent that the teeth are completely enveloped, but in the edentulous the gums are unaffected. Haemorrhage from the nose or mouth may be profuse. The total number of white cells in the blood is increased owing to an increase in the number of lymphocytes, many of which are immature; the total cell count may be raised to 100,000 cells/mm.[3]

The course of the disease may extend to several years, but in spite of remissions a fatal outcome is inevitable. At necropsy there is general lymphoid hypertrophy, with leukaemic deposits scattered throughout the body.

Deep x-ray therapy applied to the glands and spleen often controls the number of cells in the blood, but, as in other forms of the disease, a reduction in their number is not necessarily accompanied by an improvement in the clinical condition of the patient.

Glandular fever

Infectious mononucleosis

Aetiology.—Glandular fever is a disease which has come into prominence during the past three decades, although it was originally described by Pfeiffer in 1889. It occurs sporadically, but often in epidemics, and is thought to be due to a virus infection; the incubation period is from one to two weeks.

Symptoms and signs.—The onset is insidious, with general malaise, headache and pyrexia. There follows a generalized enlargement of the lymph glands, particularly those of the cervical groups, and the spleen may become palpable. In the anginose form of the disease, there is also acute pharyngitis and tonsillitis, with exudate; the patient suffers acute distress with severe dysphagia. In some cases an erythematous rash appears.

Haematology.—In the early stages there may be leucopenia or a neutrophil leucocytosis, but later there is a rise in the total white cell count, due to an increase in the number of abnormal lymphocytes.

Diagnosis.—The condition may resemble acute leukaemia, agranulocytosis, Vincent's angina, diphtheria or an overwhelming streptococcal infection, and it is often with relief that the correct diagnosis is established.

The diagnosis may be made by performing a blood count, but more certainly by a specific agglutinin reaction of the blood serum, the Paul–Bunnell reaction; this however does not become positive for several days after the onset of the disease.

It is worthy of note that false Wassermann reactions can occur. The alteration in the blood picture and serum reactions may persist for many weeks after clinical signs of the disease have disappeared.

Treatment.—The disease runs a course of a few weeks and treatment seems to exert little influence, but the mouth must be kept clean and adequate nourishment ensured, in spite of the patient's reluctance to swallow. Hot fomentations applied to the cervical glands may relieve discomfort, or cold packs may be preferred.

BEHÇET'S DISEASE

This disease was first described by Behçet in 1937; the aetiology is unknown. It runs a protracted course with periods of remission and acute relapse, when there is pyrexia, leucocytosis and raised sedimentation rate in the blood.

Pathology

The disease is characterized by massive and indolent ulceration of the mucous membranes and, sometimes, the skin. The anogenital region is commonly affected, the labia minora and cervix in women, and the uretha, glans penis and scrotum in men. There is an associated inflammation of the eye. Iritis with hypopion, conjunctivitis, choroiditis, retinitis or retinal haemorrhages are encountered. In the mouth, the manifestation consists of aphthous ulcers, rather larger and more persistent than those normally seen. Lesions in the pharynx may resemble leucoplakia, or even carcinoma. Skin lesions may resemble pemphigus or lichen planus. The central nervous system may be involved, and acute encephalitis with raised lymphocyte count and protein content of the cerebrospinal fluid may be simulated. There may be acute lesions of the brain stem or pyramidal tracts, and dementia may set in. Lesions affecting the central nervous system usually arise after several years and indicate a poor prognosis. Pain is a marked feature of the lesions, and loss of weight may be considerable. The lesions heal with gross scarring, and complications such as vesico-vaginal fistula may arise.

Diagnosis

The disease resembles any condition giving rise to ulceration in the areas referred to: syphylis, tuberculosis, carcinoma, leucoplakia, agranulocytosis and malignant granuloma, to mention a few. These may be excluded by serological tests, blood count, examination of smears from the lesion, or biopsy. In Behçet's disease these investigations do not yield any specific information, and it is usually considered that the diagnosis is confirmed when any two of the sites usually involved are affected.

Treatment

Since the aetiology of the disease is unknown, there is no specific treatment. Antibiotics have little effect, but the exhibition of steroids usually leads to an improvement in the lesions. In the mouth and pharynx, ulceration may be controlled by topical administration in the form of trochiscus hydrocortisone hemisuccinate 2·5 mg. six-hourly, but sooner or later systemic administration becomes necessary, at least 20 mg. of prednisone daily being required. The patient may survive for a number of years, but a complete cure is unlikely.

PHARYNGEAL LESIONS DUE TO NERVE DYSFUNCTION
Functional disorder

Emotion causes a variety of sensations in the pharynx and larynx, so it is natural that people who are emotionally unstable should refer symptoms to this region.

Globus hystericus

Globus hystericus is a condition in which a patient, usually a middle-aged woman, complains of the sensation of a lump in the throat, usually in the region of the thyroid cartilage. There may be other symptoms suggestive of a functional state, and the patient may admit that a relative or friend has recently succumbed to "cancer of the throat". The patient makes repeated attempts to swallow the lump which aggravate the symptoms and may lead to aerophagy and gastric discomfort. There is, however, no true dysphagia and the symptoms disappear or are improved by taking a meal. Examination of the pharynx and larynx shows no evidence of disease. The condition may be confused with chronic pharyngitis or the Paterson–Brown Kelly syndrome, but clinical examination should exclude these.

Re-assurance may serve to relieve the patient, but sedatives should be prescribed should her mental attitude require them. It may be advisable, however, to make an x-ray examination with an opaque medium, or to perform direct endoscopy, as it is only by these means that an early organic lesion in the oesophagus can be excluded.

Functional anaesthesia

Functional anaesthesia is more common than anaesthesia due to organic disease and does not give rise to any symptoms. The patient is remarkably tolerant of the spatula, and it may even be possible to perform direct laryngoscopy without an anaesthetic. The condition is of no importance, but serves to confirm the functional nature of the condition.

Neurotrophic conditions
Herpes

Herpetic eruptions may occur anywhere in the mouth or pharynx, but the soft palate is commonly involved. The lesion may occur by itself or it may complicate eruptions elsewhere, such as on the face or the eye or in the form of geniculate herpes (Hunt's syndrome). This is herpes zoster due to involvement of the spheno-palatine ganglion, and not to be confused with a local virus infection such as herpangina.

The throat is sore for a few hours before a vesicular eruption appears. The vesicles break down to form shallow ulcers similar to those seen in aphthous stomatitis. Pain is severe, and may persist after the lesions have healed. There is little constitutional disturbance save that which usually accompanies a painful lesion in the throat, leading to interrupted sleep and disinclination to take food.

Local treatment must be employed to keep the mouth clean, and local analgesics should be given before meals to ensure adequate nourishment. Sedatives are necessary to relieve the pain.

Neuralgia

Glossopharyngeal neuralgia is a rare condition similar to trigeminal neuralgia, save in the distribution of pain. There are agonizing stabs of pain, which start in the region of the tonsil and radiate towards the ear; in other cases, the pain is situated in the ear or just below it, between the angle of the jaw and the mastoid process.

The attacks are precipitated by stimulus in the trigger area. When this is situated in the throat, pain may be brought on by swallowing; temporary relief may be obtained by the application of cocaine to the posterior third of the tongue and the lateral pharyngeal wall. When the symptoms are confined to the ear, external stimulation on the ear or skin may cause an attack.

The attacks may be relieved by the administration of sedatives, but if these prove ineffectual, operation on the nerve may be necessary. The nerve may be approached within the skull, at the base of the skull, or at its periphery where it comes into relation with the tonsillar fossa.

Within the skull the nerve fibres can be divided soon after their emergence from the medulla, ensuring the relief of symptoms over the area of distribution of the nerve and its connections, notably that with the tympanic plexus. It is a formidable procedure, but with modern neurosurgical technique there is no undue risk.

Approach to the nerve at the base of the skull is difficult. The nerve is small and is lying at a considerable depth in relation to important structures. It leaves the cranium through the middle compartment of the jugular foramen lying in front of, and medial to, the vagus and accessory nerves. It passes between the internal jugular vein and internal carotid artery, crossing the latter obliquely, and passing beneath the styloid process to reach the posterior border of the stylopharyngeus muscle. When the nerve has been found it must be avulsed to remove the jugular and petrosal ganglia, otherwise the connections with the tympanic plexus remain intact, and symptoms referred to the ear are not relieved. The results of this operation are not as certain as are those of intracranial section, and there is sometimes recurrence of symptoms.

Wilson has approached the nerve through the tonsillar fossa, where the nerve can be found lying on the stylopharyngeus muscle (Wilson and McAlpine, 1946). By dividing the nerve he relieved a patient whose symptoms were confined to the throat, but he claims that it would be possible to follow the nerve to the base of the skull. Sometimes the neuralgia is associated with an abnormally long styloid process. This may be removed through the pharyngeal wall after tonsillectomy.

Loss of sensation

Anaesthesia is rarely due to organic disease, but may be due to wounds in the neck involving the sensory nerves. It may occur also in severe neuritis, that due to diphtheria being the most common. If the sensory loss is considerable, there is danger of inhalation pneumonia, and tube feeding and tracheostomy with a cuffed tube may become necessary. Many cases of anaesthesia are functional, however, when this danger does not arise.

Paralysis of the palate and pharynx

Aetiology

Toxic neuritis.—The most common form of neuritis affecting the motor nerves of the palate and pharynx is that due to diphtheria; the toxin has an affinity for neuromuscular junctions. The condition commonly arises in faucial diphtheria, and some believe that the toxin has a local action.

In the neck.—The nerves may be interrupted in their course in the neck by trauma or neoplasms. Secondary deposits from lympho-epithelioma of the nasopharynx occur at the base of the skull early in the disease and may cause pressure on any of the nerves emerging in the region of the jugular foramen.

Within the skull.—Physiological interruption of the nerves may be caused by meningitis, notably syphilitic pachymeningitis, or by pressure of cerebellopontine tumours, or other space-occupying lesions.

In the brain.—The nerves may be affected by vascular disease, thrombosis of the posterior cerebellar artery in particular, or by degenerative processes in the nuclei of the nerves or in the upper motor neurones connected with them.

Generalized nervous disease.—The motor nerves of the palate and pharynx may be involved in syringobulbia, progressive muscular atrophy (chronic bulbar palsy), disseminated sclerosis, the bulbar form of poliomyelitis and pseudobulbar palsy. In these cases, although paralysis may lead to the death of the patient from malnutrition or from inhalation pneumonia, the disease is usually well established before the onset of paralysis.

Following the removal of tonsils and adenoids.—Palatal paralysis is sometimes encountered immediately after operation, and is probably due to stretching of the muscles during manipulations. The prognosis is good, recovery taking place as a rule within a few days.

Symptoms

When the palate is paralysed, the nasopharynx cannot be shut off from the rest of the pharynx and the flow of air through the nose cannot therefore be controlled during speech. This causes the form of speech heard in cases of cleft palate, rhinolalia aperta, although the disability is not usually so marked. During deglutition, fluids and even solids may regurgitate through the nose. In spite of this, however, the patient is usually able to swallow sufficient for his needs unless the pharynx is also involved. In this case the condition is much more serious, since it is almost impossible for the patient to swallow, and also because he loses control of secretions in the pharynx, which may enter the larynx and cause inhalation pneumonia. Any attempt at swallowing results in a spasm of coughing, particularly when fluids are taken.

Signs

When the paralysis is bilateral the palate remains immobile during phonation. It may be difficult to decide whether there is any movement, but if the patient is made to gag, it is at once apparent that the palate is paralysed. The patient is unable to comply with the request to blow up a balloon or to whistle.

In cases in which the paralysis is unilateral, the symptoms are not so marked, but when the patient phonates or is made to gag, the palate is drawn up to one side like a curtain, and the uvula displaced with it.

Diagnosis

Paralysis of the palate must be distinguished from local fixation. This may be due to acute inflammatory conditions, tonsillitis or quinsy. Scarring after syphilis, lupus vulgaris, scarlet fever, or after operation for the removal of tonsils and adenoids or new growth, may also reduce the mobility of the palate.

Sometimes cases of palatal paralysis are referred to laryngologists because the symptoms are attributed to the presence of adenoids. In the case of nasal obstruction the speech defect, rhinolalia clausa, is entirely different and should not be confused, while regurgitation of fluids does not occur. The removal of adenoids in a case of palatal paralysis would, of course, be a disaster serving only to increase the disability.

Treatment

Treatment is dictated by the cause of the condition, and a paralysis of the palate is unlikely to call for any special measures, but if regurgitation is marked, swallowing may be facilitated by holding the nose during the act. When the condition is associated with pharyngeal paralysis, the passing of a stomach tube may become necessary to ensure adequate nourishment, and a sucker should be used to keep the pharynx free from secretions. It is advisable to protect the lower air passage with a cuffed tracheostomy tube. Exercises should be given to hasten the return of function when recovery is taking place.

Diphtheritic paralysis of the palate and pharynx

Pathology

Diphtheritic paralysis of the palate and pharynx is due to the action of toxin on the neuromuscular junctions. The toxin may reach the nerve endings by the blood stream, but it is possible that in cases of faucial diphtheria access is gained locally.

Paralysis occurs three or four weeks after the onset of the disease, but may occur earlier in severe cases. It may be associated with other forms of paralysis but is often the only manifestation of neuritis. It is a complication which may be expected in severe cases, but it often occurs after a mild infection, when the patient is ambulant and presents himself because of regurgitation of fluids and alteration in his speech. Such a case was seen by us, and on questioning his mother we were told that the patient had recently had a sore throat and that his brother was "in a fever hospital with diphtheria and a paralysed palate".

Pharyngeal paralysis usually occurs rather later than palatal paralysis. It is a serious complication because swallowing becomes almost impossible and there is risk of inhalation pneumonia. It complicates grave cases, and there may be respiratory paralysis as well.

Diagnosis

The diagnosis presents no difficulty when the subject is known to be suffering from diphtheria, since the paralysis is a complication which may be expected. In ambulant cases, a history of recent sore throat can usually be obtained, but the possibility of the membrane being situated elsewhere, in the nose or in a wound, must be remembered.

Treatment

Palatal paralysis calls for no treatment other than that dictated by the general condition of the patient. In cases in which the diagnosis has not already been made, the throat should be swabbed and the patient isolated until three negative results have been obtained. It is advisable to administer diphtheria antitoxin although, since the paralysis occurs late in the disease, the attack must have been mild to escape detection. Nevertheless, the patient must be kept in bed completely at rest.

When the pharynx is involved, active treatment is required to secure adequate nourishment and also to prevent inhalation pneumonia. If necessary, a stomach tube must be passed through the nose: this may be left *in situ* to avoid disturbing the patient who is likely to be desperately ill and to require absolute rest. A sucker may be used to remove pharyngeal secretions, to prevent their entry into the larynx. Diphtheria antitoxin is required in doses of up to 200,000 units/day, by the intravenous route if necessary. Tracheostomy with a cuffed tube may be necessary.

Although the paralysis always recovers spontaneously, the restoration of movement may be hastened by exercises, and the patient should be encouraged to whistle or to blow up balloons.

Prognosis

This is largely dependent upon the general condition of the patient. When the palate alone is involved, the prognosis is not unduly affected, but in the case of pharyngeal paralysis, which often occurs in grave cases, the risk of inhalation pneumonia and difficulty in feeding render recovery less certain.

Should the patient survive, the paralysis always recovers sooner or later.

Myasthenia gravis

Myasthenia gravis occurs in persons of all ages, but is usually seen in adolescents; they are sometimes referred for the removal of adenoids, when the pharynx is involved. There is a defect at the neuromuscular junction, which is believed to be due to destruction of acetylcholine depriving the junction of its activating substances. The result is a gradual loss of power in the affected muscles. Any group of muscles may be involved, commonly those in the lower limb, but occasionally the lesion is restricted to the muscles of the mouth and pharynx. There is dysarthria and dysphagia, with regurgitation of fluid through the nose, and movements of the tongue, palate and pharynx are sluggish. Disability is minimal after night's rest, but increases as the day passes.

The cause of the condition is unknown and treatment must be symptomatic. Injection of physostigmin or prostigmin brings temporary relief, and many patients are able to live a restricted life on prostigmin bromide or Mestinon, taken by mouth. Keynes (1949) has reported a large number of cases of myasthenia gravis which he has relieved by removing the thymus gland. He admits that the treatment is largely empirical, but claims that the association of dysfunction of the gland with myasthenia gravis has been established. He believes that the abnormal secretion of the gland contains some curare-like substance. The operative mortality in his early series was high, five of the first 18 cases dying, but experience has enabled him to reduce the figure to 4·2 per cent in over 100 cases. He stresses the importance of early operation if the best results are to be obtained. When a tumour of the thymus is already present, comparable results cannot be obtained.

Acute anterior poliomyelitis

This disease is of interest to the laryngologist because, when the medullary nuclei are affected (the bulbar type of acute anterior poliomyelitis), paralysis of the pharynx and larynx may occur.

97

Aetiology

The disease is due to a virus of which three principal strains have been identified. It may occur in epidemics, or sporadically. Epidemics commonly occur in hot weather, starting in midsummer and reaching their height in the autumn. Infection may be spread by people who are in the early stages of infection, or by healthy carriers who are infective for a few days. The disease is spread by faecal contamination, the portal of entry being the intestinal epithelium; at least one epidemic has been ascribed to the ingestion of infected milk.

Study of the epidemiology of the disease is difficult, because many cases do not progress to the stage at which the diagnosis is certain and, in the absence of an epidemic, cases must occur in which the true nature of the condition is not recognized. The disease occurs most regularly in children, but in the post-war epidemic in Great Britain adults formed a large proportion of the victims. The relative immunity of the adult population is probably due to previous unrecognized infection, which imparts immunity.

Motor, sensory and sympathetic axons may all be invaded by the poliomyelitis virus. The virus does not multiply in the axons but does so when it reaches the anterior horn cells. The cells invaded bear no anatomical relation to the site of inoculation, but certain groups of cells, those involved in maintaining decerebrate rigidity, appear to be more sensitive than others.

Pathology

Once the virus has gained access to the central nervous system it becomes widely disseminated throughout the brain stem and anterior horn cells of the spinal cord. The cortex and sympathetic ganglia are less severely affected. The first changes which occur are round-cell and lymphocyte collections round the vessels in relation to the nerve cells. This does not occur when the cells are degenerate, and it is assumed that this reaction is the result of the action of the virus on healthy nerve cells. Nerve cells are destroyed early in the disease, certainly within three days, and no further destruction occurs. The destroyed cells are rapidly removed by neurophages, leaving no trace. Other cells show evidence of damage by loss of Nissl granules, but these are likely to recover later. Clinical signs of paralysis are not noticeable until probably at least one-third of the cells are destroyed, and paralysis is complete when only one-tenth remain. It is very unusual for all the cells to be destroyed.

Symptoms and signs

When the disease runs its full course, there are three distinct phases.

In the first stage, there is general malaise, with either gastro-intestinal disorder or upper respiratory infection. Symptoms may be severe, with pyrexia, or so mild as to escape notice except during an epidemic. The patient is ill for a few days and then recovers; in abortive cases, health is restored and further symptoms do not appear. Within 48 hours of apparent recovery, the second stage of meningitic involvement is entered. Symptoms may be severe, with headache and neck rigidity, or they may be mild.

This stage is of short duration and the disease may be arrested or it may pass into the third stage, in which sudden paralysis of groups of muscles occurs. This is due to involvement of the anterior horn cells in the spinal cord, or more rarely of the medullary nuclei. There is pain and tenderness in the affected muscles, and although at first the paralysis may be widespread, a variable degree of recovery may be expected. The lower limb is usually involved, but the upper limb and respiratory muscles may be affected. In the bulbar type of infection, the larynx and pharynx may be paralysed; these are severe cases and the prognosis is not good.

Diagnosis

In the first stage the disease resembles a minor gastro-intestinal upset, or a mild upper respiratory infection, and it is unlikely that the correct diagnosis will be made except in the presence of an epidemic. In the second phase, of meningitic involvement, the diagnosis can be made with certainty by examination of the cerebrospinal fluid, which contains an increased number of cells, chiefly lymphocytes, and raised protein, but normal glucose and chloride concentrations. In the third stage, the sudden onset of widespread paralysis presents little difficulty in diagnosis.

Treatment

It would be out of place to discuss the treatment of all aspects of the disease, but pharyngeal and respiratory paralysis may demand our attention. In pharyngeal paralysis the main dangers are respiratory infection due to inhalation of food and secretions, and lack of nourishment; and in laryngeal paralysis, asphyxia owing to respiratory obstruction. These are treated by tracheostomy with a cuffed tube and the passage of a Ryle's tube into the stomach. This ensures adequate nourishment whilst the lower respiratory passages are protected and an adequate airway obtained. Secretions in the bronchial tree may be aspirated as often as necessary, and if the muscles of respiration are paralysed a positive pressure respirator such as a Beaver or Barnett machine may be employed.

Once the extent of the paralysis, which comes on over a period of some hours, has been established, the condition of the patient remains unchanged for a variable period, which may amount to weeks. Sooner or later, however, a period of recovery sets in which may continue for some weeks. Many are able to discard their tracheostomy tubes and regain their powers of swallowing and speech, although there may be some permanent residual paralysis. The less fortunate may be condemned to a life only made possible by the continued use of a respirator.

Immunization

Although the existence of a virus was demonstrated many years ago by its passage through filters which prevented the passage of bacteria and the production of disease by the filtrate, it is so small that it could not be observed with the aid of the most powerful magnification at that time. Its precise form and mode of life was a mystery until the invention of the electron microscope, when it could be observed. This revealed that it was an organism which required an intracellular environment, hence the lack of success with attempts to obtain cultures on the usual media. This led to the method of tissue culture on the chicken embryo and other tissues, notably the kidney of monkeys. The viruses were observed and various strains recognized. The production of vaccines followed, and in no field have the results been more dramatic than that of acute anterior poliomyelitis. It was found that three strains of virus were responsible for the disease, and Salk introduced the first vaccine by killing the three strains of virus with formalin and injecting the products of destruction systemically. Apart from one tragic episode when owing to faulty technique a batch of vaccine containing live virus was released, with consequent infection of a number of people, the method proved satisfactory. It is thought that the antigen forms a coating over the cells of the body which prevents invasion by the virus. More recently, this method has been superseded by the oral administration of attenuated live virus. It is thought that the intestinal cells are protected from invasion by the virus, but that with large doses a certain amount of antigen is absorbed into the circulation. In this method of immunization it is realized that attenuated virus is excreted in the faeces and that other individuals may become infected, but where the immunization of a community is the aim this is an advantage rather than a risk. It is not known for how long immunity is conferred by either method. There is no doubt, however, of the success of immunization since no epidemic has occurred among immunized communities since its introduction.

Spasm of the pharynx

This is a rare condition and consequently may present some difficulty in diagnosis. Frequently it is one of the signs of a well-established neurological condition, but occasionally it is the presenting feature.

Aetiology

Spasm of the pharynx is seen in tetanus, hydrophobia, spastic diplegia, and in some conditions affecting the medulla.

Symptoms

Owing to spasm, the co-ordination necessary to swallow solids, and particularly liquids, is lacking, and the patient finds himself unable to eat or drink. He refuses to take more than a sip of fluid owing to his previous experience, when its entry into the larynx threw him into a spasm of coughing. The spasms induced by attempts to swallow cause the patient great distress and his condition is pitiable. There is a very real danger of secretions in the pharynx entering the bronchial tree and causing bronchopneumonia.

Signs

Examination of the throat may be extremely difficult owing to spasm induced by the spatula.

Nystagmus of the palate

This is a condition of unknown origin in which there are rhythmical movements of the palate. The movements may be slow, or they may reach a frequency of a hundred or more per minute. There is often a clicking sound audible to the patient and to those around him. There is no disability, and treatment is not necessary, but sedatives may help to abolish the rhythmic movements.

REFERENCES AND BIBLIOGRAPHY

Ayers, M. S. (1965). *Obstet. Gynec.*, **26**, 575.
Barber, H. S. (1941). *Lancet*, **1**, 71.
Behçet, H. (1937). *Derm. Wschr.*, **105**, 1152.
— (1938). *Bull. Soc. Franc., Derm. Syph.*, **45**, 420.
— (1939). *Bull. Soc. Franc., Derm. Syph.*, **46**, 674.
Cohen, H. (1937). *J. Laryng.*, **52**, 527.

REFERENCES AND BIBLIOGRAPHY

Coll, J. R. (1969). *Gen. Practnr.*, **18,** 38.
Cunning, D. S. (1946). *Ann. Otol. etc., St. Louis*, **55,** 583.
Hamilton, P. M. (1947). *Ann. Otol. etc., St. Louis*, **56,** 61.
Keynes, G. (1949). *Brit. med. J.*, **2,** 611.
Morrison, A. W. (1959). *J. Laryng.*, **73,** 833.
Pfeiffer, E. (1889). *Jb. Kinderheilk.*, **22,** 257.
Wadia, N. L., and Williams, E. (1957). *Brain*, **80,** 59.
Walshe, F. M. R. (1941). *Diseases of the Nervous System* (5th ed.). London; Livingstone.
Wilson, C. P., and McAlpine, D. (1946). *Proc. R. Soc. Med.*, **40,** 81.

6

DISEASES OF THE TONSILS AND ADENOIDS (EXCLUDING NEOPLASMS)

S. Mawson

The word tonsil derives from the Latin *tonsilla* a mooring post, and there are three so-named anatomical structures forming part of Waldeyer's ring of lymphoid tissue encircling the entrance from the mouth and nasal passages to the pharynx; *palatine* (faucial) *tonsil* situated, one on each side, between the folds of the palato-pharyngeus and palatoglossus muscles; *lingual tonsil*, one on each side between base of tongue and vallecula; and a single *nasopharyngeal tonsil* (adenoids: Greek *aden*, gland; *eidos*, form) in the roof of the nasopharynx (epipharynx).

The palatine tonsil is a subepithelial lymph node with prominent germinal centres concerned in the production of lymphocytes and plasma cells, penetrated by branching crypts from the medial surface; the lateral surfaces being separated from the pharyngeal wall by a distinct capsule of condensed connective tissue. Surface epithelium and crypt linings are of stratified squamous epithelium. Efferent lymphatics pass to the jugulodigastric lymph node behind the angle of the mandible, and thence to the cervical chain. The lingual tonsils are similar subepithelial nodes but with smaller crypts and without a capsule. The subepithelial nasopharyngeal tonsil has neither crypts nor capsule, but prominent folds lined by respiratory epithelium (for anatomy, *see* Vol. 1).

Nomenclature

In British otolaryngology the word tonsil(s) has long been understood as referring, in practice, exclusively to the palatine (faucial) tonsil(s). The nasopharyngeal tonsil is customarily called (the) adenoids, while the two lingual tonsils retain their full title. This has the merit of avoiding confusion. The traditional terms, tonsils, adenoids and lingual tonsils will therefore be retained and hereafter used in the sense defined.

Function

Antibody level in the tonsils has been studied (Malecki, 1958) and the results obtained have indicated the capability of the parenchyma to produce antibodies with the active participation of the local plasma cells. The evidence points to the tonsils as playing some part in the defence mechanism against inspired and ingested organisms, but their precise immunological role has still to be determined.

At birth the tonsils are without germinal centres and usually quite small in relation to the oropharyngeal inlet, but coinciding with the loss of maternal source antibody there is an enlargement of the tonsils and adenoids, and to a lesser extent the lingual tonsils, further exacerbated it would seem by the exposure to infection that occurs on entry to nursery school at the age of three and primary school at the age of five. Enlargement of tonsils and adenoids is therefore normal in early childhood and probably an index of immunological activity. There are however considerable individual variations within this general trend, often related to familial tendencies or to other factors such as severe respiratory infections in infancy. Occasionally children are born with tonsils and/or adenoids of such size as to constitute an embarrassment to respiration from the start.

At or before the onset of puberty there would appear to be a decline in functional activity accompanied by a marked involution of these organs. While the tonsils and lingual tonsils remain still visible, the adenoids may completely disappear, so that indirect nasopharyngoscopy in the adult commonly reveals a roof as smooth as in those who have had the adenoids removed. Once the whole lymphatic system is mature it is unlikely that ablation of any small part, for example tonsils or adenoids, or even the thymus, will compromise immunological integrity (Malcomson, 1967), but in the present state of our knowledge it is generally agreed that the tonsils and adenoids should be conserved as probable immunological assets unless by their size they are causing severe embarrassment to respiration, eustachian tube function, speech or feeding, or unless they have become the seat of a disease the best remedy for which is excision.

OBSTRUCTIVE ENLARGEMENT

As stated above, children may be born with tonsils and especially adenoids of such a size as already to cause some obstruction to the upper respiratory tract. In the case of adenoids difficulty may very occasionally arise with feeding, as in congenital choanal atresia, and in this event it will be necessary to differentiate between the two conditions by passing a soft rubber catheter through the nose. It is most unusual for such a catheter not to be able to find a way past the adenoids and become visible in the oropharynx. But in cases of doubt a firmer instrument (e.g. eustachian catheter) or instillation of a radio-opaque contrast medium should resolve the problem.

Obstruction of a serious nature, however, seldom occurs much before the end of the first year and is more usually seen between the ages of three to five.

While it is a simple matter to assess the size of the tonsils by direct inspection, it is not so easy clinically to determine the size of the adenoids. The degree of obstruction is related to and may be inferred from the symptoms of mouth-breathing and snoring. Obstruction may also be inferred from the appearance of the tympanic membranes which may be retracted, due to absorption of air, if the tubal orifices are blocked. An attempt should always be made to try to see the adenoids with a nasopharyngeal mirror in any child who can be persuaded to keep the mouth open and tolerate a tongue depressor. Provided the approach is unhurried and careful, a rewarding view may be obtained in a surprising proportion of young patients.

Treatment

Attempts have been made to reduce the size of the adenoids by radiotherapy but this treatment is too uncertain, both in terms of adenoid response and latent effects, to be recommended. When the obstruction is interfering seriously with respiration and feeding especially, or with hearing and speech, then relief by adenoidectomy will come under consideration as the best treatment at present known.

The operation, however, is not without disadvantages, especially in the younger child (*see* "The Operation of Adenoidectomy" p. 136).

(1) Risk of haemorrhage. Depletion of blood volume reaches a more critical stage more quickly the smaller the child.

(2) Risk of recurrence. It is impossible to remove every vestige of adenoid tissue with a curette. The earlier adenoids are removed the more likely are remnants and other subepithelial deposits in the nasopharynx to undergo compensatory hypertrophy, due to the natural tendency towards tonsil tissue hypertrophy in the first five years of life.

(3) Technical difficulty is greater in the very young child.

Thus, unless hypertrophy of adenoids is causing serious retardation of the physiological functions mentioned, it is nearly always better to avoid operation until a child has at least reached the age of two, and preferably postpone it until the fourth year. Very occasionally it will be necessary to accept the disadvantages and operate earlier.

On occasions it is wise to precede a decision to operate by taking of a soft-tissue lateral radiograph of the postnasal space. In expert hands this is a most valuable procedure, as a good shadow outline of the adenoids can be obtained and the degree of encroachment upon the airway assessed.

The tonsils by size alone seldom give rise to the same degree of obstruction as the adenoids and, again, it is preferable whenever possible to postpone operation until the age of four.

ACUTE TONSILLITIS

The tonsils, being covered by the mucous membrane common to the oropharynx, may become inflamed as part of a general pharyngitis, usually concurrent with an acute upper respiratory infection. Such an inflammation has, in the past, been called *acute catarrhal or superficial tonsillitis*. In these cases there is little or no swelling of the tonsils, the surface merely appearing inflamed in continuity with the rest of the pharyngeal mucosa. Clinically true acute tonsillitis presents in three main forms: *acute follicular tonsillitis* (cryptic tonsillitis, lacunar tonsillitis) when inflammatory exudation from the crypt marks the reddened surface with whitish or yellow spots; *acute parenchymatous tonsillitis*, when the whole tonsil is uniformly congested, presenting as a definitely abnormal red swelling—the phlegmon of older textbooks; and *acute membranous tonsillitis*, in which the exudation from the crypts may coalesce to form a confluent membrane over the surface.

While acute tonsillitis can present in any one of these forms the clinical distinction between them is not of great importance, and is often blurred.

Aetiology

Acute tonsillitis is predominantly a disease of childhood with a peak incidence in the fifth and sixth years of life. But it occurs relatively frequently in adolescence and early adulthood, often as periodic exacerbation of an underlying chronic tonsil infection. It is rare in infancy and after the age of 50.

It may occur as a primary infection, that is to say infection originates with the tonsil, or as a secondary infection derived from a general infection of the upper respiratory tract. In the latter case the initial infecting organism is most likely to be a virus. Important members of the group of viruses responsible for causing local upper respiratory disease by multiplication in the epithelium are the following (Dudgeon, 1969): influenza A, B and C; para-influenza 1, 2, 3, and 4; adenoviruses (over 30 different members identified); respiratory syncitial virus; common cold or rhinoviruses (over 80 varieties classified). Of these the adenoviruses are the most commonly identified in relation to the tonsils.

While an attack of acute tonsillitis may be initiated by a local upper respiratory virus infection the typical follicular, parenchymatous or membranous appearance results from bacterial action. Virus growing in mucous membrane cells quickly renders them liable to secondary invasion by streptococci, staphylococci and pneumococci which can be present in the mouth in health. These bacteria may be responsible for a primary local acute tonsillitis if the patient's resistance is low or if the tonsils themselves are at a disadvantage through previous infections, accumulation of debris in the crypts or incomplete attempts at removal. However, there is one organism with a predilection for the tonsils and which is cultured in over 50 per cent of throat swabs, namely the haemolytic streptococcus. Most attacks of acute tonsillitis are caused by this agent and the attacks usually present clinically as the acute follicular type of infection. The process of inflammation originating within the tonsil is accompanied by hyperaemia and oedema, with conversion of lymphoid follicles into small abscesses which discharge into the crypts.

Streptococcal tonsillitis occurs in epidemics, especially where spread of infection is encouraged by overcrowding or inadequate ventilation. In institutions, such as hospitals, it may present a quite serious problem of cross-infection. Carriers of the streptococcus may initiate infection in others while remaining symptom-free themselves.

Symptoms and signs

A patient developing acute tonsillitis from an upper respiratory infection may, at first, only complain of the dry throat, general malaise, slight fever and thirst common to the latter. Sore throat is not an invariable symptom, especially in children in whom diagnosis may only be apparent on inspection of the throat during a routine search for the cause of unexplained pyrexia or refusal to eat, or in some cases abdominal pain. But once acute tonsillitis has developed it is usual for sore throat exacerbated on swallowing to be the predominant symptom. A typical primary tonsillitis due to haemolytic streptococcal infection is accompanied by a sense of fullness in the throat, severe dysphagia, often acute, with pain radiating to the ears and anorexia (largely due to the dysphagia). The voice has a plummy quality. There are pains in the neck, which is held stiffly, due to the swelling of regional lymph nodes; headache, and sometimes pains in the back and limbs. The patient feels shivery due to fever, and generally unwell.

On examination there may be some circumoral pallor. The tongue is furred and dry and the breath foetid. The tonsils are swollen and red and spotted with purulent exudate from the crypts or in severe cases covered with a purulent membrane. There is an accumulation of viscid mucus due to the patient's dislike of swallowing. In the parenchymatous type of tonsillitis the livid swelling of the tonsils, accompanied by oedema of the uvula and soft palate, may appear quite to occlude the oropharyngeal inlet, with consequent increase in dysphagia. However, dysphagia severe enough entirely to prevent the patient swallowing his own saliva seldom occurs unless a quinsy (peritonsillar abscess: see p. 113) has formed. The jugulo-digastric (tonsillar) lymph nodes behind the angles of the mandible are enlarged and tender. The temperature is raised, varying from 37·8°C (100°F) to 40·5°C (105°F).

Differential diagnosis

Acute tonsillitis is a disease of sudden onset with a typical clinical triad of sore throat, fever and malaise running, even if untreated, a relatively benign course within a week to ten days. Response to antibiotic treatment is usually rapid, at times dramatic, and it is rare for the condition of the patient, in uncomplicated cases, to give cause for anxiety. Suspicion of the presence of some other condition will be prompted by departure from this clinical pattern, or by some unusual appearance of the tonsils themselves.

Scarlet fever is a streptococcal tonsillitis with general disturbances due to the production of soluble toxins, one of which causes a punctate erythematous rash in susceptible subjects. Apart from the rash, there is tachycardia out of proportion to the pyrexia, a stippled palate, a "strawberry tongue", and an intensely red appearance of the tonsils. Sometimes the tonsils are covered with a yellowish exudate which is usually readily removable. The blood picture shows a polymorphonuclear leucocytosis and eosinophilia.

Glandular fever (infectious mononucleosis) (*see* p. 141) may be seen in the so-called anginose form as clinically, at least in the initial stages, indistinguishable from a severe attack of acute tonsillitis. It is today not too uncommon and should always be considered whenever an apparent attack of acute tonsillitis, especially in a young adult, persists, with fever, despite antibiotic therapy, with extreme local discomfort and an alarmingly swollen, membrane-covered pair of tonsils.

There is a total lymphocytosis of at least 4,500/mm.³ in the peripheral blood with at least 51 per cent lymphocytes in the differential leucocyte count, of which a significant number are atypical.

Serum heterophile antibody (sheep's cell agglutinin) titres rise during the first 2–3 weeks in nearly all adult patients. Demonstration of the presence of these antibodies by the Paul Bunnell–Davidson or ox cell haemolysis tests is diagnostically specific for infectious mononucleosis. Other signs of the infection, such as lymph node enlargement elsewhere as well as in the neck, and a palpable spleen, should always be looked for.

Vincent's angina (*see* pp. 23, 141). This is essentially a subacute tonsillitis with ulceration. It is of slower onset and accompanied by less sore throat and lower fever than acute tonsillitis. A sloughing membrane forms on the ulcer, and the patient's breath is characteristically foetid. It is rare in children. The characteristic organisms, Vincent's fusiform bacillus and *Spirochaeta denticola*, may be cultured from a throat swab.

Diphtheria, now rare in the United Kingdom, is unlikely to be confused with acute tonsillitis but must be considered whenever there is a membrane on the surface of the tonsil. Diphtheria is slower in onset, and is at first accompanied by less constitutional disturbance and less local discomfort. The membrane, which may extend beyond the surface of the tonsil onto the palate (Plate I), is dirty grey in colour. It is adherent and removal causes bleeding. The identification of the Klebs–Löffler bacillus in the membrane is diagnostic.

Granulocytopaenia and leukaemia may be accompanied by necrosing lesions of the tonsils resembling those seen in glandular fever and may present with acute sore throat. Ulceration is usually present elsewhere in the mouth and oropharynx, noticeable for absence of surrounding inflammatory reaction. The obvious severity of the patient's condition in these blood diseases renders them unlikely to be confused with typical tonsillitis.

Treatment

It is a generally accepted principle of medical practice that antibiotics should not be given for minor conditions because of the risk of the development of resistant strains of organisms or of allergic reactions on the part of the patients, which may limit the use of the antibiotic in the possible event of a future major illness. Since many cases of acute tonsillitis naturally run a relatively short, mild course, it is advocated that antibiotics should be withheld in the early stages unless or until it is clear that the patient has a major attack not to be assuaged by symptomatic treatment or is known to have had complications with previous attacks Successful antibiotic treatment moreover depends on the achievement of adequate concentration, adequately maintained at the site of infection. It is therefore also advocated that if the decision is made to administer antibiotic (and penicillin is the most appropriate in most cases) it should initially be given in relatively high dosage by intramuscular injection, reserving oral therapy for maintenance, which should never be discontinued, even in apparently rapid cure, within less than five days.

These principles of treatment being established the management of acute tonsillitis can be considered as follows.

General and symptomatic

Patients should be put to bed, isolated and encouraged to drink plenty of bland fluids. The temperature and pulse should be recorded every eight hours. If possible a throat swab should be taken and sent for culture of organisms and antibiotic sensitivity tests. If the patient's disinclination to eat solid food results in constipation a mild aperient may be given but purging, as such, is of no therapeutic value. For the sore throat aspirin taken in soluble form, dissolved as a drink, is preferred, e.g. aspirin soluble tablets BP, 1–3 tablets up to four times daily (1 tablet three times daily in children 6–12 years old: half a tablet three times daily if under 6 years). Lozenges containing antibiotics are of no benefit in true tonsillitis, and only encourage the overgrowth of monilia. Pain in the neck due to tender lymph nodes can to some extent be helped by warmth; a cotton wool collar held in place with a sock or handkerchief is an old-fashioned but comforting remedy.

Antibiotic therapy

If despite general and symptomatic treatment the temperature remains high and there is marked toxaemia, and where the exudation from the tonsil crypts, or the tonsillar swelling, is marked it is advisable to administer antibiotic, preferably according to laboratory indications. Antibiotic should also be given if previous attacks of tonsillitis have been associated with complications, especially quinsy, rheumatic fever, acute glomerulonephritis or chorea. Since, however, swab results may not be returned for several days and about 40 per cent will be sterile or show only normal commensals it is often necessary to proceed on the assumption that the infection is due to a streptococcus against which penicillin, at the time of writing, remains the most universally effective agent. If the choice, by laboratory test, lies between a new and an old agent, both equally safe and effective, then the old agent should be used. In this way emergence of bacterial resistance to the new agent will be delayed. A short course of a narrow-spectrum agent in a high dosage is better than a prolonged course of a broad-spectrum agent in low dosage. The course of treatment for acute infections should be 5–7 days, depending on the extent and severity of symptoms (British National Formulary, 1968). These considerations endorse the choice of penicillin in acute tonsillitis, which may be administered as follows to patients who have not had allergic reactions to it previously.

Initial

Intramuscular injection of 300 mg. (300,000 units) of procaine penicillin combined with 60 mg. (100,000 units) of benzylpenicillin (procaine penicillin injection, fortified BP). In severe cases the injection (in all ages over six years) should be repeated in 12 hours; and continued once or twice daily according to age, until the patient is able or willing to take phenoxymethylpenicillin (penicillin V) by mouth every six hours.

Maintenance

Penicillin V is available in tablet, capsule or elixir form. Doses of 250 mg. (125 mg. in children aged 1–5) every six hours produce adequate blood levels, but it cannot be said too often that success depends on a rigid adherence to the six-hourly regime, and to the continuance of antibiotic in those cases who really need it for a full week.

Complications

These are classified as local and systemic.

Local

Chronic tonsillitis (*see* p. 111).—The tonsil does not always return to as tate of complete health after an attack of acute tonsillitis, especially after the follicular type where minute abscesses have formed in the lymphoid follicles surrounding the crypts and possibly become walled off by fibrous tissue. Inadequate antibiotic therapy especially reveals this tendency as following apparent subsidence of an acute attack there may be recurrence after as short a time as 10 days, clearly a recrudescence of latent, inextinguished infection rather than fresh infection acquired from an outside source. This process of apparent cure followed by relapse may go on for some weeks; while in other cases the patient settles into a pattern of recurrent acute tonsillitis every 3–4 months, where the frequency of attacks points to some predisposing factor such as chronic tonsil infection or failure of local immunity.

Quinsy (peritonsillar abscess, paratonsillar abscess. *See* p. 113).—Spread of infection from the tonsil with formation of pus in the areolar space between the tonsil capsule and the tonsil bed may occur as a complication of acute tonsillitis, especially in a patient with chronic infection who suffers from repeated acute exacerbation.

Parapharyngeal abscess (*see* p. 116).—Infection may spread from tonsil or quinsy through the superior constrictor muscle and give rise to pus formation between the muscle and deep cervical fascia.

Suppurative cervical adenitis.—Occasionally suppuration may occur in the regional lymph nodes (jugulodigastric) as a result of acute infection in the tonsil.

This complication is much less commonly seen than in the pre-antibiotic era, and, as in the case of quinsy and parapharyngeal abscess, generally results from infection with a penicillin-resistant *Staphylococcus aureus.*

Acute otitis media.—Acute otitis media is a less common complication in acute tonsillitis than the anatomical proximity of the eustachian tube orifice in the pharynx would predict. However, some children appear to have a special susceptibility and suffer a regular sequence of tonsillitis followed by otitis media which if too often repeated, constitutes one of the accepted indications for prophylactic tonsillectomy.

Systemic

Systemic complications are seen principally in association with Group A beta-haemolytic streptococcal infections:

Rheumatic fever.—This occurs as frequently in patients who have had their tonsils removed as in those who have not. But the tonsil is undoubtedly the portal of entry in some cases with close incidental association between the onset of acute streptococcal tonsillitis and the rheumatic fever.

Acute glomerulonephritis.—Urine is not infrequently scanty, highly coloured and charged with urates during an attack of acute tonsillitis, but seldom contains albumen. Albuminuria may presage acute nephritis which, together with all systemic complications, is less commonly seen since the advent of antibiotics.

Chorea.—Sydenham's rheumatic chorea may be derived from tonsil infections but is, again, rare.

Subacute bacterial endocarditis.—In patients with a pre-existing valvular lesion of the heart infection of the tonsil with *Streptococcus viridans* may, through systemic infection, initiate an attack of *subacute bacterial endocarditis.* Acute tonsillitis in such at-risk patients should always be treated with antibiotics.

ACUTE LINGUAL TONSILLITIS

This is a rare condition arising from the same causal factors as acute tonsillitis. It tends to be unilateral with one-sided dysphagia as the leading symptom. It may otherwise be accompanied by the same symptoms as acute tonsillitis. On examination there is more pain on tongue depression than in the case of acute tonsillitis, and tongue protrusion is more inhibited. A mirror must be used to view the lingual tonsil, which appears swollen and inflamed. It may be distinguished from Ludwig's angina by the absence of swelling of the floor of the mouth.

Treatment

As for acute tonsillitis except that antibiotics should be administered immediately on diagnosis.

Complications

Lingual quinsy.—Pus formation within the lingual tonsil may call for surgical drainage.

Epiglottitis and laryngitis.—These structures are liable to involvement by contiguity of infection. Oedema of epiglottis or larynx may be dangerous.

ACUTE ADENOIDITIS

Acute superficial adenoiditis may be presumed to occur in every case of acute upper respiratory infection, but acute adenoiditis, as such, does not exist as a clinical diagnosis. "Infected adenoids" will be considered under the heading "Chronic Adenoiditis" (p. 133).

CHRONIC TONSILLITIS (NON-SPECIFIC CHRONIC TONSILLITIS)

To pass through childhood without an attack of acute tonsillitis is rare. To suffer one or two attacks of acute tonsillitis a year between the ages of four to nine is normal. Undue susceptibility to acute tonsillitis may arise from poor immunological defences or environmental exposure to excessive bacterial populations. But in many cases it arises because local defences are reduced by the establishment of chronic infection in the tonsils themselves.

Aetiology

Following an attack of acute tonsillitis, the tonsil may or may not return to a state of complete health. In the latter event (as shown by post-operative histological studies) minute abscesses, having formed in the lymphoid follicles, may become walled off by fibrous tissue and surrounded by a zone of inflammatory cells. It is also possible for inflammatory debris to become trapped in crypts by fibrous occlusion of the openings, and for such debris to expand into neighbouring crypts. Germinal centres can become markedly hyperplastic with notable thickening of fibrous septa.

It is possible for these histological changes to be found in tonsils which have not been associated with local symptoms of sore throat, and for there to be no direct relation between polymorphonuclear cell infiltration or fibrosis and the frequency or severity of clinical attacks of sore throat or tonsillitis. But the existence of the histological changes points to chronic infection in the tonsils through lowering of local tissue resistance as a probable cause of unusual susceptibility to acute tonsillitis. That it is indeed a principal cause has been shown by the beneficial results of tonsillectomy in countless well selected cases.

Chronic tonsillitis is usually a complication of acute tonsillitis, but may also become established more insidiously by subclinical tonsil infections manifested only as sore throat. A "feed-back" system becomes established until, in severe cases, attacks of acute tonsillitis may occur once every six weeks or so with the throat feeling constantly sore or uncomfortable in between attacks. While chronic tonsillitis, as inferred from the frequency of attacks of sore throat or acute tonsillitis, has its highest incidence in childhood between the ages of five to eight, it is by no means uncommon in teenagers and young adults, but is rare after the age of 50.

Symptoms and signs

Minor symptoms of chronic tonsillitis are a bad taste in the mouth (cacagus), halitosis and discomfort in the throat, all due to accumulation and discharge of infected cryptic debris. These symptoms alone in some cases have led to the designation of a *chronic follicular (lacunar) tonsillitis* specifically diagnosed by the demonstration of such debris in the crypts on inspection. Similarly when the tonsils are much enlarged giving rise to a "thick" voice and some embarrassment of respiration and deglutition, with perhaps snoring and food faddism, the tonsillitis has been called *chronic hypertrophic (parenchmatous) tonsillitis*. But at the other end of the scale severe symptoms of sore throat and dysphagia may well be associated with small fibrotic tonsils, harmless in appearance, so-called *chronic fibroid tonsillitis*. None of these definitions have much significance. The symptom *par excellence* of chronic tonsillitis is sore throat, grading from a mild discomfort to the severe dysphagia of acute tonsillitis, and this may occur in relation to tonsils of varying shape, size and appearance; with combined elements of cryptic infection, fibrosis or hypertrophy sometimes occurring in the same cases.

Neck tenderness from enlarged regional lymph nodes may be present, and, in children, chronic tonsillitis may be associated with enlargement of mesenteric lymph nodes, the child complaining of recurrent abdominal pain, accompanied perhaps with vomiting. Chronic tonsillitis may occasionally give rise to other distant symptoms, such as headache, muscle and joint pains or dyspepsia. The whole question of secondary effects due to focal infection in the tonsils is considered below under "Complications".

There is no definitive appearance of the tonsils on inspection on which to base an unequivocal diagnosis of chronic tonsillitis. As indicated above, the tonsils may be hypertrophic or fibrotic, or there may be debris in the crypts. The latter is a sign of some significance, but size alone is no reliable indication of the health or otherwise of these organs. If chronic infection is present it is usual for the tonsils, and especially the anterior pillars of the fauces, to appear more hyperaemic than the adjacent mucus membrane. The tonsils may also be comparatively tender on finger palpation. One of the most reliable signs of chronic tonsil infection is enlargement of the regional (jugulodigastric) lymph nodes. These become enlarged in association with attacks of acute tonsillitis and do not normally remain palpable once the tonsil has returned to a healthy state. Persistently enlarged regional lymph nodes point therefore to a continuance of infection.

The polymorphonuclear white cell count may be raised and the erythrocyte sedimentation rate prolonged.

Diagnosis

Unilateral enlargement commonly seen in quinsy, may, especially in an adult, also have more serious implications, as the first indications of developing malignancy. Lymphosarcoma, in particular, is prone to declare itself as an insidious swelling. Ulceration or membrane formation does not occur in non-specific chronic tonsillitis and will suggest, for example, glandular fever or Vincent's angina. Necrosing lesions of the tonsils may point to granulocytopoenia or leukaemia.

Chronic non-specific tonsillitis is a diagnosis based chiefly on the history of recurrent sore throats or acute tonsillitis. When such a history is accompanied by chronic enlargement of the regional lymph nodes and hyperaemia of the tonsils or anterior pillars of the fauces, and *nothing else* in the upper respiratory tract can be found to account for the symptoms, the diagnosis may be considered well substantiated.

PLATE I

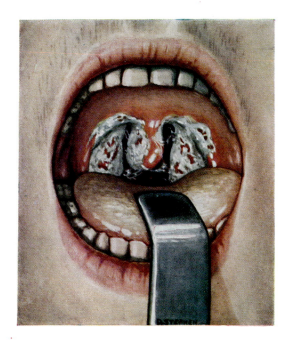

Diphtheria of the fauces.

Treatment

At the time of writing there is no medical treatment known that will eradicate chronic tonsillitis. Fibrosis within the tonsil barricades microscopical septic foci against effective concentration of antibiotic. Gargles, mouth washes and suction of crypts are at best palliative. Acute exacerbations can be treated with antibiotic without sterilizing the tonsil for the reason given above. Long term administration of antibiotic may be helpful in children who for some good reason are not suitable for surgery. But radical enucleation of the tonsils is the only certain cure for chronic tonsillitis and the only certain prophylaxis against recurrent acute tonsillitis. The effectiveness of tonsillectomy in these conditions has been shown in controlled clinical trials (McKee, 1963; Mawson, 1967; Roydhouse, 1969) in which the post-operative attack rate of sore throat has been compared with randomly matched patients whose operation had been postponed. It would hardly seem necessary to substantiate the rationale for operation by these expensive trials, since it is difficult to see how a patient who has had the tonsils properly removed could again suffer from tonsillitis. But the operation has tended at times to fall into disrepute because of bad selection, bad preparation, bad operative techniques and bad post-operative management of some cases (these are considered on pp. 118–121 under "Tonsillectomy"). The question of operation is best approached from a standpoint of preferential conservancy, modified by knowledge of the undoubted benefit that may be conferred by removal of the tonsils when the indications are favourable.

Indications for tonsillectomy

Chronic infection.—(*a*) Repeated acute tonsillitis, more than three attacks a year; (*b*) repeated sore throats, not necessarily amounting to clinical acute tonsillitis but occurring 4–6 times a year or more; (*c*) chronic enlargement of regional lymph nodes in association with sore throats or acute tonsillitis, the attacks not necessarily being as frequent as in (*a*) or (*b*); (*d*) quinsy (*see* p. 115); (*e*) recurrent middle-ear infection in association with sore throats or acute tonsillitis; (*f*) chronic infection with beta-haemolytic streptococci or diphtheria organisms in carriers, not necessarily associated with symptoms; (*g*) secondary effects in other organs. Infected tonsils may occasionally provide a provocative focus from which may be derived inflammatory or allergic reactions in distant organs (*see* "Complications", p. 109). Decision when to remove the tonsils in these cases will depend mainly on whether there is an adequate local basis for a diagnosis of chronic tonsillitis; i.e. history of sore throats, hyperaemia, pus in crypts and enlarged regional glands; (*h*) tuberculous cervical adenitis is adversely affected by superadded chronic infection. Tonsillectomy is generally helpful.

Chronic enlargement.—Chronic infection may be associated with gross hypertrophy of the tonsils which if sufficient to interfere significantly with respiration, swallowing or speaking may require removal to restore normality of these functions.

Complications

Quinsy (peritonsillar abscess, paratonsillar abscess)

Infection in the tonsil, especially the lacunar type involving the large crypt in the upper pole, may spread through the capsule into the potential space between the tonsil capsule and the tonsil bed. Here pus may quickly form and give rise to a peritonsillar abscess. In 90 per cent of cases the accumulation is anterosuperior to the tonsil, so that it lies behind the anterior pillar of the fauces, but pus can also

113

form lateral to the tonsil or posteriorly in relation to the posterior pillar and the lower pole.

While a quinsy rarely if ever arises except as a local complication of tonsil infection it sometimes forms without any preceding symptoms of acute or chronic tonsillitis. As a rule, however, abscess formation is preceded by some indication of active tonsil infection, and is most commonly seen in young adults.

Quinsy (from the older term "cynanche": Greek *cyon*, dog; *anchein*, throttle) has become less frequent since the use of antibiotics in tonsillitis. But whereas cultures of pus used to grow a mixed bacterial flora of streptococci, staphylococci or pneumococci, the tendency recently is for the appearance of pure growths of staphylococcus aureus (pyogenes) often insensitive to penicillin. Although acute and chronic tonsillitis have their highest incidence in childhood, quinsy is not often seen before the age of 12. Occasionally a latent quinsy is discovered as a symptomless collection of pus during a routine tonsillectomy.

Symptoms and signs.—Save in the rare cases of bilateral quinsy, the leading symptom is increasing unilateral pain in the throat developing after a few days of generalized sore throat due to tonsil infection. The pain is severe, maximal behind the angle of the jaw and radiating to the ear; it may be so intense as to prevent the patient swallowing anything at all, including saliva, which accumulates, dribbles out of the mouth, and confers a phlegmy quality upon the speech. Muscle spasm causes trismus and neck fixation with lateral inclination to the side affected. The patient feels ill, miserable and apprehensive. Dysphagia results in thirst and dehydration, toxaemia, weakness, and, in extreme cases, prostration.

On examination the anxious facies and stiffly held head may be evident. Trismus increases *pari passu* with pus formation so that it may be difficult to look in the mouth. But depression of the dry furred tongue reveals the typical appearance of a manifest quinsy and puts the diagnosis beyond doubt. There is gross, unilateral swelling of the palate and anterior pillar of the fauces. The uvula is displaced across the midline towards the opposite side and the tonsil is displaced downwards and medially, so that the oropharyngeal inlet may be quite occluded. Mucus hangs from the immobile palate which is discoloured an angry dusky red. The cervical lymph nodes on the side affected are large and tender, and the tissues of the neck feel thickened. The pulse rate is increased and temperature raised.

In peritonsillitis, before pus formation, the clinical features are those of severe tonsillitis without trismus and without displacement of the tonsil. Pus formation is associated with increasing oedema of the surrounding soft tissues and in advanced cases the tonsil itself may not be visible.

Treatment.—Natural resolution follows spontaneous discharge of pus either through the tonsil or the anterior pillar of the fauces, but such an outcome may take as long as a week or 10 days during which time the patient is in extreme pain and some danger. Extension of the infection into the parapharangeal space can result in thrombosis of the internal jugular vein, or rupture of the vein or one of the carotid arteries with fatal haemorrhage. Prolonged dehydration and toxaemia, if occurring in the elderly, may also prove fatal. Oedema may spread downwards to the supraglottic areas with risk of asphyxia. If the abscess ruptures spontaneously into the mouth during sleep pus may enter the trachea with, again, possible fatal consequences. For these reasons it is necessary to perform a drainage operation as soon as there is reasonable certainty of the presence of pus in the pericapsular space. At the same time, if the patient is seen before pus is thought to have formed, he should be given large doses of penicillin by intramuscular injection in the hope of aborting the abscess. The distinction may be a nice one, but patients generally fall into one of three groups: (1) pus is not suspected; (2) pus is suspected but the abscess does not look ripe for incision; (3) the examiner is in little or no doubt that pus is present and should be drained.

For patients in groups (1) and (2), any antibiotics being given by the oral route should be discontinued and benzylpenicillin injection BP 0·6 g. (1 mega-unit) should be given intramuscularly every six hours (0·3 g. six-hourly in children aged 5–12). Bed rest, analgesics and mouth washes will be ordered, while the patient will be encouraged to drink as much bland fluid as he will. Progress will be carefully observed. Response to antibiotic will usually be presaged by a gradual fall in temperature. Many patients will then slowly, sometimes dramatically, improve and become symptom free. Once response is assured the six-hourly injections may be discontinued and a twice daily injection of procaine penicillin 300 mg. (300,000 units) given until the patient has been free of all symptoms and signs for 24 hours. If pus is present in a group (2) patient there may be initial improvement which then ceases. In such a patient abscess tonsillectomy (see below) may be considered as a means of treatment.

Incision.—When pus is present or believed to be present and accessible for drainage into the pharynx the safest course to pursue to make an incision, without general anaesthetic, through the anterior pillar of the fauces. The pain of the quinsy is already intense and pain does not summate so that a sharp stab through the mucosa and muscle is not as brutal as it may seem. The patient sits holding a basin under his chin and his mouth open as far as possible. The most prominent part of the swelling is selected (if this is not obvious a site of election is chosen half way between the base of the uvula and the upper third molar tooth) and a pledget of wool moistened with 10 per cent cocaine gently applied to the area. While the patient closes his mouth and waits for a few moments the surgeon selects a sharp scalpel (e.g. size 15 Bard–Parker) and leaving 6 mm. of the tip only uncovered protects the rest of the blade with adhesive tape. He then takes a tongue depressor, instructs the patient to open his mouth, depresses the tongue and, without more ado, stabs the knife into the chosen site. He then thrusts a pair of sinus forceps through the incision, opens them widely, closes them, withdraws them and tells the patient to spit the pus into the basin. When pus is found the relief is so immediate that any distress occasioned by the operation is soon forgotten.

There is a tendency for quinsy to recur in the same patient. In view of the disagreeable nature of the condition and the risk of possible serious complications it is wise permanently to prevent further attacks by removing the tonsils. An *interval tonsillectomy* is therefore advised and usually performed six to eight weeks after the resolution of the quinsy.

Abscess tonsillectomy.—The tonsil forms the medial wall of a peritonsillar abscess. It has in many cases been separated from its bed by pus except for the mucosal margins and pedicle. It is therefore a reasonable procedure to drain the abscess by removing the tonsil. This has the merit of avoiding the later necessity for an interval tonsillectomy, and, being performed under general anaesthesia, of sparing the patient the ordeal of the standard incision.

Logical though this procedure may seem, however, it is not without risk. Criticism has been levelled against it because of a theoretical risk of spread of infection through opening of tissue planes. But the only tissues that need to be incised are the mucosal attachment of the tonsil to the margins of the anterior and posterior pillars of the fauces. The real risk lies elsewhere, in the administration of a general anaesthetic and in the removal of the other tonsil which is nearly always inflamed in these cases. If during the induction of anaesthesia in a semiconscious or unconscious patient the mouth is forced open, as it is likely to be for the purposes of intubation, muscular action may compress the abscess and cause it to burst prematurely into the mouth. There is then a grave risk of the pus being inhaled, giving rise to a lung abscess and a possible fatal outcome. This complication may be avoided by a skilled anaesthetist keeping the patient's head *below* the level of the laryngeal inlet during induction, and an electrical sucker at hand to aspirate pus should the abscess burst. The second tonsil, however, being usually inflamed *may* give rise to excessive haemorrhage during dissection. This is not by any means always the case. But the risk exists and should be recognized.

Abscess tonsillectomy may be of value in selected cases, especially those where pus is suspected, perhaps in relation to the lower pole, where antibiotics have been given with some improvement, and where the chance of finding pus by a standard stab incision does not seem high, that is to say in group (2) cases. But before embarking on this operation, three conditions must be fulfilled: (*i*) there must be a *reasonable* expectation of finding pus; (*ii*) the patient must have been on high dose penicillin by injection for at least 24 hours, and shown some response (i.e. lowering of temperature); (*iii*) a skilled anaesthetist must be available, confident in his ability to induce anaesthesia in such a way as to avoid aspiration of pus into the trachea.

Parapharyngeal abscess

This is a rare but serious complication of tonsillitis or quinsy. Pus forms in the deep substance of the neck between the pharyngeal wall (superior constrictor muscle) and the investing layer of the deep cervical fascia, in close proximity to the jugular and carotid blood vessels.

Symptoms and signs.—The patient experiences symptoms of pain in the throat and neck, as in quinsy, with marked dysphagia. Toxaemia is more severe and rigors may occur.

On examination there is a diffuse tender swelling of the neck below the angle of the mandible. Inspection of the oropharynx may reveal a quinsy or an apparently localized infection of the tonsil which, however, will be somewhat displaced medially. There is a swinging temperature typical of an abscess, with peaks in the region of 39·4 C (103° F) to 40·5 C (105° F). The patient is obviously ill and in need of hospital treatment.

Treatment.—A parapharyngeal abscess is a dangerous condition because, apart from the toxaemia, the inflammatory process may cause thrombosis in the internal jugular vein or necrosis of the wall of the vein or carotid artery with resultant massive fatal haemorrhage. Treatment therefore demands early external drainage of the abscess through an incision in the neck combined with administration of benzylpenicillin by intramuscular injection, 0·6 g. (1 mega-unit) four-hourly.

Intratonsillar abscess

This is an uncommon complication of chronic follicular (lacunar) tonsillitis, where communications form between enlarged crypts, and a collection of pus declares its presence by a constant trickle from the surface of the tonsil, sometimes in association with a protruding granulation.

Treatment.—The only satisfactory cure for this condition is removal of the tonsils.

Tonsillolith (*calculus of the tonsil*)

Chronic infection in the tonsil crypts is often accompanied by accumulation of caseous inflammatory debris which may be expressed on swallowing (or with a spatula). On occasion, however, the phosphates or carbonates of calcium and magnesium also become deposited, forming harder chalky concretions. These gradually increase in size and may eventually become quite large, up to 28 g. in weight.

The patient generally complains of discomfort in the area, but may seek advice because of having noticed, fortuitously, the appearance of something unusual in the tonsil. The dirty white, hard matter may give rise to suspicion of malignancy but the differential diagnosis is usually resolved by probing.

Treatment.—Sometimes the tonsillolith can be hooked out with an instrument and, if other indications are lacking for removal of the tonsils, further calcareous depositions may be discouraged by gargling daily with warm phenol gargle BPC. In cases where the stone has become incarcerated in the substance of the tonsil the only satisfactory treatment is tonsillectomy.

Tonsil cyst

Debris accumulating in the tonsil crypts may become sealed off by fibrous occlusion of the surface openings. This results, in some cases, in the formation of a cyst which presents as a visible white or yellowish swelling on the tonsil. The cysts are often multiple, usually quite small and frequently symptomless. Occasionally a larger cyst may give rise to discomfort due to tension.

Treatment.—In the absence of symptoms no treatment is required. Patients with discomfort or who are worried lest they have some serious condition may benefit from incision of the cyst or cysts after topical application of 10 per cent cocaine solution to the surface. The contents, expressed with a spatula, are usually sterile on culture.

The cysts have a tendency to recur and, if local incision has failed to relieve the patient of symptoms, the question of tonsillectomy may arise. Since the cysts may be indicative of a low grade chronic tonsillitis there may be good grounds for advising operation. But in the elderly, in whom the cysts seem more prone to occur, unless the symptoms are marked it is advisable to depend on local incisions, topical applications of iodine paint (Mandl)* and reassurance.

Focal infection

Rheumatic fever and glomerulonephritis.—The theory that a septic focus in some part of the body could give rise to disease in a distant part of the body has been substantiated in the past mainly by observing the effects of removing such a suspected focus. As is the tendency in medicine when a new theory seems to offer hope in difficult cases the removal of suspected septic foci, in particular teeth and tonsils, has sometimes been practised in excess of reasonable expectation of benefit and thus fallen into disrepute. But reports (Bunyard, 1969) of recent investigations would seem to confer a more respectable scientific status upon the theory. For example, there is evidence that a group A haemolytic streptococcus, which is

* Mandl's paint: iodi puri 0·4 g.; pot. iod 1·3 g.; ol menth pip 0·3 cm³; glycerine 30·0 cm.³

generally recognized to be the agent of rheumatic fever, causes permanent structural damage to the heart because the streptococcus has certain antigens in common with glycoproteins from the heart valve. Also, an extract of the cell wall of a nephrotoxic strain of group A streptococcus has been found which shares an antigenic factor in common with human kidney. Antibody–antigen reactions which destroy the glomerular basement membrane are believed to be the probable cause of glomerulonephritis.

That the tonsil can be a source of group A haemolytic streptococcus is certain, and that the two systemic diseases, rheumatic fever and acute glomerulonephritis can result from "allergic" reactions to the streptococcus from the tonsil seems beyond doubt. If eradication of foci of infection was much overdone in the past there is now some danger that it is being too much neglected.

Tonsillectomy does not help established cases of rheumatic fever or nephritis, but is indicated under antibiotic cover in persistent streptococcal infection of the tonsils of children who have had rheumatic fever, or when attacks of acute nephritis occur with recurrent tonsillitis.

Eye conditions.—Episcleritis, recurrent conjunctivitis and choroiditis have been shown to improve after the removal of infected tonsils. Iritis and retrobulbar neuritis have not been favourably influenced (Collins, 1965).

Skin conditions.—Exacerbations of psoriasis occurring in relation to attacks of tonsillitis will almost certainly respond to tonsillectomy. Other conditions which may have a relation to focal sepsis are erythema multiforme, chronic urticaria and purpura.

Other conditions.—Apart from rheumatic fever some chronic rheumatic conditions may come under consideration as stemming from a septic focus. But the classification is still very imperfect. Infective arthritis and fibrositis may well benefit from removal of infected tonsils. Rheumatoid arthritis, on the other hand, will not, as irreversible changes have taken place in the joints.

In all cases of suspected focal infection decision to remove the tonsils must be based on an adequate probability of chronic tonsillitis. Unless there have been local symptoms or there are some signs of chronic infection or a pathogen such as a haemolytic streptococcus has been cultured from the throat it is unlikely that operation will prove helpful. Decision should furthermore be jointly taken by surgeon and physician concerned after full discussion of the merits of each case.

THE OPERATION OF TONSILLECTOMY

In children between the ages of four and eight adenoidectomy is often combined with tonsillectomy, when hypertrophy and chronic infection of these organs tend to coexist. Approximately 200,000 operations on the tonsils and adenoids, combined or separate, including all ages, are performed in the United Kingdom annually. This is an unnecessarily large number in the opinion of some, and the operation is currently undergoing criticism as being not only performed too often without adequate indication but as also subjecting too many children to unnecessary risk and suffering.

The figures which the General Register Office have issued as representing the deaths associated with tonsillectomy and/or adenoidectomy are:

1959	20	1964	3
1960	16	1965	11
1961	12	1966	7
1962	21	1967	6
1963	13	1968	7

The operation figures show that in the last five years the average annual number of deaths has been a little less than seven (compared with a little more than 16 in the previous five years) which gives a mortality figure of less than 1 in 28,000.

In 1968 there were three deaths attributable to disease of the tonsils and adenoids in which no operation had been performed. Two were certified by coroners and the other was certified after a post-mortem examination. Of these three deaths one was due to a generalized septicaemia following acute tonsillitis and the other two were due to respiratory obstruction in young children associated with gross hypertrophy of the tonsils and adenoids exacerbated by an acute infection.

It is thus apparent that possession of the tonsils and adenoids is not without risk, and that considerable progress has been made in recent years through improved management in reducing the risk of operation to extremely small proportions.

As to suffering, if an adult is questioned after operation (adults complain more of post-operative pain than children) and asked to compare the soreness of the throat with an attack of acute tonsillitis the answer nearly always is "about the same". Certainly the post-operative pain of tonsillectomy does not compare with that of quinsy, and can be rendered quite tolerable with analgesics. It is therefore fair to say that the suffering from operation in terms of physical pain or discomfort is not more than the pain that will be suffered from the next and subsequent attacks of tonsillitis which the operation is calculated to prevent.

Psychological suffering is another matter. Young children especially will feel anxious and insecure if removed from their parents and placed in a hospital without explanation. To those under the age of four it is difficult to give such an explanation. For this reason it is advisable to try to postpone operation until this age, or to arrange for the mother to be admitted to hospital with the child. Skilful anaesthesia with adequate premedication is also necessary to ensure that this, often first, experience of surgery does not lay foundations for future fears.

Frequency of an operation, in itself, does not merit criticism as long as benefit results. That benefit does result has been shown in the controlled studies already mentioned (p. 113). But the responsibility incurred in operating upon a child is very great. Otolaryngological surgeons with a proper sense of responsibility will not operate unless they are convinced the child's health requires it, and are satisfied that all facilities, such as operating theatre and nursing care, are entirely adequate.

Selection of cases

Having satisfied himself that tonsillectomy is indicated for one or more of the reasons given on p. 113 it then becomes incumbent upon the surgeon to determine whether any contra-indication exists to the performing of this operation. The tonsils should not be removed if the patient is likely to be exposed to greater risk than the really extremely small one normally inseparable from this form of surgery, when carried out by a competent surgeon with the help of a competent anaesthetist in a proper operating theatre on a fit patient with skilled nursing assistance. This is not to say that having recognized a special risk the patient may not come to deferred operation once the necessary steps have been taken to provide against it. Even patients suffering from haemophilia, if there are exceptional reasons for removing the tonsils, may be safely operated upon with the right safeguards (see below), but the additional risks *must* be eliminated and these fall into three main categories:

(1) Additional risk from haemorrhage.
(2) Additional risk from anaesthetic.
(3) Additional risk from infection.

Haemorrhage

The average adult blood volume is about 5 l. A close approximation may be calculated from the ratio of 70 ml./kg. of body weight. Up to 1 l. may be lost without serious risk but if more is lost transfusion replacement is required. It is rare for an adult or child to lose much blood during tonsillectomy as vessels can at once be clamped and tied. The real risk comes in the immediate post-operative period from reactionary haemorrhage when a lot of blood may be lost in a relatively short time.

In a small child, whose total blood volume is proportionally less, rapid blood loss becomes more serious much sooner. His compensatory mechanism is liable to sudden failure and his heart is more susceptible to arrest from anoxia. If the natural mechanisms of haemostasis or the oxygen-carrying power of the blood are already impaired then the stage is set for disaster. The surgeon must be certain therefore that the patient is not suffering from a constitutional haemostatic defect or from anaemia. This necessitates a careful enquiry to exclude bleeding tendencies in patient *and* family, and to discover possible causes of anaemia such as recent blood loss (e.g. epistaxis, menorrhagia) or debilitating or inherited illness. Where these enquiries encounter the slightest suspicion of such tendencies or causes, appropriate blood investigations must be carried out.

Constitutional haemostatic defects.—These fall into two main groups, capillary contraction defects and coagulation defects. If capillary contraction is defective there will be immediate and continuous oozing from the small vessels of the tonsil bed which can be controlled by pressure, provided it is maintained long enough for the clotting mechanism to operate to seal the vessels. On the other hand if there is a coagulation defect, bleeding will occur two to four hours after operation when capillary contraction has relaxed, and no amount of pressure will control it. For the absence of clot means further bleeding as soon as pressure is again relaxed, while the pressure itself will cause bruising of the tissues and extend the field of bleeding. The management of bleeding which is due to a coagulation defect depends on tracing the missing factor and replacing it, not only at the time of operation but also throughout the period of healing.

If careful enquiry has raised the slightest doubt in the surgeon's mind about the possible existence of a haemostatic defect the following laboratory *screening tests* should be performed:

(1) Bleeding time (Duke's method)	Normal: less than 5 min.
(2) Platelet count	Normal: 200,000–500,000/mm³.
(3) One-stage prothrombin time	Normal: 12–14 sec. (Quick's method)
(4) Partial thromboplastin time	Normal: 30–40 sec.

(The exact figures for normal may vary from laboratory to laboratory).

If these tests are normal the patient may be considered not to be suffering from a constitutional haemostatic defect. But if the patient fails to pass one of these tests, or if doubt still exists because of a positive personal or family history of bleeding, further laboratory blood tests should be carried out in consultation with a haematologist.

Of patients with coagulation defects 88 per cent are deficient in Factor VIII which is antihaemophilic globulin (A HG). In 8 per cent the deficiency is of Factor IX (Christmas disease); the remaining 4 per cent include all other very rare deficiencies. Von Willebrand's disease is due to a double haemostatic defect with poor capillary contraction *and* a deficiency of Factor VIII. Operation in all these patients is a major undertaking depending entirely for success upon close co-operation between surgeon, haematologist, anaesthetist and physician. The investigation and supervision of the replacement materials and the surgery demand the exceptional facilities of an experienced unit (Livingstone, 1965).

Anaemias.—Iron deficiency anaemias are not uncommon among children and it is essential to insist on a pre-operative haemoglobin estimation in every case. Allowance must be made for the possibility of haemorrhage, and to start operation with a depleted haemoglobin is an additional, avoidable risk to the patient. Every effort should be made to raise the haemoglobin level to upwards of 11·5 g./100 ml. before operation. If anaemia does not respond to simple iron therapy further investigations should be carried out to find the reason.

The sickle trait has a normal haemoglobin and apart from an occasional target cell the peripheral blood film is normal. It can only be detected by a combination of the sickling test and haemoglobin electrophoresis. These patients only suffer from the presence of the abnormal haemoglobin under conditions of low oxygen tension such as may occur in anaesthesia. Therefore steps should be taken to detect such cases before operation. The giving of bicarbonate before and after operation aims to prevent the development of acidosis which tends to increase the risk of intravascular sickling. Special care must be taken during anaesthesia to avoid low oxygen tension at any time.

Hb–S sickle cell disease presents a more difficult and dangerous problem of operation. Cases with this disease are always anaemic with a haemoglobin level of only 6 to 8 g./100 ml. If it is essential to operate very careful preparation is required. Apart from giving bicarbonate, a transfusion will be necessary. There are two ways of doing this: by repeated small transfusions to raise the haemogbloin level slowly and depress the patient's bone marrow, thereby reducing the proportion of cells capable of sickling in the circulation, or by carrying out some form of exchange transfusion.

HbS–C disease and rarer combinations involving an HbS gene occupy an intermediate position. They usually have some degree of anaemia and may or may not require transfusion.

The sickle trait and diseases occur almost exclusively in patients of African Negro descent. As the sickle cell trait may appear normal without complete laboratory investigation, any patient of such descent who requires an emergency operation must be assumed to carry the S gene unless already excluded.

Anaesthesia

The anaesthetist should be regarded as the physician to the surgical team. All patients prior to operation should, wherever possible, be examined by the anaesthetist. If this is not practicable, the examination should be delegated to a responsible qualified medical practitioner. The object of such an examination will be to exclude any condition affecting the patient that might, by increasing the risk, contra-indicate the administration of an anaesthetic. Common conditions falling within this category include: (*a*) cardiac; (*b*) respiratory; (*c*) haematological (some already considered above); (*d*) laryngeal; (*e*) metabolic.

Infection

(1) A patient with an acute upper respiratory infection is at double risk from operation. First, administration of anaesthetic is accompanied by additional risk of spreading the infection to the lower respiratory tract. Second, there is greater risk of bleeding from acutely inflamed tissues. Thus operation is contra-indicated within at least two weeks of a patient having contracted such an acute upper respiratory infection.

(2) It is also most undesirable for operation to be performed on a patient who has been in contact with one of the infectious diseases of childhood, especially measles. If measles develop in the post-operative period the attack may not only be more severe owing to decreased resistance, but may be a cause of secondary haemorrhage from the tonsil bed.

(3) The bulbar type of poliomyelitis has been observed to occur with relatively greater frequency in patients who have recently had tonsils removed. It was at one time the practice to cease all such operations during an epidemic of poliomyelitis, and should such an epidemic recur it would be wise to do so again. But some years have passed since the last epidemic occurred in the U.K. The question that now commonly arises is in connection with the administration of polio vaccine. In general it is advised that all children should have been immunized before they undergo operation for removal of tonsils (and/or adenoids), and that operation should not be performed within less than six weeks of the last administration of vaccine.

Pregnancy and menstruation

If tonsillectomy must be performed at all in a pregnant patient it should be carried out during the middle trimester, that is between the thirteenth and twenty-fifth weeks. In general it is best to avoid operation as administration of general anaesthesia cannot yet be said to be entirely without risk to the foetus. Menstruation is traditionally thought to be associated with a greater risk of bleeding from the operation site. There is as yet no really convincing evidence that this is true, nor that menstruation should be considered a contra-indication to operation. It may be more convenient and comfortable however from the patient's point of view to select the intermenstrual period.

Voice changes

Professional singers may enquire whether removal of the tonsils is likely to alter the voice. Recurrent tonsillitis in itself is associated with a greater risk of laryngitis, while removal of the tonsils, provided the dissection is carried out with meticulous avoidance of damage to the palatal muscles, is not in itself associated with changes in the range and power of the voice. The change that may occur is in quality or timbre and usually this is for the better. Indifferent singers may sometimes seek an excuse for their lack of success and find a recent tonsillectomy a ready one. Intubation anaesthesia carries a recognized risk of vocal cord granuloma and this must be weighed in the anaesthetist's mind against other considerations, such as safety.

Hypernasality may occur in children after removal of adenoids (*see* p. 140).

Preparation of patient

Examination

It is advisable to admit the patient the evening before operation. This allows sufficient time for preliminary examination to be carried out by the anaesthetist or his deputy and for haemoglobin estimates and blood grouping to be performed. It also ensures a good night's rest (with the help of sedatives if necessary) and the opportunity for two preliminary (night and morning) temperature readings. In the event of the examination or the readings being unsatisfactory the surgeon can be informed well in advance, and a decision taken whether operation should be deferred. In the case of a non-lifesaving procedure such as tonsillectomy it is always right to postpone operation if the *slightest* doubt arises as to the patient's fitness.

Apart from a full clinical examination the following check list should be applied and cleared:

(1) No bleeding tendency in patient or family.

(2) No recent (within two weeks) upper respiratory or other infection.

(3) No recent contact with an infectious disease to which the patient is not immune.

(4) Is the patient allergic to any antibiotic? It may be necessary to administer one.

(5) Has the patient been immunized against anterior poliomyelitis?

(6) Has the patient ever received steroid therapy?

Premedication

The purpose of premedication is to counteract the rise of metabolic rate associated with fear and apprehension, to help to prevent cardiac inhibition and to suppress the secretory activity of the mucous glands of the upper and lower respiratory tract. Most premedications, therefore, are a combination of a sedative drug and a drying agent. Choice and dose rest with the anaesthetist, who will decide according to the age of the patient and anaesthetic to be administered at operation. To avoid risk of post-anaesthetic inhalation of vomit the patient must have taken nothing by mouth for six hours before the anaesthetic is due to be given.

Induction of general anaesthesia and intubation

This is the province of the anaesthetist, and it is generally agreed that intubation of the trachea is desirable when anaesthetizing a patient for any operation on the head and neck as it gives more certain control of the airway, both with regards to oxygenation and protection against inhalation of blood, mucus, or stomach contents. If the tonsils alone are being removed the tube may conveniently be introduced by the nasal route. But an oral tube may be effectively kept out of the operation field by employing a Doughty fenestrated tongue piece in the conventional Davis gag, and this apparatus is recommended for routine use for the removal of tonsils and adenoids (singly or combined).

From the surgeon's point of view the overriding requirements are an absolutely safe technique; a still, relaxed patient; the minimum of bleeding; and a non-explosive anaesthetic agent.

123

Local anaesthesia

Local anaesthesia is rarely employed for tonsillectomy in the U.K. Patients and surgeons who have had experience of a really good, safe general anaesthetic rarely remain in doubt of its advantage. With local anaesthetic there may be less bleeding at the time of operation but the overall strain on surgeon and patient is much greater. A suitable local anaesthetic is prilocaine hydrochloride 0·5 per cent with adrenaline 1 in 250,000. Prior to injection the tonsil areas may be lightly sprayed with a 5 per cent solution of cocaine hydrochloride (or 4 per cent lignocaine). The patient lies on the operating table with the head raised. The tongue is depressed and the pillars of the fauces and tissues external to the tonsil capsule are infiltrated as shown in Fig 28, 2 ml. into each site. Ten minutes are allowed to elapse before starting the dissection.

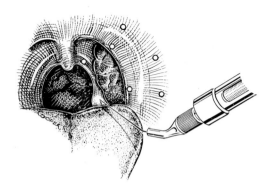

Fig. 28.—Injection sites for local anaesthesia.

Dissection of the tonsils

There are several satisfactory methods employed for removing the tonsils by dissection, each with its own minor variation of technique according to the preference of the individual surgeon. Basically it is necessary:

(1) To divide the mucous membrane where it leaves the margins of the pillars of the fauces to invest the tonsil.

(2) To dissect the areolar tissue off the tonsil capsule by which it is held lightly to the lateral wall of the oropharynx, except near the lower pole where a condensation of fascia, the falciform ligament, attaches it firmly.

(3) To divide the pedicle, or lingual attachment.

In good hands tonsillectomy is a rapid and relatively bloodless procedure that may appear deceptively easy. In the hands of the inexperienced it can be traumatic and bloody, and never should be first attempted except under the tutelage of an expert. It cannot be learned from textbook descriptions. There is no substitute for operating theatre instruction.

The method of removal of the tonsils with the guillotine is not favoured. With it the tonsils can be removed very quickly, but it will not succeed where the tonsils are attached firmly to the lateral oropharyngeal wall by fibrous tissue, as is not infrequently the case where there has been much recurrent tonsillitis. Moreover, since the advantage of speed can only be realized with a light anaesthetic, from which the patient recovers almost at once in order to cough out blood (no ligatures having been applied), there is neither sufficient palatal relaxation nor the time for a careful and unhurried curettage of the adenoids, so often required in children at the same time as the tonsils.

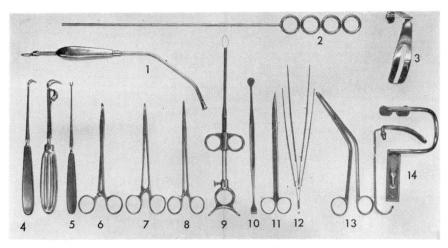

FIG. 29.—Instruments for tonsillectomy.

1. Yankauer's tonsil suction tube
2. Draffin suspension apparatus (one of two bipods)
3. Doughty's slotted endotracheal tongue plate
4. St. Clair Thomson adenoid curettes (guarded and unguarded)
5. Negus knot tier and ligature adjuster
6. Negus tonsil artery forceps
7. Birkett's fine tonsil artery forceps (curved)

8. Birkett's fine tonsil artery forceps (straight)
9. Eve's tonsil snare
10. Mollison's semi-sharp enucleator
11. Wilson's tapered and round-ended scissors
12. Waugh's tenaculum dissection forceps
13. Denis Brown's tonsil-holding forceps
14. Davis gag and Boyles's tongue plate

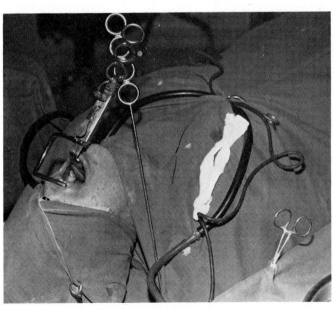

FIG. 30.—Position of Boyle–Davis gag for tonsillectomy under general anaesthesia.

Technique

Stage I—insertion of gag

The patient lies on his back, shoulders slightly raised on a small pillow or sand-bag and the head slightly extended. A Davis gag with Doughty tongue piece of suitable size is inserted, care being taken to avoid damaging the teeth or lips.

When the anaesthetist is satisfied that the anaesthetic tube has not been compressed or displaced and there is full control of the airway, the gag is held open in position by a "jack" or other device (Figs. 29 and 30).

Stage II—dissection

(1) The tonsil is grasped firmly with a Denis Browne's tonsil-holding forceps near the upper pole and retracted medially. With the point of a Waugh's tenaculum

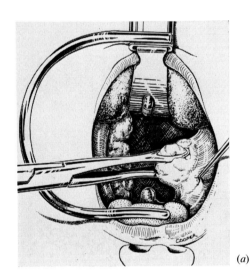

(a)

FIG. 31.—Tonsillectomy: (a) first penetration of the mucosa of the anterior pillar; (b) defining the plane of dissection.

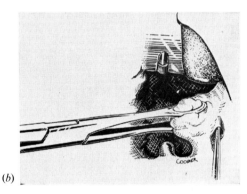

(b)

dissection forceps the mucous membrane is penetrated over the upper pole (Fig. 31a). The closed forceps may then be used to tunnel beneath the membrane, between it and the tonsil capsule, so that a narrow plane of separation is made between the tonsil and margin of each pillar of the fauces as far as the lingual attachment

(Fig.31b). One blade of a pair of Wilson's tapered round-ended scissors is slipped, along each tunnel and the membrane is snipped (Fig. 32a).

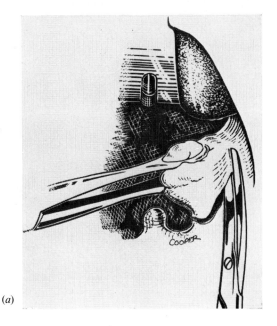

FIG. 32.—Tonsillectomy: (a) division of mucosal attachments; (b) releasing the upper pole.

(a)

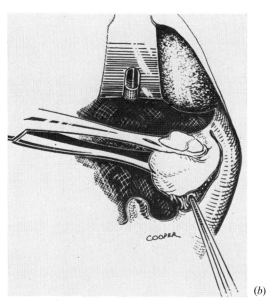

(b)

(2) Still using the Waugh's forceps, areolar tissue is stripped from the upper pole of the tonsil (Fig. 32b) until it has been freed sufficiently to change the grip of the tonsil-holding forceps so that the upper pole is held between the blades. This grip is

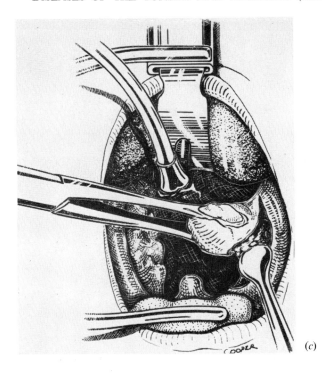

(c)

FIG. 32 (*continued*).—Tonsillectomy: (c) blunt dissection frees the body of the tonsil towards the lower pole; (d) application of Eve's snare.

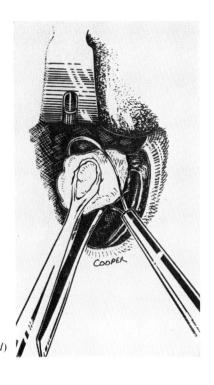

(d)

then maintained while the fibrous areolar tissue is dissected from the tonsil capsule with Mollison's semi-sharp enucleator (Fig. 32c). Significant bleeding may be encountered at this stage. If profuse the bleeding point must be picked up with Birkett's fine tonsil artery forceps. If not profuse the blood may be aspirated by an assistant using a Yankauer's tonsil suction tube while the dissection continues.

(3) When the tonsil has been freed from its bed it will then be necessary to divide the pedicle or lingual attachment. The wire loop of an Eve's tonsil snare is slipped over the tonsil (Fig. 32d) and then closed firmly and divided by the crushing action of the snare, and the tonsil is removed (Fig. 33).

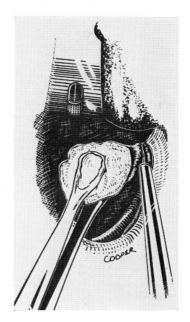

Fig. 33.—Tonsillectomy. Severance of lower pole by closure of snare.

Stage III—arrest of haemorrhage

While the second tonsil is being dissected the first fossa is packed with gauze. Unless there is much bleeding from a large vessel this will generally prove sufficient to control bleeding by compression. At the conclusion of the second dissection the first pack is removed and the tonsil bed meticulously examined for bleeding points, using the other, specially designed end, of the Mollison enucleator to retract the anterior pillar of the fauces. Any bleeding point that has not ceased bleeding after 10 minutes of packing must be controlled by other means. Small vessels may be coagulated with diathermy, but large vessels, such as the paratonsillar vein should always be tied. The point is grasped with a Birkett's forceps and lifted slightly to allow the curved blades of a pair of Negus' or Wilson's tonsil artery forceps to be passed between the end of the Birkett's forceps and the tonsil bed and closed on the vessel. Birkett's forceps are then removed and a thread is passed around the tip of the curved forceps and tied, using a Negus knot tier and ligature adjuster (Fig. 34).

129

Stage IV—removal of gag and anaesthetic tube

When the surgeon is satisfied that each tonsil bed is completely dry the naso-pharynx will be emptied of blood (which will have accumulated during the operation due to the deliberate positioning of the patient's head to drain blood away from the larynx). This may be best achieved by passing a soft catheter attached to

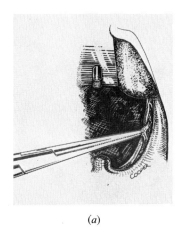

(*a*)

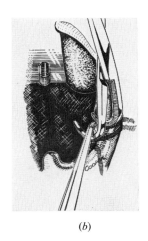

(*b*)

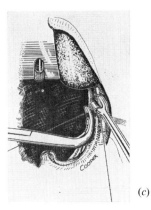

(*c*)

Fig. 34.—Tonsillectomy. Haemostasis: (*a*) bleeding point taken; (*b*) application of curved forceps across the tissue to be ligated; (*c*) ligature of bleeding point with use of Negus ligature adjuster.

the suction apparatus down one nostril. The gag and tongue piece are then carefully removed and an airway inserted. The patient's mandible, which can be dislocated by over-opening of the gag, is tested for normal mobility, then the anaesthetic tube may be removed, and the patient turned onto one side; to remain in such a position on table, trolley or bed until return of consciousness.

Post-operative care of the patient

Protection of airway

Retain patient in operating theatre area until conscious.

(1) Until patient has recovered sufficiently to cough spontaneously and protect his own airway, the laryngeal inlet must be kept clear of blood or vomit.

(*i*) Turn patient on side immediately after operation without a pillow so that larynx is higher than operation site.

(*ii*) Insert artificial airway in mouth.

(*iii*) Hold mandible forwards, closed on airway to keep base of tongue clear of posterior pharyngeal wall.

(*iv*) Have electrical suction apparatus near patient with catheter that will pass down the artificial airway, together with a Yankauer's suction tube.

(2) Relief of laryngeal spasm. If patient goes into spasm and cyanosis develops:

(*i*) Make sure artificial airway is in correct position with mandible held forwards and closed. If this fails:

(*ii*) Apply oxygen mask and attempt manual inflation with bag. If this fails:

(*iii*) Insert laryngoscope. Aspirate clot, mucus, or other matter from larynx (usual cause of spasm). If spasm continues inject suxamethonium (10 mg./6·5 kg. (1 stone)) intubate and artificially respire.

Control of reactionary haemorrhage

Recurrence of bleeding soon after the return of the patient from the operating theatre, although relatively uncommon, may constitute a grave danger if unrecognized. Blood may be swallowed and not dribble, as a warning, from nose or mouth. The utmost skilled nursing vigilance is necessary, with:

(1) Quarter-hourly pulse recording for first two hours. Half-hourly pulse recording for next four hours. Hourly pulse recording for subsequent six hours, and four-hourly pulse recording for following 12 hours. Thereafter the pulse should be taken six-hourly.

A pulse that remains high or is rising should be regarded as a sign of bleeding until proved otherwise by inspection of pharynx.

(2) Close watch for swallowing movements. A semiconscious patient may betray the presence of bleeding by repeated swallowing movements.

(3) Listen for "rattle" in the breathing. Air passing in and out through blood in the pharynx cannot have the desirable quiet dry quality.

If bleeding is suspected, the tonsil beds must be properly inspected. A headlight and tongue depressor must always be readily available, together with Luc's forceps (for removing clot) and Birkett's artery forceps. If suspected bleeding is obscured by a blood clot the latter is removed with the Luc's forceps. This alone may allow the tissues to retract and the bleeding to stop spontaneously. If the bleeding continues it may be sufficient to apply pressure with a small gauze roll held in the Birkett's forceps. If the bleeding still continues it is possible for a skilled surgeon to pick up the bleeding point with the Birkett's forceps and ligature the vessel (as described previously under "Technique"). The tonsil bed is relatively insensitive for a few hours after operation and these measures can be carried out in a co-operative patient without undue discomfort. A slight ooze may not merit such action and may stop if the patient is given ice to suck and a sedative.

If all measures taken to arrest the bleeding prove unavailing it will be necessary to return the patient to the operating theatre and tie off the bleeding point under general anaesthetic. The administration of a second anaesthetic, necessary in these circumstances, demands the service of a skilled and experienced anaesthetist. In the rare event of inability to identify a bleeding point or control the bleeding with ligatures a roll of gauze may be held in the fossa by stitching the pillars of the fauces over it. The stitches and the gauze will need to be removed in 24 hours.

Arranging the return of the patient to the theatre may take time. It should be as short as possible as continuing blood loss is a mounting hazard to life. The patient should, while awaiting removal, be cross-matched for transfusion and a request made for the correct blood. If rising pulse rate indicates failing compensatory mechanism to lowered blood volume an intravenous drip of dextran BP should be set up. If needed blood can then be readily substituted.

Control of secondary haemorrhage

Secondary haemorrhage generally occurs between the fifth and tenth post-operative day, either associated with separation of ligatures or infection of the tonsil bed with softening of clot, or both. Such bleeding is seldom severe and usually stops if the patient is given ice to suck, a sedative, and injections of penicillin. In very rare cases it may be necessary to tie a bleeding point as in reactionary haemorrhage.

General care

A soft diet, with plenty of fluids, is administered for the first few post-operative days. Pain is controlled by analgesics. A warm phenol gargle BPC every four to six hours is soothing and cleansing to the healing areas. Children must not be allowed to become overtired but will often be ready to be got up and dressed on the second post-operative day. Adults require longer to recover from the operation and generally require five to seven days in hospital before going home.

Complications of tonsillectomy (other than those already described)

Unusual haemorrhage

Alarming haemorrhage may occur through accidental injury of aberrant vessels. This is less likely to occur if a careful method of dissection is employed. The internal carotid artery is mainly at risk and special care must be taken if pulsation is visible behind the posterior pillars of the fauces.

Pulmonary complications

Operation on the tonsils and/or adenoids is nearly always accompanied by inhalation of some blood, despite every precaution taken against it but, although the presence of blood in the lungs can give rise to atelectasis, bronchitis, pneumonia or lung abscess, these complications, with the exception of atelectasis, are extremely rare.

Inhalation of blood is most likely to occur in the immediate post-operative period when the patient is recovering from anaesthesia. Symptoms of atelectasis are cough, dyspnoea, raised respiration rate and, if massive, cyanosis. All patients should have their chests examined post-operatively and before discharge from hospital. Abnormal physical signs must receive the appropriate investigations and treatment.

Focal infection

Transient bacteraemia occurs after operation in a high percentage of cases. Serious complications including meningitis, brain abscess and cavernous sinus thrombosis have been reported. Exacerbation of existing infections in the heart, kidney and joints may also occur post-operatively (Gibb, 1969). These complications are, considering the number of operations performed annually, very rare. Patients with such existing infection should have the tonsils removed under antibiotic cover. If the temperature rises post-operatively antibiotic should be administered as a precaution. But it is not considered necessary to perform every operation under an antibiotic umbrella.

Surgical trauma

Lack of skill (preventable by proper training) may result in damage to the uvula, soft palate, tongue, teeth or pharyngeal wall. Accidental breakage of a snare wire may occur at any time but it is usually a simple matter to recover the wire. Not so with the breakage of a needle. If a surgeon decides to undersew a bleeding point and the needle breaks it may prove extremely difficult to find the fragment. It is best to avoid this procedure wherever possible.

CHRONIC LINGUAL TONSILLITIS

The pathology of chronic lingual tonsillitis resembles that of chronic tonsillitis. Lingual tonsillitis is however comparatively rare but more likely to be encountered in patients who have already had the tonsils removed. The lingual tonsils may undergo compensatory enlargement and come to occupy the lower part of the tonsil fossa, giving an illusion of an incomplete tonsillectomy.

Symptoms

The throat feels "thick" and uncomfortable but the patients seldom complain of dysphagia to the same extent as in tonsillitis. There is a constant desire to clear the throat and the voice may take on a "plummy" quality. On inspection with a laryngeal mirror the enlargement of the lingual tonsils is easily seen, sometimes unilateral, and the surface may be covered with exudate. Regional cervical lymph nodes may be palpable.

Treatment

Not infrequently the patients' complaints seem out of proportion to the pathological appearances. Owing to the position of the lingual tonsils it is not an easy matter to remove them surgically and such an operation is seldom undertaken. If surgery should be contemplated due to gross hypertrophy it is best confined to attempts at reduction in size by diathermy coagulation or cryosurgery. Most patients respond to medical treatment with gargles, sprays, throat paints or lozenges.

CHRONIC ADENOIDITIS

Chronic infection of the adenoids is seen most frequently in children between the ages of three to six years. The adenoids at the same time are usually enlarged and, more often than not, the tonsils in these cases are chronically infected, giving rise to an overall clinical picture of chronic upper respiratory infection and obstruction —which has been called the T's and A's syndrome. While it is frequently necessary to consider removal of the tonsils and adenoids at the same operation, either because of infective symptoms or obstructive symptoms, or both, there are never-the-less, distinctive symptoms and signs of chronic adenoiditis which may point to the advisability of adenoidectomy on its own merits. T's and A's has come to appear on operating lists as a convenient shorthand for tonsillo-adenoidectomy. It should not become a symbol of short thinking about the precise indications for surgical treatment of the tonsils and/or the adenoids in every individual case.

Symptoms and signs

The child with chronic infection of the adenoids *may* exhibit one or more of three classical symptoms:

(1) Postnasal or anterior nasal catarrhal discharge.

(2) Nocturnal cough.

(3) Headache.

The catarrh takes the form of mucopurulent discharge. Parents often describe it as a cold that has never cleared up. The child is always blowing his nose or sniffing. Sometimes, especially in the mornings, overnight accumulation of discharge in the pharynx causes nausea, even vomiting, and the child has a poor appetite for breakfast. Nocturnal cough results from the chronic postnasal drip. Headache is presumably due to the infected material in the roof of the nasopharynx. It is frontal in type but at the age when chronic adenoiditis occurs the frontal sinuses have not developed and it is always a mistake to attribute frontal headache in young children to frontal sinusitis. The maxillary sinuses, however, may become chronically infected due to the dam-back effect of the adenoids on ciliary drainage. Chronic infection of these sinuses often coexists with chronic adenoiditis and, especially where catarrhal symptoms are prominent, an x-ray should be taken in case treatment of the sinuses is required at the same time as, or independently of, the adenoids.

Other symptoms of chronic adenoiditis are recurrent earache, mouth breathing and snoring. These may result more from enlargement of the adenoids than from infection, but where the earaches develop into acute otitis media infection of the adenoids is a likely cause.

Chronic adenoiditis may also be present without giving rise to anything more than an enhanced susceptibility to colds, as evidenced by the diminution in the number of colds that may follow removal of adenoids in some cases. But susceptibility to colds involves immunological factors as yet not fully determined and frequent colds are not to be regarded, *per se*, as symptomatic of chronic adenoiditis or an indication for adenoidectomy.

On examination of the postnasal space indirectly with a mirror, the adenoids may be seen to be invested with a lacing of mucopus or mucus. Sometimes there is so much of this catarrhal matter as to obscure the view completely. There may be visible enlargement of glands behind the pharyngeal wall on one or both sides of the midline, and cervical nodes may be palpable. There is generally some obstruction of the nose, and inspection of the tympanic membranes may show retraction due to eustachian tube obstruction.

If a mirror view of the postnasal space has not been obtained (although it is usually possible in children who will tolerate a tongue spatula) a soft-tissue lateral x-ray of the postnasal space will give a good radiographic shadow of the adenoid mass, and its size in relation to the space.

Complications

Recurrent acute otitis media

Proximity of the infected adenoids to the eustachian openings constitutes a ready pathway of infection to the middle ear. Children are frequently seen with acute otitis media which relapses as soon as antibiotic is discontinued. While this may be due to some otological cause such as retained middle ear effusion, the adenoids should also come under suspicion. Where there are confirmatory symptoms and signs of adenoid infection, especially with enlargement, adenoidectomy may well be the one measure required to terminate the attacks.

Chronic maxillary sinusitis

This has already received mention above. Where radiographic investigation suggests the possibility of antral infection, the adenoids should receive consideration of treatment *before* the sinus. It is almost impossible to cure chronic antral infection in children whose adenoids are also infected and enlarged until the adenoids have been removed. Removal of adenoids in itself may be curative of the sinus infection. It is usual however to take advantage of the anaesthetic required for removal of the adenoids to treat the sinus by a single lavage or by temporary indwelling polythene tube for daily lavage post-operatively.

Retention cysts of the adenoids

Chronic infection may result, as in the case of the tonsils, in the formation of retention cysts. These retention cysts occasionally reach quite a large size being usually seen in adults in whom involution of the adenoid tissue itself leaves the cyst more easily visible. Similar cysts described by Tornwaldt may form in the pharyngeal bursa (pouch of Luschka) and secrete sticky mucus but distinction is difficult on clinical examination. Cysts of the adenoids or Luschka's pouch may be treated by uncapping and thorough aspiration under general anaesthetic. Simple incision or needle aspiration will almost certainly be followed by recurrence. In the case of the adenoid cyst curettage may be required. If the cysts are symptomless (not associated with postnasal catarrh) they may be left untreated.

Mental lethargy

While the adenoids should not be blamed for backwardness when the cause may lie in hereditary, developmental, or environmental factors, there is no doubt that, other things being equal, a child with infected and enlarged adenoids shows reduced mental alertness and less physical energy. This is not surprising in view of the universal adult experience of mental dullness when the nose is blocked, for example, during a cold.

Impaired speech

Nasal obstruction due to adenoids results in rhinolalia clausa or closed-nose voice. While this is likely to cure itself in time, it is unpleasing and productive of bad speech habits.

High arch palate

Constant mouth breathing may be associated with impaired development of the nasal airways so that the floor of the nose (roof of palate) fails to descend. This in turn results in orthodontic disturbance and the so-called adenoid facies; a pinched nose, open mouth, and narrow maxillary alveolar arch with crowded and protruding teeth.

Treatment

When adenoids are both so enlarged as seriously to interfere with nasal respiration and/or middle ear ventilation and are thought to be chronically infected there is no better treatment than adenoidectomy. While enlargement and chronic infection are more often found to be present at the same time, there are some cases where symptoms suggest chronic infection but inspection or x-ray study does not reveal significant enlargement. In these cases a regime of medical treatment is advisable before undertaking surgery.

Medical treatment will aim at (*i*) reducing the adenoid size still further by the use of decongestant nasal drops (ephedrine 0·5 per cent in normal saline is appropriate); (*ii*) reducing infection by systemic antibiotics based on laboratory culture of nasal swabs. Swabs often will fail to grow pathogenic organisms, when a course of broad spectrum antibiotic must perforce be tried; (*iii*) reducing volume of mucus secretion by antihistamine therapy (e.g. chlorpheniramine malleate 2–4 mg. twice daily). Such medical treatment may be given in courses. There is no point in prolonging treatment if no improvement has been obtained after three weeks. But some patients respond and relapse, and it is for these that repeated courses may be helpful. Others may benefit from prolonged daily oral antibiotic therapy if response has been good. But the advisability of prolonged antibiotic therapy, which carries a risk of induced organism resistance or patient allergy, must be questioned when a probability exists of cure by surgery.

THE OPERATION OF ADENOIDECTOMY

The operation is indicated, as previously discussed (*i*) when the size of the adenoids is interfering with nasal or eustachian tube ventilation, speech or feeding; (*ii*) when chronic infection is considered to be the cause of repeated upper respiratory infection, repeated otitis media, chronic catarrh, headache, nocturnal cough or lethargy; (*iii*) especially when obstructive and infective symptoms coexist.

Removal of adenoids may be required independently of removal of the tonsils, but in practice the indications are more often present for removal of both. Whether the tonsils alone, adenoids alone, or both, are being removed the overall considerations set out under "The Operation of Tonsillectomy" on pp. 118–123 are of equal relevance. Safety, depending on appreciation of the risks involved, selection of cases, contra-indications, preparation of patient, surgical technique and postoperative care, is the overriding factor of importance. *These pages should be read before the technicalities of the operation of adenoidectomy (below) are studied.*

In order that removal of adenoids may be as complete as possible the anaesthetic should provide a relaxed palate and superior constrictor muscle, and time for adequate exploration and clearance of the retrotubal fossae of Rosenmüller. Oral intubation is desirable with the use of a Doughty split tongue piece and Davis gag. If the tonsils are being removed at the same operation the adenoids are most conveniently removed first. The postnasal space may then be packed with ribbon gauze while the tonsils are being dissected, and in the majority of cases all bleeding will have ceased from the adenoid bed when the pack is removed at the end of the procedure.

As with the tonsil operation there are several methods of adenoid removal, using different types of curettes which may be equally successful in expert hands. The importance lies in learning one good method well. The method to be described has given satisfactory results over many years.

Technique

Stage I—engagement of curette

(1) The patient lies on his back. The surgeon stands at head of table, which is tilted 20 degrees head-down below the horizontal. The mouth is held open with the Davis gag, with the head and neck in a straight line. Head is slightly flexed to abolish convexity of upper cervical vertebrae (electrical suction *must* be available).

(2) The nasopharynx is palpated and adenoids identified together with eustachian cushions. With the examining finger, adenoid tissue lying in the fossae of Rosen-müller is displaced towards the midline. This should be no more than a gentle scraping action with the glove-protected finger-nail.

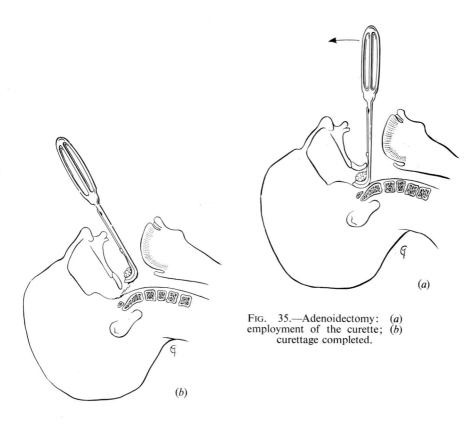

Fig. 35.—Adenoidectomy: (*a*) employment of the curette; (*b*) curettage completed.

(3) A St. Clair Thomson's adenoid curette of suitable size, fitted with a cage to "catch" the adenoids as they are scraped off, is passed strictly in the midline behind the soft palate until brought into contact with the posterior edge of the nasal septum.

Stage II—curettage

(1) The curette, in contact with the nasal septum, is pressed against the hard roof of the nasopharynx. This action pushes the adenoids through the fenestration of the curette and engages the cutting edge correctly (Fig. 35*a*).

(2) The curette is firmly kept in contact with the roof and posterior wall of the pharynx as it is swept downwards to a level just short of the curved lower edge of the soft palate, when it is moved sharply away from the posterior pharyngeal wall to break the adenoid mass free from the mucosa (Fig. 35*b*). If the last movement is not brisk the mucosa may not be torn through cleanly but stripped off the pharynx in unsightly ribbons. If the actions have been correctly performed the curette can be removed easily from the mouth with the main mass of adenoids caught in the cage. If the mass has not been cleanly removed a second stroke of the curette in the midline may succeed. If the mass still remains attached to mucosa it must be grasped in Luc's forceps and the attachment cut with scissors. Care should be taken not to injure the uvula in the process.

Stage III—removal of remnants

The examining finger is again inserted and the area searched for remnants. These will generally be found in the fossae of Rosenmüller or where the nasal septum joins the roof of the nasopharynx. The finger may again be used to scrape these areas clean. It is safer than exploring the lateral recesses with a curette which may either injure the superior constrictor muscle and cause unnecessary bleeding or scarring, or else damage the eustachian entrance with the possibility of post-operative disturbance of function. The use of adenoid tag forceps or punch forceps to remove remnants can be the cause of excessive and possible dangerous bleeding.

After care

Protection of airways

This is the same as in tonsillectomy (p. 130).

Control of haemorrhage

Primary haemorrhage (during operation).—To control bleeding occurring at the time of operation a length of folded gauze with a tape attached is packed into the nasopharynx and left in position for 10 minutes. In many cases this coincides with the time taken for removal of the tonsils and the adenoid bed is dry when the pack is removed (it is always wise to attach a tape to the pack and lead it out of the mouth so that the pack cannot possibly go out of mind during the tonsillectomy).

If removal of the pack is followed by brisk haemorrhage the cause may lie with a remnant preventing proper contracture of vessels. A second curettage and packing often succeeds in arresting bleeding. If removal of the pack is repeatedly followed by bleeding a pack may be left in for 12–24 hours (attached to two tapes led one through each nostril and tied in front of the nose to hold it in position, and a third tape led through the mouth and strapped to cheek to facilitate removal when the nasal tapes are untied). If the pack is not held in position by nasal tapes it may subsequently displace downwards, impact on the larynx and cause asphyxia. If left in too long a pack will lead to local sepsis which in turn may provoke further bleeding or give rise to acute otitis media. Any patient in whom it is deemed necessary to leave a pack for over 12 hours should be given antibiotic.

Reactionary haemorrhage (*see also* p. 131).—If bleeding occurs in the post-operative period turn patient on his side, raise the head slightly and attempt to control:

(1) Place ice cold packs across bridge of nose and on back and sides of neck for reflex vasoconstriction. If the child is very restless give sedation (i.m. injection papaveretum (Nepenthe) 0·06 ml. (1 minim) for every year of life up to a maximum of 0·6 ml. (10 minims)).

(2) If bleeding persists an inflatable postnasal tampon may be inserted (Mawson, 1956). This is a rubber balloon attached to a fine rubber catheter which is introduced through a nostril and inflated with 20 ml. of air in the postnasal space. It is then pulled against the posterior choana and the tension maintained by strapping the catheter to the cheek, a roll of wool or gauze protecting the corner of the nostril from pressure.

(3) If bleeding still persists a postnasal pack must be inserted. This can sometimes be done in a co-operative child without anaesthetic, but usually it is necessary to return the patient to the theatre and re-anaesthetize. *It must here be emphasized that at this stage the child may be in a position of imminent danger.* It is not always easy to decide whether to wait expectantly for bleeding to stop spontaneously, especially if it appears to be diminishing, or whether to re-anaesthetize with the risks that attend re-intubation through a field obscured by blood, and of anoxia in a patient with depleted red cells. But the risks of re-anaesthetizing increase greatly with waiting, and if the child's compensatory mechanism is showing signs of failure with approaching shock there will be need not only for a hurried second anaesthetic and insertion of a postnasal pack to arrest the haemorrhage, but also for blood transfusion. *The object of treatment will be to prevent the child ever entering this dangerous stage* and an early decision to re-anaesthetize and repack is *always* safer than delaying.

When the child is anaesthetized intravenous infusion of dextran BP may be set up. This assists in restoration of blood volume and allows rapid substitution with blood transfusion if required. The second anaesthetic demands greater skill than the first and it is essential for it to be given by an experienced anaesthetist. The surgeon will palpate the postnasal space with a finger. If any tags or remnants are apparent they may be reduced by morcellement with the finger or a midline recurettage may be performed. Curettage of the lateral recesses is more likely to increase bleeding. A postnasal pack will be inserted and held in position with tapes as described above (*see* "Primary haemorrhage"). Postnasal packs should normally be removed not later than 24 hours after insertion. The presence of the pack promotes sepsis which in turn may promote further bleeding tendency or otitis media. Children with packs in should be given systemic penicillin.

Secondary haemorrhage.—Infection of the adenoid bed may lead to secondary haemorrhage between the fifth and tenth post-operative days. Such bleeding usually stops with nasal ice packs, sedatives and penicillin injections. It is extremely rare for postnasal packing to be required.

General care.—It is very rare for reactionary bleeding to occur later than 12 hours after operation, and most small children are ready for discharge from hospital the day following. Analgesics are not required and a normal diet may be taken as soon as the child feels like it. Antibiotics are not given routinely, but a rise in temperature may indicate secondary infection when medical advice should be sought.

Other complications of adenoidectomy

Unusual haemorrhage

As in the case of tonsillectomy alarming haemorrhage may very rarely occur through accidental injury of aberrant vessels. The internal carotid artery has been encountered in a dangerous looped position in relation to the nasopharynx as a congenital anomaly (McKenzie and Woolf, 1959).

Pulmonary complications (*see* p. 132)

Surgical trauma

A badly performed adenoidectomy may result in:

(1) Damage to the eustachian cushions with subsequent scarring. Such scarring may interfere with eustachian tube function with liability to otitis media and deafness.

(2) *Subluxation of atlanto-axial joint.* A traumatic operation followed by infection may lead to decalcification of the vertebrae and laxity of the anterior ligament between the atlas and the axis. Muscle spasm then results in stiff neck and torticollis. The spinal cord is at risk of compression. The deformity must be reduced by traction (after radiographic confirmation of the displacement) and an immobilizing collar worn for at least 10 weeks after the adenoid bed is healed (Gibb, 1969).

(3) Damage to the palate. This occurs less rarely than with tonsillectomy.

(4) Cicatricial stenosis of the nasopharyngeal aperture has been reported (Guggenheim, 1963).

Hypernasality (*rhinolalia aperta*)

The gradual involution of the adenoids that occurs in later childhood or early adolescence is not accompanied by hypernasality. But the sudden operative removal of a large adenoid mass may result in incompetence of the velopharyngeal isthmus with escape of air from the nose during speech. The adenoids because of their size facilitate nasopharyngeal closure. The palate becomes habituated to moving only a short distance. The tonsils may also push the posterior pillar of the fauces backwards and aid closure. If palatal movement is also subsequently hindered by postoperative scarring a serious problem of hypernasality may arise.

Some assessment of speech and palatal function should be made before operation, and parents should be warned that removal of the adenoids may result in hypernasality, but also that the effects are usually temporary. The writer has only seen one serious case of hypernasality in 18 years of practice. But Gibb (1969) considers it probably occurs in a serious form once in every 2,000 operations.

Treatment consists of remedial exercises to increase palatal movement under a speech therapist. In serious cases some form of plastic surgery to narrow the isthmus may be required.

THE ANGINAS

Angina is an ancient term (Greek *anchein*; Latin *angere*, throttle) used by Hippocrates to signify sore throat. Under it are traditionally grouped some diseases of the tonsils which, while having sore throat in common, differ in aetiology. These are

Vincent's angina, monocytic angina, aphthous angina, agranulocytic angina and leukaemic angina.

Vincent's angina

This is a subacute ulcerative, usually unilateral, tonsillitis of insidious onset liable to appear, as in the trenches in World War I, in overcrowded, insanitary and unhealthy conditions. Vincent's angina as originally described was confined to the tonsils, but in so-called "trench mouth" the ulcerating lesions more often affect the gums, and oral mucous membrane (*see* p. 23). The disease is attributed to the symbiotic action of two organisms, *Bacillus fusiformis* and *Spirochaeta denticolata*, always present in the lesions.

Clinical features

Following a short incubation period the patient begins to feel generally unwell with headache and loss of appetite and energy, soon to be aggravated by discomfort in the throat and tender enlargement of the jugulodigastric lymph nodes (frequently unilateral).

On examination the breath is characteristically foetid, glandular enlargement is confirmed, the temperature is slightly raised and the tonsil shows a typical appearance according to the stage of the disease reached when examined.

At first the affected surface is partly covered with an exudate or an easily removable membrane. Soon the membrane thickens into a slough derived from an underlying excavating ulcer, with irregular edges. If the membrane or slough is removed in the early stages it will quickly reform. But after a week or two, the slough tends to separate permanently and the ulcer to heal.

In some cases the ulcerating process may involve the whole tonsil and extend to adjoining tissues, with subsequent scarring and loss of part of fauces or uvula. Although complications are very rare the disease has been known to spread to larynx and bronchial tree.

Treatment

At the time of writing the standard treatment for Vincent's angina is administration of penicillin (e.g. penicillin V elixir or tablets 250 mg. six-hourly) to which the responsible organisms are normally sensitive. Should the patient be debarred from receiving penicillin because of allergy an alternative antibiotic must be selected on laboratory findings. Mouth washes or gargles (phenol gargle BPC or sodium perborate 5 g. in 250 ml. of warm water), isolation and bedrest until the ulcer heals are advisable. Feeding utensils should be sterilized during the disease and toothbrushes discarded after recovery.

Monocytic angina (infectious mononucleosis, glandular fever, anginose glandular fever)

The term glandular fever came into use in 1889, infectious mononucleosis in 1920, anginose glandular fever (from which monocytic angina was coined) in 1934. Today infectious mononucleosis is the widely considered term of choice to describe the not very common, usually benign, self-limiting disease in which there is a high incidence of sore throat and, sometimes alarming, tonsillitis. Virological investigations suggest that the herpes-like Epstein–Barr virus may prove to be the causative agent but diagnosis still depends on the clinical, haematological and serological characteristics of the condition (Carter and Penman, 1969).

Infectious mononucleosis principally affects young patients between the ages of 15 to 30 years. The method of transmission is still not known for certain, although oral contagion through kissing or sharing of drinking vessels is suspect.

Clinical features

Early symptoms include general malaise, fatigue, feverishness, anorexia, nausea and headache and a curious sudden distaste for cigarettes but the most consistent complaint is the sore throat (angina). Sore throat develops at some stage of the disease in 80–85 per cent of patients and, although in the majority is mild, can be severe, reminiscent of quinsy, with inability even to swallow saliva.

Signs of infectious mononucleosis are, commonly, slight pyrexia (occasionally peaking to 40°C (104°F)), bradycardia, posterior cervical adenopathy, splenomegaly, pharyngitis and tonsillitis. Less commonly patients develop a palatal enanthem in the form of small petechiae, peri-orbital oedema, and a skin rash resembling rubella.

The appearance of the pharynx varies from a mild hyperaemia and congestion to gross oedema with ulceration and membrane formation. When the tonsils are involved the otolaryngologist is often called in consultation because a diagnosis has been made of acute tonsillitis, and the medical practitioner is disturbed because of failure to respond to antibiotics with alarming persistence of red swollen tonsils covered with patches of dirty grey membrane.

Haematological and serological findings

There is a total lymphocytosis of at least 4,500/mm³. in the peripheral blood with at least 51 per cent lymphocytes in the differential leucocyte count, of which a significant number are atypical.

Serum heterophile antibody (sheep's cell agglutinin) titres rise during the first two to three weeks in nearly all adult patients. Demonstration of the presence of these antibodies by the Paul Bunnell–Davidson or ox cell haemolysis tests is diagnostically specific for infectious mononucleosis.

Treatment

There is no cure for this disease, from which patients generally recover spontaneously albeit sometimes very slowly, taking several weeks. Antibiotics are useful only to prevent or treat secondary infection with bacteria (e.g. beta-haemolytic streptococcus). Treatment is symptomatic. For the relief of sore throat sodium perborate gargle (5 g. in 250 ml. of warm water) and lozenges containing chlorhexidine dihydrochloride and benzocaine (hibitane lozenges ICI) are useful.

Complete airway obstruction is extremely rare but can occur and may require temporary tracheostomy. Tonsillectomy may be indicated if the tonsils remain uncomfortable or enlarged after the infection, or if, as not infrequently occurs, the patient subsequently becomes susceptible to recurrent attacks of tonsillitis.

Aphthous angina

This is probably the same condition as the angina ulcerosa benigna of older text books. Aphthous ulcers may appear anywhere in the oral cavity or oropharynx. They are common on the anterior pillar of the fauces and occur on the tonsil. The ulcer is usually small, solitary and quite superficial. The aetiology is uncertain but the lesions are self-curing. Healing and relief of pain may be assisted by allowing a betamethasone lozenge BPC (containing betamethasone sodium phosphate equivalent to 0·1 mg. betamethazone) to dissolve slowly in the mouth near the lesion four times a day.

Agranulocytic angina

In agranulocytosis the total white cell count is low and the polymorphonuclear cells may be reduced to 5 per cent or less. As a result of this the patients have diminished resistance to infection and frequently suffer from severe ulcerative and necrotic lesions in the mouth, on the pillars of the fauces and on the tonsils. The sore throat or mouth is an incidental symptom in a rapidly prostrating febrile illness of obvious severity that prompts further urgent investigation. The blood count is diagnostic and serves to differentiate from acute leukaemia or monocytic angina with which it may be initially confused. Treatment is the province of a physician.

Leukaemic angina

Ulcerating lesions similar to those seen in agranulocytosis and glandular fever may be seen on the tonsils of patients suffering from acute leukaemia. In the commoner myelogenous type nearly all the circulating white cells are myeloblasts and there is a severe and progressive anaemia usually of a microcytic type. A leukaemic angina may simulate agranulocytic angina with a total white count below 1,000. But the high proportion of immature forms on differential count serves to distinguish from the latter.

KERATOSIS PHARYNGIS

This is a curious disease where the epithelium overlying aggregations of lymphoid tissue in the pharynx undergoes hypertrophy and keratinization with the production of discrete greyish-white horny spicules. These horny growths are found on the lingual tonsils, adenoids and on the lymphoid nodules that frequently become apparent on the posterior pharyngeal wall, as well as on the tonsils.

The tonsil crypts are the most frequent site of origin. In an advanced case the tonsil appears dotted with miniature cow-horns. Where the excrescences are small the condition may be confused with the caseous debris of chronic follicular (lacunar) tonsillitis but the keratotic spicules are more adherent and there is no surrounding inflammation.

The condition was formerly considered to be a mycosis because of the presence of numerous leptothrix filaments among the cornified epithelial cells. But the cause has still to be positively determined.

The excrescences cause little in the way of symptoms. But a patient looking for a source of discomfort or irritation in the throat may be alarmed at the appearance of the tonsils or pharynx. In fact the disease is benign and usually disappears spontaneously in time.

Treatment is symptomatic. There is no known specific cure. Excrescences recur if removed but it may increase comfort to scrape off all excess from the tonsil surfaces and treat with iodine (Mandl's) paint. An improvement in general health achieved by diet, holiday and exercise may have a beneficial influence.

FOREIGN BODY IN TONSIL

Apart from tonsillolith (p. 117) the only foreign bodies found in the tonsil with any degree of frequency are fish bones. Bones, or rather the fine cartilaginous filaments, from a herring or similar fish are especially liable to enter a crypt during swallowing and become impacted. If a patient complains of a bone stuck in the throat after eating such a fish the surgeon should pay particular attention to the tonsil area and inspect meticulously with a good headlight and mirror. It is an easy matter to extract a bone once located.

ELONGATED STYLOID PROCESS

In some cases ossification in the stylohyoid ligament prolongs the length of the styloid process until it comes into relation with the palatopharyngeus muscle. Occasionally it may penetrate the muscle and the tonsil. Such elongations are not infrequent but are of no importance unless giving rise to symptoms.

If a patient complains consistently of pain in the tonsil area, unilateral or bilateral, on swallowing, referred to the ear, and if the tonsils appear perfectly healthy without enlargement of regional lymph nodes and if nothing can be found on palpation of the neck or inspection of the pharynx to account for the dysphagia, an x-ray should be taken to exclude this condition. If the x-ray confirms the presence of elongated styloid process or processes and if finger pressure on the tonsil in a backward and downward direction reproduces the pain, a diagnosis of styloid neuralgia may be made.

Treatment

The necessity for treatment depends on the severity of pain. The only effective cure is to perform tonsillectomy, locate the tip of the elongated process and amputate a sufficient length to remove it from contact with the pharynx.

Technique

(1) Tonsillectomy (*see* p. 124).

(2) Finger palpation of the posterior half of the posterior wall of the tonsil fossa to locate the tip of the process.

(3) Delivery of the process through the muscle of the fossa palatopharyngeus by blunt separation of muscle fibres with non-toothed dissection forceps.

(4) Incision of periosteum over tip of process and careful stripping of periosteum from tip towards base of skull. As long as the plane of dissection is subperiosteal there is no risk of damage to adjacent structures.

(5) Amputation of exposed bony tip with bone forceps.

In unilateral cases it is advisable to remove the other tonsil in the interest of oropharyngeal symmetry.

REFERENCES

Bunyard, P. (1969). *Wld Med.*, **5**, 36.
Carter, R. L., and Penman, H. G. (1969). *Infectious Mononucleosis.* Oxford; Blackwell.
Collins, E. G. (1965). *Diseases of the Ear, Nose and Throat* (2nd ed., Vol. 2, p. 135). Ed. by W. G. Scott-Brown, J. Ballantyne and J. Groves. London; Butterworths.
Dudgeon, J. A. (1969). *Proc. R. Soc. Med.*, **62**, 1.

REFERENCES

Gibb, A. G. (1969). *J. Laryng.*, **83,** 1159.
Guggenheim, P. (1963). *Arch. Otolaryng.*, **77,** 13.
Livingstone, G. (1965). *Proc. R. Soc. Med.*, **58,** 65.
Malcomson, K. G. (1967). *Practitioner*, **199,** 777.
Malecki, J. (1958). *Arch. Otolaryng.*, **67,** 28.
Mawson, S. R. (1956). *Lancet*, **1,** 486.
— Adlington, P., and Evans, M. (1967). *J. Larying.*, **81,** 777.
McKee, W. J. (1963). *Brit. J. prev. soc. Med.*, **17,** 49.
McKenzie, W., and Woolf, C. I. (1959). *J. Laryng.*, **73,** 596.
Roydhouse, N. (1969). *Lancet*, **2,** 931.

145

7

TUMOURS OF THE PHARYNX

R. S. Lewis

INTRODUCTION

The pharynx runs from the base of the skull downwards to its junction with the oesophagus opposite the sixth cervical vertebra. Opening into it anteriorly are the cavities of the nose, the mouth and the larynx; hence these three regions are named the nasopharynx, oropharynx and laryngopharynx. Wood-Jones (1940) pointed out that morphologically and functionally the nasopharynx is a posterior extension of the nasal cavities and is not a part of the pharynx at all, but since no other generally acceptable name has been proposed the terms nasopharynx or postnasal space will continue to be used.

The pharynx contains tissues derived from all germinal layers and so theoretically almost any form of neoplasm may appear in it. Certain types, as will be seen, are far more common than others. Tumours of developmental origin and cysts will also be described though they are not true neoplasms.

The neoplasms of course may be benign or malignant and there are those which shade imperceptibly from one group into the other.

PATHOLOGY

Benign neoplasms

These are rare in the pharynx except for the soft palate and faucial areas. Papillomas are the commonest and, more rarely, pedunculated fibromas from the tonsils have been reported.

Scattered throughout the mucosa of the mouth and pharynx are numerous glands variously called mucinous, seromucinous or minor salivary glands. Simple adenomas can arise in them but appear to be extremely rare. Pleomorphic tumours, resembling the pleomorphic tumour of the major salivary glands, are more common and occur in these glands in all three of the pharyngeal regions, but again most commonly on the soft palate. They range in type from the completely benign mixed tumour to the frankly malignant carcinoma. The percentage of malignant cases is higher than in tumours of the major salivary glands.

Chondroma occurs occasionally, usually in the nasopharynx, and it is sometimes difficult to distinguish it histologically from low grade chondrosarcoma. It may arise from the cartilage of the intervertebral discs or of the eustachian tube.

Osteomas, myxomas and rhabdomyomas have been described but are seldom seen.

Malignant neoplasms

These are much more common than the benign growths. They are classified according to the tissue from which they arise.

Malignant neoplasms of epithelial origin

(a) Squamous cell carcinoma. Except for the upper part of the postnasal space the pharynx is lined by squamous epithelium and squamous cell carcinoma occurs throughout the region even in those areas of the postnasal space which are lined by ciliated columnar epithelium. All degrees of cellular differentiation may be found from the well differentiated growth to the completely undifferentiated one.

A special variety of epithelioma, to which the name lympho-epithelioma has been given, occurs in the nasopharynx and oropharynx where there are collections of subepithelial lymphoid tissue. Clinically it is characterized by its more frequent occurrence in young subjects, its tendency to early and widespread metastasis and its sensitivity to irradiation. Histologically there are masses of lymphocytes interspersed with which are columns and sheets, often syncitial, of epithelial cells with large pale vacuolated nuclei. This growth has caused confusion because some authors have classified it among the sarcomas and hence reports of the relative frequency of carcinoma and sarcoma in the pharynx are often not comparable.

Yeh (1962) extensively reviewed a series of 1,000 cases of carcinoma of the post-nasal space seen on the island of Formosa (Taiwan). He concluded that the lympho-epithelioma was not a separate entity but was an anaplastic carcinoma modified in appearance by arising in intimate association with subepithelial lymph tissues. This opinion is being generally endorsed by other pathologists. Its clinical characteristics, however, make it a useful subgroup to retain. The transitional cell carcinoma is another variety of epithelioma.

(b) Adenocarcinoma. Varieties of adenocarcinoma are muco-epidermoid carcinoma, adenoid cystic carcinoma, often called cylindroma, and acinic cell carcinoma. They metastasize late and are slow growing but infiltrate locally, particularly the adenoid cystic carcinoma, and are therefore difficult to eradicate. They are relatively radio-insensitive.

(c) Malignant pleomorphic tumours. These and adenocarcinomas are discussed more fully in the chapter on tumours of the salivary glands.

Malignant neoplasms of mesodermal or connective tissue origin

(a) Fibrosarcoma.

(b) Osteosarcoma.

(c) Rhabdomyosarcoma.

(d) Chondrosarcoma.

Since fibrous tissue, bone, muscle and cartilage are all present in the pharynx it is to be expected that sarcomatous change will take place in them but this occurrence is very rare.

Chordoma.—In man a few vestiges of the notochord may remain in the adult spinal column, particularly in the basioccipital and sacrococcygeal regions; in these vestiges the tumour known as chordoma may develop. Beaugié, Mann and Butler (1969) state that 41 per cent of chordomas occur in the basioccipital region. Histologically they consist of irregular groups of cells separated by fibrous tissue. The tumour cells contain mucus which sometimes pushes the nucleus to one side or is present as multiple vacuoles giving the bubbly appearance of the characteristic physaliphorous cell. Mucus also appears in the intercellular spaces. The tumour is locally malignant, widely infiltrating the surrounding tissues and invading bone and nerves. Reports of the occurrence of metastases vary from 5 to 43 per cent.

Malignant neoplasms of reticulo-endothelial origin

The naso- and oropharynx contain a good deal of lymphoid tissue and it is therefore not surprising that malignant lymphomas occur. McNelis and Pai (1969) report that of 153 cases of malignant lymphomas of the head and neck 16·3 per cent were found in these regions, most commonly on the faucial and lingual tonsils. The monocellular types. i.e. lymphosarcomas and reticulum cell sarcomas, greatly predominate but it is difficult to ascertain their frequency relative to the epitheliomas because of the histological confusions in the past. Lambert (1960) reported 133 carcinomas to 41 lympho- or reticulum cell sarcomas in the nasopharynx but this high incidence of sarcomas may be due to histological nomenclature rather than to basic pathology. MacComb and Fletcher (1967) report an incidence of 8·9 per cent and this may be nearer the mark in white races. Malignant lymphomas are rarer in the Chinese where their incidence in the nasopharynx is only 0·8 per cent of malignant tumours in this region (Yeh, 1962).

Extramedullary plasmacytoma

These are rare solitary tumours occurring in the upper respiratory and alimentary tracts. They are indistinguishable histologically from multiple myeloma but there are no Bence Jones proteins in the urine and the plasma proteins are unchanged. Metastasis to lymph nodes sometimes occurs and after many years true multiple myeloma may develop but this is not inevitable. The condition is said to be radiosensitive and the writer's experience confirms this.

Tumours of developmental origin

There are two main varieties.

(*a*) Branchiogenic cysts.
(*b*) Hamartomas or teratoid tumours of the nasopharynx (*see* p. 151).

Tumours of uncertain origin (juvenile angiofibroma)

Since this occurs only in the nasopharynx it will be described in that section.

Retention cysts

These are common on the tonsils but also occur occasionally throughout the pharynx, notably on the anterior surface of the epiglottis.

Tumours of the pharynx may be classified as in Table I.

TABLE I

TUMOURS OF THE PHARYNX

BENIGN	
Of epithelial origin	*Of mesodermal origin*
Papilloma	Lipoma
Adenoma (including the pleomorphic adenoma)	Fibroma
	Chondroma
	Osteoma
	Myoma

MALIGNANT	
Of epithelial origin	*Of mesodermal origin*
Squamous cell carcinoma (including transitional cell carcinoma and lympho-epithelioma)	Fibrosarcoma
	Rhabdomyosarcoma
	Chondrosarcoma
Adenocarcinoma	Osteosarcoma
Mucoepidermoid carcinoma	Chordoma
Adenoid cystic carcinoma	
Acinic cell carcinoma	
Malignant pleomorphic carcinoma	
Of reticulo-endothelial origin	
Lymphosarcoma	
Reticulum cell sarcoma	
Hodgkin's disease	
Giant follicular lymphoma	
Plasmocytoma	
Tumours of developmental origin	
Branchiogenic cysts	
Hamartomas	
Tumours of uncertain origin	
Juvenile angiofibroma of the nasopharynx	
Other tumours	
Simple retention cysts	

TUMOURS OF THE NASOPHARYNX

ANATOMY

The nasopharynx or postnasal space is a cavity, the roof of which is formed by the basisphenoid and basiocciput which slope downwards and backwards to merge with the posterior wall formed by the arch of the atlas and upper part of the body of the second cervical vertebra. The lateral part of the roof, over the pharyngeal recess, consists of the foramen lacerum and tip of the petrous temporal bone.

Laterally the space is bounded by the superior constrictor muscle and between the upper border of this muscle and the base of the skull (the sinus of Morgagni) pass the eustachian tube and levator palati muscle. Behind the opening of the eustachian tube is a lateral recess known as the pharyngeal recess or fossa of Rosenmüller. Anteriorly the space opens into the anterior choanae of the nose and inferiorly into the oropharynx. Its mucous membrane lining is of ciliated columnar epithelium above and squamous below. The exact proportion between the two types is very variable.

150

There is an extensive submucosal plexus of lymph vessels. Rouvière (1938) describes lateral and medial retropharyngeal lymph nodes into which this plexus drains. The medial retropharyngeal lymph nodes lie on either side of the midline posteriorly but are inconstant and often disappear in adult life. The main lymph node station is the lateral retropharyngeal nodes which lie high up in the parapharyngeal or lateral pharyngeal space near the base of the skull in front of the lateral mass of the atlas (Fig. 36). They are in relation posterolaterally with the

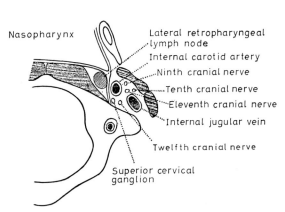

Nasopharynx

Lateral retropharyngeal lymph node
Internal carotid artery
Ninth cranial nerve
Tenth cranial nerve
Eleventh cranial nerve
Internal jugular vein
Twelfth cranial nerve
Superior cervical ganglion

FIG. 36.—Section through the nasopharynx showing its relationship to the parapharyngeal space and its contents. Note the lateral retropharyngeal lymph node (*adapted from Rouvière*).

internal carotid artery, jugular vein and the ninth, tenth, twelfth cranial nerves and the superior sympathetic ganglion. The nodes drain into the upper deep cervical nodes which also receive vessels direct from the postnasal space.

A knowledge of this anatomy helps greatly in understanding the symptoms of disease in this area.

DEVELOPMENTAL TUMOURS

Branchiogenic cysts

These are situated laterally and are derived from the inner end of the second branchial cleft. They are lined by ciliated columnar epithelium. Midline cysts from Rathke's pouch may also occur (Mills, 1955). They cause no symptoms until they are large enough to interfere with respiration. They have to be diagnosed from retention cysts and antrochoanal polyps and are best treated by excision; complete excision may not be necessary and removal of the anterior wall so as to marsupialize the cyst may be enough. Excision by the transpalatine route and aspiration and injection of sclerosing solutions have also been recommended.

Hamartomas or teratoid tumours

These result from an error of growth early in foetal life resulting in some cells being freed from the restraints of orderly physiological development. They grow concurrently with the host forming a mass of recognizable but unorganized tissue which contains examples of structures derived from two or more of the germinal layers. They are not true neoplasms but it is possible for neoplasms to develop in them at any period.

The most common are bidermal in origin and form the dermoid or hairy polyp of the postnasal space. They are covered with skin, contain fat and sometimes other mesodermal tissue and are usually pedunculated. Foxwell and Kelham (1958) found 89 reported in the literature. More complex hamartomas are much rarer; Howarth found six cases in the literature in 1938 and added one of his own. The writer has seen two solid sessile complex hamartomas (reported by Foxwell and Kelham) in the postnasal space of two new-born children, one of which contained well-formed tissues derived from all three germ layers.

Clinical aspects.—The majority of hairy polyps are pedunculated so that the symptoms of dyspnoea, cyanosis, and coughing may be intermittent and the polyp is sometimes visible in the mouth.

Large sessile tumours will not only completely obstruct the normal airway but will depress the soft palate and impede mouth breathing as well. The danger of asphyxiation and difficulties in feeding may therefore be much greater than in congenital choanal atresia.

The diagnosis rarely presents difficulty since the tumours can usually be seen projecting below the level of the soft palate on oral examination. A lateral soft tissue radiograph will usually show a mass in the nasopharynx.

Treatment.—In newly-born infants this should be delayed when the symptoms are not severe, but occasionally immediate operation is needed because of respiratory obstruction. A general anaesthetic is advisable; pedunculated polyps are removed with a snare but sessile tumours may be seized with grasping forceps passed behind the soft palate and avulsed. The amount of bleeding after this manoeuvre in the writer's two cases was slight and both children recovered without any sequelae.

BENIGN NEOPLASMS

These are exceedingly uncommon in the nasopharynx. Those most often seen are chondromas and pleomorphic tumours. They should be removed and Wilson's transpalatine approach is useful for this purpose, but in both instances complete removal may be impossible and malignant change may supervene.

MALIGNANT NEOPLASMS

Squamous cell carcinoma, in its varying degrees of differentiation, is by far the most common; next come lymphosarcoma and reticulum cell sarcoma. Adenocarcinoma, chondrosarcoma and chordoma are rare. Stout and Kenney (1949) collected from the literature 24 cases of plasmacytoma arising in the nasopharynx but more have been added since. Other malignancies have been reported. Differentiation of these lesions depends upon microscopic examination and so the following description will be based almost entirely on the carcinomas and lymphomas.

Aetiology

Squamous cell carcinoma of the nasopharynx has an interesting racial distribution. Sturton, Wen and Sturton (1966) report that it is common in Cantonese population of the Kwantung province of China, Hong Kong and Macao. In

Hong Kong it accounts for 13 per cent of all deaths from cancer as compared with about 0·5 per cent in most other countries. They say that as far as they know this high incidence does not occur in the rest of China. However, it is also prevalent in the Chinese of Singapore and Taiwan (Formosa). California has a large Chinese population, mainly derived from the Kwantung province. According to Buell (1965) the incidence of postnasal carcinoma in the Chinese who have emigrated to California is as high as that in Kwantung, and a male native born Chinaman in California is 40 times more likely than a white Californian to develop this neoplasm. In the first generation of Californian born Chinamen this ratio drops to 20 to 1. At first sight this would seem to indicate that environment plays a large part in causing this growth but Buell thinks that a genetic tendency is the more important factor and points out that immigration to California could create a genetic selectivity which would account for the drop in frequency seen in the first generation Chinese. There may also be a genetic–environmental interaction. Sturton, Wen and Sturton suggest that environment is the more important factor and from statistics compiled from Hong Kong bring some evidence to show that exposure to the smoke of incense burning may play a part.

Other races such as the Malays and Kenya Africans also have a high incidence of postnasal cancer.

Males are more commonly affected than females and the growth is more common after the age of 40. Lympho-epitheliomas however arise in younger patients and it is not uncommon to find them in patients under the age of 20.

Site of origin

This is difficult to determine in the majority of cases since by the time they are seen the growths already occupy a large part of the postnasal space. When the growth has been small enough to determine its site of origin, in the writer's experience this has been in most cases on the vault of the nasopharynx just above and behind the posterior margin of the septum. It also often arises from the fossa of Rosenmüller or the lip of the eustachian tube.

Spread

The more differentiated carcinomas tend to be ulcerative in type while the anaplastic ones, the lympho-epitheliomas and sarcomas are exophytic and often form massive outgrowths. Spread posterolaterally takes place through the sinus of Morgagni to the parapharyngeal space (Fig. 36) where lie the great vessels, the last four cranial nerves and the sympathetic chain. Paralysis of the nerves may follow but involvement of the vessels is rare. More direct lateral spread will involve the mandibular nerve as it emerges from the foramen ovale. More commonly, however, the fifth and sixth nerves are involved intracranially by spread of the growth through the foramen lacerum, which forms part of the roof of the fossa of Rosenmüller. This spread accounts for the many cases of intracranial nerve involvement in which there is no radiological evidence of bone destruction.

The carcinomas, but not the malignant lymphomas, may involve bone and erosion of the tip of the petrous part of the temporal bone and of the basisphenoid and basiocciput occurs (Fig. 37). The sphenoid sinus may also be invaded and lateral spread will destroy the pterygoid plates and the foramina ovale et spinosum.

The eustachian tube is of course very vulnerable to the spread of postnasal growths.

153

Invasion of the orbit with proptosis and involvement of the optic nerve is rare and is more suggestive of a growth arising from the posterior ethmoid region.

Downward extension to the oropharynx and forwards into the nasal cavities is seen in very large growths.

Lymphatic spread.—It is a characteristic of postnasal carcinomas and sarcomas to give rise to early and widespread lymph node metastases and the great majority of cases have palpable nodes when first seen. Bilateral invasion is more frequent than unilateral. These nodes are usually the upper deep cervical nodes but the

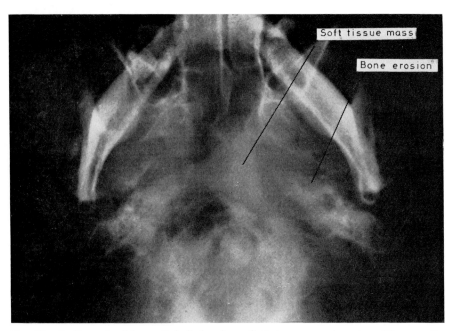

Soft tissue mass

Bone erosion

FIG. 37.—Radiograph of base of skull showing soft tissue mass and erosion of bone on the left side in a case of carcinoma of the nasopharynx.

middle and lower deep cervical and the accessory and supraclavicular nodes are also often enlarged. The submaxillary and sublingual nodes are frequently involved and the high lateral retropharyngeal nodes, which may well be the first affected in the majority of cases, are beyond the reach of the examining fingers. More than one group of nodes are commonly enlarged.

Distant spread to the lungs, bones and other viscera eventually occurs.

Symptoms

It can be readily understood from the anatomy and mode of spread that malignant disease in the postnasal space can cause a variety of symptoms which may be grouped into four main categories.

(*a*) Cervical (lymph node enlargement)

(*b*) Nasal

(*c*) Otological

(*d*) Neurological.

The first symptom may come from any of these categories but the most commonly presenting one is enlargement of cervical lymph nodes. The others follow in the above order of frequency but only too often symptoms from two or more of the categories are already present when the patient is first seen.

Cervical symptoms

The clinical character of the enlarged lymph nodes can be very varied; they may of course be hard and fixed with infiltration of the surrounding tissues so that their malignant nature is obvious but before this stage is reached they may be small, soft, mobile and discrete. In between these extremes any degree of hardness and fixation may be encountered. It must be emphasized that any enlarged lymph node—or other similar swelling of the neck at any age—must be regarded with suspicion and a thorough search made for a primary infective or malignant focus before resorting to excision for biopsy (Fig. 38).

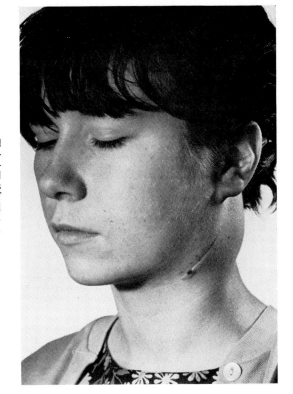

FIG. 38.—Biopsy of enlarged cervical lymph nodes. The pathologist reported lympho-epithelioma and suggested examination of the postnasal space where the primary growth was found. This examination should of course be done as a routine in all cases of cervical swelling and would have made this biopsy unnecessary.

Although the upper deep cervical nodes are the ones most commonly palpable the whole neck on each side must be carefully examined and with the malignant lymphomas the question of involvement of the superior mediastinal nodes should also be considered.

Nasal symptoms

Partial nasal obstruction is first noticed, then slight nose bleeds or blood stained nasal discharge. Hawking of blood into the mouth also occurs.

Otological symptoms

Extension to the eustachian tube will cause conductive deafness with a retracted tympanic membrane or a serous exudate in the middle ear and these signs demand a careful examination of the postnasal space.

Neurological symptoms

Clinically it has been shown that the second division of the fifth is the first cranial nerve to be involved, followed by the abducens nerve. This is consistent with the position of these nerves above the foramen lacerum through which the growth reaches them. Theoretically, however, as Flatman (1954) has pointed out, the nerve of the pterygoid canal should be involved first by this route of spread but tests for its function (i.e. Schirmer's test) are seldom carried out and so clinical proof is as yet lacking. Pain in the cheek and region of the maxillary sinus and upper teeth, paraesthesias such as irritations and mild burning sensations and anaesthesia in these areas should all arouse suspicion of a nasopharyngeal neoplasm.

Paralyses of the oculomotor nerves and of the last four cranial nerves are easily detectable on routine examination but perhaps Schirmer's test should be more frequently employed. Homonymous hemianopia through involvement of the optic tract which lies close to the foramen lacerum is another possibility and might be looked for since patients often do not complain of this symptom even when it is present.

Diagnosis

It would seem therefore that the diagnosis of the presence of a malignant growth in the nasopharynx should be a relatively easy matter and indeed this is so in the majority of cases. However, when the presenting symptoms are cervical or neurological the patient may be first referred to a general physician or surgeon, a neurologist or an ophthalmic surgeon. Neurologists and ophthalmic surgeons are aware of the importance of nasopharyngeal tumours in causing otherwise unexplained ocular, other cranial nerve palsies and "neuralgias" and usually call in the otolaryngologist. The others still too often remove a node for histological examination before examining the postnasal space. This perhaps occurs more frequently in patients in the younger age groups where the nodes are fairly soft and discrete and where the diagnosis of Hodgkin's disease or tuberculous adenitis is thought likely (Fig. 38). The condition is not uncommon in teenagers and should not be discounted on age alone.

The final diagnosis depends upon histological examination of a biopsy from the nasopharynx.

Examination

Indirect examination with a postnasal mirror is satisfactory in the majority of cases and will reveal the tumour as an ulcerated area or a fungating mass of friable rather vascular tissue. It is usually difficult to determine its exact site of origin. Large lesions may extend downwards, depressing the soft palate and appearing in the oropharynx either in the midline or on the lateral wall behind the tonsil, sometimes lying underneath an intact mucosa.

There are a few patients, adults as well as children, who cannot tolerate examination with a postnasal mirror, even after thorough local analgesia. The nasopharyngoscope may help in some of these. It is built on the lines of a small cystoscope and gives a right-angled view. The examination is conducted under local analgesia with the patient in a semi-recumbent position. The instrument is warmed and gently slid along the floor of the nose under visual control. The middle turbinate and posterior edge of the septum are guides on the way to the nasopharynx where the orifices of the eustachian tubes are other landmarks. By rotating the nasopharyngoscope most of the postnasal space can be brought into view but it must be admitted the instrument does not give as much help as might be expected. However, it may help to decide, in doubtful cases, whether a patient need be admitted for examination under an anaesthetic or not.

Biopsy

This is necessary to confirm the diagnosis and to demonstrate the type of growth, since knowledge of its histology is essential for planning treatment and estimating prognosis. Often the biopsy can be carried out under local analgesia without admitting the patient. If the growth is large and low it can be done through the mouth with a biopsy forceps inserted up behind the soft palate. Otherwise the nose should be anaesthetized and a Grunewald's or cupped forceps passed along the floor of the nose to the postnasal space. If necessary its direction can be controlled with a postnasal mirror.

Radiological examination

Lateral soft tissue radiographs and sagittal tomographs will help to show the size and spread of a neoplasm and may possibly even demonstrate one that had not been detected clinically. The submentovertical view (*see* Fig. 37) is useful in showing the extent of bony involvement which may include destruction of the pterygoid plates, the foramina at the base of the skull and walls of the sphenoid sinus. Beside destructive lesions osteoblastic reactions may occur. Coronal tomograms will also show bony lesions of the base of the skull.

Examination under anaesthesia

This may be necessary to take a biopsy and to visualize the space when posterior rhinoscopy is impossible or fails to show a strongly suspected lesion.

The patient lies supine with the head extended and anaesthesia is administered through an oral armoured endotracheal tube which is lifted out of the way with a Doughty blade in a Davis Boyle gag, as in tonsillectomy. The soft palate is retracted with small retractors or with fine rubber catheters passed through the nose and brought out through the mouth. A large laryngeal mirror placed in the oropharynx will then enable a close inspection to be made of all parts of the nasopharynx. A biopsy can be taken from any suspected area under visual control through the mirror, the forceps being passed down one of the nostrils. A magnified view and photographs of the nasopharynx can be obtained by using a Zeiss microscope with a 300–400 mm. objective.

Additional information can be obtained by palpation with the forefinger but this examination should be left to the last since it may cause bleeding. The writer has never found Yankauer's postnasal speculum to be of much help.

Exploration of the nasopharynx

The nasopharynx is notorious as being a region where it may be very difficult to demonstrate a primary neoplasm even though it may be strongly suspected. Wilson (1957) reported five cases where the mucosa of the pharyngeal recess after surgical exposure looked normal and yet a deep biopsy showed a carcinoma to be present, and others have had similar experiences.

To explore the nasopharynx a slightly forward-curved incision is made 0·5 cm. in front of the posterior border of the hard palate. Laterally it turns backwards to the inner side of the tuberosities and the greater palatine foramina. The projecting spine of the palate is removed and the mucosa of the upper surface incised so that the postnasal space is entered. The incisions are carried backwards along the pterygomandibular raphé until the soft palate is mobilized enough to drop back exposing the space. This may entail division of the hamulus of the internal pterygoid plate or of the tendon of the tensor palati muscle. If carefully stitched this incision heals well.

A permanent opening for inspection or treatment of the space can be obtained by omitting the posterior prolongations of the incision and adding a midline incision on the hard palate. These mucosal flaps are elevated. The bone of the hard palate is removed with hammer and gouge without damaging the mucosa on its upper surface and the posterior part of the septum is excised submucosally. The mucosa of the floor of the nose is incised in such a way that it can be turned laterally and sutured to the mucosa of the inferior surface of the palate to cover the raw areas. A dental obturator must be made to close the defect.

Cases needing this type of exploration are very rare and careful examination will reveal the growth in the great majority. A deep biopsy through normal mucous membrane, either blind through the nose or by the transpalatine approach, should be considered, however, when suspicion is directed to the nasopharynx: for example when there is an enlarged upper deep cervical lymph node and an unexplained cranial nerve palsy.

Differential diagnosis

This depends finally upon the biopsy. Cysts and antrochoanal polypi are smooth, pale and grey in appearance and their nature is usually obvious. Chondromas and chordomas present as firm smooth swellings covered by intact normal epithelium. Juvenile angiofibromas and hamartomas are discussed elsewhere in this chapter. If the biopsies of a granulomatous or ulcerating area are constantly negative Wegener's type granuloma must be thought of, though its limitation entirely to the postnasal space must be very rare indeed. One source of trouble may be the condition known as Thornwaldt's bursitis; in this there is an area of pus and crusting on the roof of the postnasal space. It is said to be due to infection in the pharyngeal bursa. The crusts may prevent a proper view of the mucosa so examination under anaesthesia may be needed.

Persistence of adenoid tissue into adult life can cause confusion and adenoidectomy may have to be considered to obtain tissue for section.

Treatment

External irradiation is the treatment of choice and it is agreed that the properties of supervoltage radiation make it very suitable for its use in nasopharyngeal carcinomas, though orthovoltage may be adequate for the malignant lymphomas.

The anatomy of the nasopharynx makes a complete surgical resection impossible and intracavity irradiation gives an insufficient depth-dose and should be used only for some cases of recurrence. The results of chemotherapy with cytotoxic drugs are disappointing and this method can be regarded only as an adjuvent to radiotherapy in a few selected cases.

In planning treatment consideration of the extent of the primary growth and its histological character is of paramount importance. A large tumour with bone destruction and cranial nerve involvement has such a poor prognosis that a palliative course of treatment may be the wisest thing to offer. If during this treatment the response of the tumour is better than expected, it can be extended to a full course.

The primary growth and all its possible areas of local spread should be included in the treatment field but, owing to the risk of injury to the central nervous system, the middle cranial fossa is omitted unless there is evidence of its involvement. The field is checked radiographically.

These tumours metastasize so readily to the lymph nodes on both sides of the neck that, although no nodes may be palpable, the probability of microscopic deposits being present is high. The submental and submaxillary nodes are rarely involved, but with these exceptions the whole lymphatic areas of the neck should therefore also be irradiated on both sides.

In general, a tumour dose of 6500–7500 rad. in about six to seven weeks is desirable in all varieties of carcinoma. The malignant lymphomas and plasmocytomas respond to a smaller dose and 4000–5000 rad. in four to five weeks is usually enough.

The high dose and large fields recommended for the carcinomas are often more than can be tolerated and when this is so, the dose to the lower cervical lymph fields may be reduced to 5000 rad. or less if there are no nodes palpable. The response of both normal tissue and growth to radiotherapy is unpredictable.

For recurrences Snelling (1954) says that another full course of treatment will give a worthwhile, though temporary, regression. The nasopharynx seems to be very tolerant of irradiation but the risk of severe radionecrosis and transverse myelitis must not be forgotten.

Intracavity irradiation through a palatal fenestration by means of an intra-oral x-ray cone or by the implantation of seeds, and even surgical removal through the fenestration have all been tried, but it is doubtful whether the results justify the discomforts and the post-operative defects of the operation.

Intra-arterial infusion of cytotoxic drugs may be considered when pain cannot be relieved by simpler methods.

If, after treatment has been finished and the primary growth has apparently healed, operable enlargement of lymph nodes appears in the neck there should be no hesitation in performing a radical neck dissection. It is not often that such a situation arises but it should be accepted since operation gives a good chance of eradicating the disease.

Results

The prognosis is very much influenced by the histological type of the neoplasm. Lederman (1961) reported the following five-year survival rates:

Epithelioma	13 per cent
Lympho-epithelioma	20 per cent
Sarcoma of lymphoid tissue	33 per cent

The better prognosis for the lympho-epitheliomas and lymphomas is confirmed by most other writers.

CHORDOMA

The majority of chordomas presenting in the nasopharynx are probably downward extensions from cranio-occipital tumours but some may be primarily naso-pharyngeal. They cause headache, nasal obstruction and, later, cranial nerve palsies. They are slow growing and present as a smooth non-ulcerated swelling in the naso-pharynx; diagnosis depends on biopsy.

Radiographs and tomographs (Fig. 39) are useful to show the size of the tumour and extent of bone destruction.

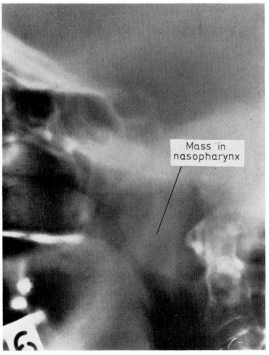

Mass in nasopharynx

FIG. 39.—Tomograph showing a large smooth mass in the nasopharynx. Biopsy showed it to be a chordoma.

Treatment

Wright (1967) in a wide survey of the subject states that complete surgical removal is usually not possible because of the bone involvement. In purely nasopharyngeal cases bone may not be affected and an attempt at removal through a transpalatine approach is probably justifiable. Chordoma is said to be radio-insensitive but it is not completely so (Windeyer, 1959) and radiotherapy is worth trying when removal is not possible. Even though the lesion may not disappear it may get smaller and its growth rate may be diminished so that some palliation is achieved.

JUVENILE ANGIOFIBROMA

This is a tumour which occurs in the nasopharynx of males between the ages of 10 and 20. It is doubtful whether it is a true tumour and Willis (1953) looks upon it as a form of immune response. Osborn (1959) suggests it is an overgrowth of erectile tissue in the postnasal space following the hormonal changes of puberty. Hayes Martin claimed that many of the cases showed evidence of delayed sexual development but most other reports fail to confirm this.

It has a broad base of origin in the nasopharynx and will gradually fill the space and grow into the nose, the pterygopalatine fossa, the temporal fossa and even into the cranial cavity. It may form new attachments in these areas.

There is said to be a tendency to spontaneous regression around the age of 25 but it is rarely possible to wait for this event. However, gradual disappearance of tumour remaining after incomplete removal, without further treatment, has been recorded on several occasions.

Cases apparently occurring in females and adults should be regarded with some doubt.

Pathology

The tumour has two main components: vascular and fibrous, the former being probably the basic one. Härmä (1959) recognizes two types of blood vessels: the first consists of arterial and venous channels, some of which are deficiently developed, and the second, of thin walled vessels which may form large lacunae or smaller channels of capillary size. The more slowly growing tumours show a larger number of blood vessels of wide calibre with relatively few proliferating phenomena in the vessel walls.

Symptoms and signs

Gradually increasing nasal obstruction and recurrent severe epistaxis lead to inspection of the postnasal space where a red, vascular, lobulated, non-ulcerated swelling will be seen. It is firm and bleeds readily and the patient is often therefore very anaemic. In advanced cases there is gross deformity of the nose and face and the tumour may be visible in the nose.

Lateral radiographs and tomographs confirm the presence of the tumour and angiograms will show its very vascular nature. The angiogram is so typical that many authors advise against biopsy because of the risk of severe haemorrhage. If it is done it should be carried out under general anaesthesia with full facilities for stopping bleeding and for giving a blood transfusion.

An antrochoanal polyp is softer and greyer while malignant neoplasms are more friable and ulcerated.

Treatment

Many cases are far advanced when first seen and a successful result may be difficult to achieve. The mortality rate appears to be about 6 per cent.

After correction of the anaemia and the patient's general condition as far as possible there are three lines of treatment to choose from.

161

Surgical removal. Access is through the transpalatine approach but this may need to be supplemented in extensive growths by the Caldwell–Luc or Denker's incisions or even lateral rhinotomy. Removal of the posterior part of the hard palate will allow access to intranasal extensions.

The mucous membrane should be incised down through the periosteum around the tumour and with strong periosteal elevators and gauze dissection it can often be separated without severe haemorrhage. Diathermy and cryosurgery will also help to limit bleeding.

Radiotherapy has had mixed results. Recently Fitzpatrick (1967) reported six cases treated with a dose to the midline of 3500 rad. in three weeks. There was little immediate response but gradual diminution in size took place over the following months till finally the tumours disappeared altogether, though in some cases not till a whole year had elapsed. The writer has seen two cases treated at Mount Vernon Hospital in a similar manner. In the first 6000 rad. were given with complete disappearance of the tumour in seven months. In the second gradual reduction in size was also taking place satisfactorily after 4000 rad. in four weeks, but the surgeon in charge was impatient and removed the residual mass. The final result in both cases was complete eradication of the angiofibroma.

Hormonal therapy. The results of this form of treatment have also been variable. Both oestrogens and testosterone have been used with success, though failure to influence the lesion is much more common. Improvement can occur in patients who show no evidence of hormonal imbalance (Henderson and Patterson, 1969).

Summary of treatment

Small tumours should be treated by surgery. Capps (1961) reports success in six cases.

When extension into the nose or elsewhere is present radiotherapy on the lines indicated should be given a trial; any residual tumour, after a long interval for observation, being treated surgically.

Hormonal treatment is worth trying if the above methods fail to control the lesion.

TUMOURS OF THE OROPHARYNX

ANATOMY

The oropharynx is that part of the pharynx which is situated behind the mouth. The soft palate forms its upper limit but there is no anatomical lower boundary. This is usually defined as being at the level of a horizontal line drawn through the hyoid bone. The anterior pillar of the fauces, the tonsils, the lateral and posterior pharyngeal walls and the base of the tongue complete the oropharynx. The anterior pillars and soft palate are often referred to as the palatine arch and the retromolar trigone is usually included. This trigone is a small triangular area, the base of which lies behind the last lower molar tooth with its apex pointing towards the tuberosity of the maxilla. The oropharynx is lined by non-keratinizing squamous epithelium which contains seromucinous glands of the salivary type and small subepithelial collections of lymphoid tissue. The faucial and lingual tonsils form larger masses of this tissue.

The free part of the epiglottis projects upwards into the oropharynx but this, with the valleculae and aryepiglottic folds, will be considered as the marginal zone in the section on the laryngopharynx.

Functionally the oropharynx is concerned with swallowing and it allows the passage of air as well as food and drink.

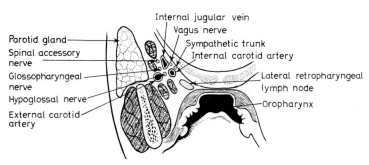

FIG. 40.—Section of neck showing the relationship of the parapharyngeal space to the oropharynx (*adapted from St. Clair Thomson and Negus*).

The lymphatic vessels of the oropharynx are numerous and drain mainly into the jugulodigastric node but the upper deep cervical nodes and the lateral retropharyngeal nodes also receive afferents from this region.

Laterally, it is in relationship with the great vessels and nerves of the neck in the parapharyngeal space (Fig. 40).

BENIGN NEOPLASMS

Except for the papillomas and pleomorphic tumours these are extremely rare. The papillomas arise on the soft palate or anterior faucial pillars and form soft mobile warty growths. They are usually small and are discovered as a rule by accident. They are easily removed under topical analgesia with scissors or a snare.

Pedunculated fibromas on the tonsils have been reported and the writer has seen only one simple adenoma in this region.

Neoplasms arise in the glands of the mucous membrane of the soft palate and are usually of the pleomorphic salivary gland type which are considered fully elsewhere.

Plasmacytomas have been recorded in the tonsils and haemangiomas on the soft palate (Eggston and Wolff, 1947). Osteomas and chondromas may bulge into the oropharynx from the anterior surface of the vertebral column.

MALIGNANT NEOPLASMS

Pathology

Malignant disease occurs in each of the subdivisions of the oropharynx and there are some differences in behaviour and prognosis in each site. The growths however are in the main similar and will be considered together, the more important differences being pointed out when indicated.

The most common malignant neoplasm is the squamous cell carcinoma. It may occur in any degree of differentiation, the more highly differentiated ones appearing as a rule on the soft palate and fauces. Carcinomas of the tonsil and base of the tongue are nearly always anaplastic.

Lympho-epithelioma is uncommon and even more rare are the various types of adenocarcinoma and the malignant pleomorphic tumour. Lymphosarcoma and reticulum cell sarcoma arise in the faucial and lingual tonsils.

Malignant mesodermal tumours are so rare as hardly to deserve more than passing mention.

Aetiology

Squamous cell cancer is uncommon before the age of 50 but increases in frequency thereafter. Men are about five times more often affected than women. Keratosis with dysplasia is well recognized as a pre-cancerous condition in the mouth but it seldom occurs in the oropharynx except on the palatine arch. As with oral cancer, there is strong evidence that tobacco smoking and chewing are important causal factors: Wynder, Bross and Feldman (1957) incriminate cigars and pipes more than cigarettes. Alcohol usually in the form of spirits may also be a predisposing cause but nearly all heavy drinkers are heavy smokers and it is difficult therefore to determine its true importance. The mucosal atrophy associated with iron deficiency anaemia seems often to be the precursor of oropharyngeal cancer in women. Syphilis and dental sepsis are no longer important factors in this country. Another primary growth in the upper alimentary tract or lung is found in about 10 per cent of cases of squamous cell carcinoma of the mouth and oropharynx.

Lymph node involvement

According to MacComb and Fletcher (1967) and Terz and Farr (1967) about 70 per cent of carcinomas of the base of tongue and tonsil present with nodal involvement. The growths arising from the palatine arch are less aggressive and enlarged nodes are present in about 50 per cent of cases when first seen. Bilateral involvement is common from base of tongue and central soft palate lesions.

The jugulodigastric node is the one most frequently involved but deposits may occur in any node of the cervical field. This possibility, together with the fact that the metastasis may skip intervening nodes (Toker, 1963) makes anything less than a complete neck dissection an uncertain method of eradicating the disease. Distant metastases may be more common than has been suspected in the past and an incidence of up to 57 per cent of distant metastases has been reported in patients dying of head and neck cancer by Gowen and de Suto-Nagy (1963). Arons and Smith (1961) put the incidence lower at 23 per cent. In most of these cases local disease was still present.

Staging

It is difficult to devise satisfactory staging in the T.N.M. notation for these lesions. Since the size of the primary growth has been shown to correlate well with the prognosis the following scheme has been suggested:

T_1—Tumours less than 2 cm. in diameter.
T_2—Tumours between 2 cm. and 4 cm. in diameter.
T_3—Tumours more than 4 cm. in diameter.
T_4—Massive tumours.

Symptoms

A growth in the oropharynx may become quite large before attracting attention. The first symptom is usually a disturbance of swallowing variously described as a soreness or pain or a pricking sensation as the food is passing down. Occasionally blood is spat up or the growth may be seen by a dental surgeon or the patient himself. Not uncommonly the appearance of a lump in the neck is the only abnormality noticed by the patient. Pain referred to the ear, via the tympanic branch of the glossopharyngeal nerve, excessive salivation and foetor are late symptoms.

Examination

Two main clinical types of squamous cell carcinoma may be recognized: the exophytic (Fig. 41) and the ulcerative (Fig. 42). The exophytic type tends to spread superficially and the ulcerative type infiltrates deeply, but exceptions occur. An adenocarcinoma presents as a smooth non-ulcerated swelling and the malignant lymphomas as enlargements in the tonsillar fossae or base of the tongue. Ulceration supervenes eventually.

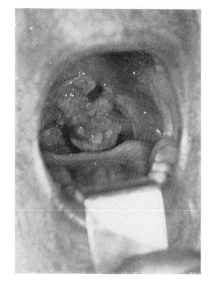

Fig. 41.—Carcinoma of the soft palate and uvula. Exophytic type.

Provided good lighting is used the growths can be seen easily, though for those originating in the base of the tongue a laryngeal mirror is needed. Note should be made of any fixation of the palate or tongue and palpation with the forefinger will help in estimating the extent of infiltration. Palpation is especially important when the base of the tongue is suspected because the growth may start deep in the crypts of the lymphoid tissue and be invisible in the early stages. A postnasal mirror should be used to detect extension into the nasopharynx or on to the upper surface of the soft palate.

The importance of careful palpation of the neck must not be forgotten. It is done from behind and the lymph node areas should each be examined in turn, first lightly with the tips of the fingers and then deeply by picking up the tissues deep to the sternomastoid muscle with the fingers and thumb. It cannot be too strongly emphasized that one must not wait until a node is stony hard and fixed before diagnosing a metastasis; in the earlier stages of involvement the node in most cases remains discrete and mobile and may be no more than firm to the touch. In a few cases the enlargement and fixation of a node may be so rapid as to suggest a subacute infection.

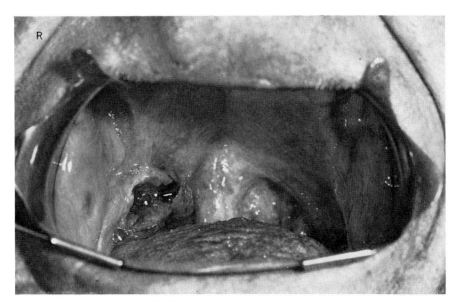

FIG. 42.—Carcinoma of the right tonsil, ulcerative type.

Radiology is of help only in tumours of the base of the tongue and of the posterior pharyngeal wall (Fig. 43).

Diagnosis

This is usually not difficult since most chronic ulcerative or proliferative lesions in the oropharynx turn out to be malignant. A biopsy, however, is necessary to confirm the diagnosis and to establish the histology of the growth, since this is of importance in planning treatment. In most cases the biopsy can be done under topical analgesia but a general anaesthetic may be needed in base of the tongue lesions. The anaesthetic will also help in determining the extent of the growth by allowing deep palpation in this region. Small smooth non-ulcerated lesions should be dealt with by wide excisional biopsy. In larger lesions of this kind a piece should be taken for section after reflecting healthy mucosa which is then sewn up again. Since these swellings often turn out to belong to one of the radio-insensitive adenocarcinoma groups needing wide surgical excision it is advisable to have this information beforehand, so that the patient can be prepared both mentally and physically for an extensive and possibly mutilating operation.

On the soft palate, keratosis and nicotine stomatitis raise problems as to whether malignant change has supervened. Cytological examination of scrapings from suspected areas may be helpful in these cases. Similarly, if the lesion is cleaned, dried and painted with toluidine blue 2 per cent aqueous solution and examined after the area has been washed with water any malignant change will be shown up as a deeply staining area. The writer has not found this a very reliable test but it may be occasionally helpful.

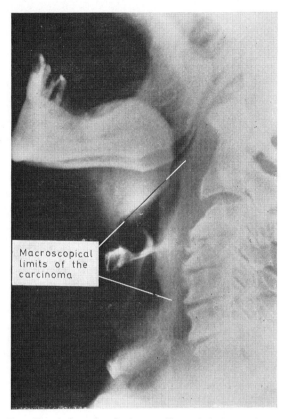

Fig. 43.—A lateral soft tissue radiograph helps to show the extent of a carcinoma of the posterior wall of the oropharynx.

Chest radiographs and blood examinations, including serological tests for syphilis, should be routine and will eliminate tuberculosis, syphilis and the blood dyscrasias from the diagnosis. A double pathology is of course always possible. A gumma before breaking down may resemble an adenocarcinoma or sarcoma and very occasionally an indolent quinsy may look like a lymphosarcoma of the tonsil. In more acute ulcers a throat swab may demonstrate Vincent's organism.

Neurilemmomas of the vagus nerve or sympathetic chain, mixed tumours of the deep portion of the parotid gland and glomus tumours sometimes form a smooth bulge in the lateral pharyngeal wall behind the tonsil pushing it forwards and medially. Secondary deposits in the tonsils have been described from bronchial carcinoma and testicular seminoma. Tonsiloliths may be deceptive and bilateral lymphosarcomas of the tonsils sometimes occur.

If biopsies are consistently non-specific the possibility of Wegener's type granuloma must be considered.

Every attempt must be made to get an immediate diagnosis: it is never justifiable to wait and see.

Treatment

The treatment of malignant growths of the oropharynx is difficult and should be carried out in a clinic where informed surgical and radiotherapeutical opinion is available and where a planned policy for all the types of malignancy has been decided upon. The cure rates in such clinics are higher and improve as knowledge and experience accumulates.

As in most cancer of the head and neck, treatment may be by radiotherapy or surgery or by a combination of the two. Cytotoxic drugs may also have a place in certain cases.

In planning treatment the size, site and histology of the growth and the state of the lymph nodes are important factors. The age, general condition, habits, mental stability and occupation also need consideration.

In small (i.e. less than 1 cm. in diameter) well differentiated carcinomas trans-oral resection and radiotherapy give about equal rates of cure but radiotherapy is usually preferred. However, radiotherapy has its drawbacks: it is a prolonged treatment often causing dysphagia and pain during the treatment and an uncomfortable dryness of the mouth and loss of taste afterwards. In these small lesions therefore resection may be considered, especially when the patient is frail or elderly or in alcoholics who are said to stand irradiation poorly, provided the resection can be done without disturbing the function of swallowing.

Since the small well-differentiated lesions we have just been discussing nearly all arise from the palatal arch from which lymph node metastases are relatively uncommon an elective neck dissection need not be done.

All varieties of adenocarcinomas are relatively radio-insensitive and should be treated by excision. The excision should be particularly radical for adenoid cystic carcinoma which infiltrates widely along perineural spaces.

Apart from these exceptions radiotherapy is the most generally accepted form of treatment for all malignant disease of the oropharynx and radiotherapists are agreed on the superior merits of supervoltage irradiation. Exophytic growths respond better than infiltrative ones; for the more extensive infiltrative lesions MacComb and Fletcher (1967) recommend reviewing the position after 5000 rad. have been delivered in five weeks. If the response has been poor the irradiation is stopped and radical surgical excision undertaken in five or six weeks' time.

Of equal importance to the primary growth in planning treatment are the cervical lymph node areas. Even when there is no palpable enlargement the possibility of a microscopic deposit remains high, and bilateral involvement is common in anaplastic and lymphomatous growths of the base of tongue and midline soft palate.

Radiotherapists vary in their approach to this problem and only a rough approximation of dosage and fields can be given. For details special works on the subject should be consulted.

For T_1N_0 and T_2N_0 *well differentiated* carcinomas the field is designed to irradiate the primary growth and an adequate surrounding area of healthy tissue. From its very nature the field will include the immediate lymph drainage areas, but no attempt is made to treat the whole neck. A tumour dose of 6500 to 7000 rad. in about 6–7 weeks using supervoltage is aimed at.

In larger carcinomas and in poorly differentiated growths, whether lymph nodes are palpable or not, the whole neck should be irradiated as well. Some patients are unable to tolerate the high dose to such a large field and if the state of the nodes allows it the last 1000–1500 rad. can be given through reduced fields to the primary growth only. When the primary tumour approaches the midline and in all base of tongue tumours both sides of the neck should be included.

For the malignant lymphoma group complete coverage of the cervical lymph node field is necessary but the total dose need not be so high—4000–5000 rad. in 4–5 weeks being usually considered enough. Lympho-epitheliomas should be treated as anaplastic carcinomas, not as lymphomas.

There are some advocates, chiefly in the United States (Terz and Farr, 1967), of primary radical surgery in nearly all cases but it is doubtful whether the results are better than carefully planned and executed treatment on the above lines and it certainly results in much more morbidity and deformity as well as having a higher initial mortality.

Prognosis

This depends very much on the site of the growth, its size and the presence of metastases. Pharyngeal wall and base of tongue lesions have the worst prognosis. For small growths, under 3 cm. in diameter, of the tonsil and palatine arch without nodal involvement a 50 per cent five year cure rate has been reported (Schultz, 1965). The results fall off sharply for more extensive lesions and when lymph nodes are involved. The overall five year survival rates for oropharyngeal cancer in most centres ranges from 20–30 per cent.

Attempts have been made to improve on these results by using cytotoxic drugs either by intra-arterial perfusion or by the mouth before going on to radiotherapy.

Friedman and Daly (1967) reported significant regression of squamous carcinoma of the head and neck after two weeks of oral methotrexate (7·5 mg. a day) and believe that it led to improved results from the subsequent irradiation. There has been little confirmation of this observation and it must always be borne in mind that the systemic administration of cytotoxic drugs may affect the immune reactions of the body and allow of widespread dissemination of the growth.

The use of hyperbaric oxygen with radiotherapy is considered elsewhere.

The place of surgery in the treatment of malignant disease of the oropharynx

Muco-epidermoid carcinoma, adenoid cystic carcinoma and acinic cell carcinoma are relatively radio-resistant and require wide primary surgical excision.

Trans-oral surgery may be considered as the primary treatment for small *well differentiated* carcinomas particularly in the elderly and in alcoholics.

Surgery is needed to deal with recurrent or residual growth, either in the primary site or in the lymphatics of the neck. It is sometimes needed to remove areas of necrosis of soft tissue or bone following radiotherapy.

The surgical techniques available are:

The transoral route.—This is suitable for small primary, residual or recurrent carcinomas in the tonsillar, posterior pharyngeal wall and soft palate regions. It has been claimed that up to half the soft palate can be removed with little subsequent disability. The remaining raw areas may be sutured or left to heal as do the tonsillar beds after simple tonsillectomy. Most of these cases will have had radiotherapy so that split skin grafts are unlikely to take. An attempt may be made to cover raw areas with a flap of mucous membrane raised from the dorsum of the tongue (Klopp and Schuster, 1956). Local removal of a growth of the base of the tongue is rarely indicated by this route though total glossectomy can be carried out.

Median translingual pharyngotomy.—Sir Wilfred Trotter (1929) devised this operation as an approach to the base of the tongue, epiglottis and pharynx. The lower lip, mandible, tongue and floor of mouth are split in the midline and the two sides widely retracted (Fig. 44). The section of the tongue is continued posteriorly until the lesion can be resected with a wide margin of healthy tissue. The operation was condemned by Negus but was resurrected by Hayes Martin, Tollefsen and Gerald (1961). It may be used for small well differentiated growths on the midline of the base of the tongue, and tip of epiglottis. A temporary tracheostomy is necessary post-operatively.

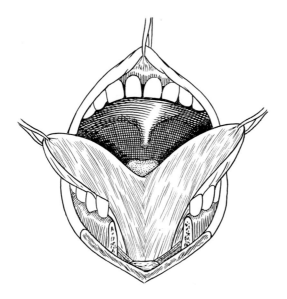

Fig. 44.—Median translingual pharyngotomy.

Median pharyngotomy.—In this operation the pharynx is opened by a horizontal incision through the thyrohyoid membrane. Part of the hyoid bone may be resected to give more room but access is very limited and only small lesions of the base of the tongue or posterior pharyngeal wall can be dealt with adequately. It carries the risk of damage to the superior laryngeal nerves.

The lymph node areas will have already been irradiated in most of the cases that can be treated by these three routes so a radical neck dissection is done only if nodes are palpable.

Lateral trans-thyroid pharyngotomy.—This operation also originated in the fertile mind of Trotter. It has been modified and extended by Alonso, Ogura and others. It gives access to the laryngopharynx as well as to the base of the tongue, valleculae and epiglottis and will therefore be described in the next section.

Composite resection.—This is often called the commando operation because of its formidable nature. In its full form it includes resection of nearly half the mandible, the lesion in the oropharynx with a margin of at least 2 cm. of healthy tissue around it and a radical neck dissection (Fig. 45). If a full course of irradiation has been given to the primary growth and neck areas it is advisable to limit the neck dissection to the suprahyoid region only. If any of the nodes in the resected area are positive the rest of the neck can be cleared when the first operation has healed soundly. The full operation after radiotherapy carries a grave risk of wound breakdown and secondary haemorrhage from the carotid arteries.

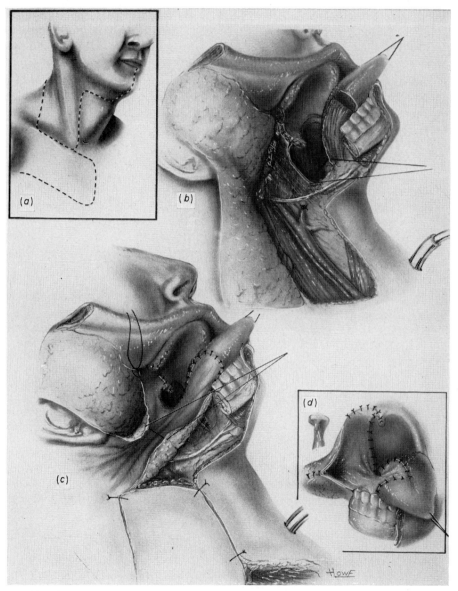

FIG. 45.—Composite resection for carcinomas of the tonsillar area and lateral margin of the tongue. (*Reproduced with permission from Hoffmeister and Bakamjian (1967).*)

This operation is suitable for quite extensive carcinomas of the tonsillar area and retromolar trigone, soft palate and lateral margin of the tongue. Base of tongue lesions must not extend across the midline and there must be an adequate margin of healthy tissue between the growth and the epiglottis if laryngectomy is to be avoided. Tracheostomy is necessary for 7–10 days after operation.

The large raw area left after operation is often difficult to cover adequately with mucosa. As before suggested a tongue flap may be tried or a pedicled skin flap used. The technique suggested by Bakamjian (1964) is a useful way of using a skin flap to cover raw surfaces inside the mouth. The proximal part of the flap is tubed in reverse to keep its epithelial surface from coming into contact with raw surfaces along its entry to the mouth (Fig. 45). Alternatively, a forehead flap may be preferred because of its superior viability. The flap is turned down and passed into the mouth through an horizontal incision in the cheek.

Laryngectomy and partial or total glossectomy.—Resection of the whole base of the tongue interferes so much with the function of swallowing that the larynx should be removed as well in all except the younger group of patients. Laryngectomy may also be necessary when the growth extends from the base of the tongue to the epiglottis and vallecula but some of these growths may be dealt with by the lateral trans-thyroid pharyngotomy approach as described by Ogura (1965). A pharyngostome should be made in post-irradiation cases.

The surgeon should always keep in mind that though many of these operations are technically possible the final cure rate for the extensive carcinomas for which they have been devised is low. The patients are usually elderly and the operation often only adds to the burden of misery they have to bear, without offering much hope of a reasonable, dignified existence.

TUMOURS OF THE LARYNGOPHARYNX

ANATOMY

The laryngopharynx extends from the hyoid bone down to the entrance to the oesophagus opposite the sixth cervical vertebra. The larynx projects into it from in front (Fig. 46) so that grooves are formed on either side which are known as the *pyriform fossae* or lateral food channels. These are shallow above and are separated from the valleculae by the pharyngo-epiglottic folds. Lower down the pyriform fossae become deeper and more cleft-like. The upper shallow part of the pyriform fossa is bounded laterally by the thyrohyoid membrane and medially by the aryepiglottic fold. The lower deeper part of the fossa is in relation laterally to the thyroid cartilage and medially to the cricoid cartilage. The *postcricoid* region runs from the upper border of the cricoid cartilage to its lower border where the oesophagus begins and is seen as a paler area of mucosa in the figure. The laryngopharynx is completed by its *lateral and posterior muscular walls*.

These clinical subdivisions of the laryngopharynx merge into each other and have no strict delimitation. The aryepiglottic folds and the free portion of the epiglottis are often called the *marginal zone* since they separate the laryngopharynx from the larynx and oropharynx respectively.

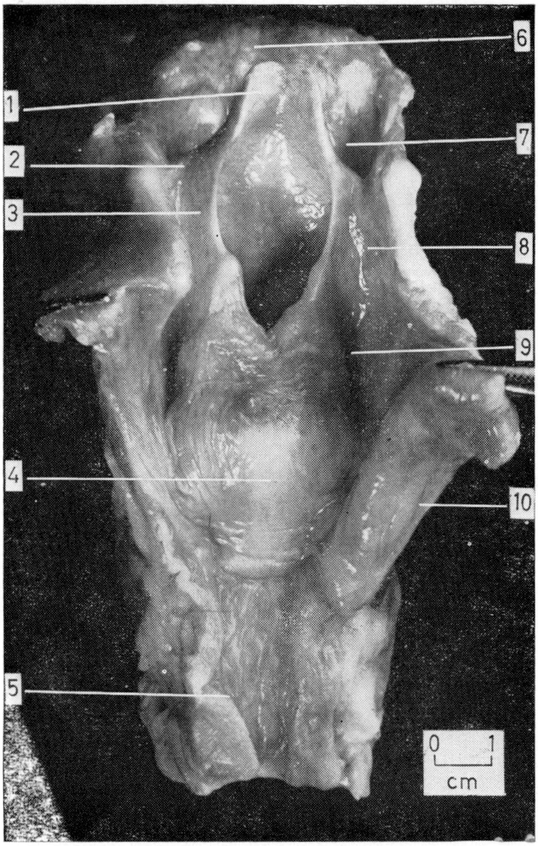

FIG. 46.—The normal pharynx and larynx opened up from behind. The contrast between the shallow upper and deep lower parts of the pyriform fossa is well shown.

1. Epiglottis
2. Pharyngo-epiglottic fold
3. Aryepiglottic fold
4. Postcricoid region
5. Cervical oesophagus
6. Base of tongue
7. Vallecula
8. Upper pyriform fossa
9. Lower pyriform fossa
10. Posterolateral pharyngeal wall

BENIGN TUMOURS

Papillomas and adenomas are very rare indeed; mesodermal neoplasms are a little more common and lipomas, fibromas and leiomyomas are occasionally reported.

These benign tumours grow very slowly and form smooth, well-defined, mobile (sometimes pedunculated) masses. They can seldom be confused with malignant tumours though their true nature can be shown only by microscopic examination. Small ones may be removed by endoscopy but larger ones need excision through the lateral pharyngotomy approach.

Cysts of the anterior surface of the epiglottis are more frequent. They are yellow in appearance and seldom grow large enough to cause symptoms. It is usually sufficient to remove most of the cyst wall endoscopically and recurrence is rare. The lining membrane consists of squamous epithelium.

MALIGNANT NEOPLASMS

Pathology

Malignant growths of the laryngopharynx are nearly all squamous cell carcinomas. Adenocarcinomas, malignant lymphomas, mesodermal tumours and

173

metastatic deposits from elsewhere in the body are very rare and need only be mentioned. Their structure will be shown by the biopsy which should always be taken.

The squamous cell carcinomas are most often moderately well differentiated and macroscopically present as either exophytic or ulcerative growths. The exophytic form occurs most commonly in the upper piriform fossa and aryepiglottic fold regions and the ulcerative in the remaining areas of the laryngopharynx. Atrophic mucosal changes elsewhere in the pharynx and oral cavity may be seen, especially in women with postcricoid cancer, and a second primary growth is not uncommon.

It is customary to group squamous cell carcinomas of the laryngopharynx according to the anatomical subdivisions of the region, i.e.

(1) Marginal (or epilaryngeal)
(2) Pyriform fossa
(3) Posterolateral wall
(4) Postcricoid (+ upper cervical oesophagus = epi-oesophageal).

Some systems of classification place the marginal zone carcinomas with the laryngeal growths but their behaviour, symptomatology and mode of spread is such that the writer prefers to include them with the laryngopharyngeal tumours. Upper oesophageal carcinomas are difficult to separate from the postcricoid ones and are often grouped with them. This combined group is sometimes termed epi-oesophageal (Lederman, 1962).

Frequently the growth is so advanced when first seen that it is difficult to determine its site of origin and placing it in one of the above categories is rather a matter of guesswork. This may account in part for the reported variations in frequency with which each area is involved, but there is undoubtedly a wide geographic variation.

Dalley (1968) gives the incidence at the Royal Marsden Hospital, London, for the years 1945–1965:

Marginal (epilaryngeal)	185 (22 per cent)
Pyriform fossa	334 (39 per cent)
Posterolateral wall	47 (6 per cent)
Postcricoid	208 (24 per cent)
Cervical oesophagus	74 (9 per cent)

MacComb and Fletcher's (1967) figures from Houston, Texas, differ markedly even allowing for differences in classification.

Pyriform fossa	182 (75 per cent)
Pharyngeal wall	26 (10 per cent)
Postcricoid	5 (2 per cent)
Cervical oesophagus	32 (13 per cent)

Bryce (1967) reports that of 230 cases in Toronto there were:

Pyriform fossa	61 per cent
Postcricoid	24 per cent
Pharyngeal wall	15 per cent

It is generally agreed that the pyriform fossa is the most common site of origin and that, except for the postcricoid area, men are more frequently affected than women.

174

Spread

Both the exophytic and ulcerative forms spread submucosally well beyond the macroscopic limits of the growth, especially in the poorly differentiated lesions, but the ulcerative form has a greater tendency to infiltrate deeply. Deep spread forwards and laterally leads to invasion of the thyroid cartilage and gland; medially the aryepiglottic fold and ventricular band become infiltrated and swelling and fixation of one half of the larynx develops. Paralysis of a vocal cord may also arise from direct involvement of the recurrent laryngeal nerve behind the cricothyroid joint. Postcricoid growths tend to spread circumferentially, as well as vertically, thus producing stenosis.

The collecting vessels from the lymphatics of the mucous membrane of the laryngopharynx converge on the thyrohyoid membrane and pass through it alongside the superior laryngeal artery. Some empty into the jugulodigastric node but others spread up and down so that almost any node in the deep cervical chain may be the first to be enlarged and when one node has been involved the distribution may be even more eccentric.

Lymphatic vessels from the lower part of the laryngopharynx pass directly to the lower nodes of the deep cervical chain and to the paratracheal nodes.

Since the lymphatic network freely crosses the midline bilateral lymph node metastasis occurs; this is particularly common of course when the growth itself crosses the midline as in postcricoid carcinomas.

Lymph node involvement is early and there may be a large lymph node in the neck while the primary growth in the laryngopharynx is still minute. The majority of patients already have palpable cervical lymph node involvement when they are first seen and Dalley (1968) puts the incidence of this as follows:

Marginal (epilaryngeal)	57 per cent
Pyriform fossa	66 per cent
Posterolateral walls	55 per cent
Postcricoid	42 per cent
Cervical oesophagus	31 per cent

Other writers have reported a similar incidence. Of more importance to the surgeon, however, would be the ability to estimate the likelihood of occult metastases in a case in which there are no palpable nodes, but there are not many figures available. Ogura and Mallen (1965) showed that of 39 cases of carcinoma of the superior and inferior hypopharynx (corresponding to our marginal and piriform fossa divisions) 15, or 38 per cent, had microscopic involvement although clinically no nodes were palpable. The numbers are small but they conclude that this figure is high enough to justify an elective neck dissection.

Distant metastasis to bones and viscera occurs and are becoming increasingly recognized, possibly because patients are surviving their primary lesion for longer (Arons and Smith, 1961).

Aetiology

The relative frequency of laryngopharyngeal cancer is difficult to assess, since official mortality statistics of cancers of the larynx and pharynx are often combined. In the Bulletin No. 4 of the South Metropolitan Cancer Registry (1966) the total number of cases of cancer of the "hypopharynx" registered during 1961–63 is given as 540 while during the same period there were 860 cases of laryngeal cancer.

Since 1957 postcricoid cancers have been classified separately by the Registrar General and about 250 deaths a year are recorded in Great Britain: this should correlate well with the total incidence of the disease since few are cured.

The incidence of postcricoid cancer is higher in Great Britain and Scandinavia than elsewhere. Even within Britain the incidence varies and it is low in south-east England and high in North Wales. Jacobs (1963) pointed out the distribution is similar to that of gastric carcinoma but could offer no explanation for this similarity. Wynder, Bross and Feldman (1957) think there is a significant association between laryngopharyngeal carcinoma and smoking though, in contrast to cancer of the lung, the association is with pipes and cigars, rather than with cigarettes. They also note an association with the heavy drinking of spirits but since most heavy drinkers are heavy smokers it is difficult to disentangle the effects of the two habits.

There is also a strong relationship between postcricoid cancer in women and the Paterson–Brown Kelly syndrome. In this syndrome there is dysphagia, often with a web or stricture of the cervical oesophagus, and sideropenic anaemia. Richards (1969) reported that 35 per cent of 266 cases of postcricoid carcinoma treated at Cardiff had a history of dysphagia for five years or more before the diagnosis of carcinoma was made. He also stated that a benign postcricoid stricture was known to have existed in 9 per cent of these cases before the onset of malignancy. The cause of the syndrome and ensuing carcinoma is unknown. Iron deficiency is probably only one factor and other factors may be gastric mucosal atrophy, vitamin B_{12} malabsorption and pyridoxine deficiency. Many of the phenomena associated with the syndrome such as glossitis and angular cheilitis are non-specific.

A few cases of carcinoma of the laryngopharynx have resulted from previous irradiation of the neck, usually for thyrotoxicosis. Kapur (1968) reviewed the subject and points out that there is a latent period of 10–35 years between the irradiation and the appearance of a tumour. In the English literature 52 post-irradiation malignancies of the larynx, pharynx and oesophagus have been reported. Of these 45 were epithelial tumours most of which occurred in the "hypopharynx and postcricoid region".

Symptoms

A carcinoma in the laryngopharynx will first affect swallowing, except for the marginal growths which may first produce a thickening or muffling of the voice. Since the laryngopharynx is a fairly capacious structure and since carcinoma is at first painless, symptoms may not arise until the growth is well advanced. The symptoms at the start may be indefinite but discomfort or pain on swallowing develop, at first with solid foods only. The discomfort begins simply as a soreness or slight pricking sensation as solid food is going down, but it gradually progresses to pain, which may be referred to the ear via Arnold's nerve, and to obstruction with all acts of swallowing.

Carcinomas of the postcricoid region and below cause obstructive symptoms earlier than those at a higher level but discomfort and pain are not so evident. In early cases the patient may say that she feels as though the food is passing over a ledge or ridge while fluids go down without difficulty. In most cases, however, obstructive symptoms are quite severe by the time the patient first seeks advice and loss of weight is usually more marked than in carcinomas arising in the other sites.

As has already been pointed out, an enlarged lymph node may appear in the neck while the primary growth is still small, before it has given rise to any throat symptoms.

In males the growth is usually seen in the sixth and seventh decades but in females postcricoid lesions often appear earlier and cases are not uncommonly met with in the late twenties and the thirties.

The feeling of a "lump in the throat" or the sensation of a foreign body being present, like a hair or a small pip, causing the patient to swallow constantly is not suggestive of an organic lesion. In these cases food and drink go down without difficulty and the symptoms are intermittent as against the gradually increasing severity of those caused by carcinoma.

Examination

The possibility of a malignant cause should be considered in all cases of dysphagia and investigations must be pursued until a diagnosis is arrived at.

While the history is being taken the general appearance of the patient should be observed and any suggestion of loss of weight, anaemia or cachexia noted. The mouth might also give suggestive evidence such as glossitis, mucosal atrophy or angular cheilitis.

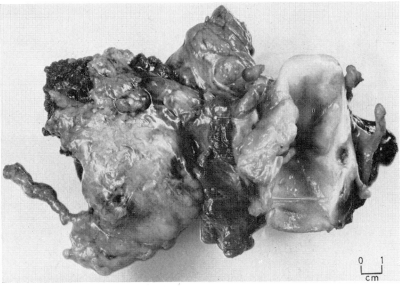

Fig. 47.—Laryngopharyngeal carcinoma, marginal type. The growth involves the aryepiglottic fold and upper pyriform fossa and is proliferative. A radical neck dissection in continuity has been done. There was a palpable node which proved positive on section.

The laryngopharynx can be seen by indirect pharyngoscopy but surface analgesia may have to be used to get a satisfactory view. All regions of the laryngopharynx are visible except the deeper parts of the pyriform fossae and postcricoid area (Fig. 46). Any ulcerative or proliferative lesion is almost certain to be a carcinoma since other conditions affecting this region are extremely rare. A growth in the

177

deeper part of the piriform fossa or postcricoid area may not be visible in the mirror but may cause pooling of saliva or oedema of the arytenoid eminence. The larynx may be fixed and swollen by infiltration but sometimes a vocal cord is paralysed simply by involvement of the recurrent laryngeal nerve alone.

Marginal carcinomas and those of the upper pyriform fossa often form large granular masses (Fig. 47) but the lower growths are more ulcerative and spread deeply fixing the larynx and surrounding tissues (Fig. 48).

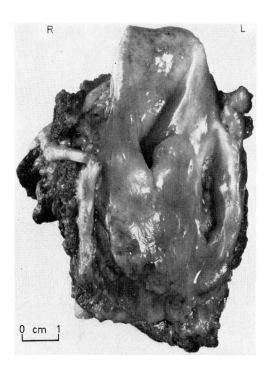

FIG. 48.—Laryngopharyngeal carcinoma. Deep ulcer in right pyriform fossa persisting after a full course of radiotherapy.

The next step in the investigation is to examine the whole neck carefully for enlarged lymph nodes. Ideally this should be done in a good light with the patient stripped nearly to the waist. The absence of the grating feeling on moving the larynx is suggestive and large pharyngeal growths may be palpable as thickenings.

These examinations can eliminate the possibility of carcinoma in many cases with vague symptoms such as a "lump in the throat" but if there is any doubt further investigations must be done because the postcricoid and epi-oesophageal regions are not completely visible on mirror examination and a small growth may be missed.

Radiology

A simple lateral soft tissue radiograph is particularly useful in postcricoid carcinomas and should not be omitted even though more elaborate investigations are also planned. A postcricoid or epi-oesophageal carcinoma will show up as a thickening of the soft tissue shadow between the lower cervical vertebrae and the trachea. Normally this should be less than the width of the vertebral bodies

Dysphagia with anaemia should always necessitate direct pharyngoscopy even though radiological investigations have been normal or have shown a simple stricture only. Very early carcinomatous changes can be missed radiographically.

It sometimes helps in assessing dysphagia to observe the patient eating or drinking.

Staging

Staging in carcinoma of the laryngopharynx is not so satisfactorily achieved as in laryngeal carcinoma.

The American Joint Committee for Cancer Staging and End Results Reporting proposes the following definitions.

Stage I T_1, N_0, M_0.

Stage II T_2, N_0, M_0. T_3, N_0, M_0.

Stage III T_1, N_1, M_0. T_2, N_1, M_0. T_3, N_1, M_0.

Stage IV   All more advanced lesions.

Treatment

Carcinoma of the laryngopharynx was for long regarded as almost incurable. Many of the early laryngectomies were done for this type of growth, which was then called extrinsic carcinoma of the larynx, but recurrences were early and operative mortality high. Reconstructive operations were difficult and often failed to enable normal swallowing to be regained. It is little wonder that McKenty, quoted by St. Clair Thomson and Colledge (1930), said that this cancer was hopeless and was not amenable to surgery. However they also stated that "of recent years Soerensen and Gluck have performed such operations extensively for growths of the pyriform fossa and neighbouring regions". Gluck was strongly against attempts at peeling the tumour off the larynx and emphasized that the one chance of permanent cure lay in the sacrifice of the larynx and diseased portion of the pharynx. In spite of this St. Clair Thomson and Colledge favoured lateral pharyngotomy without total laryngectomy for growths on the epiglottis, aryepiglottic folds and lateral pharyngeal wall. Like Trotter, they reported cures by this method "in a fair proportion of cases". For extensive lesions they employed irradiation, mainly for its palliative effect, which was slight, and rarely used pharyngolaryngectomy.

This attitude held the field till after World War II when the improvements in anaesthesia and blood transfusion and the use of antibiotics enabled surgeons to tackle the problem again in a more aggressive way and yet with a much diminished mortality and morbidity. The emphasis was with Gluck, and total extirpation of the larynx with radical neck dissection was advocated notably by Owen and Negus. Later Alonso, Ogura, and others, enlarging the scope of lateral pharyngotomy, devised operations which would remove the carcinoma with an adequate margin of tissue and yet preserve a functioning larynx.

At the same time radiotherapy was also developing and hopes of improving results rose with the advent of supervoltage machines such as the linear accelerator and cobalt–60 bomb. There are also high hopes for irradiation under hyperbaric oxygen but its true value has not yet been established.

Cytotoxic drugs have not yet established a place in the treatment of laryngopharyngeal carcinoma.

In spite of these changes results are still on the whole poor and many clinics are now planning to combine radiotherapy and radical surgery in an attempt to improve matters.

Radiotherapy

This may be used with intent to cure, for palliation only, or planned to be combined with surgery.

Curative treatment

As with all carcinomas the primary growth, manifest secondary deposits in the cervical lymph nodes and the possibility of occult metastases in these nodes are of primary importance in planning treatment. Other factors to be considered are the histology of the carcinoma, distant metastases and the age and general condition, mental and physical, of the patient.

Since all laryngopharyngeal carcinomas have such a strong tendency to metastasize to the cervical lymph nodes, ideally in all cases the primary growth and the lymph node area in the neck, on both sides when the growth has crossed the midline, should be irradiated. This is usually not possible even with supervoltage therapy and a compromise has to be worked out as has been indicated for carcinomas of the postnasal space and oropharynx.

For *well differentiated* carcinomas a large field covering the primary growth and adjacent lymph node area and of course any enlarged nodes is used and a dose using supervoltage of 6500–7000 rad. in 6–7 weeks is given. The remaining lymph node areas where no nodes are palpable are left untreated, and if a node appears after treatment is completed it can be dealt with by radical neck dissection.

For *undifferentiated or anaplastic* carcinomas prophylactic irradiation of the cervical fields is advisable. This should include the paratracheal nodes in the superior mediastinum for low pyriform fossa and postcricoid carcinomas. The submental and submaxillary nodes are rarely involved and can be omitted from treatment with the advantage that the salivary glands in these areas will help to the mitigate mouth and pharyngeal dryness caused by the irradiation. Both sides of the neck should be treated in postcricoid cases.

It will be realized that most patients will be unable to tolerate the full course to such large fields and after about 5000 rad. the fields can be reduced in size and the remaining 1500–2000 rad. given to the manifest growth only. It is believed that 5000 rad. in five weeks is likely to destroy any microscopic deposit of cancer cells in a lymph node (Goldman, Friedman and Bloom, 1968).

Many of the carcinomas of the lower part of the laryngopharynx are invisible on mirror examination and so their response to treatment is difficult to assess. It is therefore advisable to perform a direct examination about eight weeks after treatment has been completed and, later, at the slightest suggestion of return of pain and obstruction to swallowing, of increasing oedema of the aryepiglottic folds, or of cord fixation.

Palliative treatment

Small doses are ineffective and treatment almost up to the curative level, though with smaller fields, must be used. If the response is better than expected the case can be reconsidered and a full curative course arranged. In very advanced cases with fixed nodes attempts at palliation fail and suffering is only prolonged or made worse. It is then probably wiser to withhold radiotherapy altogether.

Surgical treatment

The primary growth and secondary deposits in the neck area are both amenable to resection and this, in most cases, means pharyngolaryngectomy and neck dissection. However, as Trotter has said, an operation for cancer should be to remove a disease not an organ, and it may be possible in rare instances to remove the carcinoma with a wide margin of healthy tissue around it and still preserve enough of the pharynx or larynx for them to function satisfactorily afterwards.

The operations for carcinoma of the laryngopharynx may be classified into four groups.

(1) Total laryngectomy and total pharyngectomy (pharyngolaryngectomy)
(2) Total laryngectomy and partial pharyngectomy
(3) Partial pharyngectomy
(4) Partial pharyngectomy and partial laryngectomy.

Pharyngolaryngectomy.—Since the pharynx is to be removed plans must be made beforehand for replacing it. Until recent years the removed segment was reconstituted by the creation of a full thickness skin lined tube and to do this two or more operations were necessary. This would have been more acceptable if a satisfactory cure or repair rate could have been achieved but too often recurrence took place before swallowing could be restored. Even when this had been done local recurrence of the growth often led to stenosis again and so little had been gained by the treatment. However, in carefully planned series lasting cures can be achieved in 20–25 per cent of cases with restoration of normal swallowing after a comparatively short stay in hospital (Lewis, 1965). This tends to be forgotten in the search for more speedy results.

Negus in 1953 used a split-skin graft over a rubber or plastic mould to refashion a pharynx in one stage but this was only partially successful because stenosis was common and multiple operations were often necessary.

Som (1956) and Simpson (1960) advocated the laryngotracheal graft but many cases are not suitable for this technique. The success of thoracic surgeons in replacing the oesophagus with abdominal viscera was noted and in 1954 Goligher and Robin reported replacement of the pharyngo-oesophageal segment with the left colon. Since then the colon, jejunum and stomach have all been mobilized and brought up into the neck by various routes to reconstitute a pharynx.

Som had some success with a re-vascularized free graft of jejunum but has since abandoned the operation and Stuart (1966) has recommended bridging the gap between pharynx and oesophagus with a plastic tube only.

(*a*) Pharyngolaryngectomy and reconstitution with skin flaps.

First stage. The incision is shown in Fig. 51. The vertical incision is offset to the side on which the neck dissection is to be done to avoid imperilling the blood supply to the skin. If the growth is a long one the vertical diameter of the flap can be increased by placing the upper incision nearer the mandible and covering the raw area of the exposed tongue with a split-skin graft. It is paradoxical that it does not help to place the inferior incision any lower than indicated in the figure even if a low transection of the oesophagus is necessary. This is because the bridge of skin between the flaps and trachea has also to be stitched to the oesophagus and if the tracheal incision is placed over the sternum it cannot be mobilized sufficiently to allow this.

The operation proceeds as for laryngectomy (with radical neck dissection if indicated—see later) until all the strap muscles have been divided, the superior laryngeal vessels tied and the hyoid bone freed from the tongue. If the growth is predominantly unilateral only the thyroid lobe on that side is removed but a total thyroidectomy is necessary for postcricoid carcinoma. This usually means that the parathyroid glands are also removed. While the thyroid gland is being mobilized, it is possible to dissect up the paratracheal and upper mediastinal glands from behind the manubrium sterni. Standing at the head of the table, and using a headlight are aids to this manoeuvre. Harrison (1969) prefers to remove the manubrium for this purpose.

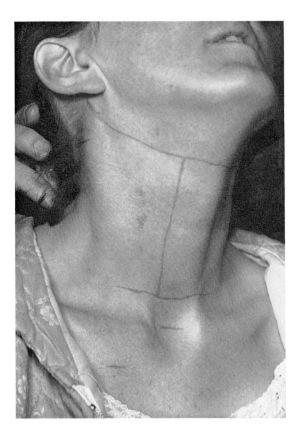

Fig. 51.—Incision for two-stage pharyngolaryngectomy. (*From Lewis* (1965), *reproduced by courtesy of the Editor of* Journal of Laryngology.)

After this has been done, the pharynx is separated from the vertebral column behind from the level of the hyoid bone down to the cervical oesophagus, which is also mobilized freely. It is convenient now to transfer the endotracheal anaesthetic tube to the trachea, making the opening at the level at which the trachea will eventually be transected. The pharynx is opened laterally just below the tip of the greater cornu of the hyoid bone and the growth inspected through this opening. This inspection is important to assess the limits of the growth and extent of the resection needed.

The posterior wall of the pharynx is divided at least 2 cm. above the carcinoma and anteriorly the pharynx is separated from the base of the tongue through the valleculae. The specimen now remains attached to the oesophagus and trachea only. The oesophagus is cut across, also at least 2 cm. below the growth. It is difficult to estimate this level and sometimes a further piece of the oesophagus has to be removed to achieve adequate clearance.

The trachea is now completely divided at a level below any possible involvement by the carcinoma and brought through the small transverse skin incision in the manubrial notch and stitched to it, forming the permanent tracheostome.

The skin flaps are stitched together forming an upper pharyngostome and a lower oesophagostome (Fig. 52). It is important, to avoid later stenosis, to make the oesophagostome as large as possible. This can be done by placing the stitches close together in the oesophagus but wider apart on the skin so that when they are tied, the mouth of the oesophagus is splayed open. Conversely, the pharyngostome should be reduced in size to aid reconstruction.

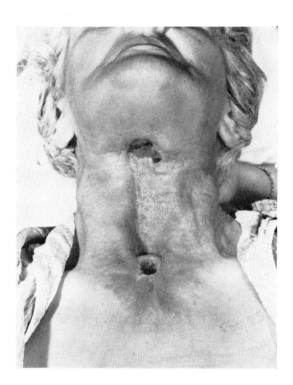

FIG. 52.—Twenty days after pharyngolaryngectomy, first stage. A full therapeutic course of radiotherapy had been completed eight weeks previously. Good healing except for a small granulation at the upper stoma. (*From Lewis* (1965), *reproduced by courtesy of the Editor of* Journal of Laryngology.)

A drain, either open, or closed suction, is placed in the neck dissection area and a feeding tube into the oesophagus. A large dressing giving firm pressure over the neck dissection, but allowing free escape of saliva through the pharyngostome, is arranged by a combination of Elastoplast and crepe bandages. A Lombard's tube or cuffed tracheostomy tube is placed in the tracheostome.

Post-operative care is as for laryngectomy but with 10 ml. of 10 per cent calcium gluconate added to each bottle of intravenous fluid. When tube feeding starts 50,000 units of calciferol are given twice a day with one tablet of calcium sandoz four times daily. Frequent checks on serum calcium levels must be made during the ensuing months because some recovery of parathyroid function may occur and the dose of calcium and calciferol have to be altered. Thyroxin 0·1 mg. b.d. is also given after 2–3 weeks.

The operation is done under cover of a broad spectrum antibiotic such as ampicillin and provided it has been possible to sew up the wound without undue tension anywhere, it should heal and be ready for the second stage in 5–7 weeks. This applies not only to the cases which have not been irradiated but also to those whose radiotherapy has been completed less than 8–10 weeks previously. The longer the delay following irradiation, the more likely is the wound partially to break down. It is however in the second stage in post-irradiation cases that serious failures in healing mainly occur (Lewis, 1965).

Second stage: if healing has been uneventful, this may be undertaken 5–7 weeks after the first operation. Irradiated cases may need a longer interval to consolidate healing of the wound and occasionally recurrences appear so rapidly that repair cannot be attempted.

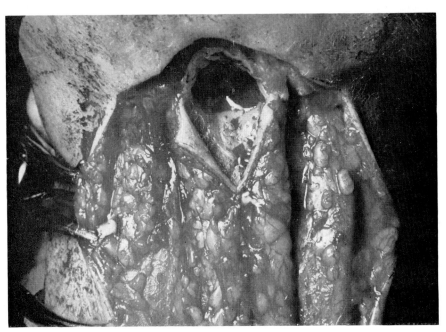

Fig. 53.—Closure showing inversion of the skin flaps to create a skin-lined tube. A vertical mattress stitch should be used and the knots tied in the lumen. (*From Lewis* (1965), *reproduced by courtesy of the Editor of* Journal of Laryngology.)

The pharynx is reconstructed by fashioning a tube from the skin of the neck between the pharyngeal and the oesophageal stomata. A flap is outlined and the margins elevated as atraumatically as possible, just sufficiently for them to be stitched together in the midline without any trace of tension (Fig. 53). An inverting mattress stitch with 00 Mersilk on an atraumatic needle is used. The tongue can be easily mobilized to assist closure above but the lower end can be very difficult unless a bridge of skin at least 2 cm. wide has been preserved between the tracheal and oesophageal openings. If this bridge is inadequate, reconstruction is complicated and entails a series of plastic operations.

The formation of this skin tube leaves a large raw area in front of the neck to be covered. It is tempting to use a Thiersch graft to cover it and some success has been reported but most writers feel that it is safer to use full thickness skin with a good blood supply.

If the case has not been irradiated or if the treatment has been given not more than 8–10 weeks before the first stage, the flaps illustrated in Fig. 54 are effective, the remaining raw areas being covered with split skin grafts (Fig. 55). Alternatively, and when the radiotherapy has been given more than 8–10 weeks pre-operatively, an acromiothoracic or the versatile deltopectoral flap should be used.

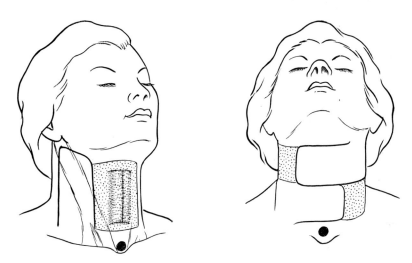

Fig. 54.—The use of local cervical skin flaps in the reconstruction of the pharynx.

If the original skin flaps have sloughed, tube pedicle flaps will have to be prepared and migrated to the neck to fashion both the lining and the cover of the new pharynx.

If bilateral radical neck dissections are indicated, the second side may be done at the same time as the repair.

The two-stage pharyngolaryngectomy should be planned with care and carried out with meticulous attention to detail. If this is done, the patient's stay in hospital need not be longer than 9–12 weeks. If a wound breakdown occurs at any time, the picture changes and a long stay in hospital ensues with probably many operations to close the defect.

The chief drawback of this operation from the curative point of view is the difficulty in getting well below the carcinoma in some instances. However, downward spread seems to be limited in many cases and out of 37 treated by the author by this method, seven have survived for five years or more, free from disease, and three others died over two years post-operatively of intercurrent disease with no sign of recurrence. It remains to be seen whether removing the whole oesophagus with the pharynx and larynx (q.v.) will increase the number of cures.

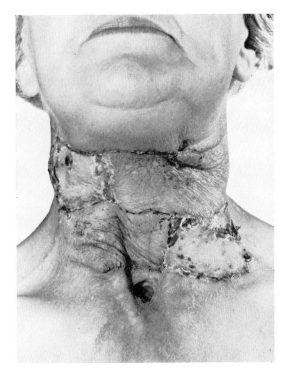

FIG. 55.—Twenty-four days after reconstruction and two and a half months after the primary laryngopharyngectomy. An acromiothoracic or deltopectoral skin flap would have been used as cover if the irradiation had been given more than three months pre-operatively.

(*b*) Pharyngolaryngectomy in one stage.

(*i*) *Reconstitution by means of a Thiersch graft.* This was advocated by Negus (1953) and consists of connecting the pharynx to the oesophagus with a moulded Latex tube and covering the tube with a Thiersch graft. The tube is withdrawn through the mouth after 2–3 weeks (Shaw, 1957). While occasionally successful, this operation is too often followed by fistulae and stenosis to be recommended.

Stuart (1966) modified this technique by using a similar but longer tube without a skin graft and leaving the tube in permanently. The method is still under trial and may be considered in some cases for palliation.

(*ii*) The laryngotracheal graft. Acting on a suggestion by Asherson (1954), Som (1956) and Simpson (1960) have used the front half of the larynx and trachea to reconstruct the pharynx. A U-shaped skin incision is recommended and after division of the inferior strap muscles, the thyroid gland is defined and the greater part of the muscles removed. The lateral lobes of the gland are then divided longitudinally, while the superior thyroid arteries and veins are preserved. The thyrohyoid membrane must be defined posteriorly and the superior laryngeal artery and vein identified and carefully preserved since it is mainly on these vessels that the nourishment of the graft depends. The pharynx is freed from the front of the verte-brae, from the level of the hyoid bone down to the cervical oesophagus and an esti-mate of the position of the lower end of the carcinoma is made. Two centimetres or more below this level, the trachea is cut across and the anaesthetic tube inserted in the lower end. Vertical incisions are made upwards on each side of the trachea so that it is divided into two roughly equal longitudinal halves. These incisions are

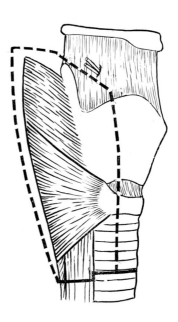

FIG. 56.—Tissues removed by the laryngotracheal graft technique. Note the preservation of the superior laryngeal artery and vein.

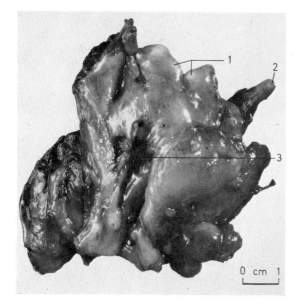

FIG. 57.—Specimen removed by the laryngotracheal graft technique. The pharynx and oesophagus have been opened up posteriorly. It is by no means a limited resection; the patient lived for three years free from recurrence and died of a breast carcinoma.

1. Arytenoid eminences
2. Superior cornu of thyroid cartilage
3. Infiltrating carcinoma

189

continued upwards through the cricoid and thyroid cartilages and larynx to enter the pharynx in front of the arytenoid eminences. The anterior half of the larynx and trachea can now be lifted upwards and the posterior half with the pharynx and its growth can be removed (Fig. 57). The raw surface in front of the vertebrae is covered with a split-skin graft which is stitched to the pharynx above and the oesophagus below. The anterior laryngotracheal segment is now swung back into position and the lower hemi-circle of the trachea with its cartilaginous ring sutured to the anterior half or two-thirds of the oesophagus. The lateral margins of the skin graft are stitched to the larynx and trachea so that a complete tube, consisting of the lumen of the trachea in front and the split skin graft behind, is formed leading from the oropharynx to the oesophagus. A feeding tube is passed through it via the nose, a tracheostome is made, the wound is sewn up and a firm dressing applied. After 10–14 days, the patient should be radiographically screened while swallowing gastrograffin and, if there is no fistula, normal feeding may be started.

(c) Replacement with abdominal viscera.

Colon and stomach have been used. Brain and Reading (1966) recommended bringing up the colon subcutaneously in front of the thoracic cage; this is a safe procedure since it avoids extensive intrathoracic manipulations but swallowing is not always satisfactory. Fairman and John (1966), having used the anterior mediastinal route now recommend removing the oesophagus and bringing up the colon through the posterior mediastinum. This is a severe operation needing two intra-abdominal anastomoses and the writer prefers to use the stomach as recommended by Le Quesne and Ranger (1966). A pharyngolaryngectomy, with or without neck dissection, is carried out in the usual way, except that the oesophagus is not divided, but is freed as far down as possible in the mediastinum. At the same time, the abdominal team has mobilized the stomach by dissection outside the anastomotic arcades of the two curvatures, leaving intact only the right gastric and right gastro-epiploic vessels; the duodenum and head of the pancreas are also mobilized, and pyloroplasty performed.

The lower oesophagus must now be freed from below until the operator's fingers meet with those freeing it from above. This can be difficult and must be done with great care to avoid tearing the pleura. When free, gentle traction on the oesophagus will pull the stomach up into the neck where its fundus is stitched to the pharynx. A feeding tube is passed into it through the nose and the neck wounds closed with drains, and a firm dressing. If all goes well, feeding can be started in 7–10 days or earlier (Fig. 58).

Post-operatively, a watch must be kept for pneumothorax and pleural effusion and it is advisable to take a radiograph of the chest before the patient leaves the theatre.

A further development of interposition of viscera to the pharynx is the use of a re-vascularized free intestinal graft. Special techniques for the anastomosis of the small vessels involved are required and this method has yet to prove its value.

Although visceral replacement operations restore swallowing almost immediately, this advantage must be offset against their much higher mortality rate and the need for more intensive immediate post-operative management. These difficulties, however, are being overcome gradually and with careful selection of cases the mortality and morbidity will diminish to acceptable proportions.

A great advantage of replacement techniques with stomach or colon is that they can be used without fear of wound breakdown in cases which have been irradiated.

Laryngectomy and partial pharyngectomy.—In many cases of pyriform fossa and marginal carcinomas it is possible to preserve enough mucous membrane of the pharynx on the opposite side, to reconstruct the pharynx from it alone. If a mucosal lined pharynx the size of an ordinary pencil can be made, it will suffice.

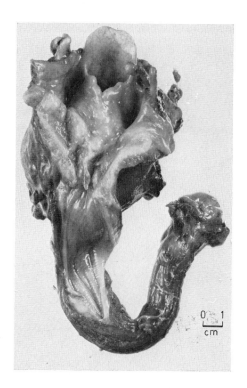

FIG. 58.—Pharyngolaryngo-oesophagectomy. The patient was a man aged 29 and there was a rapid recurrence of the growth.

Partial pharyngectomy and partial laryngectomy.—The operation of lateral trans-thyroid pharyngotomy (Trotter, 1929) provides an exposure through which tumours can be removed from the pharynx and upper part of the larynx. It can be used without neck dissection to deal with innocent tumours and cysts of the larynx, pharynx and base of the tongue or with a radical dissection for malignant lesions.

When a neck dissection is not indicated the incision may be either a vertical one over the posterior border of the thyroid cartilage, or a curved one starting from near the mastoid tip passing downwards to just below the greater cornu of the hyoid bone and then forwards and upwards to the midline above the body of the hyoid (Fig. 59). The skin flaps are reflected and the anterior margin of the sternomastoid muscle freed. The common facial vein and other small vessels are ligated and the carotid sheath and its contents retracted backwards exposing the pharyngeal constrictor muscles. Retraction and rotation of the larynx to the other side helps in this exposure, and division of the superior thyroid or external carotid artery is usually necessary to get adequate access.

191

The sternohyoid, omohyoid and thyrohyoid muscles are freed from the hyoid bone and turned downwards, and depending on the extent of the exposure needed the greater cornu of the hyoid bone and posterior half of the thyroid cartilage are

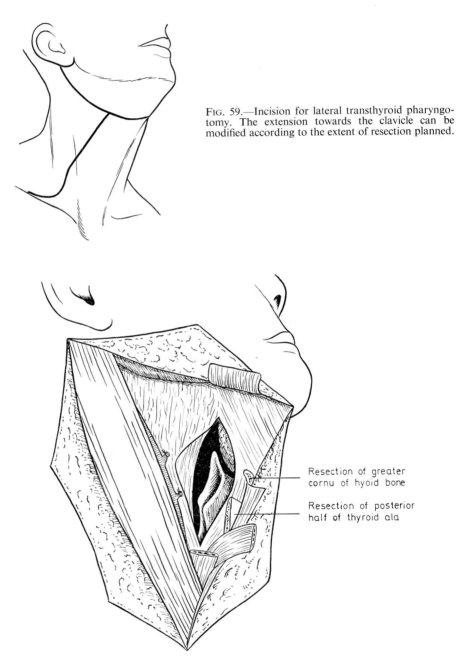

FIG. 59.—Incision for lateral transthyroid pharyngotomy. The extension towards the clavicle can be modified according to the extent of resection planned.

Resection of greater cornu of hyoid bone

Resection of posterior half of thyroid ala

FIG. 60.—Lateral transthyroid pharyngotomy. The pharynx has been opened, showing the larynx but a radical neck dissection has not been done.

resected subperiosteally and subperichondrially. The pharynx can now be entered at the chosen point and the incision enlarged as necessary to deal with the lesion (Fig. 60).

When a radical neck dissection is indicated an incision downwards from the midpoint of the curved incision to the midpoint of the clavicle is added and the neck dissection performed as usual. If it is difficult to remove it *en bloc* with the lesion it may be removed separately since involvement of the nodes is by embolism, and permeation of the lymphatic vessels between the primary growth and the nodes is a late phenomenon.

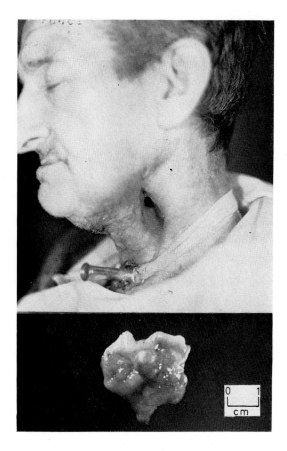

FIG. 61.—Pharyngostome formed after removal of a small carcinoma of the lateral pharyngeal wall. There were palpable nodes and a radical neck dissection was also done. The patient lived for more than eight years without recurrence.

If all raw areas can be covered with mucosa and if the incision in the pharyngeal mucous membrane can be closed easily without tension, satisfactory healing is likely and the wound can be closed completely. This is possible sometimes even when the neck has been previously irradiated but in the majority of these cases it is wiser to stitch skin to mucous membrane to form a pharyngostome which may be closed a few weeks later (Fig. 61).

A tracheostomy should always be done because of the laryngeal oedema which usually follows the operation.

D.E.N.T.(VOL.4)—14

Although Ogura and Mallen (1965) have obtained good results using a modified form of this approach (extended supraglottic subtotal laryngectomy) to remove upper pyriform fossa and marginal carcinomas these carcinomas are also the ones which are likely to respond to radiotherapy. Apart therefore from the rare adeno-carcinoma or pleomorphic tumour of the base of the tongue this operation is needed only when irradiation has failed. In these circumstances a laryngectomy or pharyngolaryngectomy is more usually indicated but with careful selection a few cases can be saved from this mutilation.

Combined treatment

The results of treatment in laryngopharyngeal carcinoma have been poor. Surgery seldom gives a higher five year survival rate than 20–25 per cent and a certain amount of selection must be involved in most series. For radiotherapy the figures are nearer 10–15 per cent. Consequently many clinics are now combining the two methods hoping thereby to improve the results. The majority favour pre-operative irradiation but there is as yet no general agreement of the dose and size of the fields to be used. Reported results have been promising but are not yet conclusive.

The purpose of the irradiation in planned combined treatment is not to eradicate the growth entirely but to circumscribe it by destroying proliferating cells in the periphery of the growth and in metastatic nodes and to render the remaining cells less active, so that the subsequent operation is more likely to eradicate the carcinoma completely. A full cancericidal dose may therefore not be necessary and healing after the operation is consequently less likely to be affected.

Various schemes of treatment have been devised and mention will be made of a few results. Strong and his colleagues (1966) claim that 2000 rad. in five days followed immediately by radical neck dissection reduces the number of glandular recurrences after both elective and therapeutic neck dissection. Goldman, Friedman and Bloom (1968) believe that 5500 rad. in five weeks can destroy carcinomatous deposits in lymph nodes which are not palpable. They therefore recommend irradiating the primary tumour and the neck nodes, whether palpable or not, to a dose of 5500 rad. in five to six weeks using cobalt-60. Except for very large tumours (T_4, N_0, M_0) they feel that when the primary lesion is removed about five weeks later an *elective* neck dissection need not be done. Skolnik and his colleagues have also reported that 5000 rad. in four weeks completely eradicated cancer cells from some lymph nodes although complete eradication of the tumour from the primary or metastatic sites was not obtained in any case. There was an increased post-operative morbidity rate. Strong and his colleagues (1966) quote laboratory evidence supporting the value of pre-operative irradiation. No agreement on the most effective way of carrying this out has been reached.

Post-operative irradiation has not found much favour in Great Britain or the United States though it has been extensively used in Europe. Simonetta (1962) and Leroux-Robert (1956) irradiate the lymph node areas after laryngectomy if no nodes are palpable and claim results as good as those who practice elective neck dissection in these cases. Shaw (1967) recommends radical surgery followed by radiotherapy for postcricoid and upper oesophageal lesions.

Choice of treatment

Marginal and upper pyriform fossa carcinomas

T_1, N_0 and T_2, N_0 cases often respond well to radiotherapy and should be treated by a full curative course using supervoltage with inclusion of the lymphatic fields. A careful monthly follow-up is instituted and failures or recurrences are treated by laryngectomy and partial pharyngectomy. In a few cases the residual growth may be removed by the lateral pharyngotomy approach.

In more advanced cases where fixation of a vocal cord has occurred and also in those with enlarged but operable lymph nodes planned pre-operative radiotherapy, as outlined below, followed by laryngectomy and partial pharyngectomy and radical neck dissection is advisable.

Pyriform fossa, postcricoid and upper oesophageal carcinomas

These tumours are usually advanced when they first present and are extremely difficult to cure. It is hoped that the combination of radiotherapy and surgery will improve results.

Since the optimum dose of irradiation for this form of treatment has yet to be determined the following scheme is put forward tentatively as a rationalization of the present evidence and it will certainly need modification as more information accumulates.

It is suggested that 4000–5500 rad. be given to the primary growth and lymph nodes (bilaterally for postcricoid carcinoma) in 4–6 weeks and the case be then reviewed by the radiotherapist and surgeon. In rare instances the response may be deemed so satisfactory that it will be decided to continue with radiotherapy to the full dose of 6500–7500 rad., but in the majority of cases treatment is stopped and pharyngolaryngectomy planned for 4–6 weeks later. Pharyngogastric or colonic anastomosis is recommended because it is less affected by previous irradiation than other methods. Since there is some evidence that irradiation of this order can eliminate non-palpable metastases an elective neck dissection need not be done but it should not be omitted if there had been or are palpable nodes. This eases the problem in postcricoid carcinomas where, in non-irradiated cases bilateral neck dissection is indicated. However, in all cases careful dissection of the paratracheal nodes should be carried out.

The laryngotracheal autograft should not be used after irradiation unless the dose has been in the order of only 2000 rad. in two weeks. If this method is used consideration should preferably be given to post-operative radiotherapy to the lower deep cervical and upper mediastinal nodes.

It is sometimes suggested that removal of the cervical lymphatic system by radical neck dissection may interfere with the patient's immune response to his carcinoma. At present the practical benefits of the operation undoubtedly outweigh the theoretical objections to it. Griffiths (1968) in his investigations into this problem found no justification for preserving regional lymph nodes in immunologically competent patients with carcinoma under the assumption that they control local and regional malignant cell propagation.

REFERENCES

Arons, M. S., and Smith, R. R. (1961). *Ann. Surg.*, **154**, 235.
Asherson, N. (1954). *J. Laryng.*, **68**, 550.
Bakamjian, V., and Littlewood, M. (1964). *Brit. J. plast. Surg.*, **17**, 191.
Beaugié, J. M., Mann, C. V., and Butler, E. C. B. (1969). *Brit. J. Surg.*, **56**, 586.
Brain, R. H. F., and Reading, P. V. (1966). *Brit. J. Surg.*, **53**, 933.
Bryce, D. P. (1967). In *Proceedings of the International Workshop on Cancer of the Head and Neck*
  (Ed. by J. Conley). Washington; Butterworths.
Buell, P. (1965). *Brit. J. Cancer*, **19**, 459.

Capps, F. W. (1961). *J. Laryng.*, **75**, 924.
Dalley, V. M. (1968). *J. Laryng.*, **82**, 407.
Eggston, A. A., and Wolff, D. (1947). *Histopathology of the Ear, Nose and Throat*. Baltimore; Williams and Wilkins.
Fairman, H. D., and John, H. T. (1966). *J. Laryng.*, **80**, 1091.
Fitzpatrick, P. J. (1967). *Clin. Radiol.*, **18**, 62.
Flatman, G. E. (1954). *Proc. R. Soc. Med.*, **47**, 555.
Foxwell, P. B., and Kelham, B. H. (1958). *J. Laryng.*, **72**, 647.
Friedman, M., and Daly, J. F. (1967). *Amer. J. Roentgen.*, **99**, 289.
Goldman, J. L., Friedman, W. H., and Bloom, B. S. (1968). *Laryngoscope*, **78**, 539.
Goligher, J. C., and Robin, I. G. (1954). *Brit. J. Surg.*, **42**, 283.
Gowan, G. P., and de Suto-Nagy, G. (1963). *Surgery Gynec. Obstet.*, **116**, 603.
Griffiths, C. O. (1968). *Amer. J. Surg.*, **116**, 559.
Harma, R. A. (1959). *Acta. Otolaryng. Stockh.* Suppl., 146.
Harrison, D. F. N. (1969). *Brit. J. Surg.*, **56**, 95.
Henderson, G. P., and Patterson, C. N. (1969). *Laryngoscope*, **79**, 561.
Hoffmeister, F. S., and Bakamjian, V. (1967). In *Proceedings of the International Workshop on Cancer of the Head and Neck* (Ed. by J. Conley). Washington; Butterworths.
Jacobs, A. (1963). *Brit. med. J.*, **1**, 1373.
Kapur, T. R. (1968). *J. Laryng.*, **82**, 447.
Klopp, C. T., and Schuster, M. (1956). *Cancer*, **9**, 1239.
Lederman, M. (1961). *Cancer of the Nasopharynx*. Springfield, Ill.; Thomas.
— (1962). *J. Laryng.*, **76**, 317.
Leroux-Robert, L. (1956). *Ann. Otol., etc., St. Louis*, **65**, 137.
Lambert, V. (1960). *J. Laryng.*, **74**, 1.
Le Quesne, L. P., and Ranger, D. (1966). *Brit. J. Surg.*, **53**, 105.
Lewis, R. S. (1965). *J. Laryng.*, **79**, 771.
MacComb, W. S., and Fletcher, G. H. (1967). *Cancer of the Head and Neck*. Baltimore; Williams and Wilkins.
MacNelis, F. L., and Pai, V. T. (1969). *Laryngoscope*, **79**, 1076.
Martin, H., Tollefsen, H. R., and Gerold, F. P. (1961). *Amer. J. Surg.*, **102**, 753.
— Ehrlich, H. E., and Abels, J. C. (1968). *Ann. Surg.*, **127**, 513.
Mills, C. P. (1955). *J. Laryng.*, **69**, 215.
Negus, Sir V. E. (1953). *Brit. J. plast. Surg.*, **6**, 102.
Ogura, J. H., Saltzstein, S. L., and Sputz, H. J. (1961). *Laryngoscope*, **71**, 258.
— and Mallen, R. W. (1965). *Proceedings of the Eighth International Congress of Otolaryngology*. Excerpta Medica Foundation.
Osborne, D. A. (1959). *J. Laryng.*, **73**, 295.
Richards, S. H. (1969). Meeting of the A.H.N.O. of Great Britain, Cardiff (Unpublished).
Rouvière, H. (1938). *Anatomy of the Human Lymphatic System*. Ann Arbor, Mich.; Edwards.
Schultz, M. D. (1965). *Laryngoscope*, **75**, 958.
Shaw, H. J. (1957). *Ann. R. Coll. Surg.*, **21**, 290.
— (1967). *J. Otolaryng. Soc. Aust.*, **2**, 1.
Simonetta, B., and Guiacci, F. (1962). *Arch. Otolaryng.*, **76**, 451.
Simpson, J. F. (1960). *J. Laryng.*, **74**, 300.
Snelling, M. (1954). *Proc. R. Soc. Med.*, **47**, 549.
Som, M. L. (1956). *Arch. Otolaryng.*, **63**, 474.
— (1967). In *Proceedings of the International Workshop on Cancer of the Head and Neck* (Ed. by J. Conley). Washington; Butterworths.
Skolnick, E. M., Tenta, L. T., Comito, J. N., and Jerome, D. L. (1966). *Ann. Otol., etc., St. Louis*, **75**, 336.
Stout, A. P., and Kenney, F. R. (1949). *Cancer*, **2**, 261.
Strong, E. W., Hensche, V. K., Nickson, J. J., Frazell, E. L., Tollefsen, H. R., and Hilaris, B. S. (1966). *Cancer*, **18**, 1509.
Stuart, D. W. (1966). *J. Laryng.*, **80**, 382.
Sturton, S. D., Wen, H. L., and Sturton, O. G. (1966). *Cancer*, **19**, 1666.
Terz, J. J., and Farr, H. W. (1967). *Surgery Gynec. Obstet.*, **125**, 581.
Thomson, St. Cl., and Colledge, L. (1930). *Cancer of the Larynx*. London; Kegan Paul.
— and Negus, V. E. (1955). *Diseases of the Nose and Throat*. London; Cassell.
Toker, C. (1963). *Ann. Surg.*, **157**, 419.
Trotter, W. (1929). *Brit. J. Surg.*, **16**, 485.
Willis, R. A. (1953). *Pathology of Tumours*. London; Butterworths.
Wilson, C. P. (1957). *Ann. Otol., etc., St. Louis*, **66**, 5.
Windeyer, B. W. (1959). *Proc. R. Soc. Med.*, **52**, 1088.
Wood-Jones, F. (1940). *J. Anat. Lond.*, **74**, 147.
Wright, D. (1967). *J. Laryng.*, **81**, 1337.
Wynder, E. L., Bross, J. J., and Feldman, R. M. A. (1957). *Cancer*, **10**, 1300.
Yeh, S. (1962). *Cancer*, **15**, 895.

8

HYPOPHARYNGEAL DIVERTICULUM (PHARYNGEAL POUCH)

JOHN BALLANTYNE

The relatively common type of pharyngeal pouch, correctly known as a hypopharyngeal diverticulum, is a posterior pulsion pouch which occurs between the upper thyropharyngeal fibres and the lower cricopharyngeal fibres of the inferior constrictor muscle.

The inferior constrictor muscle arises from the oblique line on the lamina of the thyroid cartilage, and from the side of the arch of the cricoid cartilage (Fig. 62). It has two parts; an upper oblique part, the thyropharyngeus; and a lower circular part, the cricopharyngeus.

The fibres of the thyropharyngeus are inserted into the median raphe of the pharynx. Its upper fibres are supported by the overlapping fibres of the middle and superior constrictors, but its lower fibres lack this support below the level of the vocal cords and are, furthermore, thinned out. This leaves a potentially weak area above the cricopharyngeus (*Killian's dehiscence*).

The cricopharyngeus is thicker than the other pharyngeal muscles and it extends around the pharynx, without interruption, from one side of the cricoid arch to the other. There is no raphe here. The muscle acts as a sphincter at the lower extremity of the pharynx and it is continuous with the circular muscle coat of the oesophagus. It is normally closed, except for momentary relaxation during the act of deglutition, and it has a different nerve supply from the other constrictors.

All the nerve fibres to the constrictor muscles, except those destined for the cricopharyngeal sphincter, leave the brain stem in the cranial root of the accessory nerve, and pass thence to the vagus. Most of these fibres pass in its pharyngeal branch to the pharyngeal plexus, whence the constrictor muscles are innervated. However, the sphincter derives its nerve supply from the recurrent laryngeal nerve and the external laryngeal branch of the superior laryngeal nerve.

The rare congenital pouches arising in the sites of the branchial clefts were discussed by Wilson (1962) in his Semon Lecture.

Aetiology

There is still much controversy about the cause of hypopharyngeal diverticula.

Negus (1950) believed that tonic spasm of the cricopharyngeus muscle prevented the downward passage of the bolus and that the relatively weak area of the posterior pharyngeal wall (Killian's dehiscence) gave way to the long-continued pressure within the pharynx above the sphincter, with eventual herniation.

A more commonly held theory is that of a neuromuscular inco-ordination. This postulates that there is a delay or failure of relaxation of the cricopharyngeal sphincter at the end of the second stage of swallowing, that is, that the diverticulum results from an achalasia rather than a spasm.

Kodicek and Creamer (1961) were unable to find any evidence to support a theory of faulty relaxation or achalasia of the cricopharyngeal sphincter as a cause of pharyngeal pouch. They measured the intraluminal pressures of the pharynx and the sphincter in five patients with pouches, through fine water-filled polythene tubes attached to manometers; the resting tone of the sphincter was normal and, on swallowing, normal relaxation was recorded.

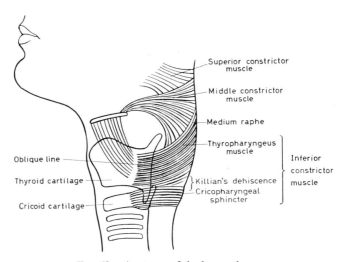

FIG. 62.—Anatomy of the lower pharynx.

As Korkis pointed out in 1958, neither of these theories explains the absence of diverticulosis in this area in cases of long-standing stenosis of the upper oesophagus; nor do they explain how it is that the condition appears to be permanently cured by adequate excision of the pouch, even though the alleged cause remains.

Wilson (1962) agrees with this view and goes further by saying there is no dehiscence above the cricopharyngeal sphincter; indeed, in many dissections of the pharynx, he has found that the lower fibres of the thyropharyngeus are transverse and usually overlap the cricopharyngeus. "To produce a pouch", he adds, "there must certainly be increased hypopharyngeal pressure, and this can only be produced by a descending peristaltic contraction of the inferior constrictor when the upper sphincter of the gullet is closed."

He further states that, in examining the barium radiographs of patients with these pharyngeal pouches, there are two constant features: in the first place, there is always some residual barium after the act of swallowing has been completed; and secondly, the pharynx is usually larger than normal (megapharynx). In some patients with a megapharynx, according to Wilson, there is a "primary swallow" which is initiated by the tongue, with elevation of the pharynx, peristaltic contraction of the constrictors and relaxation of the upper sphincter of the gullet; but these patients take large mouthfuls and leave a residue of food, and also of air, in the pharynx after the sphincter has closed. Then, in these patients a "secondary swallow" takes place—a voluntary act—not initiated by the tongue at all, but a consciously initiated contraction of the constrictor muscles immediately after the primary swallow, while the sphincter is closed; that is to say, increased pressure is produced between the contracting portion of the inferior constrictor above and the closed gullet below. This, so Wilson believes, gives rise to the herniation which subsequently becomes a pouch.

Ardran, Kemp and Lund (1964), in a cine-radiographic study, have emphasized that all the above theories are based on studies of established pouches and not on pouches in the process of formation. The swallowing abnormalities noted by those authors may therefore be the result rather than the cause of a pouch. Their cine-radiographs were taken on 35 mm. film at 25 frames per second.

In normal subjects, the films showed a wave of peristalsis in the pharynx produced by the contracting pharyngeal constrictors. This wave, which includes the sphincter, sweeps down the upper digestive tube in a progressive fashion, squeezing the bolus from top to bottom "like squeezing the toothpaste out of a tube".

The common factor in all patients with pouches, from very small to very large, was the early closure of the cricopharyngeal sphincter, usually but not invariably in association with weakness or inco-ordination of the pharyngeal peristaltic wave.

Continuing their analogy, these authors show that, if one starts to squeeze a tube of toothpaste from the bottom, and then suddenly (with the other hand) squeezes it near the top, a bulge will occur in the tube between the two flattened parts. The squeeze near the top produces the same effect as the sudden early contracture of the sphincter; the bulge represents the pouch. Thus the pouch is formed when the sphincter is contracting and not when it is relaxing. In fact, relaxation is usually adequate.

It is difficult to say whether these diverticula are caused by the early contraction of the cricopharyngeal sphincter or by the late arrival of the peristaltic wave in the pharynx, but Ardran, Kemp and Lund believe it is most likely that the fundamental upset is the early contraction of the cricopharyngeus muscle ahead of the expressor action.

In contradistinction to Wilson's view that a "secondary swallow" against a closed sphincter is responsible for the formation of a pouch, Ardran, Kemp and Lund have emphasized that, except in one case in their series, the pouch (in the earliest stage of development) was always visualized during the first swallow, never as the result of an obstructed second swallow.

Pathology

The pouch is composed usually of mucosa and fibrous tissue only. As it enlarges, the pouch sags downwards behind the oesophagus and may reach the mediastinum. The opening of the pouch becomes more and more a direct continuation of the pharynx and the oesophageal opening becomes concealed in front of the mouth of the pouch. As more food enters the pouch, pressure is exerted on the oesophagus from behind to cause oesophageal obstruction.

Originating posteriorly, the pouch usually passes down to the left of the oesophagus, much less commonly to the right.

A hypopharyngeal diverticulum may be complicated by carcinoma within the pouch, usually in its lower two-thirds. A carcinoma confined to the neck of the pouch is very rare but has been reported.

The recurrent laryngeal nerve may be implicated by a large pouch, especially when it is complicated by neoplasia.

Clinical features

Pharyngeal pouches occur most commonly in late middle age, and they are three or four times more common in men than in women.

Their cardinal symptoms are dysphagia, often of long standing, and regurgitation of undigested food, often foetid; this causes bad breath.

Discomfort may be caused by the excessive collection of saliva in the pouch, and as the sac grows the patient takes longer and longer to complete a meal. This is a source of growing social embarrassment.

A swelling in the neck may be present, usually on the left side. It may gurgle and empty on external pressure.

Cough may be caused by overflow of fluids from the diverticulum into the larynx, or rarely by compression of the recurrent laryngeal nerve, the latter also causing occasional hoarseness, especially when the pouch contains a carcinoma.

Emaciation will eventually result from oesophageal obstruction or from neoplastic changes, the latter diagnosis being always suggested when there is blood in the regurgitated material. Small pouches are not uncommonly asymptomatic.

Diagnosis

In most cases, radiography with a barium swallow will show a characteristic retort-shaped swelling, which may extend into the mediastinum. It will also demonstrate the septum between the gullet and pouch (Fig. 63).

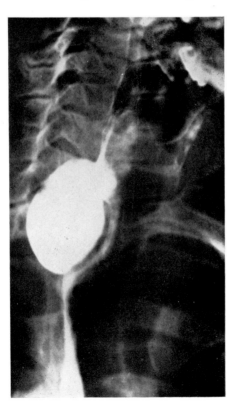

FIG. 63.—Barium swallow—pharynx and upper oesophagus. The radiograph demonstrates a pharyngeal pouch of moderate size. The septum between the pouch and the oesophagus is well demonstrated.

Cine-radiography may demonstrate the earliest tendency to herniation and is useful in demonstrating the results of treatment.

Turner (1963), reporting the radiographic findings in two cases of hypopharyngeal diverticulum with carcinoma, emphasized that when an interruption is found in the normally smooth outline of a barium-filled pouch, and when this is continuous with a filling defect in the interior of the pouch, the diagnosis is very likely to be that of a carcinoma. If such an appearance is quite constant after an interval of one or more days, the diagnosis is practically certain.

Treatment

No treatment is necessary for very small pouches, but if symptoms persist dilatation of the cricopharyngeal sphincter may give relief of varying duration. More lasting results may be effected by the use of a hydrostatic bag (Negus, 1950). However, such methods rarely give permanent relief.

If it be accepted—and it probably can be accepted—that the site of obstruction in cases of hypopharyngeal diverticula lies at the cricopharyngeal sphincter, then it would seem rational, at least in early cases, to divide the circular muscle fibres of the cricopharyngeal sphincter by an external route. This may be compared with Heller's operation for achalasia of the cardia or Ramstedt's operation for infantile pyloric stenosis, and such a procedure has been supported by Spencer Harrison (1958), who advises that this should be followed by inversion of the sac by means of a purse-string suture, bringing together neighbouring tissues over the gap in the posterior pharyngeal wall.

Myotomy of the cricopharyngeus muscle would seem to be a simple, safe and successful alternative to excision or endoscopic diathermy in small pouches, especially when a prominent cricopharyngeus muscle is shown in the x-ray. After the myotomy, the cricopharyngeal and oesophageal muscles should be dissected from the underlying mucosa for about half the circumference of the mucosal tube, to allow the mucosa to protrude freely through the incision. Ellis and his colleagues (1969) have reported 18 cases in which a myotomy was performed; in four it was combined with excision, in another four with suspension, of the pouch. Fourteen patients became symptom-free; three had only occasional symptoms of dysphagia; and only one, who had a large pouch, had no relief at all.

More radical surgical procedures are difficult and unsatisfactory at this stage, but they offer the only hope of permanent relief in more advanced cases.

Excision of the pouch

The one-stage excision of a large pouch is undoubtedly the most satisfactory form of treatment when the patient's general condition permits it, and a complete cure of symptoms with the return of normal radiographic appearance is to be expected in the majority of such cases.

The sac is first emptied by suction through an oesophageal speculum and the upper oesophageal opening identified. This opening may be pulled backwards by the pouch, making its identification very difficult. However, once found, the opening should be dilated and a plastic oesophageal feeding tube inserted through it. The pouch is then lightly packed with 2·5 cm. ribbon gauze impregnated with an aqueous solution of flavine. This fills the pouch and makes it more readily identifiable through the external approach.

The speculum is withdrawn and an incision is made along the anterior border of the sternomastoid muscle, from the hyoid bone above to the sternum below, usually on the left side of the neck when the sac projects to this side.

After separation and retraction of the skin, fascia and platysma muscle, the omohyoid is found and divided (Fig 64a). Blunt dissection and separation of the tissues between the larynx, trachea and lateral lobe of the thyroid gland medially, and the sternomastoid muscle and great vessels of the neck laterally, will usually bring into view the inferior thyroid artery and some inferior thyroid veins. These must be ligatured and divided as required, and the neck of the sac is soon brought into view (Fig. 64b).

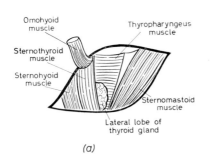

(a)

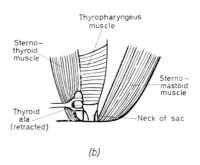

(b)

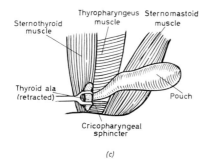

(c)

FIG. 64.—Excision of a pharyngeal pouch: (a) omohyoid muscle divided; (b) neck of sac exposed; (c) pouch mobilized.

The fundus of the sac is identified and freed by gentle dissection; grasping it lightly with tissue forceps, the surgeon gradually delivers it into the wound by further blunt dissection until the neck is clearly seen (Fig. 64c).

At this stage, the flavine gauze must be removed through the mouth, the neck of the sac clamped with curved forceps and the pouch excised. The defect in the pharynx is closed by a continuous suture passed round the forceps, and the forceps gradually withdrawn as the suture is closed. A second invaginating layer passes through the outer muscular coat of the pharynx and surrounding tissues, and the cricopharyngeal sphincter is divided down to the mucosa.

Finally, a corrugated rubber drain is inserted down to the suture line and the wound closed in layers. In fit subjects, the feeding tube may be removed on completion of the operation and the patient fed intravenously for four or five days. This encourages quick healing and there is much less discomfort, but it is wise to leave a tube in position in debilitated patients.

Systemic antibiotic cover is given for five days, the drain removed in 48 hours and the oesophageal feeding tube removed (if it has been retained) after four days.

The main complication of excision in the days before antibiotics was infection in the deep cervical tissues, and mediastinitis was responsible for many deaths; but the incidence of this fatal complication has been very greatly reduced.

Post-operative stricture results from the removal of too much of the pharynx at the neck of the pouch, or too tight suturing. It may require repeated dilatations. Pouches may recur if too much of the neck is left behind.

Fistulae can be extremely troublesome, but will usually heal spontaneously if an oesophageal feeding tube is re-inserted and left in position until healing is complete.

Paralysis of the recurrent laryngeal nerve is a rare complication.

In cases of carcinoma within a pharyngeal diverticulum, Garlock and Richter (1961) recommend a wide local excision when the growth is confined to the pouch, but recommend radical excision of the upper oesophagus together with the pouch when extension has occurred to the neighbouring oesophagus.

Endoscopic diathermy

Under certain circumstances, especially when the barium swallow suggests that the sac is adherent to the adjacent oesophageal wall, division of the septum between the gullet and the pouch, after the method originally described by Dohlman, has gained favour with many laryngologists. It may be particularly useful in patients who have become emaciated by prolonged dysphagia or are unfit (by reason of some general disease of poor or uncertain prognosis) for major surgery, but it is also applicable to many large or medium-sized pouches. It is not to be recommended for a small sac, nor for a very large one extending well down into the thorax, nor when it is very difficult to find the opening into the oesophagus.

Dohlman and Mattson (1960) reported the results of treatment by the endoscopic operation is nearly 100 cases, without mortality or serious complications; and more recently White (1968) has reported a small series of nine cases treated satisfactorily by this method, emphasizing that excision can be carried out subsequently without undue difficulty if the diathermy operation fails to relieve symptoms or is followed by recurrence. Spencer Harrison (1958) stated that, at that time, no case had yet been reported of a carcinoma arising within the pouch in patients who had been treated by this technique; but Juby (1969) has reported one case, in a total series of 17 cases treated by him and his colleagues over a period of 12 years, in which neoplastic changes developed (in 1965) at the junction of the pouch and the oesophagus, five years after the last of a series of six treatments with diathermy; and he regards this as a very important reason for advocating radical excision whenever the patient is fit for it.

Dohlman uses a bivalved oesophageal speculum (Fig. 65a). The anterior blade enters the oesophagus, the posterior blade entering the pouch. As the instrument is advanced, the "septum" between gullet and pouch forms a bulky horizontal mass which contains the cricopharyngeal sphincter (Fig. 65a). This is grasped with the jaws of the diathermy forceps (Fig. 65b) and a coagulating current is applied until the tissues held by the forceps become blanched. The forceps are withdrawn, and an insulated spatula (Fig. 65c) introduced into the pouch. Finally the coagulated tissues are divided by a cutting current applied through the insulated knife (Fig. 65*d*).

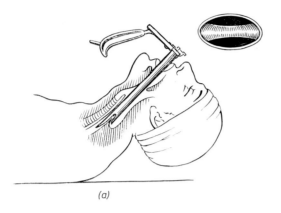

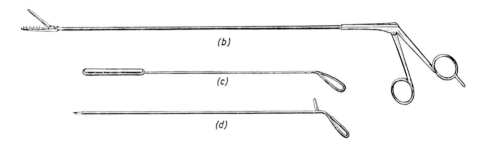

FIG. 65.—Dohlman's operation: (*a*) the Dohlman bivalved speculum in position. Inset shows the horizontal "septum"; (*b*) diathermy forceps; (*c*) spatula; (*d*) diathermy knife.

Simpson (1964) has devised an improved modification of Dohlman's diathermy forceps (Fig. 66) which can be introduced through the ordinary oesophageal speculum of Negus. The spatulate end enters the pouch as the cutting part is introduced carefully into the oesophagus. The jaws are opposed only when the cutting "knife" has passed beyond the sphincter. The instrument is withdrawn in the closed position, whilst a cutting current is applied.

An oesophageal feeding tube should be left in position for four or five days, and systemic antibiotic cover is given for the same period.

A barium swallow after diathermy division of the septum will, of course, show that the pouch is still present; but it also shows in successful cases that the barium is no longer held up and there is no regurgitation.

Despite the report of an isolated instance of carcinoma following a Dohlman operation, it is known that such a lesion may develop spontaneously in one of these diverticula; and the procedure, or one of its modifications, has given very satisfactory symptomatic relief in many cases, including some in which the lesion has been present for so long that the patient's general condition precluded radical excision.

Division of the septum may have to be repeated several times, an average of three in Juby's series, and mediastinitis has been known to occur.

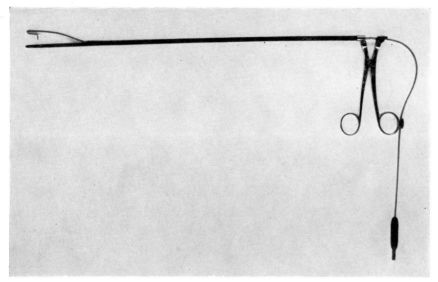

Fig. 66.—Simpson's diathermy forceps. (*Reproduced by courtesy of Mr. J. F. Simpson and the Photographic Department, St. Mary's Hospital, London.*)

Diverticulo-oesophagostomy

Jackson, Slack and Williams (1960) have recorded a case of a very large pouch occurring in a man 57 years of age, who had had a history of regurgitation of food for five years. The pouch was so large and descended so far into the thorax that they regarded the case as unsuitable for excision through the neck or diathermy division through the endoscope.

The pouch was therefore exposed in the chest and the lower end of the pouch was anastomosed to the oesophagus, by an end-to-side anastomosis.

Two weeks later, the patient was swallowing well and had gained 4·5 kg. in weight and the barium swallow demonstrated a good stoma; ten weeks after the operation, he was still swallowing well and had gained 12·5 kg.

REFERENCES

Ardran, G. M., Kemp, F. H., and Lund, W. S. (1964). "The Aetiology of the Posterior Pharyngeal Diverticulum: A Cineradiographic Study". *J. Laryng.*, **78**, 333.

Dohlman, G., and Mattson, O. (1960). "The Endoscopic Operation for Hypopharyngeal Diverticulum." *Arch. Otolaryng.*, **71**, 744.

Ellis, F. H., Schlegel, J. F., Lynch, V. P., and Payne, W. S. (1969). "Crico-pharyngeal Myotomy for Pharyngo-oesophageal Diverticulum". *Ann. Surg.*, **170**, 340.

Garlock, J. H., and Richter, R. (1961). "Carcinoma in a Pharyngo-Oesophageal Diverticulum: A Case Report." *Ann. Surg.*, **154**, 259.

Jackson, J. W., Slack, W., and Williams, R. A. (1960). "Pharyngeal Pouch Treated by Diverticulo-Oesophagostomy." *Lancet*, **1**, 470.

Juby, H. B. (1969). "The Treatment of Pharyngeal Pouch". *J. Laryng.*, **83**, 1067.

Kodicek, J., and Creamer, B. (1961). "A Study of Pharyngeal Pouches." *J. Laryng.*, **75**, 406.

Korkis, F. Boyes (1958). "The Aetiology, Diagnosis and Surgical Treatment of Pharyngeal Diverticula." *J. Laryng.*, **72**, 509.

Negus, Sir Victor (1950). "Pharyngeal Diverticula. Observations on their Aetiology and Treatment." *Brit. J. Surg.*, **38**, 9.

Simpson, J. F. (1964). Personal communication.

Spencer Harrison, M. (1958). "The Aetiology, Diagnosis and Surgical Treatment of Pharyngeal Diverticula." *J. Laryng.*, **72,** 523.

Turner, M. J. (1963). "Carcinoma as a Complication of Pharyngeal Pouch." *Brit. J. Radiol.*, **36,** 206.

White, I. L. (1968). "Endoscopic Treatment of Hypopharyngeal Diverticula". *Calif. Med.*, **109,** 374.

Wilson, C. P. (1962). "Pharyngeal Diverticula, Their Cause and Treatment." (Semon Lecture.) *J. Laryng.*, **76,** 151.

9

OESOPHAGEAL CONDITIONS IN THE PRACTICE OF EAR, NOSE AND THROAT SURGERY

E. H. MILES FOXEN and JOHN GROVES

GENERAL CONSIDERATIONS

Symptoms of disease of the oesophagus

Dysphagia

Difficulty in swallowing will usually lead the patient quickly to his doctor. Few discomforts are as alarming or distressing. In the presence of this symptom clinical examination, radiography and endoscopy will be promptly undertaken. In the absence of dysphagia, however, the possible oesophageal significance of the other symptoms discussed below is all too easily overlooked. Investigation and diagnosis then will be unnecessarily late.

Since dysphagia can be caused by virtually any abnormality or disease affecting the tongue, pharynx or oesophagus, there is little point in compiling or memorizing a "list of causes". It is helpful, however, to consider some categories of causes, particularly in that they may cause characteristic patterns of difficulty in swallowing.

Inflammations of the throat give rise to painful difficulties at the beginning of the act of swallowing. In the upper oesophagus they cause a feeling of obstruction with pain which may necessitate a second voluntary act of deglutition to get the bolus down. At the lower end of the oesophagus they cause discomfort for a few seconds, subsiding spontaneously as the bolus is first checked by muscular spasm and then slowly moved through into the stomach.

Organic stricture (fibrous or neoplastic) causes obstruction (but seldom pain), whose severity depends upon the "tightness" of the stricture. If it is high in the oesophagus or in the hypopharynx a sensation of choking is felt during swallowing, a double effort may be necessary, and coughing and choking result from spill-over into the laryngeal inlet. The patient quickly learns to restrict each swallow to the small amount that can be contained above the stricture without rising above the watershed of the arytenoid eminences. Strictures in the middle or lower oesophagus do not usually cause bronchial tree spill-over unless associated with recurrent laryngeal nerve paralysis or tracheo-oesophageal fistula, but the patient may localize the subjective feeling of obstruction behind the sternum or in the root of the neck. An obstruction in the lower oesophagus may be localized by the patient at any level from the epigastrium upwards.

Neuromuscular disorders of deglutition as a rule cause greater difficulty with liquids, either because of regurgitation into the nose (past a paralysed palate) or by laryngeal spill-over if the laryngeal sphincters are paralysed. Often such patients can manage better with soft solid food, in contrast to those with an organic stricture, who swallow liquids more easily than solids.

When the oesophagus is compressed or distorted by a lesion outside its wall dysphagia is usually not very severe, and localization by the patient of the level of the hold-up is often rather vague. Liquids may be swallowed quite freely, while solids will go down if well chewed and given sufficient time to pass.

If dysphagia develops only slowly or is of long standing (for example, in some cases of Paterson–Brown Kelly disease) it may come to be accepted and tolerated so that the patient only mentions it when specifically questioned on the point. Conversely the rapid onset of a similar degree of narrowing (e.g. due to a neoplasm) causes great distress and rapid loss of weight due to insufficient food intake.

Regurgitation

Painless regurgitation of undigested food is indicative of a dilated viscus above an obstruction. In its most marked form, due to achalasia of the cardia, regurgitation occurs when the patient lies down. In contrast, the regurgitation due to lesions of the upper oesophagus happens during a meal. When it is due to the emptying of a pharyngeal diverticulum the act of regurgitation relieves temporarily the dysphagia caused by the distension of the pouch with food.

Acid regurgitation from the stomach into the throat is associated with a bitter taste, or a burning sensation in the precordium and back, and is caused not by obstructive lesions but by failure of the cardiac sphincteric mechanism (as in hiatus hernia).

Pain

When caused by oesophageal disease pain may be felt in the epigastrium, in the substernal region, in the back (particularly in the left scapular region) or in the root of the neck. Referral of pain to the vagus nerve territory of the ear is rare, and may originate even from the lowest part of the oesophagus, as in reflux oesophagitis.

If the pain is associated with, or aggravated by, swallowing its significance is readily appreciated. If dysphagia is slight or absent, however, oesophageal pain may be erroneously attributed to diseases of the heart, lungs or stomach.

Bleeding

Gross haemorrhage from the oesophagus is rather uncommon and is usually due to varices. A few patients with neoplasms or inflammatory disease may vomit or regurgitate blood-stained fluid. Fresh blood appearing in quantity in the throat without effort may arise from lesions near the upper end of the oesophagus.

Respiratory symptoms

Recurring attacks of bronchitis or bronchopneumonia complicate the progress of any disease of the oesophagus associated with laryngeal spill-over, or tracheo-oesophageal fistula. Progressive deterioration of pulmonary function may be so severe that it dominates the clinical picture. The underlying oesophageal cause may even be missed altogether. *Hoarseness*, whether due to an obvious cord paralysis,

208

or to laryngitis, or to the simple weakness of cachexia, should always arouse suspicion of an oesophageal lesion.

General symptoms

Loss of weight is the most important of these, and occurs rapidly in the presence of oesophageal obstruction. General malaise and the symptoms of anaemia are frequently observed and justify suspicion of oesophageal disease if their cause is not readily apparent on clinical examination.

Physical examination

When symptoms suggest the possibility of an oesophageal lesion a routine physical examination of the patient's chest, abdomen and cardiovascular and nervous systems must be followed by attention to the following special points:

(1) Evidence of wasting and dehydration must be noted.

(2) Inspection and palpation of the neck (for thyroid enlargement, palpable lymph nodes and inflammatory or neoplastic masses arising from the pharynx or oesophagus). Absence of laryngeal crepitus against the vertebral column is noted in some cases of carcinoma of the postcricoid or upper oesophageal region.

(3) Mirror examination of the pharynx and larynx (for palatal or vocal cord paralysis, ulceration or tumour). Even though all of these visible regions may be normal, pooling of saliva in the pyriform fossa of one or both sides is strongly suggestive of a lesion at a lower level.

(4) In completing his special examination the laryngologist will inspect the mouth and tongue for clinical evidence of anaemia, in the form of glossitis, atrophy of lingual papillae, and cracks or healed fissures at the corners of the mouth.

The patient should then be given something to drink, and his performance of deglutition is observed. This simple test should never be omitted. Coughing, choking, pain, "double-effort", and regurgitation are much easier to assess in the clinic than by hearsay. If swallowing is repeated while the examiner palpates the root of the neck a typical gurgling sensation will be felt under the hand in cases of pharyngeal pouch.

Laboratory investigations

(1) Blood examination is always indicated to determine the presence of anaemia associated with Paterson–Brown Kelly disease, carcinoma, or oesophageal bleeding. Occasionally serological tests for syphilis will be necessary.

(2) Bacteriological investigations are seldom helpful, but in rare conditions such as diphtheria, fungus infections or tuberculous disease of the oesophagus, examination of a throat swab, specimens of sputum, or oesophageal washings may assist diagnosis.

(3) Exfoliative cytology has been shown to be of value in carcinoma of the oesophagus (Klayman, 1955). A Ryle's tube is passed to the level of the lesion and through it saline lavage and suction are performed. The aspirated fluid is centrifuged and the residue is suitably fixed, stained and examined microscopically.

(4) Examination of the stools for occult blood will usually give positive findings in the presence of malignant or other bleeding disease of the oesophagus, but the test has only slight diagnostic value.

209

Radiographic examination

Routine plain films

Routine plain films must include:

(1) Postero-anterior views of the chest and mediastinum, to show pulmonary fibrosis or tumour, enlargement or displacement of the mediastinum, aortic aneurysm, and the size and shape of the heart.

(2) Lateral soft-tissue views of the neck to show the outlines of the larynx, trachea, vertebral column, and the vertical band of soft tissues representing the postcricoid area and cervical portion of the oesophagus (Fig. 67*a*). Pathological widening of this band may indicate a tumour or cellulitis. Surgical emphysema, a fluid level within an abscess cavity or a persistent gas bubble in the upper oesophageal lumen are all significant abnormalities detectable in this projection.

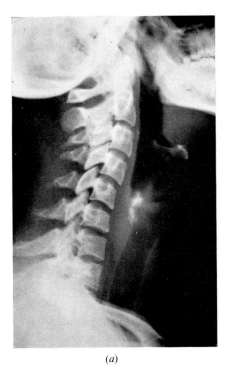
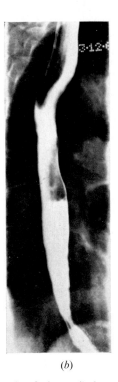

(*a*)   (*b*)

FIG. 67.—(*a*) Lateral radiograph of the neck. Note the normal soft-tissue shadow between the trachea and vertebral column; (*b*) normal barium swallow appearances of the thoracic part of the oesophagus.

Fluoroscopic screening and contrast studies

These are normally done together and permanent records of the radiologist's observations are made by means of "still" exposures and cine-photography. The latter technique is finding an increasing usefulness, especially in cases where slow-motion study of abnormal deglutition can contribute to the analysis of neuro-muscular disorders.

The technique of conducting these examinations is not described here. The clinician must always try to indicate to the radiologist the likely level of the lesion, so that the examination can be as brief and informative as possible. This is particularly important in patients who are weak and ill. It is also very important to warn the radiologist of the possibility of inundation of the bronchial tree in cases with laryngeal "spill-over" or suspected broncho-oesophageal fistula. In these cases the examination should begin with the swallowing of a small amount of iodized oil which would do no harm if it were to "go the wrong way".

In screening these cases the radiologist will follow the passage of a mouthful of barium and use it to indicate the outlines of the oesophageal lumen, its mucosal folds, the form and position of physiological and pathological constrictions, and the rate and smoothness of the peristaltic waves. The lower end of the oesophagus, the cardia and the stomach are all observed. When sufficient barium has collected in the stomach the patient is placed in Trendelenburg's position and manual pressure is applied to the stomach. This manoeuvre demonstrates the presence of hiatus hernia, and the competency or otherwise of the cardiac sphincteric mechanisms. The normal barium swallow appearances are shown in Fig. 67b, and are described in more detail in Volume 1.

Fig. 68 (pp. 212 and 213) illustrates some typical deformations of the normal oesophagus by extrinsic lesions. These deformations are best shown radiographically, are important in the differential diagnosis of dysphagia, and some of them may be contra-indications to oesophagoscopy. Their importance to the oesophagoscopist is therefore very great.

Oesophagoscopy

Direct endoscopic inspection of the oesophagus by means of a straight rigid tube was reported in 1868 by Kusmaul, who used professional sword-swallowers as subjects. Really satisfactory instruments and techniques were only developed, however, with the invention of electrical lighting systems. In more recent times the Jacksons and many other oesophagologists have established the clinical applications of the method. During the last 30 years oesophagoscopy has come to be taken for granted as a simple diagnostic routine, practised more or less regularly and uneventfully by non-specialists, such as thoracic surgeons and physicians, as well as by laryngologists. This facilitation has been accelerated by modern anaesthetic techniques which have reduced the difficulties and hazards. Oesophagoscopy nevertheless is still potentially one of the most dangerous of all procedures, and the laryngologist bears a great responsibility to maintain the highest possible standards both in the performance and in the teaching of the technique. Oesophagoscopy should only be done when definite indications are present, and these must always be assessed in terms of likely benefit to the patient. Mere confirmation of diagnosis is no justification if no advantage can accrue to the patient by it.

Flexible fibre-optic oesophagoscopes are currently being developed for use under topical anaesthesia, permitting safer inspection, biopsy and photography. Without doubt, when these tools are adopted in general use many advantages will be gained, but at the time of writing the standard techniques about to be described are not superceded, nor are they likely to be in the foreseeable future in any cases requiring intra-oesophageal manipulations.

Common sense should dictate who should perform a given oesophagoscopy. Clearly, the thoracic surgeon should inspect lesions of the middle or lower oesophagus, such as carcinoma or hiatus hernia, when transthoracic surgical treatment may be envisaged. Lesions of the hypopharynx and upper oesophagus are primarily the laryngologist's concern. An impacted foreign body should be removed by the most competent endoscopist available at the time—almost invariably this person is a laryngologist. Specific indications for oesophagoscopy emerge later in this chapter. Some contra-indications must now be considered.

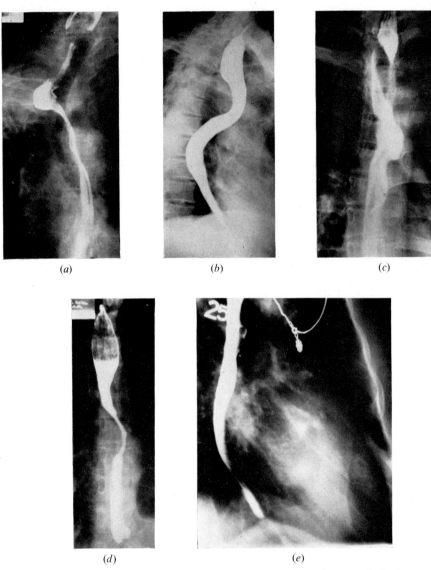

(a) (b) (c)

(d) (e)

FIG. 68.—Deformations of the oesophagus by lesions outside its wall, as seen in barium swallow radiographs: (a) extreme displacement and kinking caused by the traction of fibrosis in the right upper lobe of the lung (healed pulmonary tuberculosis); (b) distortion due to a large aortic arch aneurysm; (c) spiral filling defect due to aberrant right subclavian artery passing behind the oesophagus (*dysphagia lusoria*); (d) compression of the middle third of the oesophagus by mediastinal lymph node metastases (carcinoma of the breast); (e) cardiac enlargement. The gullet is compressed by the dilated left atrium.

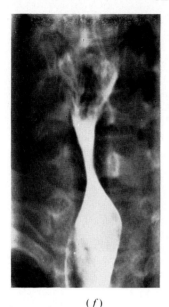
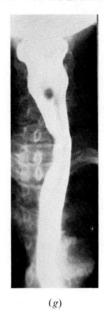
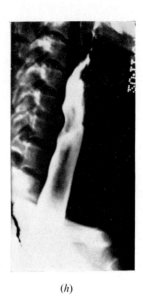

(*f*)   (*g*)   (*h*)

FIG. 68.—(*f*) Symmetrical indentation of cervical oesophagus by pressure of a diffuse goitre; (*g*) sideways displacement of cervical oesophagus by neoplasm of right lobe of thyroid; (*h*) scalloping of posterior outline of oesophagus due to cervical osteophytes.

Contra-indications to oesophagoscopy

(1) Aneurysm of the aorta.

(2) Severe spinal deformities, such as kyphosis or advanced osteophytosis of the bodies of the cervical vertebrae.

(3) Advanced "general" disease such as heart, kidney or liver failure.

Other factors may make oesophagoscopy difficult. These are prominent upper teeth, a narrow mandibular arch, a stiff, short and thick neck, and moderate degrees of kyphosis. Such difficulties can usually be overcome with patience and skill, but they may occasionally dictate the abandonment of the investigation.

Instruments

The oesophagoscope is basically a rigid metal tube. Lighting may be distal (as in the Jackson type), proximal through obliquely-placed side tubes (Negus), or proximal in the form of an external light source directed down the tube by a mirror or prism (Bruning, Killian, Haslinger). The most effective lighting is undoubtedly the recently-introduced remote source applied by a flexible fibre-optic cable, and the Negus type of instrument lends itself particularly well to this improvement.

The different types vary considerably in the design of their distal ends. These differences are seen in the obliquity of the mouth of the tube, and in the thickened "rolled" leading edge of some patterns. In cross-section types range from a very flat oval to a virtually circular shape. Several lengths are available in each of the various patterns, so that the endoscopist can operate at the shortest practicable working distance whatever the level of the lesion. An extremely useful short tube is the so-called oesophageal speculum, which allows inspection of the upper 10–12 cm. of the oesophagus as well as the hypopharynx.

Other essential equipment includes: (*a*) metal suction tubes in various lengths to suit the oesophagoscopes to be used; (*b*) various grasping and biopsy forceps; (*c*) bougies in a series of graduated sizes.

In addition, special devices will be needed for particular cases. These may include foreign body forceps, hydrostatic dilators, equipment for the introduction of metal or plastic tubes, snares, or special syringes.

The operating table must be versatile in its tilting arrangements, and the section supporting the head must be easily raised and lowered, ideally by the operator himself. Some surgeons favour the special Negus head rest, which facilitates movement from side to side as well as up and down.

Anaesthesia

Preparation of the patient includes examination of the teeth. Any which are decayed or loose must be noted. Elaborate and fragile dental works such as "jacket crowns" are easily overlooked and may be damaged if the patient is not questioned on this point. Mirror laryngoscopy is required to detect any oedema which might be aggravated by endoscopic manoeuvres. Retained food, as in diverticula or achalasia should be cleared away as well as possible by lavage through an oesophageal tube.

A general anaesthetic is almost invariably preferred nowadays. The fasting patient receives suitable pre-anaesthetic medication. The surgeon requires complete relaxation of the jaws, neck and pharyngeal muscles, easily attained with modern drugs. A cuffed orotracheal tube guarantees the airway and permits assisted respiration when necessary. Passed through the mouth, the tube obtrudes less upon the oesophagoscopist's field than does a nasotracheal tube.

It is difficult to imagine circumstances in which a local anaesthetic would be unavoidable for oesophagoscopy today. The skilful anaesthetist required to give a "general" is far more ubiquitous than the well-equipped oesophagoscopist. The patient himself is probably safer under a modern general anaesthetic.

Technique

The patient is placed on the operating table, and his head is supported either by an assistant or by a special head-rest. The head must be lifted so that the cervical spine is flexed and the occipito-atlantoid joint is extended. A piece of gauze is placed so as to protect the upper lip and teeth, and the lubricated oesophagoscope is passed through the mouth and backwards over the tongue. From this stage onwards all landmarks must be plainly seen through the oesophagoscope and the instrument may only be advanced when the lumen of the gullet is clearly in view, and in line. Utmost gentleness is essential, otherwise the pharynx or oesophagus will be perforated. The epiglottis is first seen and behind it the anaesthetist's tube. About 4 cm. lower and more posteriorly the arytenoids are next defined. The beak of the oesophagoscope is then passed behind the larynx and lifted so as to open the hypopharynx. Very gentle progress strictly in the midline for a further 2 cm. or so will bring into view the cricopharyngeal sphincter which opens to receive the oesophagoscope if the patient is completely relaxed. This is the most dangerous and difficult step, and the surgeon must take time to be absolutely sure of the entrance to the oesophagus. Often the sphincter will open after a short wait, or additional relaxant may be needed before progress can safely be made. Some surgeons advocate the insinuation of a fine bougie which defines the lumen and can then be followed through the "narrows" of the pharyngo-oesophageal junction.

Beyond this point progress is usually easier, but the oesophageal lumen must always be directly in view, and in line, each time the instrument is advanced. Below the aortic arch the oesophagus swings forwards and the head of the patient must be progressively lowered. When the cardia is reached the head will be lower than the shoulders, and the oesophagoscope will be pointing towards the left anterior superior iliac spine.

Every part of the oesophageal wall is closely examined. Small areas can be magnified with a suitable lens attached to the proximal end of the oesophagoscope. The cardia is recognized by the appearance of a redder mucous membrane.

Removal of the instrument is done slowly and the walls of the oesophagus are re-examined. "On the way out" the unfolding mucosal pattern may reveal small abnormalities or a foreign body overlooked during introduction of the oesophago-scope. The head must again be positioned throughout so that the oesophagoscope is properly aligned at all stages during its withdrawal.

Hazards

Apart from damage to the lips and teeth due to rough technique, the chief danger in oesophagoscopy is perforation of the oesophagus. Strict observance of the rules outlined above will prevent this accident in most cases. The danger arises chiefly when force is used to overcome difficulties. Awkward jaws and teeth, a short stiff neck, and vertebral osteophytosis multiply the dangers.

In children there is some danger of compression of the trachea by the oesophago-scope. This can cause anoxia, despite the endotracheal anaesthetic technique. Adequate theatre lighting is essential so that the onset of cyanosis can be noted immediately if this complication arises. It cannot be emphasized too strongly that if the patient becomes "blue" and there is no apparent reason for it, the oesophago-scope must be completely withdrawn and the anaesthetist must be given sole access to the mouth.

Surgical exposure of the oesophagus

Throughout its length the oesophagus is very deeply placed, and surrounded by vital structures. Its blood supply is segmental, not longitudinal, and is jeopardized if more than about 5 cm. of the viscus is mobilized. An outline is given below of the usual routes by which the oesophagus may be approached at operation.

In the neck

An incision is made along the anterior border of the sternomastoid muscle from the level of the clavicle to the level of the hyoid bone. The deep cervical fascia is opened in the same line, and the carotid sheath is displaced laterally. The thyroid gland is displaced anteromedially by blunt dissection and the middle thyroid vein is ligated and divided. The thyroid gland is then further displaced forwards and the vertebral column is palpated. The prevertebral fascia is then identifiable and immediately anterior to it the visceral compartment of the neck enclosed in the parapharyngeal fascia. The latter must be opened to expose the oesophagus, and the inferior thyroid artery may first require division if it impedes access. In this region the recurrent laryngeal nerve must be carefully preserved.

By means of this approach localized strictures and tumours of the cervical oesophagus can be removed. Oesophagotomy for removal of a foreign body (when endoscopic removal has failed), the repair of an oesophageal perforation, or the drainage of a para-oesophageal abscess are carried out by the same route. By blunt (finger) dissection downwards alongside the oesophagus an upper mediastinal abscess may be opened and drained.

In the chest

Transpleural thoracotomy on the right side gives access to the entire thoracic oesophagus, after division of the azygos vein. Left thoracotomy exposes the oesophagus from the aortic arch downwards, and provides in addition wide access to the abdominal contents through the left half of the diaphragm.

Extrapleural access can be gained by posterior mediastinotomy. This is the preferred route for drainage of a para-oesophageal abscess, but it does not give sufficiently wide exposure for surgical attack upon the oesophagus itself.

In the abdomen

Left upper laparotomy exposes the lowest 3 or 4 cm. of the oesophagus and the gastro-oesophageal junction.

In the operation of total oesophagectomy blunt finger dissection from the abdomen and from the neck can mobilize the entire viscus prior to its withdrawal through the neck wound, without the necessity for a transthoracic exposure.

PATHOLOGY AND TREATMENT OF DISEASES OF THE OESOPHAGUS

Congenital abnormality of the oesophagus

In order to understand the congenital anomalies of the oesophagus it is necessary to recall its development. It is formed from that part of the primitive foregut immediately caudal to the pharynx, and three salient features should be noted:

(1) At about the fourth week of intra-uterine life, the median laryngotracheal groove appears in the ventral aspect of the foregut. As the groove deepens, its lips approximate and fuse, forming the laryngotracheobronchial tree ventrally, and the oesophagus dorsally (Fig. 69). Incomplete fusion explains the presence of a fistula between the oesophagus and trachea, which usually occurs at the level of the bifurcation of the latter.

(2) In the early stages of the developing oesophagus there is such proliferation of its lining membrane that the lumen is almost obliterated, but later the wall becomes thinner and the normal lumen is restored. Interference with this latter stage may result in atresia.

(3) Again, early in its development, the oesophagus is exceedingly short, but later it has to undergo rapid lengthening, for the developing lungs push the stomach caudally. This may explain some cases of short oesophagus, although it is probable that reflux oesophagitis is more often responsible for this condition.

Types of abnormality

(1) Atresia (see Vogt's classification below).

(2) Tracheo-oesophageal fistula without atresia.

(3) Congenital oesophageal stenosis.

(4) Short oesophagus.

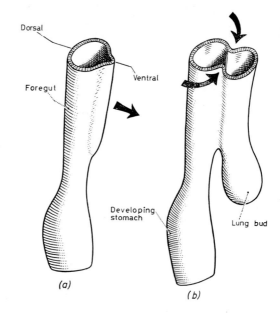

Fig. 69.—The development of the oesophagus and trachea: (*a*) the median laryngotracheal groove is appearing in the ventral aspect of the foregut; (*b*) the lips of the groove are closing in and separating the developing lower respiratory tract from the alimentary canal.

Atresia

Vogt (1929) classified congenital atresia of the oesophagus as follows:

Type I. Absence of the oesophagus.

Type II. Cases in which both upper and lower segments of the oesophagus end in blind pouches.

Type III. Atresia of the oesophagus with tracheo-oesophageal fistula: (*a*) fistula is between upper oesophageal segment and trachea; (*b*) fistula is between lower oesophageal segment and trachea; (*c*) fistulae are between both oesophageal segments and trachea.

According to Belsey and Donnison (1950) the incidence of oesophageal atresia is distinctly greater than 1 in 800, and much the most common type of malformation is atresia, in association with a fistula between the trachea or left main bronchus and the lower segment of the oesophagus (Fig. 70). The upper segment of the oesophagus ends blindly. This type—Vogt Type III (*b*)—accounts for approximately 80 per cent of all congenital oesophageal abnormalities, a fact of supreme importance to all medical personnel associated with the newly born. All the other types of congenital abnormality are much less common.

Diagnosis of congenital oesophageal atresia.—Excessive salivation, cyanosis and inability to swallow fluid soon after birth constitute the triad, which should suggest the possibility of congenital oesophageal atresia to the medical or nursing attendant, and the infant should be immediately transferred to a unit fully equipped to

217

deal with this emergency. A lubricated rubber catheter passed through the nose or mouth will be held up in the upper oesophageal segment, and the diagnosis is often confirmed by introducing 1–2 ml. of iodized oil into the catheter and taking

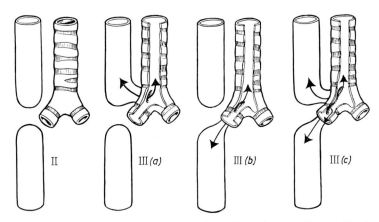

II   III (a)   III (b)   III (c)

FIG. 70.—The types of congenital oesophageal atresia according to Vogt's classification (*see* text). Type III (*b*) is the most common.

x-ray films (Fig. 71). The blind end of the upper oesophagus is seen to be pear-shaped and regular in outline. A pencil-line airway may be demonstrable leading from the bifurcation of the trachea to the stomach and is said to represent air in the lower oesophagus. Barium must not be used under any circumstances, as its entry into the lungs would be disastrous—in fact, Nixon and Wilkinson decry the use of any opaque medium, for there is likely to be some spillage into the lungs, predisposing to bronchopneumonia. If the x-ray films suggest the presence of gas in the stomach and the passage of a catheter has been arrested in the upper oesophageal segment, the diagnosis of atresia of the oesophagus, with tracheo-oesophageal fistula, may be made with confidence.

Management.—Once the diagnosis has been established it is essential to commence supportive therapy, including intravenous fluids and oesophageal suction, although these measures do not obviate the infant's chief hazard—the passage of gastric juice up the lower oesophageal segment and through the fistula into the tracheobronchial tree.

Operation is usually by the right transpleural route, although in some circumstances the approach may be extrapleurally or from the left side. Ideally, the two oesophageal segments are defined, the fistula is closed and anastomosis between the two segments is completed, but many cases are fraught with difficulty. Other anomalies, such as imperforate anus, may be present, further handicapping the infant, and it is necessary to search for these. There is not infrequently some degree of prematurity. It may be possible only to perform cervical oesophagostomy and gastrostomy, and to delay reconstitution of the oesophagus until a later date. Intensive post-operative care is necessary and involves special positioning of the infant, oxygen therapy, pharyngeal aspiration, antibiotics and meticulous attention to fluid balance (Benson and colleagues, 1962). Yet, in spite of the hazards attending these procedures, results have continued to improve and impressive series of anastomosing operations have been placed on record, as for example that of Ty, Brunet and Beardmore (1967) in which no less than 15 cases of repair are quoted with "zero operative mortality".

The entire subject of oesophageal atresia and tracheo-oesophageal fistula is covered in very great detail by Freeman (1969) who gives an exhaustive bibliography.

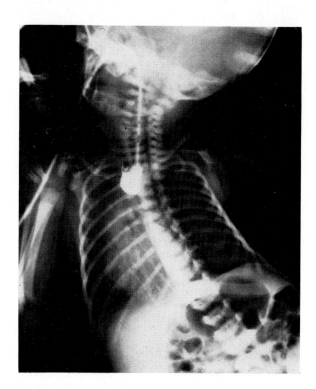

FIG. 71.—Radiograph showing oesophageal atresia. (Mr. David Levi's case.)

Tracheo-oesophageal fistula without atresia

This is a condition of exceeding rarity, but the case histories described are of great interest: Negus (1929); Imperatori (1939); Helmsworth and Pryles (1951); Robb (1952–3); Mullard (1954); and Franklin (1959).

It is important to remember that it is by no means necessarily inconsistent with life as, for example, is the Vogt Type III (*b*) deformity and, consequently, diagnosis is sometimes delayed for a very long time. The condition must be considered if feeding the infant causes choking and cyanotic attacks, and these symptoms may be more pronounced when fluids are administered and the infant is placed in certain positions. Recurrent pulmonary infections are likely to occur.

The diagnosis is confirmed by radiography using contrast media, and by bronchoscopy and oesophagoscopy.

The approach used by the thoracic surgeon in order to effect closure of the fistula varies according to the site of the latter, and the surgery is fraught with difficulty. However, gratifying cases of cure have been reported.

Congenital oesophageal stenosis

Congenital strictures and cases of stenosis of the oesophagus are very rare. In the past the term has, without doubt, often been applied where the stenosis has been the result of reflux peptic oesophagitis. This error is less likely to be made if it is recalled that, in the acquired type of stricture, dysphagia gradually increases in severity, particularly after the infant commences to take solids, whereas in true congenital stenosis dysphagia is present from birth. If, on oesphagoscopy, as a result of finding normal mucosa below the site of the stricture, a diagnosis of true congenital stricture is made, the treatment consists of dilatation with gum-elastic bougies over a long period.

Short oesophagus

There has been much confusion on this subject in the past, but it is now considered that cases of true congenital short oesophagus are extremely rare, and Barrett (1954), who has made a detailed study, considers that the term congenital short oesophagus should be reserved for those cases which are true anomalies. The confusion has arisen from the fact that cases of short oesophagus, although dubbed "congenital", have in fact been produced after birth by reflux of gastric juice. The oesophagitis caused by this reflux leads to fibrosis and, eventually, shortening of the viscus.

Olsen and Harrington (1948), in a review of 220 cases of short oesophagus, considered that of these only 4 per cent were really congenital, and Sweet (1954), Allison, Johnstone and Royce (1943), and many others, have found a similar state of affairs.

Injuries of the oesophagus

External wounds

External wounds may involve the cervical oesophagus as a result of suicidal "cut-throat", gunshot wounds, or very rarely as a surgical accident in the course of a tracheostomy operation. If the patient survives the immediate wounding the oesophagus must be exposed surgically and repaired over an indwelling oesophageal feeding tube. The neck wound may require debridement and free drainage to forestall the dangers of mediastinitis. Systemic broad-spectrum antibiotics must be given in large doses. Associated injuries to the larynx, recurrent laryngeal nerves, or trachea will necessitate tracheostomy in most cases.

Spontaneous rupture

Spontaneous rupture of the oesophagus is rare. It occurs in the lowermost part of the thoracic oesophagus and is caused by sudden localized distension during vomiting. Mediastinitis always results, and often empyema as well. The condition is rapidly fatal if not recognized and treated. Diagnosis depends upon the history of vomiting, severe pain in the chest or epigastrium, and the radiographic evidence of mediastinal emphysema and pleural effusion. Perforation of a gastric or duodenal ulcer requires consideration in differential diagnosis, while in some cases coronary thrombosis, pulmonary embolus, or dissecting aneurysm of the aorta may need to be excluded.

Immediate treatment consists of intravenous fluids and systemic antibiotics. Nothing is allowed by mouth. As soon as possible thoracic surgical treatment must be given. Early drainage of the infection and repair of the oesophageal wall offer the best hope of recovery.

Accidental perforation

Accidental perforation of the oesophagus from within its lumen results from penetration by metallic pointed foreign bodies such as an open "safety" pin, or by spicular fish or meat bones.

Perforation is also a complication of oesophagoscopy and the danger is greater when the oesophagus is abnormal. The risk is especially great during the removal of foreign bodies, dilatation of strictures, and when biopsy material is being taken.

Symptoms and signs develop quickly, but at first the patient is not as desperately ill as would be the case with the massive contamination of the mediastinum caused by spontaneous perforation during vomiting (*see above*). If the perforation is in the upper oesophagus crepitus due to surgical emphysema in the neck may be detectable within an hour or so of the accident. *After every per-oral endoscopy the neck should be routinely palpated one to two hours later for this reason.* A plain radiograph (Fig. 72a) confirms the diagnosis. If the oesophagus is perforated near its lower end clinical signs of surgical emphysema in the neck and over the chest wall are slower to appear, and the first indication of disaster will then be severe substernal or epigastric pain, which the patient notices as soon as he recovers from the anaesthetic.

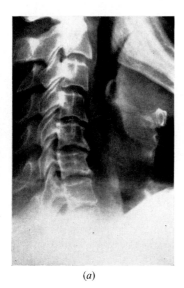
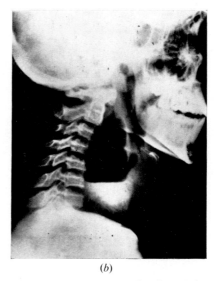

| (a) | (b) |

FIG. 72.—(a) Surgical emphysema in the soft tissues of the neck, following perforation of the cervical oesophagus; (b) retro-oesophageal and retropharyngeal abscess, with fluid level and gas above, due to infection after an upper oesophageal perforation.

As soon as the diagnosis is clear, the patient is forbidden to take anything whatsoever by mouth. A small dose of morphine may be necessary for relief of pain. Intravenous fluids and systemic antibiotics are given. Operative treatment may be deferred for a few hours, since in many cases a gradual improvement in the local and general condition is seen.

Indications for operation are: (*a*) increasing surgical emphysema; (*b*) abscess formation (Fig. 72*b*); (*c*) evidence of pleural effusion; (*d*) progressive worsening of the general condition.

If the site of perforation is likely to be at a level above the arch of the aorta a cervical approach is made (p. 215). The oedematous tissues of the visceral compartment of the neck are explored and drained. In early cases a gush of saliva may be released but, later, pus will be found. Goligher (1948) advocates the earliest possible intervention and immediate repair of the torn viscus. However, this is only possible if the tear can be found, and if the tissues are as yet not oedematous and friable. In most cases only drainage can be achieved. If necessary saliva or pus must be sought in the mediastinum by finger dissection downwards along the oesophageal wall. At the end of the operation a small oesophageal tube is passed gently from the nose into the stomach.

If the perforation is known to be below the level of the aortic arch, or the early development of pleural effusion makes this seem likely the aid of a thoracic surgeon is essential since posterior mediastinotomy or possibly a transthoracic repair of the torn oesophagus is urgently required.

The management of any case of perforation of the oesophagus presents very great difficulties. If the site and cause of the perforation are known it becomes much easier to decide what to do, but these patients quickly become very ill and a second oesophagoscopy to locate the tear is not likely to give positive findings and may be very dangerous. Massive dosage of broad-spectrum antibiotics, and shrewd decision as to the timing and route of surgical drainage are the two essentials in treatment. The mortality of this complication is less than in the pre-antibiotic era, but it is still formidable.

Corrosive injury of the oesophagus

The swallowing of corrosive poisons is usually accidental in children and suicidal in adults. Strong solutions of caustic alkali are a rare household commodity in England, while the strong acids, such as sulphuric, nitric and hydrochloric, are only found in industry. The greatest damage when these poisons are swallowed is seen in the mouth and in the lower third of the oesophagus. While the mouth burns contribute largely to the patient's agony it is the injury to the oesophagus which determines the long-term outlook. The immediate question of survival hinges upon the acute disturbance of acid–base equilibrium and renal function, and upon the incidence of laryngeal oedema and bronchopneumonia. The last-named respiratory complications are more serious in cases due to ingestion of corrosives which give off injurious fumes such as strong ammonia, hydrochloric acid and fuming nitric acid.

Immediate treatment is directed towards the relief of shock and pain, and the neutralization of the corrosive by an appropriate weak acid or alkali given by mouth. Intravenous fluids and systemic (parenteral) antibiotics are commenced as soon as possible. Careful watch is kept for signs of laryngeal oedema which may call for tracheostomy. In close collaboration with the chemical pathologist the acid–base equilibrium and renal function must be studied and controlled by suitable regulation of the intravenous fluid–electrolyte input.

Prevention of stricture formation.—An impassable stricture, usually of the lower oesophagus, is extremely likely to occur if burning penetrates the muscular wall of the viscus. Modern therapy is aimed at preventing this by means of the insertion of an indwelling nasogastric tube within the first day or two of the illness. This, if done gently, is not as dangerous as it was once thought to be. Some authorities recommend oesophagoscopy at the earliest possible moment, although there seems to be little therapeutic advantage in this. The main thing is to get a tube down and keep it there until two or three weeks later when the patient is ready for solid food. (A good bolus of well-chewed solid food is the best dilator of all if there is a lumen for it to pass through, and some muscle to drive it down.)

Systemic steroid therapy, if begun in the first two or three days of the illness, is considered to be effective in keeping fibrosis (and therefore stenosis) to a minimum.

In recent years cervical oesophagostomy has been found useful, especially in children, in permitting early and well-tolerated oesophageal intubation. It has also the advantage later that if stenosis threatens, frequent passage of bougies is possible without the necessity for either training the patient to swallow them, or frequent general anaesthetics.

Delayed stenosis may develop after two or three months or even longer. It is less likely if the patient perseveres with a normal diet, but in all cases regular surveillance and repeated barium swallow examinations should be maintained for at least six months. The treatment of an established stricture is discussed in more detail on pp. 237 and 238.

Foreign bodies in the oesophagus

A complete study of foreign bodies in the oesophagus and upper respiratory tract was made by Jackson and Jackson (1936), who published records of over 3,000 patients who had ingested foreign bodies. This is by far the largest series of cases. Each case history is described in detail with endoscopic findings, description of the foreign body and the type of forceps used for removal. Schlemmer (1920), Holt, Diggle (1932), Alpin (1934), Mosher (1935), Phillips (1938), and later Flett (1945), reported on similar but smaller series.

Aetiology

Statistics show that coins and bones are the most common foreign bodies to lodge in the oesophagus. Open safety-pins and lumps of meat are the next in order of frequency. Jackson says that poor children who are not given individual attention and who are left to feed themselves at an early age are more liable to swallow a foreign body (Jackson and Jackson, 1936). The incidence of foreign bodies rises in old people who get lumps of meat impacted in the oesophagus; this may be due to the lack of propulsion efficiency or to the fact that the patient is often edentulous and therefore unable to masticate his food properly.

Dental factor.—A patient who has an artificial denture is unable to detect a fish or meat bone in the mouth as easily as a person with a normal palate, and is therefore more likely to swallow a foreign body. Tough meat, if improperly chewed, may become impacted. If the denture or plate is ill-fitting or broken it may itself be swallowed and this occasionally occurs whilst the patient is drunk or asleep.

Oesophageal factor.—Local conditions of the oesophagus may determine the impaction of a foreign body. A stricture of the oesophagus is more likely to occlude the passage of a small foreign body which would normally pass through. In a carcinomatous stricture the first sign of this disease may be the lodging of a foreign body, with the sudden onset of dysphagia or even aphagia.

Type of food.—Carelessness in the preparation of food is a factor in the lodging of a foreign body. Certain types of food are eaten very rapidly because the patient does not suspect the presence of bones. Stews and soups may contain meat with splinters of bone attached if the meat has been prepared with a chopper. Fish cakes may also contain bones which may become impacted in the alimentary tract.

Voluntary swallowing.—Foreign bodies are swallowed voluntarily by patients who attempt suicide, by prisoners and by mentally ill patients.

Type of foreign body.—Foreign bodies may lodge in the oesophagus by reason of the nature of the foreign body. Coins and disc-shaped objects which pass through the mouth and pharynx of a child may then lodge in the upper part of the oesophagus. Open safety-pins stay in the oesophagus because of the resilience of the pin when the point is uppermost or by penetration of the oesophageal wall when the point is downwards.

Site

Coins lodge usually in the upper end of the oesophagus. Meat and soft foreign bodies may lodge above a stricture, and sharp foreign bodies, such as meat bones, may lodge anywhere but most commonly in the upper end of the oesophagus.

Pathological changes caused by the foreign body

Coins may stay in the oesophagus for many months and cause only a slow ulceration of the oesophageal wall, but meat and fish bones will very soon give rise to ulceration, peri-oesophagitis and other complications.

History

The patient, if an adult, may be able to give a very accurate account of the type and shape of the foreign body swallowed. He is very often able to point to the exact site of the obstruction, particularly if the foreign body is lodging in the upper part of the oesophagus. When the foreign body is in the middle or lower third of the oesophagus localization is not so accurate and the pain is referred to the back or behind the sternum. The pain is of a sharp, "cutting" nature, is worse with attempts to swallow, and occurs at the same place every time the patient swallows. A smooth foreign body may give rise to only a vague sensation of discomfort and not to actual pain. In children who cannot give a history, the presence of a foreign body may be unsuspected for several months. Dysphagia is nearly always present and is due to the size of the foreign body or inflammatory reaction and spasm caused by its presence. At first there is only slight difficulty in swallowing but later the difficulty becomes more pronounced. There is also regurgitation of food and later regurgitation of blood-stained saliva and mucus. In the later stages when the obstruction is complete there may be pulmonary symptoms produced by the overflow of the oesophageal contents, which suggests the presence of a foreign body in the respiratory tract.

Examination

The patient must be observed during the act of swallowing. When a sharp foreign body is lodging in the upper part of the oesophagus, in the larynx or in the postcricoid region, swallowing gives a definite expression of pain. Examination of the neck may show a tender swelling in the lower part of the neck medial to the sternomastoid muscle; this swelling is usually caused by the inflammatory reaction around the foreign body, to actual abscess or to surgical emphysema which is recognized by the accompanying crepitus. Wright (1934) and Tucker (1925) stressed the importance of tenderness on pressure on the trachea, and the latter observer considers it pathognomonic of the presence of a foreign body in the cervical oesophagus if, on movement of the trachea and larynx towards the point of maximum tenderness, there is marked exacerbation of pain.

The mouth, pharynx, tonsillar region and base of the tongue must be examined with the use of a headlight and spatula. A small sharp foreign body, such as a fish bone, may lodge in the base of the tongue or tonsillar crypt, although the patient may be convinced that the foreign body has actually been swallowed. The area around the foreign body is bruised and inflamed.

Indirect pharyngoscopy and laryngoscopy must be extremely thoroughly carried out. Each part of the pharyngeal wall must be minutely studied in the mirror, otherwise the tip of a small fish bone almost completely buried in the tissues will be overlooked. If the patient can localize his pain to one side or the other, then the foreign body, or the laceration caused by its passage, must be above the cricoid level and should be visible in the mirror. Most foreign bodies which can be seen with the mirror can be removed without recourse to general anaesthesia. After receiving careful explanation of what is to be done, the patient co-operates by holding his own tongue in a piece of gauze, leaving the surgeon free to hold his mirror in his left hand and a pair of suitably angled grasping forceps in his right. The forceps are guided down the throat until the foreign body can be grasped and withdrawn. There must of course be no blind "grab"—every step must be clearly observed in the mirror. There is no greater reward in all laryngology than to see the relief and gratitude of a patient who, in a matter of moments, is relieved of a fish bone in the pharynx. The technique, which requires a little practice, is well worth cultivating.

If no foreign body can be seen in the laryngeal mirror further investigations are necessary.

Radiological examination (Fig. 73)

Plain films of the neck and chest are taken. If the foreign body is not revealed the neck, thorax and abdomen are screened. If an opaque shadow is still not seen a little barium sulphate is given and its passage down the gullet observed. The opaque medium may be held up at one point and may actually outline the foreign body, or the flow of barium may be split. If the barium cannot be easily dislodged by further swallowing or washed down with water the presence of a foreign body is to be strongly suspected. An air bubble in the oesophagus in the region of the hold-up is very often indicative of a foreign body. In a difficult case a pledget of cotton-wool soaked in barium paste, or a gelatin capsule filled with barium may impact upon the foreign body, thus revealing its presence and position.

Management of a patient

The diagnosis is sometimes difficult if the foreign body is small and not opaque and if the radiological examination is inconclusive. If there is any doubt about the presence of a foreign body an oesophagoscopy is imperative. Even if the symptoms improve rapidly the patient must be kept under observation until he is completely symptom free. Abrasion of the oesophageal mucosa will give some pain and cause dysphagia but usually these symptoms disappear rapidly. Increase of pain and dysphagia indicates the presence of a foreign body or some more serious damage

225

to the oesophageal wall and warrants more active treatment, such as endoscopic examination.

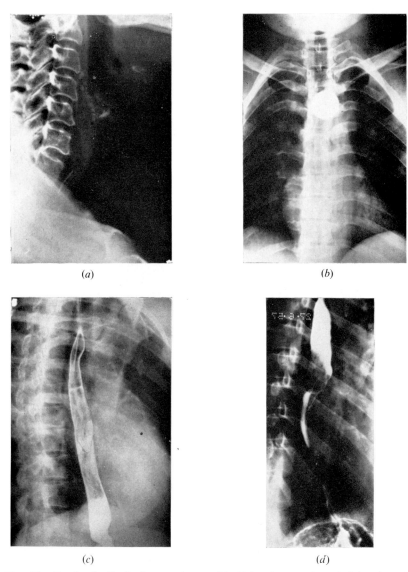

(a)　　　　　　　　(b)

(c)　　　　　　　　(d)

FIG. 73.—Foreign bodies in the oesophagus: (a) chicken bone at thoracic inlet; (b) coin in the oesophagus of a child; (c) plastic denture faintly outlined by barium in the mid-thoracic oesophagus; (d) meat bolus, impacted at level of aortic arch.

Treatment

Although oesophagoscopy for the removal of a foreign body may be an emergency operation, the surgeon must have knowledge of the nature, size and site of the foreign body, and if possible a replica should be examined.

Coin in the oesophagus of a child.—The radiological examination must be repeated immediately before the endoscopy is done because the coin may have passed into the stomach if there has been a delay between first seeing the patient and endoscopic examination. The oesophagoscope used is a small Negus type (35 cm. in length), but an oesophageal speculum or even an anterior commissure laryngoscope may be the only instrument necessary in a small child if the coin is impacted in the upper end of the oesophagus. The instrument should be passed slowly because it is very easy to over-ride the foreign body, especially if it has been in the oesophagus for some time, in which case it is coated with mucus. Any food debris is removed by suction. The operator must pass the oesophagoscope as near the foreign body as possible, making sure he does not push the foreign body ahead. The coin must be maintained in the centre of the field. Alligator forceps are then passed and the coin is seized firmly and brought out until it impinges on the end of the oesophagoscope. The forceps are fixed by the surgeon at the proximal end of the oesophagoscope so that the foreign body, forceps and oesophagoscope can be pulled out of the oesophagus together. Care must be taken, when the foreign body is passing the cricopharyngeus, that the coin is turned so that it lies in the coronal plane. Often, despite this, it slips off when being pulled over the sphincter and may be found lying in the hypopharynx; for its removal a laryngoscope is then necessary.

A sharp foreign body in the oesophagus.—A sharp foreign body such as a meat bone or fish bone may lodge anywhere in the oesophagus and, unless the position is verified by a radiograph, a full length oesophagoscope must be used.

The anaesthetist must take care not to pass the intratracheal tube blindly because it may accidentally go into the oesophagus and cause the foreign body to perforate the oesophageal wall. The oesophagoscope is passed until the foreign body is seen and the surgeon must resist any tempation to extract the foreign body quickly without noting the position of its sharp edge. The problem is not simply to remove the foreign body but to remove it with little or no risk to the patient. Mucus, food debris, and any barium which has been left after an x-ray examination, are removed by suction. If the end of the foreign body is free the forceps are passed and the end is gripped. If any bleeding occurs a swab soaked in adrenaline is introduced. If the ends of the foreign body are buried in the oesophageal wall, manipulation is necessary to try to release one end and to get a point of the foreign body into the tube, so that its long axis is parallel with the oesophagoscope.

A small bone may be extracted through the oesophagoscope, but a large one should be treated as for a coin and removed with the oesophagoscope and forceps. The patient should be kept under close observation because this type of foreign body is likely to cause complications.

Meat and soft foreign bodies.—Meat and soft foreign bodies are extracted piecemeal. If the patient refuses to undergo oesophagoscopy or if there is some contra-indication to endoscopy the method advised by Richardson (1945) should be tried. In this method papain, which contains enzymes similar to pepsin, is given by mouth. This solution acts in an acid medium and is said to digest 30 times its weight of lean meat. A 5 per cent solution dissolved in 10 per cent alcohol is used and 1 ml. is given by mouth every 15 minutes. The obstruction is said to be relieved in 2–3 hours without any reaction or complications. If no treatment at all is given the meat will be digested in time but this may take 7–14 days.

Safety-pin in the oesophagus.—An open safety-pin presents no difficulty if the sharp point is distal. If the point is proximal there is often great difficulty, and several methods have been devised to overcome it. If it is not too large it may be possible to turn the pin in the oesophagus, or alternatively to manipulate the point of the pin into the lumen of the oesophagoscope. Some endoscopists prefer to cut the pin *in situ* using endoscopic shears, or close it with Clerf's or similar forceps. If all else fails, the pin may be grasped with rotation forceps at the ring, pushed into the stomach and allowed to rotate and then be extracted through the oesphagus with the point trailing.

Denture in the oesophagus.—A denture in the oesophagus presents many hazards. The radiograph should be studied carefully with special regard to the hooks and points on the denture. During oesophagoscopy the hook should, if possible, be manipulated into the lumen of the oesophagoscope before extraction. The denture may be impacted and may have to be divided *in situ*. If there is any gross trauma of the oesophagus by the foreign body or if any previous manipulation has been performed endoscopic removal should be delayed, and it is better to wait until the inflammatory reaction has subsided and do the oesophagoscopy some days later. In the meantime the patient should be treated as for a peri-oesophagitis or perforation of the oesophagus with systemic antibiotics.

External operation for removal of foreign body

The majority of foreign bodies which lodge in the oesophagus can be removed endoscopically. Guisez, in a series of 530 foreign bodies, had only to remove three, or 0·6 per cent, by the external route. There are instances, however, in which an external operation is preferable.

The majority of foreign bodies are situated in the upper or cervical part of the oesophagus. Large and irregular foreign bodies, such as dentures, may present great difficulty in removal. Oesophagoscopy may so injure the oesophagus as to cause great damage and complications.

The following types of foreign bodies may require removal by the external route:

(1) An impacted foreign body.

(2) A foreign body producing peri-oesophagitis after unsuccessful attempts at removal through the oesophagoscope.

(3) A peri-oesophageal abscess with a foreign body lodging in the abscess itself.

Inflammation of the oesophagus

Aetiology

Apart from the inflammatory changes which result from corrosives and foreign bodies, inflammation can occur from a number of other causes.

Diphtheritic, tuberculous, and syphilitic oesophagitis are all rare today. Each occurs as a complication of its "parent" disease, and will be recognized by its characteristic type of ulceration at oesophagoscopy, presence of membranous exudate, bacteriological investigations and, where appropriate, biopsy findings. Treatment is that of the causative disease.

Fungal infection occasionally causes oesophagitis with marked dysphagia. It may complicate a thrush (monilial) infection of the mouth and pharynx in infants and young children. It can also occur in elderly or debilitated patients, causing the acute onset of severe dysphagia with considerable pain. Very occasionally fungal oesophagitis is a complication of broad-spectrum antibiotic therapy. Treatment consists of correction of dehydration, parenteral administration of vitamins, and a suspension of nystatin given by mouth every 2–3 hours. In very severe cases a nasogastric feeding tube may be needed for a few days.

Non-specific types of oesophagitis.—Gastric juices in the oesophagus set up chronic inflammatory changes, with ulceration, pain, dysphagia and sometimes bleeding. The condition may occur as a result of protracted vomiting, or very rarely may be due to secretion of gastric acid and enzymes by islets of gastric mucosa in the walls of the oesophagus. As a congenital condition these islets are considered to be a rare curiosity. The most common cause of lower oesophagitis is hiatus hernia (*see below*), in which derangement of the cardiac sphincteric mechanism allows frequent regurgitation. Gastric contents are especially likely to rise in the oesophagus when the patient lies down. In late cases chronic inflammation is followed by fibrosis and stricture formation.

Localized inflammation of the wall of the oesophagus may be caused by the pressure of an oesophageal feeding tube if it is retained for long periods. Oesophagitis is invariably present above strictures, and in achalasia of the cardia, due to stagnation of undigested food particles. Inflammatory changes, with superficial erosions, are commonly observed in relation to large varices of the lower oesophagus in cases of portal hypertension. Reflux oesophagitis is a frequent complication of oesophagogastric anastomosis when this technique is used to restore continuity after partial oesophagectomy. At its upper end the oesophagus is sometimes involved in the inflammatory changes of Paterson–Brown Kelly disease (*see* p. 88).

Leucoplakia.—Long-continued irritation of the oesophageal lining can result in the formation of areas of leucoplakia and the risk of carcinoma. Localized patches of hyperkeratosis and pre-malignant change are seen in chronic oesophagitis due to almost any of the above-mentioned causes.

Diagnosis

The diagnosis of oesophagitis is usually evident after scrutiny of the history, barium swallow and oesophagoscopic findings.

Treatment

The cause is removed whenever possible. The gullet is rested by restriction of diet to soft foods and fluids. Gastric acidity is reduced by appropriate alkalis taken by mouth. Gastric reflux is prevented as far as possible by the avoidance of bending and stooping, avoidance of "indigestible" foods, and over-eating, and by persuading the patient to sleep propped up in a sitting position. In cases of hiatus hernia successful weight reduction helps a great deal, while the failure of medical treatment indicates surgical repair of the diaphragmatic hiatus.

Hiatus hernia

Hiatus hernia may be defined as a displacement of the stomach into the lower mediastinum through the oesophageal opening of the diaphragm. Two main types are recognized (Fig. 74).

Para-oesophageal hernia.—A peritoneal sac leads from the abdominal cavity upwards alongside the oesophagus. Within the sac a varying amount of the stomach is found, but the cardia lies at or below the level of the diaphragm. Flavell (1963) states that this type of hiatus hernia is always congenital, although the more usual view has been that in most cases it is an acquired condition.

Sliding hernia.—Laxity of the hiatal orifice permits the entry of the gastro-oesophageal junction into the thorax whenever intra-abdominal pressure is raised. This process is almost literally the "thin end of the wedge", and once it has begun to occur, the hiatus becomes more and more widely stretched, and more and more of the stomach follows the cardia into the chest. The angulation between the oesophagus and stomach is lost, and with it muscular control of the gastro-oesophageal junction. Reflux oesophagitis is then inevitable, and may lead to fibrous stenosis and shortening of the oesophagus.

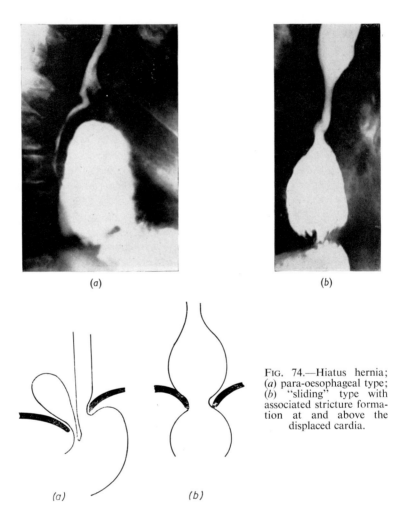

(a) (b)

Fig. 74.—Hiatus hernia; (a) para-oesophageal type; (b) "sliding" type with associated stricture formation at and above the displaced cardia.

(a) (b)

Although this kind of hernia occurs in infants and children, it is common in middle-aged and elderly patients. It is probably due to the well-known causes of raised abdominal pressure—obesity, flatulence, constipation, pregnancy and corsets. Most of these factors beset humanity when the muscles, including the diaphragm, are somewhat past their prime. Flavell points out that crush injuries of the abdominal region may cause hiatus hernia, even in young patients with good muscles.

Management

In the *para-oesophageal* cases oesophagitis is absent, and diagnosis may therefore be long delayed. Breathlessness on exertion if the herniation is large, or anaemia secondary to ulceration and bleeding in the thoracic portion of the stomach, may be overlooked or attributed to other causes, unless a barium swallow is done. Treatment is surgical. The stomach is replaced in the abdomen and the hiatus is repaired.

Sliding hiatus hernia is characterized by the symptoms of reflux oesophagitis, in addition to breathlessness if the hernia is large. Complications such as bleeding and stricture formation are common, and are pressing indications for surgical repair of the diaphragm. Thoracic surgeons, naturally enough, advocate surgical treatment as the principal line of attack in hiatus hernia. The hardships and hazards endured by the elderly patient, in whom many years of conservative treatment have merely served to postpone operation until he is no longer fit to undergo it, are a grim warning. Each individual case will be assessed carefully on its merits. In very early cases, in the very old and in infants, it will usually be best to adopt medical treatment (*see* p. 229). Severe cases, those with complications, and those becoming worse despite conservative treatment, should be advised operation. The newer techniques of gastroplication (Nissen, Rossetti and Markman, 1965; Belsey, 1966; Logan, 1967) in which effective valvular action is restored at the lower end of the oesophagus, are reported to give satisfactory results and a very low recurrence rate.

Achalasia of the cardia or cardiospasm

In considering the various causes of dysphagia, achalasia of the cardia or "cardiospasm", although not commonplace, is by no means rare, and is therefore of importance to the laryngologist.

Aetiology

The term cardiospasm, although more often used than the term achalasia, is perhaps somewhat inaccurate, for the great dilatation of the oesophagus in these cases is probably caused by an abnormality of the upper segment of the oesophagus associated with failure of relaxation of the cardiac sphincter, rather than by true spasm, although what underlies this disorder of function is a matter of conjecture. Numerous theories have been advanced.

Chronic inflammation, causing stasis and degeneration of Auerbach's plexus, has been said to be a cause although, in fact, it is probably an effect of the condition. There is, however, indisputable evidence of degeneration of Auerbach's plexus (Hurst, 1943), though recent histological work of Chesterman (1965) has shown that in some cases of achalasia there is no loss of ganglia.

Psychological disorders have been blamed. They may, in fact, be associated with air-swallowing, and it is of interest to note that Negus (1955) has given strong support to the theory that air-distension may play an active part in the initiation of the process.

Crural spasm, or the so-called diaphragmatic pinchcock, was suggested by Chevalier Jackson (1922), who coined the term "phreno-oesophagospasm", in the supposition that the underlying cause lay in the diaphragmatic crura rather than in the oesophagus but, as Negus (1955) has pointed out, division of the phrenic nerve should improve matters but does not.

Vitamin B₁ deficiency was postulated as a possible cause by Etzel (1942), but the cases described were natives of Brazil who also had megacolon and mega-ureter. It is not considered that vitamin deficiency is a likely contributory cause of cardio-spasm as seen in Europe.

Recent valuable work has been carried out by Ellis and his colleagues (1957, 1960, 1962), showing the effect of cholinergic and adrenergic drugs on strips of oesophageal muscle in the laboratory.

It was found that in the normal oesophagus the autonomic response of the circular muscle of the lower end is primarily adrenergic, but that the longitudinal muscle is mainly cholinergic in response. At higher levels the response of both circular and longitudinal muscle is the same—cholinergic.

On the other hand, in muscle strips removed from patients with achalasia evidence was found that the cholinergic mechanism is defective in the upper segment, and the defect is likely to be in the post-ganglionic nerves.

It is possible, though not yet conclusively proven, that the adrenergic mechanism may be normal, and if this should be so it is suggestive that achalasia is primarily a *defect of mobility of the upper segment of the oesophagus only, and that failure of relaxation of the lower segment may be secondary to a properly conducted stimulus failing to reach it from above.*

Clinical picture

The condition is of more frequent occurrence in men than in women. It may occur at any age, but is most often seen between the ages of 30 and 60, a common early symptom being epigastric discomfort, or a feeling of fullness in the upper abdomen.

Later dysphagia occurs, but unlike the unrelenting and slowly progressive dysphagia of malignant disease of the oesophagus, it may be marked by temporary remissions. After these early symptoms have been present for many months or even years regurgitation is noticed. The volume regurgitated is at first slight, but after a time becomes more bulky, until eventually enormous quantities of frothy mucus mixed with swallowed food and fluids may be brought back. Loss of weight is moderate and, as a rule, by no means so pronounced as in oesophageal malignancy.

In advanced cases pulmonary complications, due to inhalation, are common, and pulmonary osteo-arthropathy is described in association with the condition.

Diagnosis

Radiological examination and oesophagoscopy confirm the diagnosis (Fig. 75a). In the earliest stages the lower oesophagus is spindle-shaped, and the meal passes in a narrow ribbon-like stream into the stomach. Later, the obstruction and dilatation become more marked and no barium enters the stomach. A fluid level may be demonstrated, and in advanced cases the oesophagus will hold as much as 500 ml. of fluid.

The oesophagus may be fusiform, spindle-shaped, pear-shaped or S-shaped; fusiform dilatation is most common. At first there is spasm involving the cardia and cardiac ampulla; Allison (1943) has demonstrated that the mucosal junction lies above the constricted portion. In the earliest stages there is only moderate dilatation in the plain muscle segment above the constriction, up to the level of the aorta, and above this the dilatation is much greater. Later, the lower segment becomes more dilated, but the upper segment still remains the wider portion.

No normal peristalsis occurs, and if waves are seen they are irregular in the lower segment or plain muscle portion. In the late stages of the disease the oeso-phagus shows no peristalsis, the muscular tissue becomes atrophic and the mucosa is thickened. This thickening is responsible for the visibility of the organ without barium. It is important to note that the outline of the lower end of the oesophagus is smooth and regular as distinct from the irregular outline often (but not invari-ably) seen in cases of malignant disease.

Oesophagoscopy is mandatory. Not only has the diagnosis to be confirmed, but a co-existing carcinoma must be carefully excluded. Oesophageal carcinoma com-plicating achalasia constitutes a well-known diagnostic trap, and Groves (1956), who reviewed the literature, himself adding two cases, drew attention to the diffi-culty of diagnosis. He emphasized that oesophagoscopy, with careful study of the entire length of the oesophagus, is called for, pointing out that even direct endo-scopy may fail to demonstrate a large tumour if the oesophageal wall is dilated and obscured by retained food and secretion. There are many parallel instances where the finding of a relatively benign condition may obscure and delay the diagnosis of a co-existing sinister lesion.

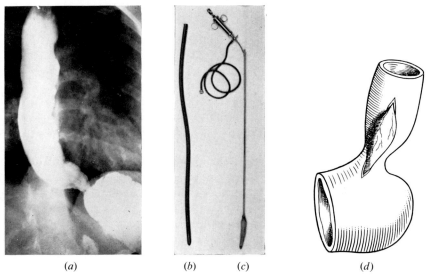

Fig. 75.—Achalasia of the cardia: (*a*) typical radiographic appearances; (*b*) Hurst's mercury-filled bougie; (*c*) hydrostatic dilator (Negus); (*d*) Heller's operation showing the incision of the muscle coats.

Prior to the administration of a general anaesthetic a gastric suction tube should be passed into the oesophagus and the latter drained of any stagnant contents which may lurk after the statutory period of fasting. The mucosa lining the dilated oeso-phagus is generally found to be unhealthy and may be ulcerated and bleed readily. Longitudinal folds can often be seen. The oesophagoscopist may have the feeling that he is groping in a strange and almost boundless territory, and it is not always a matter of simplicity to find the cardia. Once found, however, a large bougie should pass with ease; in fact, any difficulty encountered in intrumentation calls for careful exclusion of malignant stricture.

Treatment

Conservative treatment by drugs such as octyl nitrite has, on the whole, been disappointing, but one form of conservative treatment which has been used for many years and is undoubtedly of value is regular dilatation by means of a Hurst mercury bougie (Fig. 75*b*). This method has the advantage that it can be used by the patient himself, the bougie either being swallowed before each main meal, or less frequently in less severe cases. It is of importance that on the first occasion of bouginage an x-ray should be taken in order to confirm the presence of the bougie in the cardiac sphincter.

In other cases dilatation with a Negus hydrostatic bag (Fig. 75*c*) is carried out under direct vision through a wide-bore oesophagoscope. The empty bag is introduced through the sphincter, then slowly filled with water, stretching the muscle. This method of dilatation may have to be repeated several times but often affords lasting relief.

Dilatation with Starck's expanding metal dilator is hardly mentioned in any article or textbook which considers the treatment of this condition. The methods and the results of treatment are recorded by Starck (1934, 1936) and by Schindler (1956) in a total of 500–600 cases without a fatality and minor complications in less than 2 per cent.

The method is used by a few surgeons in this country, and Scott-Brown reports 30 years' experience with this dilator with no fatality, no complications in any case, and excellent results in 80 per cent of cases after one dilatation. It is important to carry out a sudden dilatation without an anaesthetic and when the cardia is in spasm. It is only in those cases where the spasm yields before rupture of the fibres takes place that a further 1–3 dilatations are necessary.

This method of treatment has also been used in a few cases of failed cardio-myotomies without any complications and with good permanent results (Scott-Brown, 1964).

Operative treatment is by Heller's operation of cardiomyotomy, first described in 1914 and again in detail by Barlow (1942).

The approach is via the abdomen or a left-sided thoracotomy, and after exposure an anterior longitudinal incision is made through the muscular wall at the cardio-oesophageal junction down to, but not through, the mucous membrane (Fig. 75*d*). Ellis (1962) has drawn attention to the remarkable propensity of the muscle to heal, with possible recurrence of symptoms, and the importance of making a long incision (at least 12 cm.) and carrying out submucous dissection. However, despite recurrence of symptoms and reflux oesophagitis in a few cases, extremely good results are claimed (Acheson and Hadley, 1958; Douglas and Nicholson, 1959; la Roux and Wright, 1960). In some cases however operations of the Wangensteen type (1951) in which portions of redundant oesophagus and stomach are excised are considered more appropriate.

Diverticula of the oesophagus

The following section refers to pouches or diverticula of the oesophagus proper and has no bearing on diverticula of the hypopharynx, which are more common and more familiar to the ear, nose and throat surgeon. Unfortunately, the term "oeso-phageal pouch" is still sometimes inaccurately used to include both the oesophageal and the hypopharyngeal variety.

It is usual to classify diverticula of the oesophagus as of the "pulsion" type or the "traction" type, and Barrett, in a classical paper on this subject in 1933, added a third variety—the "traction–pulsion" diverticulum.

Pulsion diverticula

These are due to herniation of the mucous membrane through the muscular walls of the oesophagus. The underlying cause may be a congenital weakness or defect in the muscle, and increasing pressure from retained food leads to an increase in the size of the pouch.

Most of these pulsion diverticula occur in the lower two-thirds of the oesophagus and cause, at first, dyspepsia and a sensation of fullness in the chest and, later, dysphagia due to pressure on the oesophagus below. The diagnosis is established by barium swallow and oesophagoscopy, and treatment, if called for, consists of removal of the pouch by thoracotomy. If a pouch is not causing symptoms and is discovered accidentally no active treatment is advised.

Traction diverticula

Traction diverticula occur most commonly in the middle third of the oesophagus (Fig. 76a) and are caused by adhesions between the latter and adjacent structures. This region contains numerous lymph nodes, and the most common cause of a traction diverticulum of the mid-oesophagus is fibrosis following tuberculous disease of these nodes.

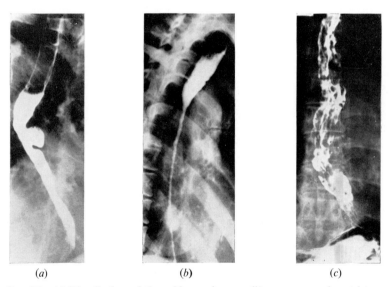

(a)　　　　　　　　　(b)　　　　　　　　　(c)

Fig. 76.—(a) Diverticulum of the mid-oesophagus;　(b) severe corrosive stricture;
(c) oesophageal varices.

In contrast to the smooth downward convexity of the pulsion diverticulum, the traction pouches, which may be multiple, tend to have an irregular outline and to be directed upwards; thus food is unlikely to collect in them, although fatal mediastinitis had been recorded as a result of perforation (Smith, 1928).

Non-malignant strictures of the oesophagus

Aetiology and pathology

Most oesophageal strictures, apart from the congenital type which is uncommon, are a complication of acute or chronic oesophagitis which has encroached on the muscular layer of the oesophageal wall. Serious damage results from the swallowing of corrosive poisons and very young children may develop a stricture after swallowing hot fluids. Damage to the muscular layers of the oesophagus by hasty removal of a foreign body or from prolonged impaction of a foreign body, causing peri-oesophagitis and abscess formation, may give rise to stenosis. Reflux oesophagitis due to hiatus hernia, or prolonged vomiting, may cause ulceration in the lower end of the oesophagus and this ulceration may give rise to a simple stricture.

At the upper end of the gullet, stricture and web formation occur in association with the Paterson–Brown Kelly syndrome. In the middle third of the oesophagus there may be a congenital narrowing and Brown Kelly (1936) considers that during adult life a superimposed infection may cause further narrowing of the oesophagus. Simple strictures may also follow external injury to the oesophagus and occur very occasionally in typhoid fever and in scarlet fever. The most common postoperative complication of operations which entail oesophageal anastomosis is a fibrous stricture at the suture line. Fibrotic stenosis of the oesophagus also occurs as a late development in scleroderma, a rare form of collagen disease.

Complications.—If an untreated stricture becomes impermeable or so narrow that it is easily blocked by food and debris, malnutrition, dehydration and starvation may result. Chronic infection of the lungs from regurgitation and aspiration of oesophageal contents can occur, especially in children; occasionally there is malignant change in the scar.

Symptoms

After the ingestion of a caustic, the patient has difficulty in swallowing caused by acute ulcerative pharyngitis, and when initial reaction has subsided there is usually a period during which the patient swallows without any apparent difficulty. The medical attendant may hope that the return of normal swallowing will indicate that no permanent damage to the oesophagus has occurred, but only too soon dysphagia re-appears with the formation of a stricture. At first the dysphagia may be only slight and intermittent owing to temporary obstruction of the lumen of the stricture caused by an irritative spasm and inflammatory reaction. In untreated patients fluids and even saliva are eventually regurgitated. The sudden onset of complete oesophageal obstruction in a patient who had previously only slight difficulty in swallowing indicates a "corking" of the lumen of the stricture by a hard foreign body such as a bolus of food.

Examination

On general examination no clinical abnormality, apart from malnutrition, may be found. Radiography with barium swallow will show the site of the narrowing.

Some observers have noted that strictures after the swallowing of corrosives are more common at the sites of normal narrowing of the oesophagus, at the crossing of the left bronchus, at the upper end of the oesophagus and at the diaphragmatic narrowing. The oesophagus is only moderately dilated above the stricture and never to the degree shown in achalasia of the cardia.

In a stricture which is caused by instrumental trauma or by a congenital defect the lumen is regular and the length of the stenosis short, but in a stricture due to corrosive poisoning the lumen of the oesophagus is irregular and the stricture is long and multiple (Fig. 76b). The differential diagnosis between simple and malignant strictures of the oesophagus by radiological methods is often difficult, especially if there is no definite history of trauma to the oesophageal wall. Above a carcinomatous stricture there is little or no dilatation of the oesophagus and the stricture itself has a more tortuous and irregular channel than the simple type.

Oesophagoscopy

Above a simple stricture the oesophageal mucosa may be normal, but if the stricture has been present for some time evidence of chronic oesophagitis will be apparent. The oesophageal lumen may be central or eccentric and if the stricture is very narrow the oesophagus above will be dilated and will contain debris and food particles. Near the stricture the mucosa is dull and thickened, and granulation tissue may be present. The stricture is recognizable by the pallor of the mucosa and by the lack of elasticity of the oesophagus. When an attempt is made to pass the oesophagoscope farther along the lumen the rosette appearance of the normal oesophageal mucosa changes to a dull white inelastic membrane.

Treatment

The stricture must be examined through the oesophagoscope and preliminary dilatation performed under direct vision. The wide Negus oesophagoscope is ideal for this method of treatment because it allows an unobstructed view of the end of the bougie. The contents of the oesophagus must be aspirated until an accurate view of the lumen of the stricture can be obtained. The stricture is dilated by the use of tapering soft fine gum-elastic bougies. These are passed in increasing sizes until difficulty is experienced. There are many types of bougies in use, the flexible gum-elastic bougie of Jackson, the olive-headed bougie of Vinson and the dilatable bougies of Tucker and Negus. There may be a small amount of bleeding after the passage of the dilator in the early stages of treatment. Care has to be taken because there is a tendency for the bougie to pass into a pocket next to the lumen of the stricture and to cause a false passage. Dilatation by bougie under direct vision is the first and principal method of treatment. Dilatation may have to be done very frequently and even when the stricture is fully dilated the patient should be kept under observation, and any return of dysphagia will necessitate further treatment. The patient should be advised to take care with food and should always masticate properly and avoid swallowing large lumps of food which may lodge in the oesophagus.

In a case requiring frequent dilatation the patient may be taught to swallow the bougie himself. No force is used. Many endoscopists maintain that blind bouginage is dangerous and quote Truman, the French clinician, who said that "a patient using a bougie would sooner or later die of the instrument". The practice of blind bouginage is not often done now but some laryngologists advise the use of a Hurst mercury tube which can be used by the patient himself.

Impermeable stricture.—An impermeable stricture is rare. If a gastrostomy has been performed and dye, taken through the mouth, cannot be found in the gastric contents, then the obstruction is said to be complete. Usually there is a pin-point opening through the stricture and, with practice, a twisted silk thread can be swallowed or a very small bougie coaxed through the lumen. Closure of the stricture occurs slowly except when it is "corked" by a foreign body. It is usually in neglected cases that an impermeable stricture occurs.

Oesophagoscopy must be done as a preliminary measure in an attempt to dilate the stricture. If no passage is found a gastrostomy should be performed. Such an operation is also necessary if an adequate and permanent dilatation cannot be maintained or if the mechanical obstruction is causing starvation. A gastrostomy gives physiological rest to the oesophagus, allows any inflammation to subside and very often enables bouginage to be re-started.

Treatment of the impermeable stricture is difficult. Among many methods which have been advised are:

(1) Establishment of the lumen by oesophagoscope: the oesophagus is ballooned from above, and forceps or a small metal bougie is pushed through the occluding membrane.

(2) Combined oesophagoscopy from above and bouginage from below.

Retrograde bouginage.—A stricture which cannot be dilated from above may still be permeable from below where the lumen narrows like a funnel towards the lesion, and the entrance to the stricture is concentrically placed. A small oesophago-scope is inserted through the gastrostomy into the lower oesophagus and bougies are then passed up through it. It is a help if the patient can swallow a thread which finds its way through the stricture and is recovered from the gastrostomy opening. The bougie can then be attached to the thread and guided up through the stomach to the stricture by gentle traction upon the upper end through the mouth. Alternatively, the ends of the thread may be joined to form an endless loop, by which olive-shaped dilators, graduated in size, can be drawn up through the stricture.

By whatever method it is achieved bouginage must be continued, daily at first, and later at longer intervals. Neglect of follow-up care all too often results in the return of severe obstruction or aphagia. Bouginage is more often successful with short annular strictures than with long tubular ones.

Surgical treatment

If bouginage fails to establish or maintain a satisfactory lumen external operation is required. The type of operation depends on the upper level at which the oeso-phagus is diseased. Strictures of the lower half may be dealt with by oesophagec-tomy, mobilization of the stomach and an oesophagogastric anastomosis above the level of the aortic arch. If the upper oesophagus is also involved the anastomosis may be made in the neck. In some cases a jejunal or colonic transplant may be preferable to bringing up the stomach. The thoracic surgeon today has a wide choice of techniques for dealing with these problems, thanks to the progress of the last 15 years in oesophageal surgery for cancer.

In frail elderly patients unfit for major thoracic surgery, the failure of bouginage to give lasting benefit justifies insertion of a Souttar or Mousseau–Barbin tube (*see* pp. 241–243).

Oesophageal varices

Cirrhosis of the liver due to any cause gives rise to portal hypertension, and this raised pressure results in varicosity wherever the portal and systemic venous systems converge. At the lower end of the oesophagus such varicosities form an irregular, tortuous mesh in the submucosa. They are subject to repeated trauma by swallowed food, and often the overlying mucosa is affected by reflux oesophagitis. Sooner or later haematemesis occurs, with grave danger to life.

The condition may be diagnosed by barium swallow (Fig. 76c) and oesophago-scopy which reveals varicosities reaching high into the oesophagus and, at the lower end, projecting into its lumen.

Treatment

When life is immediately in danger from profuse bleeding the most effective treatment is by means of a Sengstaken tube. This is passed into the stomach, the lower balloon is inflated and traction is applied so that the veins of the cardia are compressed from below. The upper balloon is then used to compress the veins in the lowest part of the oesophagus.

Some workers, notably Macbeth (1955), advocate strongly the use of sclerosing injections for the control of bleeding. A special syringe designed for use through the oesophagoscope is necessary. The method has not found much favour, despite the obvious advantages as compared with the Sengstaken tube, or external operative measures.

Definitive treatment consists of portacaval anastomosis, which can relieve the causative portal hypertension. Partial oesophagogastrectomy destroys the faulty collateral venous circulation and, by diminishing gastric secretions, lessens the risk of oesophagitis. This procedure is indicated in cases in which portacaval anasto-mosis is not feasible.

Neoplasms of the oesophagus

Benign neoplasms

Benign tumours are very rare. Leiomyoma, occurring as a tumour of smooth muscle, arises usually in the lower one-third of the oeosphagus. It may reach a large size as an encircling submucosal mass which can be completely shelled out at thoracotomy without resection.

Other benign tumours, such as fibroma, papilloma, haemangioma and cysts, can occur at any level, and rarely are pedunculated so that they can be regurgitated into the mouth. Such tumours may be suspected from the history and the barium swallow findings. Oesophagoscopy permits their diagnosis and endoscopic removal.

Malignant growths

Fibrosarcoma, leiomyosarcoma, lymphosarcoma, melanosarcoma and rhabdo-myosarcoma are exceedingly rare.

Carcinoma

Squamous-celled carcinoma is the most common tumour at any level in the oesophagus. At the lower end a fair proportion of adenocarcinomas are found. These arise from mucous glands in the oesophageal wall, or by extension of gastric carcinoma upwards, beyond the cardia.

Oesophageal carcinoma occurs most frequently after the age of 50, and is many times more common in men than in women. The cause is unknown, but predis-posing factors are recognized, such as long-standing chronic oesophagitis, fibrous stricture, achalasia of the cardia, and Paterson–Brown Kelly disease.

The tumour, usually ulcerative in form with surrounding submucosal extensions, soon encircles the oesophagus. Obstruction follows, partly from stenosis and partly from the intraluminal mass of the tumour. Less often a fungating tumour distends the lumen from within, although it fails to encircle the gut, and obstruction is then less marked.

Direct spread of the growth occurs in submucosal lymphatics and this may result in "satellite" ulcers at a distance, with apparently normal tissue intervening. Extrinsic spread involves the mediastinal contents, especially the trachea and bronchi leading to fistula formation, the recurrent laryngeal nerves causing vocal cord paralysis, and the great vessels. Metastases occur in the lymph nodes of the mediastinum, root of neck, and coeliac area. Secondary (blood-borne) deposits are common in the lungs and the liver.

Symptoms.—It must be emphasized that obstruction sufficiently marked to cause symptoms occurs late in the course of the disease. Once established, dysphagia is rapidly progressive and in a matter of weeks loss of weight and dehydration are severe. Total obstruction may occur at any time due to the impaction of a fragment of food. Dysphagia of long standing is more likely to be due to a non-malignant cause than a cancer, but it must be remembered that benign disease of the oesophagus may conceal the later onset of a carcinoma. Pain due to oesophageal carcinoma is not common, and usually is a sign of spread in the mediastinum.

Diagnosis is made as a result of the systematic investigations described at the beginning of this chapter. Some comments regarding the radiographic and endoscopic findings are now made.

Radiography (Fig. 77).—Soft tissue films are taken to show whether there is any enlargement of the visceral tissues at the root of the neck or in the mediastinum. Barium swallow is then carried out. This immediately outlines the upper end of the lesion, and if it is permeable, a trickle passes on through the stricture. An irregular filling defect, an everted upper edge to the mass, and the familiar "rat-tailed" attenuation of the barium stream are all suggestive of malignant disease. The lower

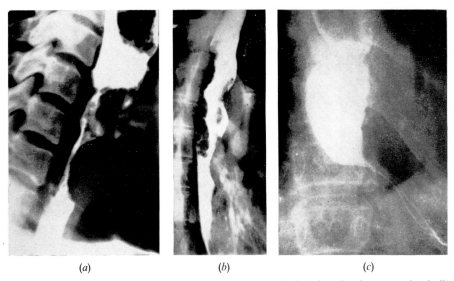

(a)   (b)   (c)

FIG. 77.—Carcinoma of the oesophagus: (*a*) growth at and below the cricopharyngeus level; (*b*) growth at mid-thoracic level—a long ragged filling defect; (*c*) carcinoma of the lower end. Differential diagnosis from benign stricture due to reflux oesophagitis may be difficult.

limit of the tumour can sometimes be roughly indicated by the use of Trendelen-burg's position, which allows barium to flow back again to the lesion. The examination must be abandoned if opaque medium enters the bronchial tree through a broncho-oesophageal fistula. Radiography can be relied upon always to show the level of the lesion (unless the latter is so small that a normal picture is produced), but differential diagnosis between benign and malignant strictures can be difficult.

Oesophagoscopy is essential in any case of suspected malignancy of the oeso-phagus, and in all cases in which abnormal radiographic appearances are noted in the gullet. The site of the ulcer or stricture is inspected and the distance of the lesion from the line of the upper teeth or alveolar margin is measured.

The type of ulceration is noted. A rough hard knobbly surface indicates the probable presence of malignancy, whereas a softer stricture with surface ulceration is more likely to result from reflux oesophagitis.

Inspection of the upper surface of a stricture will give no clue as to the length of gullet involved in the stricture, but by passing a Jackson type of bougie through the stricture and then withdrawing it until the shoulder of the upper part of the bougie is felt to be caught by the lower surface of the stricture, the surgeon may get some idea of its length.

Whenever an oesophagoscopy is carried out an examination of the main bronchial tree should be made at the same time if malignant disease is suspected. In many cases the gullet becomes involved by direct extension from an undiagnosed bronchial growth. In other cases a primary oesophageal cancer spreads into the tracheobronchial tree. If either of these complications is present it indicates that the lesion has progressed beyond all help of any treatment other than alleviation of symptoms.

Biopsy.—In all cases, a piece of tissue should be removed through the oesophago-scope for microscopic examination. Special forceps are made for this purpose and care must be taken to avoid injuring the wall of the oesophagus to such an extent that a perforation is produced.

Before advising radiotherapy or operative treatment, it may be necessary to carry out more than one biopsy. It is not possible to be certain of obtaining a positive report of malignancy from one small piece of tissue, and in suspected cases a negative microscopic report calls for a further oesophagoscopy and removal of another specimen for examination.

Palliative treatment consists of maintaining the nourishment of the patient by keeping the oesophagus permeable.

The stricture of the gullet can be prevented from becoming complete by dilatation followed by the introduction of a rigid tube (Fig. 78).

Dilatation with bougies alone produces such a short period of freedom from obstruction that it is hardly worth considering.

If the site of obstruction lies below the thoracic inlet a Souttar's tube (metal or plastic) may be inserted through the oesophagoscope. The technique is illustrated in Fig. 79. The larger plastic Mousseau–Barbin tube functions better, however, and can sometimes be inserted by sliding it over a small bougie passed through the stricture. The narrow part of the tube is of course first cut off. The oesophagoscope is removed, the bougie remaining in position to guide the tube. The latter is passed behind the larynx with a finger and then gently pushed on by the oesophagoscope which is re-inserted around the bougie. When the tube is snugly seated on the growth the bougie, and then the oesophagoscope, are finally removed. If these

241

measures fail the standard Mousseau–Barbin technique must be used (Fig. 80). A laparotomy is done and the stomach is opened. The stricture is then dilated from above, through an oesophagoscope, and a medium-sized bougie is passed through and retrieved from the stomach. The tail of the tube is fixed to the upper end of the bougie, which is then pulled through from below. The tube slides down through the mouth until its flange is seated upon the stricture. Finally the tube is cut across

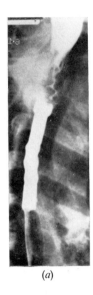 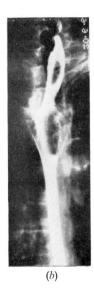

FIG. 78.—Intubation for carcinoma of the oesophagus. Barium swallow radiographs showing: (a) Souttar's tube; (b) Mousseau–Barbin tube.

(a) (b)

FIG. 79.—Technique of inserting Souttar's tube through the oesophagoscope: (a) after gentle dilatation of the lumen the Souttar's tube is passed down along the metal guide; (b) the flange of the tube is seated firmly on to the upper rim of the growth; (c) the guide is withdrawn while the tube is held in position with the ring-shaped introducer. The latter is then removed and the position of the tube finally scrutinized before withdrawal of the oesophagoscope.

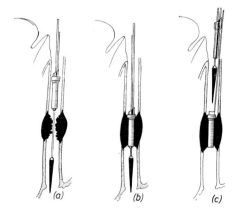

(a) (b) (c)

just below the cardia, and the stomach is closed. This technique is best done by two teams of surgeons, and is greatly improved by the use of Crossling's bougies (Crossling, 1961) (Fig. 80). Better functional results have recently been claimed for Celestin's nylon and latex tube which is more flexible, and less liable to cause pressure necrosis around the rim of the funnelled upper end.

Intubation is not well tolerated in the cervical part of the oesophagus. Here, and in the postcricoid region, severe obstruction is best managed by the insertion of a nasogastric feeding tube, pending the outcome of radiotherapy or the decision to undertake radical excision. Gastrostomy merely for the prolongation of hopeless misery should be avoided, although there may be cases in which it may be necessary to improve the general condition in preparation for an attempt at curative operation.

In cases where radiotherapy is likely to be used, plastic, and not metal, tubes should be insisted upon for all these manoeuvres.

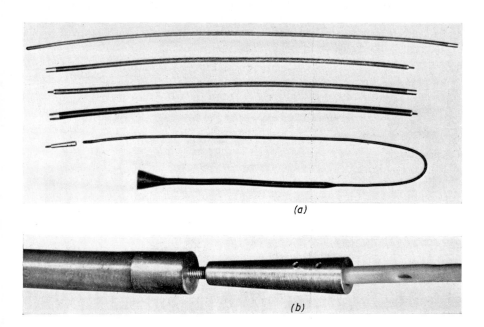

FIG. 80.—Technique for inserting Mousseau–Barbin tube: (a) Crossling's graduated screw-ended bougies (there are six in the complete set), with metal adaptor, and a Mousseau–Barbin plastic tube. The bougies are assembled as a continuous rod, passed through the mouth and drawn out at the gastrotomy wound; (b) method of attaching the tail of the Mousseau–Barbin tube to the threaded bougie; (c) three stages in pulling down the tube on to the growth (*see* text).

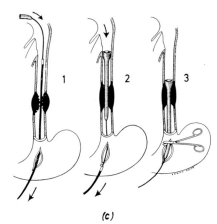

Treatment by radiotherapy.—The majority of cancers of the oesophagus are inoperable. A small proportion of them can be improved by radiotherapy, and an even smaller number may be apparently cured. Endoscopic application of radium, and interstitial radon or gold seeds, have been virtually abandoned in favour of external irradiation. The ability to deliver effective tumour doses has increased with the availability of tele-cobalt beam therapy and, in some centres, megavoltage x-ray machines.

Significant damage to the lungs is now largely avoided and even if treatment fails the patient's plight is not worsened by it. In cases of satisfactory tumour regression a fibrous stricture remains, requiring dilatation at intervals.

Cytotoxic drugs.—In malignant disease of the oesophagus regional infusion is not possible, and the use of these drugs has been restricted to general systemic administration. Up to this time there is no convincing evidence of worthwhile palliation of symptoms, but their use is justified if no other treatment is possible.

Oesophagectomy.—Thoracic surgery offers the best chance of cure, and a fair chance of palliation if cure should fail, in carcinoma of the lower and middle thirds of the oesophagus. The decisions as to operability and choice of technique are extremely complex, and outside the endoscopist's province. The present position is thoroughly reviewed, with a full bibliography, by Flavell (1963).

Inoperability is beyond dispute in cases having involvement of the bronchial tree, or recurrent laryngeal nerve, or distant metastases.

At the present time it is considered that growths above the aortic arch should be treated only by radiotherapy, but modern techniques of total oesophagectomy, with colon, jejunal or stomach transplantation may in the future provide a better line of attack.

Carcinomas of the cervical oesophagus are rarely operable, but if an adequate margin of healthy oesophagus is present between the tumour and the thoracic inlet, it is the laryngologist who must decide whether to proceed or rely upon radiotherapy. Such tumours can be excised by means of slightly modified techniques, as described for the hypopharynx in Chapter 7. In practice, simple oesophagectomy is rarely indicated here, and involvement of the trachea, larynx or recurrent laryngeal nerves will dictate oesophagopharyngolaryngectomy. The addition of total thyroidectomy increases the chances of total clearance of local spread of the disease, but inability to remove the mediastinal lymph nodes adequately is responsible for the very high failure rate for this type of operation.

REFERENCES AND BIBLIOGRAPHY

Acheson, E. D., and Hadley, G. D. (1958). *Brit. med. J.*, **1**, 549.
Allison, P. R. (1943). *J. thorac. Surg.*, **12**, 432.
— (1946). *J. thorac. Surg.*, **15**, 308.
— Johnstone, A. S., and Royce, G. B. (1943). *J. thorac. Surg.*, **12**, 342.
Alpin, M. (1934). *Mschr. Ohrenheilk*, **68**, 1172.
Barlow, D. (1942). *Brit. J. Surg.*, **29**, 415.
Barrett, N. R. (1933). *Lancet*, **1**, 1009.
— (1954). *Brit. J. Surg.*, **42**, 231.
Belsey, R. H. R. (1966). *Proc. R. Soc. Med.*, **59**, 927.
— and Donnison, C. P. (1950). *Brit. med. J.*, **2**, 324.
Benson, C. D., Mustard, W. T., Ravitch, M., Snyder, W., and Welch, K. J. (1962). *Pediatric Surgery* (Vol. 1, p. 266). Chicago; Year Book Publishers.
Chesterman, J. T. (1965). *Brit. J. Surg.*, **52**, 601.
Crossling, F. T. (1961). *Brit. med. J.*, **1**, 1032.
Diggle, F. H. (1932). *Brit. med. J.*, **1**, 277.
Douglas, K., and Nicholson, F. (1959). *Brit. J. Surg.*, **47**, 250.
Ellis, F. G. (1962). *Ann. R. Coll. Surg. Engl.*, **30**, 155.
— Kauntze, R., and Trounce, J. R. (1960). *Brit. J. Surg.*, **47**, 466.
— — Nightingale, A., and Trounce, J. R. (1960). *Quart. J. Med.*, **29**, 305.

REFERENCES AND BIBLIOGRAPHY

Etzel, E. (1942). *Amer. J. med. Sci.*, **203**, 87.
Flavell, G. (1963). *The Oesophagus.* London; Butterworths.
Flett, R. L. (1945). *J. Laryng.*, **60**, 1.
Franklin, R. H. (1958). *Proc. R. Soc. Med.*, **51**, 595.
Freeman, N. V. (1969). In *Neonatal Surgery* (Ed. by P. P. Rickham and J. H. Johnston). London; Butterworths.
Goligher, J. C. (1948). *Lancet*, **1**, 985.
Groves, J. (1956). *Brit. J. Surg.*, **43**, 413.
Heller, E. (1914). *Mitt. Grenzgeb. Med. Chir.*, **57**, 141.
Helmsworth, J. A., and Pryles, C. V. (1951). *J. Pediat.*, **38**, 610.
Hurst, A. (1943). *J. Laryng.*, **58**, 60.
Imperatori, C. J. (1939). *Arch. Otolaryng.*, Chicago, **30**, 352.
Jackson, C. (1922). *Laryngoscope*, **32**, 139.
— and Jackson, C. L. (1915). *Peroral Endoscopy and Laryngeal Surgery.* St. Louis; The Laryngoscope Co.
— — (1936). *Diseases of the Air and Food Passages of Foreign Body Origin.* Philadelphia; Saunders.
— — (1933). *Arch. Otolaryng.*, **18**, 731.
Kelly, A. Brown (1936). *J. Laryng.*, **51**, 78.
Klayman, M. I. (1955). *Ann. intern. Med.*, **43**, 33.
Logan (Quoted in *Current Problems in Surgery* (1967). Ed. by M. M. Ravitch, E. H. Ellison, O. C. Julian, A. P. Thal and O. H. Wangensteen). Chicago; Year Book Medical Publishers.
Macbeth, R. G. (1955). *Brit. med. J.*, **2**, 877.
Mosher, H. P. (1935). *Surg. Gynec. Obstet.*, **60**, 403.
Mullard, K. S. (1954). *J. thorac. Surg.*, **28**, 39.
Negus, V. E. (1929). *Proc. R. Soc. Med.*, **22**, 527.
— (1955). In *Diseases of the Nose and Throat* (6th ed.). London; Cassell.
Nissen, R., Rossetti, M., and Markman, I. (1965). *Prensa med. argent.*, **52**, 2510.
Nixon, H. H., and Wilkinson, A. W. (1963). In *Congenital Abnormalities in Infancy* (Ed. by A. P. Norman). Oxford; Blackwell.
Olsen, A. M., and Harrington, S. W. (1948). *J. thorac. Surg.*, **17**, 189.
Phillips, C. E. (1938). *J. Amer. med. Ass.*, **111**, 998.
Richardson, J. R. (1945). *Ann. Otol.*, **54**, 328.
Robb, D. (1952–53). *Aust. N.Z. J. Surg.*, **22**, 120.
le Roux, B. T., and Wright, J. T. (1960). *Brit. J. Surg.*, **48**, 619.
Schindler, R. (1956). *Ann. intern. Med.*, **45**, 207.
Schlemmer, F. (1920). *Arch. Klin. Chir.*, **114**, 37.
Scott-Brown, W. G. (1964). Personal communication.
Smith, M. K. (1928). *Ann. Surg.*, **88**, 1022.
Starck, H. (1934). *Münch. med. Wschr.*, **81**, 1794, 1805.
— (1936). *Sonderdruck aus "Knolls" Mitteilungen für Ärtze.* Jubiläuausgabe.
Sweet R. H. (1954). *Thoracic Surgery* (2nd ed.). Philadelphia; Saunders.
Terracol, J., and Sweet, R. H. (1958). *Diseases of the Oesophagus.* Philadelphia and London; Saunders.
Trounce, J. R., Deuchar, D. C., Kauntze, R., and Thomas, G. A. (1957). *Quart. J. Med.*, **26**, 433.
Tucker, G. J. (1925). *J. Amer. med. Ass.*, **84**, 511.
Ty, T. C., Brunet, C., and Beardmore, H. E. (1967). *J. Pediat. Surg.*, **2**, 118.
Vogt, E. C. (1929). *Amer. J. Roentgenol.*, **22**, 463.
Wangensteen, O. H. (1951). *Ann. Surg.*, **134**, 301.
Wright, A. J. (1934). *J. Laryng.*, **49**, 175.

PART II

DISEASES OF THE LARYNX AND TRACHEOBRONCHIAL TREE

METHODS OF EXAMINING THE LARYNX AND TRACHEOBRONCHIAL TREE

R. S. Lewis

THE LARYNX

The complete investigation of laryngeal disease may necessitate examination by external palpation, indirect laryngoscopy, direct laryngoscopy, stroboscopy and radiography, and biopsies and swabs may be taken. With all these means available it should be possible to arrive at a diagnosis in almost every case.

It is hardly possible to list all the indications for the various procedures; the experience and judgement of the examiner must determine which of the investigations are necessary.

Indirect laryngoscopy

In many cases indirect laryngoscopy, considered with the history, will be sufficient to establish a diagnosis. It is a straightforward procedure which should be within the capabilities of every practitioner; and it ought to be more frequently employed than it is. Cases would then be diagnosed earlier with consequent improvement in the results of treatment.

In order to get a satisfactory view of the larynx, the examiner must be accustomed to using frontal illumination. A good headlamp is as satisfactory as light reflected from a forehead mirror and is easier for the beginner. Several laryngeal mirrors of different sizes are needed, also a spirit lamp and a gauze square for holding the tongue. If a spirit lamp is not available the mirror can be warmed in a bowl of hot water. The examiner may wear a mask or shield to protect his face in infected cases.

The co-operation and relaxation of the patient are essential to the success of an examination, and before he begins the examiner should explain what he is going to do and how he would like the patient to help. The patient's position is important: he should sit with his body upright and his head held level; the examiner sits facing him and draws the head a little forward from the shoulders. Any dentures the patient may be wearing are removed, and the largest mirror which will conveniently fit at the back of the patient's throat is selected; a small mirror gives a less complete view of the larynx and pharynx, and may slip behind the soft palate when the mirror is raised to elevate it. The mirror is warmed by holding it, face downwards, in the flame of a spirit lamp and, before it is introduced into the patient's mouth, its temperature is tested on the examiner's hand or cheek. The patient is asked to put out his tongue and, covering it with the gauze square, the examiner takes hold of it with the thumb and middle finger of his left hand; the forefinger lifts the upper lip out of the way, and rests on the incisor teeth for steadiness (Fig. 81). At this point the patient is asked to breathe steadily in and out through his mouth in order to separate the tongue and soft palate, otherwise the mirror cannot be placed in position. The warmed mirror, held in the right hand like a pen, is passed face downwards over the tongue (with care not to touch the tongue and smear the

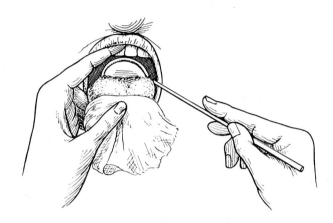

FIG. 81.—Indirect laryngoscopy. Method of holding tongue and laryngeal mirror.

surface with saliva) and placed firmly against the base of the uvula, lifting it upwards and backwards; the shaft rests against the angle of the mouth for support. The examiner focuses his light on the mirror and, by tilting the mirror in different directions, the reflected images of the various structures of the larynx and laryngopharynx may be seen.

The ease with which the larynx may be seen varies from patient to patient, but by going about it in the right way the number of difficult cases may be reduced to a minimum. Success depends to a great extent on the patient's relaxation, and gentleness in handling is therefore most important. The tongue should be held firmly in position, but not dragged upon or pinched. Too much downward pull will press the lower surface of the tongue against the lower incisor teeth, causing pain, or even laceration of the fraenum. A mirror which is placed firmly against the soft palate and deliberately tilted as required is much better tolerated than one which only just touches it and which slides about when moved to bring the laryngeal structures into view. Even so, there are many patients who retch or gag when the mirror is put into position and in these cases the soft palate must be anaesthetized by spraying with a 2·5 per cent solution of cocaine, or by the patient sucking an amethocaine or lignocaine lozenge.

It is possible to see the base of the tongue, the larynx, and the upper portions of the hypopharynx and pyriform fossae by indirect laryngoscopy, but all these structures will not appear at one time in the laryngeal mirror, and the examiner has to piece together the various images into a complete picture. Each structure should be inspected in turn, and it is advisable to keep to the same order of inspection in every case. It is only by adhering to a regular routine of inspection that one may be certain of not missing any detail. Before the examination is completed the mirror may have to be taken out and re-inserted several times to give the patient a rest.

Structures visible on indirect laryngoscopy

The first structures seen are the anterior surface of the epiglottis, the base of the tongue and the valleculae. Raising the mirror and tilting it downwards brings into sight the entrance to the larynx. It is bounded in front by the upper edge of the epiglottis, behind by the mucous membrane between the arytenoid cartilages, and on each side by the aryepiglottic folds. The epiglottis is a flattened, leaf-like structure, covered with pale mucous membrane, across which a few blood vessels arborize. Its shape varies a good deal, and it is more folded upon itself in infants and young children than in adults. It may overhang the larynx, making it almost impossible to get a good view of the interior (Fig. 82). The posterior surface of the

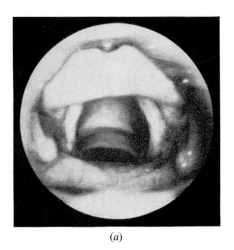
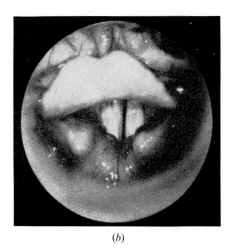

(a)   (b)

FIG. 82.—Indirect laryngoscopy: (*a*) during inspiration; (*b*) during phonation. Note how clearly the cartilages of Wrisberg stand out in the aryepiglottic folds. (*Reproduced by courtesy of Dr. Paul H. Holinger and the Editor of* Annals of Otology, Rhinology and Laryngology.)

epiglottis forms a slight elevation, known as the tubercle, just above the anterior commissure of the vocal cords. Running posteromedially from the lateral margins of the epiglottis to the arytenoid cartilages on each side is a free fold of mucous membrane. This is the aryepiglottic fold. It is thin in front, but thickens behind, where it contains the cartilages of Wrisberg and Santorini. Beneath these are the eminences formed by the arytenoid cartilages, and in between is the interarytenoid space.

The ventricular bands lie immediately above the vocal cords and appear to be in contact with them; the ventricles of the larynx cannot usually be seen by indirect laryngoscopy. The vocal cords run backwards from the angle of the thyroid cartilage to the vocal processes of the arytenoids, forming the triangular aperture of the rima glottidis. In the mirror-image the vocal cords appear as flat, ribbon-like structures with sharp, free margins. They are glistening white in colour, and there should not be any vessels visible on their surface. The motility of the cords should be determined by making the patient phonate, saying "e-e-e-e". If there is no paresis or fixation, the cords and arytenoids will approximate and the interarytenoid space will be obliterated (Figs. 82 and 83).

Below the vocal cords is the subglottic space, the walls of which are hidden from view but, farther down, the first two or three rings of the trachea may be seen anteriorly.

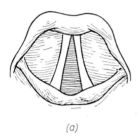 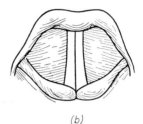

(a)   *(b)*

FIG. 83.—Indirect laryngoscopy. Diagrams of larynx: (*a*) during quiet respiration; (*b*) during phonation.

The larynx lies in contact with the posterior wall of the pharynx, and moves away from it only on deglutition; thus the lower half of the hypopharynx cannot be seen. The entrances to the pyriform fossae can be seen in the mirror and a little more of the fossae becomes visible on phonation, but complete inspection is not possible by the indirect method of examination.

The image of the larynx seen in the mirror is reversed anteroposteriorly but not from side to side. That is to say, the anterior commissure will appear to point away from the examiner and the right-hand structures will be seen on his left.

The most difficult part to bring into view is the anterior commissure, and the larynx cannot be passed as normal until this has been inspected. It is often invisible during quiet respiration, but if the patient is asked to say "e-e-e-e" the larynx elevates and the epiglottis tilts forwards, uncovering the anterior commissure. In some cases the overhang of the epiglottis may be so marked that this manoeuvre fails. Occasionally this is simply due to the nervousness and tenseness of the patient and re-examination a day or two later when he is less apprehensive may succeed. If not, the examiner will have to hook the epiglottis forward with a curved probe or special epiglottis retractor, the patient holding his own tongue to free the examiner's hand. Another obstacle to satisfactory examination is the fact that the tongue may elevate on phonation and hide the mirror, just when a view is most wanted; this can be overcome by using a tongue depressor.

Children are difficult to examine by indirect laryngoscopy and direct inspection is usually required if it is necessary to see the larynx. Sometimes, however, a sufficiently good view can be obtained if the mirror is placed almost horizontally against the hard palate, instead of the uvula, so that the cough reflex is not elicited.

Observations during examination

During examination the observer must look for, and assess the significance of, any abnormal appearances. There may be injection, swelling, oedema, proliferation or ulceration; and the movements of the vocal cords may be impaired. In those parts of the larynx and pharynx which cannot be seen in the mirror, a lesion may produce visible indications that will lead to correct diagnosis. For example, impairment of movement of a vocal cord may be due to a hidden subglottic growth, and frothy saliva in the pyriform fossae may be traced to a low laryngopharyngeal or upper oesophageal carcinoma.

Consideration of the position of the cartilage of Wrisberg in the aryepiglottic fold may be of assistance in the diagnosis of laryngeal paralysis, especially in differentiating paralysis from fixation of the crico-arytenoid joint. In the latter case, the cartilage retains its normal upright position, braced by the action of the posterior crico-arytenoid muscle. In recurrent laryngeal nerve paralysis this action fails, and the cartilage droops forward over the posterior end of the vocal cord, making it appear shorter than its fellow.

Indirect laryngoscopy is used mainly for diagnosis. In the past, various manipulations such as laryngeal biopsy, removal of innocent growths and cauterization of tuberculous ulcers, were done under indirect laryngoscopic control. They demand considerable skill and, since more accurate work can be done by direct laryngoscopy, the modern operator seldom troubles to acquire it. However, it is still sometimes convenient to take a biopsy of a large malignant growth by this method and Mackenzie's spoon-bladed forceps are recommended (Fig. 84) (Thomson and Negus, 1955).

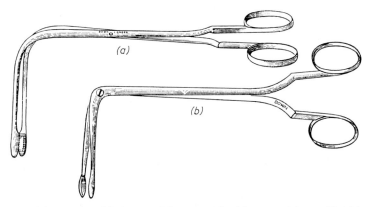

FIG. 84.—Mackenzie's laryngeal forceps: (*a*) with serrated jaws; (*b*) with scoop jaws. (*Reproduced by courtesy of Down Bros. and Mayer & Phelps Ltd.*)

The laryngeal mirror is also useful in guiding the manipulations for anaesthetizing the larynx and trachea for direct laryngoscopy and bronchoscopy, and when bronchograms are required iodized oil may be introduced into the trachea via the larynx.

The operator requires both hands free to carry out these procedures under indirect vision, and the tongue has to be held by an assistant or by the patient himself. The operator usually holds the laryngeal mirror in his left hand and the instrument in his right hand.

Direct laryngoscopy

By this method the larynx is looked at directly instead of in a reflected image. Except for injuries and diseases of the cervical spine, there are very few contra-indications to its use. When there is marked laryngeal obstruction, a tracheostomy should be done first. The examination may not be possible when severe trismus exists.

Many varieties of laryngoscopes have been devised, but the basic pattern is that of Chevalier Jackson. In his instrument the illumination is provided by a small electric bulb at the distal end. Negus (1947) has improved this laryngoscope by introducing proximal illumination by means of two small lamps set obliquely in the walls of the tube (Fig. 85). In this way the convenience and unobstructed lumen of Jackson's instrument is preserved, while an even illumination is thrown well ahead of the tube.

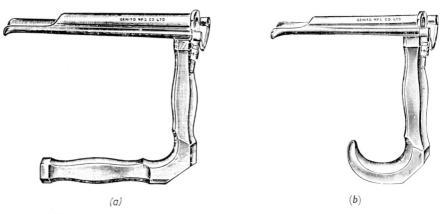

(a)   (b)

FIG. 85.—(a) Adult laryngoscope with Negus' lighting system; (b) child laryngoscope with Negus' lighting system. (*Reproduced by courtesy of the Genito-Urinary Manufacturing Company Ltd.*)

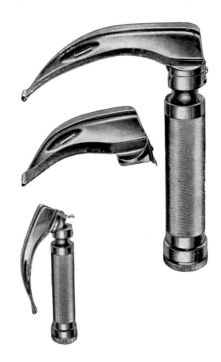

FIG. 86.—Mackintosh laryngo-scope. (*Reproduced by courtesy of The British Oxygen Company Ltd.*)

A still more recent advance is the use of light transmitted through a fibreglass cable. Instruments with distal lighting, such as Negus bronchoscopes, need no adaptation to take the fibre-optic system, but with the proximal twin-lighting system, some modifications are necessary. A brighter and more uniform field is given with this method.

The Mackintosh laryngoscope (Fig. 86) is favoured by most anaesthetists for passing endotracheal anaesthetic tubes and is also useful for removing foreign bodies arrested in the valleculae and the region of the laryngeal aditus.

Anaesthesia

With the modern developments of anaesthesia direct laryngoscopy is now usually performed under a general anaesthetic. Occasionally where there is an extensive laryngeal or pharyngeal growth and it is desired to avoid tracheostomy local analgesia may be preferable. In infants and young children Chevalier Jackson used to teach that no anaesthetic at all should be used, but it is now considered wiser and safer to give a general anaesthetic. The relaxation and control given by well administered general anaesthesia enables the surgeon to make a more thorough examination and perform his manipulations with greater accuracy than when he has to contend with a conscious patient.

Local analgesia

A preliminary talk with the patient helps to secure his co-operation and stress should be laid on his maintaining complete relaxation. The stomach should be empty when he comes to the theatre and dentures must be removed.

An injection of Omnopon and scopolamine is the most satisfactory form of pre-medication. Barbiturates such as Nembutal and Sodium Amytal are less certain in their action and sometimes cause some mental confusion and lack of co-operation. The Omnopon, 20 mg., and scopolamine, 0·4 mg., are given $1\frac{1}{2}$ hours before operation; these doses are for a normal adult and are varied according to the age, sex, build and clinical condition of the patient.

The writer has used cocaine for many years without complications but nowadays it is claimed that lignocaine is a safer drug. A 4 per cent solution is recommended and not more than 5 ml. (200 mg.) should be used. If cocaine is preferred a 10 per cent solution mixed with an equal quantity of 1:1,000 adrenaline is safe unless the patient has an idiosyncrasy to the drug. This may be tested by giving the patient a subcutaneous injection of 10 mg. cocaine a day or so before the operation. Faintness, tachycardia, nausea, vomiting, or dilated pupils indicate undue sensitivity to the drug. The pulse should be counted every five minutes for half an hour after the injection and an increase of more than 20 per cent in the rate indicates sensitivity.

The patient sits upright on the trolley with his back supported so that the drowsiness induced by the premedication is disturbed as little as possible. The mouth, fauces, base of tongue and pharynx are sprayed with the analgesic solution, particular care being paid to the upper lip and alveolus which may be heavily pressed upon during laryngoscopy. The next step is to pass a swab wrung out of the solution into each pyriform fossa in turn and to hold it there for at least half a minute. Krause's laryngeal forceps is a convenient instrument for this purpose. This manoeuvre blocks the superior laryngeal nerves as they run under the mucosa of the lateral walls of the fossae, and is best carried out under the guidance of a laryngeal mirror. Finally, 1·0 ml. of the analgesic solution is taken up in a laryngeal syringe and, again under laryngeal mirror guidance, a few drops are dropped on to the epiglottis; the rest is squirted into the interior of the larynx. This causes a spasm of coughing which spreads the lignocaine or cocaine to all parts of the larynx.

After each spraying or application the patient is instructed to spit out any excess of the solution. The analgesia wears off in about an hour and he must not eat or drink until sensation has returned.

General anaesthesia

For children from 2 to 7 years old trimeprazine tartrate is an excellent premedication. It is given by mouth 1½ hours before operation at a dose rate of 3–4 mg./kg.

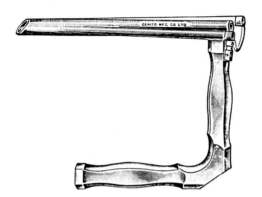

FIG. 87.—Anterior commissure laryngoscope, with Negus' lighting system. (*Reproduced by courtesy of The Genito-Urinary Manufacturing Company Ltd.*)

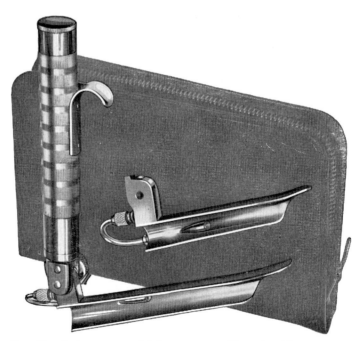

FIG. 88.—Anderson neonatal laryngoscope. (*Reproduced by courtesy o, Medical & Industrial Equipment Ltd.*)

An intramuscular injection of 0·4–0·6 mg. of atropine is also given half an hour before the operation is due to begin.

Above the age of 7 years pethidine and atropine are probably preferable to Omnopon and scopolamine because they do not depress the cough reflex so much. Pethidine 10 mg./6·35 kg. (1 stone) for children and a full dose of 100 mg. for adults is given with 0·6 mg. of atropine 45 min. pre-operatively by intramuscular injection.

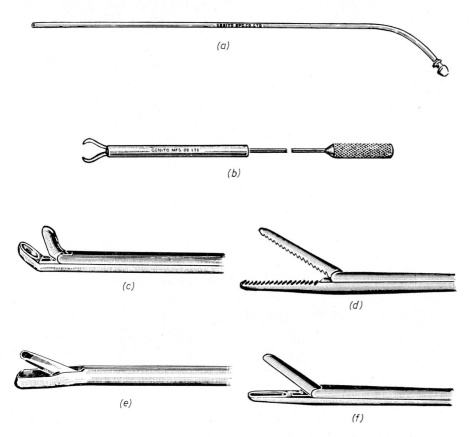

FIG. 89.—Instruments used in direct laryngoscopy: (*a*) aspirating tube, Chevalier Jackson, open end; (*b*) swab holder, Coolidge; (*c*) nodule forceps, Chevalier Jackson; (*d*) grasping forceps, Chevalier Jackson; (*e*) biopsy forceps, Taylor; (*f*) cutting forceps, Patterson. (*Reproduced by courtesy of The Genito-Urinary Manufacturing Company Ltd.*)

The introduction of the muscle relaxant drugs has been of great help in per-oral endoscopy and nowadays most laryngoscopies and many bronchoscopies are performed under their influence. Adults are induced with intravenous thiopentone followed by intravenous suxamethonium and when relaxation has been obtained a small bore (7 mm.) endotracheal tube is passed through the nose or the mouth. Anaesthesia is maintained through the tube with nitrous oxide, oxygen and halothane. The tube lies in the posterior commissure and most of the larynx can be thoroughly inspected while it is in position. It is removed or displaced by

257

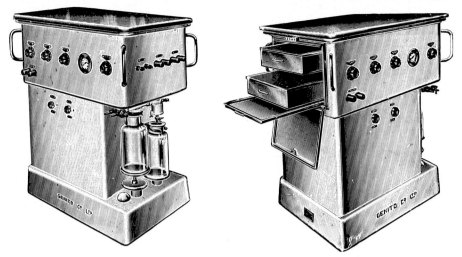

FIG. 90.—Negus endoscopic instrument table. (*Reproduced by courtesy of The Genito-Urinary Manufacturing Company Ltd.*)

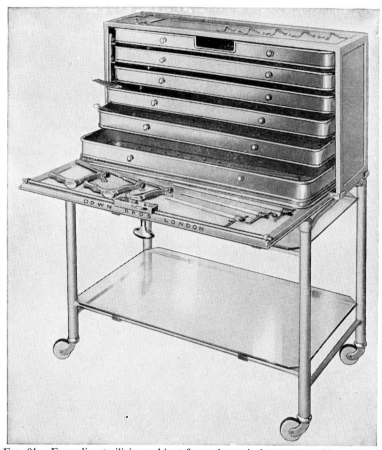

FIG. 91.—Formalin sterilizing cabinet for endoscopic instruments. (*Reproduced by courtesy of Down Bros. and Mayer & Phelps Ltd.*)

the laryngoscope to allow inspection of the posterior commissure and adjacent regions.

For the average adult, the dose of thiopentone is usually 300 mg. and that of suxamethonium 50 mg.

Instruments

Several sizes of laryngoscopes are required and the Negus type is recommended. Of the standard laryngoscope pattern two sizes, adult and child, are needed (*see* Fig. 85) but a more frequently useful instrument is the anterior commissure laryngoscope (Fig. 87). Anderson's neonatal laryngoscope (Fig. 88) is valuable for investigating laryngeal conditions in the newborn and very young infants. In addition to laryngoscopes, an aspirating tube, swab holders and laryngeal forceps of different patterns are required (Fig. 89). The lighting current is provided by a dry cell battery or a transformer, and some form of suction apparatus is also necessary. It is advisable to have instruments for bronchoscopy and oesophagoscopy at hand in case these investigations become necessary. A sterilized tracheostomy set should always be kept ready, and oxygen and carbon dioxide must be available, in case complete obstruction to the airway should develop.

It is convenient for all the instruments for per-oral endoscopy to be kept together permanently sterilized. The table illustrated (Fig. 90) contains two drawers for instruments in formalin vapour and the remaining equipment can be kept similarly sterilized in a cabinet (Fig. 91). The table incorporates a suction apparatus, cautery and low tension currents for the endoscopic lamps.

Position of the patient

If there is any likelihood of having to inspect the trachea, bronchi or oesophagus as well as the larynx, the Negus head rest is recommended (Figs. 93–94); besides giving free control of the position of the head and neck, it has the advantage of an attached quiver to hold the various instruments required. For direct laryngoscopy, however, no head rest is needed (Lewy, 1953): the shoulders are simply raised slightly on two or three folded towels or a small pillow allowing the occiput to rest on the table. When the laryngoscopy is being done to remove a foreign body, the same position is adopted but the table is tilted into the Trendelenburg position so that if the foreign body is dislodged before it can be grasped with forceps, it will not fall into the trachea or bronchi.

Examination

The examination should be conducted with full aseptic precautions to prevent the carrying of infection from one patient to another. The laryngoscopes and cables are best sterilized by keeping them in formalin vapour for 24 hours. The laryngoscopes may be autoclaved after the light bulbs have been removed.

The method of holding and introducing the laryngoscope is shown in Figs. 92–96. It is passed to one side of the tongue, which is crowded over to the opposite side. In this way the effort required to lift the laryngoscope against this muscular structure is reduced. When the posterior one-third of the tongue is reached, the laryngoscope is directed to the midline and elevated slightly, bringing the epiglottis into view (Fig. 97). Its tip is then guided behind the epiglottis, advanced about 1 cm. and elevated. This is effected by *lifting* upwards and forwards with the left hand. There must be no *levering* of the laryngoscope on the upper teeth or gums (Fig. 94).

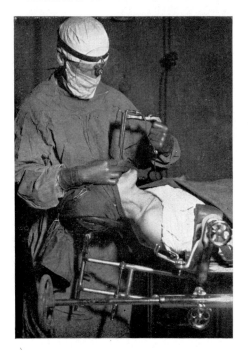

Fig. 92.—Method of holding laryngoscope and position of patient on table. The sterile towels have been drawn back and the quiver for holding instruments has been removed to give a better view. The theatre walls, towels and gowns are green, which reduces glare. The operator stands at the head of the table, to the left of the patient, and his face is protected by a glass shield. With the ring and middle fingers of his right hand he retracts the upper and lower lips, respectively. The patient lies with his head and shoulders projecting over the head of the table, the head comfortably supported at the right level by the head-rest.

Fig. 93.—Introduction of the laryngoscope. The instrument is passed to one side of the tongue and the epiglottis is brought into view (*see* Fig. 97). The ring and middle fingers of the right hand retract the lips and the thumb and forefinger help to guide the tube. If there are any incisor teeth they are protected with rubber or gauze.

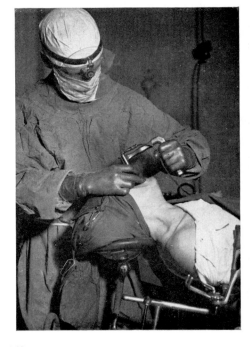

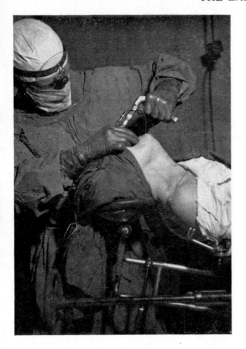

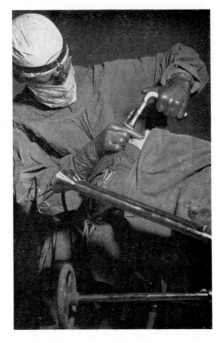

Fig. 94.—Exposing the interior of the larynx. The tip has been passed behind the epiglottis and elevated strongly without levering on the upper alveolus. As this movement alters the angle of the tube, the table is raised to keep the operator's eye in line. Alternatively he may sit. The position corresponds to the views shown in Figs. 98 and 99.

Fig. 95.—The examination with towels and instrument-holder in place. In the quiver are the sucker, biopsy forceps and swab holder, each in a separate compartment. They are conveniently placed, so that the operator may pick them out with his right hand, without looking. An assistant replaces swabs and cleans instruments at a nearby table, and the operator is not surrounded and crowded by helpers.

Fig. 96.—Lewy's laryngoscope holder in place (*Reproduced by the courtesy of the Editor of* British Journal of Surgery).

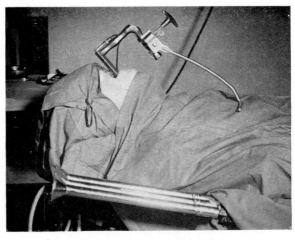

Only the posterior part of the larynx (Fig. 98) is usually seen at first, and further elevation may be necessary to bring the anterior commissure into view. If it still remains out of sight, it may be helpful to alter the position of the head by raising or lowering it a little; sometimes it is useful to get an assistant to press the thyroid cartilage back from the outside.

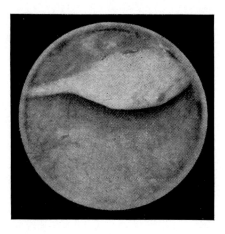

Fig. 97.—Direct laryngoscopy. Epiglottis and posterior pharyngeal wall. (*Reproduced by courtesy of Dr. Paul H. Holinger and the Editor of* Annals of Otology, Rhinology and Laryngology.)

The standard laryngoscope gives a general view of the larynx, but the anterior commissure laryngoscope is more useful for a detailed examination and for exposing the anterior commissure of the larynx. The tip of the anterior commissure laryngoscope can be used to lift up the ventricular bands, so that the interior of the ventricle is exposed and it can be passed between the vocal cords to inspect the subglottic region. When the distal end of this instrument is placed between the

Fig. 98.—Direct laryngoscopy. Posterior part of larynx. (*Reproduced by courtesy of Dr. Paul H. Holinger and the Editor of* Annals of Otology, Rhinology and Laryngology.)

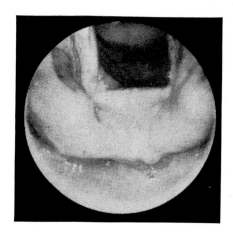

ventricular bands, it fixes the larynx and reduces all movements to a minimum, so that it is possible to remove small growths and nodules from the larynx with great care and accuracy (Fig. 99).

The leverage laryngeal holder designed by Lewy (1953) relieves the operator of a great deal of muscular strain and enables him to sit comfortably and examine the larynx at leisure, and so achieve greater accuracy in his observations and manipulations. Figure 96 shows an early model holding a pharyngeal speculum in position for the diathermy of a pharyngeal pouch.

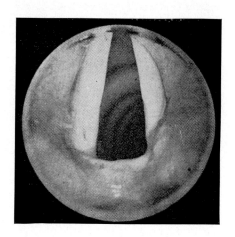

FIG. 99.—Direct laryngoscopy. Interior of the larynx; the vocal cords are fixed by passing the anterior commissure laryngoscope between the ventricular bands. (*Reproduced by courtesy of Dr. Paul H. Holinger and the Editor of* Annals of Otology, Rhinology and Laryngology.)

When the Mackintosh laryngoscope is used the tip of its blade is placed in the valleculae. Lifting the tongue upwards and forwards brings the epiglottis with it exposing the interior of the larynx. The cut-away at the side facilitates the introduction of tubes and instruments.

Comparison of direct and indirect laryngoscopic appearances

Direct laryngoscopy gives the more accurate picture of the larynx, and the student should understand the reasons why the larynx looks different in the reflected mirror image. In indirect laryngoscopy, the angle at which the mirror has to be held causes some foreshortening in the anteroposterior diameter, so that the apparent length of the vocal cords and aryepiglottic folds is reduced, and a lesion of the vocal cord will appear to be nearer the arytenoid cartilage than it really is. The line of vision also is different in the two methods. The mirror, placed posteriorly in the pharynx, reflects the light downwards and forwards into the laryngeal aperture, and thus, in effect, the examiner is looking at the larynx from above and behind. From this viewpoint it is impossible to see much of the anterior surface of the interarytenoid space (*see* Fig. 82). With the direct laryngoscope, however, the whole of the area is exposed (Fig. 98). In the mirror-image a false impression of the depth of the larynx is given and it looks much shallower than it really is. The ventricular bands appear to be in contact with the upper surface of the vocal cords, which look flat and white with sharp free margins. Direct laryngoscopy reveals the true depth of the larynx, the presence of the ventricle between the true and false cords, and the fact that the cords are actually slightly rounded and faintly pink in colour.

Microlaryngoscopy

Suspension laryngoscopy (Killian, 1911) has now been almost entirely abandoned and coming into more general use is the microscopic examination and treatment of laryngeal lesions introduced by Kleinsasser. Indeed, the majority of direct laryngoscopies could with advantage be done by this method.

Kleinsasser (1968) designed laryngoscopes of much greater diameter than had heretofore been used, which permitted more freedom for the surgical manipulations within the larynx (Fig. 100). With a 400 mm. objective on the Zeiss microscope, instead of the 200 mm. one used in ear surgery, a magnified, binocular view of the

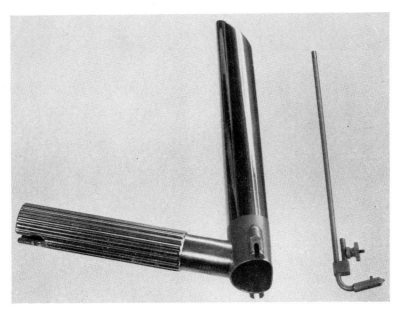

FIG. 100.—Kleinsasser's laryngoscope and light-carrier (Stortz). It is available in several different sizes.

interior of the larynx can be obtained through these laryngoscopes and photographs taken for permanent record. Fine instruments have been devised to use through the laryngoscope under magnification. Microlaryngoscopy has therefore enabled laryngeal lesions to be examined in greater detail and allows for more accurate surgical treatment of such lesions when indicated (Fig. 101).

It is carried out under general anaesthesia. Weigand recommends an armoured oral cuffed endotracheal tube with controlled respiration. We have found a 6–7 mm. nasotracheal tube with normal or controlled respiration equally satisfactory.

For the introduction of the laryngoscope, a small light-carrier is clipped to it, which provides the illumination until the tube is correctly placed in the larynx. Before removing the light, a chest holder is attached to the laryngoscope and with it the laryngoscope tip is levered up until a full view of the interior of the larynx is obtained. The microscope is now brought into use and the light-carrier removed (Fig. 102). If the lesion is in the posterior commissure, the laryngoscope can be placed behind the endotracheal tube, lifting it out of the way. This manoeuvre is easier if an oral rather than a nasal endotracheal tube is used.

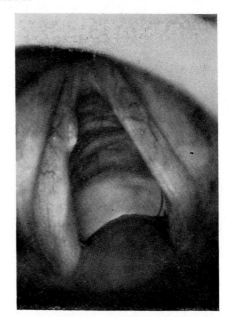

FIG. 101.—Microphotograph of a small patch of keratosis on the left vocal cord.

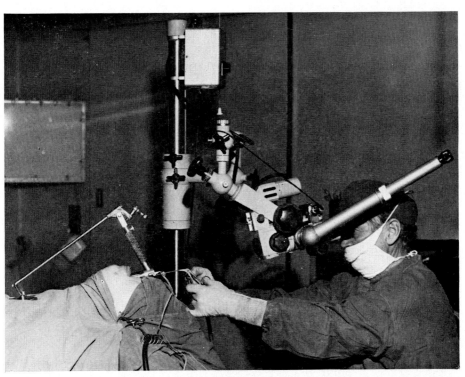

FIG. 102.—Microlaryngoscopy. Note that besides giving a stereoscopic view of the larynx, the wide laryngoscope permits bimanual instrumentation.

Stroboscopy

The vibrations of the vocal cords during phonation are much too rapid to be followed by indirect laryngoscopy, but with the stroboscope an effect of slowing down can be achieved, enabling them to be followed and analysed by the naked eye. This apparent slowing down is brought about by the use, during indirect laryngoscopy, of an interrupted source of light. The original means of producing the interruptions was by a disc with holes in it, set before the light and rotated at varied speeds by an electric motor.

If, when the patient phonates, the frequency of the note uttered corresponds exactly with the frequency of the flashes of interrupted light, the same phase of the vocal cord movement will be illuminated by each flash and the cords will appear to be motionless. If, however, the speed of the disc be so altered that there is a difference of 1 c/sec. between the frequency of the note and the light flashes, a slightly different phase of the vocal cord vibration will be illuminated by each flash, with the original phase re-appearing at the end of one second. It will appear, therefore, as though only one excursion of the vocal cords is taking place each second. This obviously greatly facilitates the study of the physiology of speech and analysis of faults of voice production.

Instruments are now commercially available which automatically adjust the frequency of the light interruptions to the note produced by the larynx. This makes the examiner's task much easier than formerly when he had to control the frequency of the light interruptions himself.

Palpation of the larynx

Palpation of the larynx may yield useful information and constant practice is necessary to acquire the skill to detect minor deviations from the normal.

Before palpating the neck sufficient clothing must be removed to give a free and unrestricted approach and the neck is first inspected in a good light.

To obtain the necessary muscular relaxation the patient should sit with his head slightly flexed; the examiner stands behind and palpates the neck and larynx with the finger tips of both hands. It is rarely necessary for the patient to lie down, and palpation from in front is unsatisfactory.

The prominence of the pomum Adami is first identified and the wings of the thyroid cartilage are carefully examined for any thickening, tenderness, or alteration of shape or position. The thyroid notch is easily found and just above this can be felt the hyoid bone; the greater cornua of the hyoid can be grasped between the fingers and thumb of one hand as they run upwards and backwards below the mandible. Below the thyroid cartilage the anterior surface of the cricoid cartilage forms an important surgical landmark. In adults it lies at the level of the sixth cervical vertebra but in children it may be as high as the lower border of the fourth cervical vertebra. Although about seven rings of the trachea are present in the neck they cannot be palpated even when the neck is fully extended. The isthmus of the thyroid gland lies over the second, third and fourth tracheal rings.

The movements of the larynx should be noted: the larynx is stationary during quiet respiration but on deep breathing and in laryngeal stenosis respiratory excursions occur, the larynx descending on inspiration and ascending on expiration. The larynx also moves upwards on swallowing and during the production of high notes. It can be moved from side to side on the vertebral column, with which it is in contact, and a peculiar grating sensation is often felt; this must not be mistaken for pathological crepitus.

Attention should also be paid to the other structures of the neck, particularly the regional lymph nodes. It should be remembered that paralysis of the sterno-mastoid and trapezius muscles may occur in association with laryngeal palsies.

Radiography of the larynx

In recent years, the use of x-rays in the study of laryngeal conditions, especially extrinsic and intrinsic carcinomas, has become increasingly common. The normal appearance of the larynx is so variable, however, that interpretation of the abnormal is difficult, and a good deal of experience is necessary before reliable conclusions can be drawn from a film. Plain films, tomography, laryngography, and cine techniques all have their value. The normal appearances are described in Volume 1.

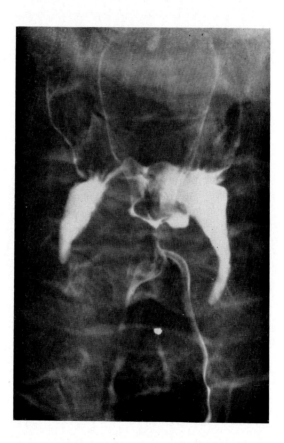

FIG. 103.—Laryngogram showing a right subglottic neoplasm.

Radiographs of the larynx are useful in conditions other than malignant disease. Foreign bodies are rare in the larynx, but those that get impacted are usually metallic and so can be easily shown. Fractures of the laryngeal cartilages may be demonstrated, and also oedema, with narrowing of the airway and surgical emphysema. The degree and extent of laryngeal and tracheal stenosis may be shown by x-ray examination, and after tracheostomy and in the treatment of stenosis a radiograph is useful to check the position of the tracheostomy tube and any intralaryngeal mould that may have been used. A retropharyngeal abscess appears as a considerable thickening of the pre-vertebral soft tissues.

Tomography

Tomograms of the larynx are often more useful than lateral skiagrams in the demonstration of growths and stenosis. The vocal cords, ventricular bands and the ventricle of the larynx can be defined, and thickening of the cords and obliteration of the ventricle are readily seen when they are involved by growths. As in ordinary radiographs, the most important point to be learnt from tomography in carcinoma of the larynx is the amount of subglottic spread that has taken place.

Laryngograms

Study of laryngograms may give additional information as to the site, size and spread of a laryngeal neoplasm (Fig. 103) and so help in deciding upon the right treatment. It is claimed that the accuracy of assessment of a growth by this method is higher than by ordinary methods but the interpretation of the films needs a good deal of study and practice (Holtz and colleagues, 1963).

THE TRACHEOBRONCHIAL TREE

Bronchoscopy

Although bronchoscopy was brought to its present state of perfection by the skill and enthusiasm of laryngologists, notably Killian in Germany, Chevalier Jackson in the United States of America and Negus in Great Britain, its practice is now passing into the hands of the chest surgeons and physicians who naturally want to see the lesions they are to treat. However, the laryngologist still has occasion to examine the respiratory passages below the larynx and he should therefore have a knowledge of the anatomy of the bronchial tree, of pulmonary diseases and of the technique of bronchoscopy.

Instruments and equipment

It is impossible to describe more than a few of the instruments that have been devised for use in bronchoscopy. Some, though rarely needed, may be essential in an emergency and it should be realized that it will not be possible to improvise or find substitutes while the operation is in progress. Each clinic must therefore carry a number of instruments which will be used very rarely or should be prepared to hand on to a larger unit all but the simplest and most routine cases. The following is a list of instruments which will meet most requirements.

1 Negus adult laryngoscope.
1 Negus child laryngoscope.
1 Negus adult bronchoscope, 11 mm. outside diameter × 40 cm. length.
1 Negus adult lower bronchus bronchoscope, 7 mm. outside diameter × 45 cm. length.
1 Negus adolescent bronchoscope, 9 mm. outside diameter × 40 cm. length.
1 Negus child bronchoscope, 8 mm. outside diameter × 30 cm. length.
1 Negus infant bronchoscope, 6 mm. outside diameter × 27·5 cm. length.
1 Negus suckling bronchoscope, 4·8 mm. outside diameter × 27·5 cm. length.
1 Negus tracheoscope.
1 direct-vision bronchoscopic telescope, 46 cm. length.
1 retrograde bronchoscopic telescope, 48 cm. length.

1 90-degree telescope for the subglottic region and trachea with spring clip adapter is very desirable but not essential.
1 extra light carrier and lamp for each lighted instrument.
1 extra flex for each lighted instrument.
1 Chevalier Jackson round-tipped forward-grasping forceps, 60 cm.
1 Chevalier Jackson forward-grasping forceps, 40 cm.
1 Chevalier Jackson fenestrated forward-grasping forceps for peanuts, 45 cm.
1 Chevalier Jackson medium-weight side-curved forceps, 40 cm.
1 Chevalier Jackson standard side-curved forceps, 50 cm.
1 Chevalier Jackson delicate dangling rotation forceps, 40 cm.
1 Chevalier Jackson delicate dangling rotation forceps, 60 cm.
1 Tucker medium-weight pin forceps, 50 cm.
1 Gordon bead forceps, 50 cm.
1 Paterson oesophageal forceps, 45 cm.
2 Chevalier Jackson aspirating tubes, open end, for 30-cm. and 40-cm. tube.
2 Chevalier Jackson aspirating tubes, open end, for 45-cm. tube.
2 Chevalier Jackson aspirating tubes, open end, for 30-cm. tube. These are particularly fine for use through the 4·8 mm. tube.
2 Negus aspirating tubes with gum-elastic ends.
2 Negus aspirating tubes with fully curved gum-elastic ends.
2 spare gum-elastic ends of each of the above.
1 Luken specimen collector.
2 Coolidge fine sponge-holders.
2 Coolidge medium sponge-holders.
2 Coolidge large sponge-holders.
2 Negus revolving eye-shields.

Bronchoscopes.—Fundamentally, a bronchoscope consists of a hollow brass tube, which is slanted at its distal end and which has a small handle at the proximal end. Accurately placed breathing-holes are situated in the side walls of the distal part of the tube, to allow respiration to take place through the bronchi which are not occupied by the bronchoscope. Various small auxiliary tubes are incorporated into the main bronchoscopic tube for the purposes of lighting and aspiration, and for insufflation of oxygen and of anaesthetic vapours.

Bronchoscopes have been designed to fit the bronchi at various developmental ages and at various depths in the bronchial tree. The bronchi will not tolerate dilatation, and bronchoscopes of greater diameter than the air passages to be explored should never be used as the results of the over-distension of a bronchus may be very serious and rupture is generally fatal.

The diameters of the bronchoscopes are limited also by the size of the glottis and of the laryngeal cavity. In an adult the glottis is a triangle measuring approximately $12 \times 22 \times 22$ mm., which permits of the passage of a tube not exceeding 12 mm. in diameter without risk of injury. Subglottic oedema may occur as a result of the passage of an instrument too large to be tolerated by this region, or by too prolonged or too frequently repeated bronchoscopic examinations in a previously normal larynx. The duration of a bronchoscopic examination in a small child should never exceed 20 min., and it should be repeated only at reasonable intervals. Other causes of subglottic oedema are trauma caused by undue force or improper direction during the insertion of the bronchoscope, rough manipulation of instruments and injury inflicted by a foreign body during its extraction.

Subglottic oedema is a serious lesion which may necessitate early tracheostomy and which sometimes may prove fatal.

The Negus bronchoscopes illustrated in Fig. 104 are to be preferred to the original Jackson ones. The proximal third of the Negus bronchoscope, which remains in the mouth and pharynx, is expanded and this affords more room for inspection and the introduction of instruments. It is also more economical of space, having a finer light carrier which is held in a groove, not a tube, so increasing the effective lumen of the bronchoscope.

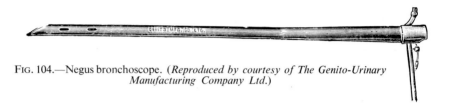

FIG. 104.—Negus bronchoscope. (*Reproduced by courtesy of The Genito-Urinary Manufacturing Company Ltd.*)

Bronchoscopic telescopes.—Bronchoscopic telescopes (Fig. 105) are of great value in the examination of the subglottic region, the trachea and the bronchi since they give a wide-angle magnified view of the area under inspection. Direct vision, 90 degree and retrograde telescopes are available. When in use they are kept standing in a vessel containing hot water and covered at the bottom with cotton wool to prevent damage to the lens. This is to prevent fogging when they are passed down the bronchoscope.

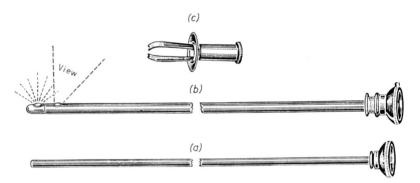

FIG. 105.—(*a*) Direct-vision bronchoscopic telescope; (*b*) retrograde bronchoscopic telescope; (*c*) spring clip adapter with shield for holding telescope in position in laryngoscope. (*Reproduced by courtesy of the Editor of* Lancet.)

Aspiration tubes.—Jackson's open ended aspirating tubes and Negus' tubes with detachable gum-elastic ends are most generally useful (Fig. 106) in the sizes given in the list of instruments for bronchoscopy (p. 268). A Luken's specimen collector (Fig. 107) is also needed. An efficient suction apparatus is necessary and is usefully incorporated in an endoscopic table (*see* Fig. 90). They must in every case be sparkproof to meet the regulations against explosion of anaesthetic vapours.

In addition to suction tubes, sponges are needed to dry the field and to clean the light of the bronchoscope. They are made from selvedge ribbon gauze in several sizes and are held in Coolidge's sponge holders.

Forceps.—Almost all bronchoscopic forceps are of a tubular type and they are so constructed that a slender tube works over a stilette which carries spring-spread jaws. The forceps are made in lengths which vary from 40 cm. to 60 cm., as required for use through the different bronchoscopes; and a very delicate or "mosquito" size is available for the infant and suckling bronchoscopes.

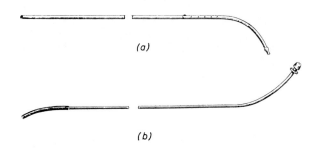

FIG. 106.—Aspiration tubes; (a) Jackson's open end aspirating tube. (*Reproduced by courtesy of W. B. Saunders, Philadelphia*); (b) Negus' aspirating tube with flexible gum-elastic end. (*Reproduced by courtesy of The Genito-Urinary Manufacturing Company Ltd.*)

(a)

(b)

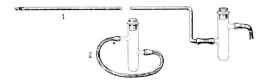

FIG. 107.—Luken's specimen collector. (*Reproduced by courtesy of W. B. Saunders, Philadelphia.*)

The stilette and tube are fixed in the handle mechanism. The Chevalier Jackson handle is illustrated in Fig. 108; the Negus modification of this, which gives more steadiness to the tip of the forceps, is also shown. A ratchet handle may be substituted for the above if it is desired to lock the forceps on to a foreign body or tumour.

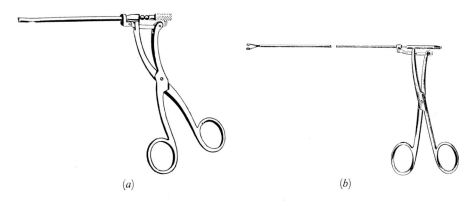

(a)   (b)

FIG. 108.—(a) Chevalier Jackson's bronchoscopic forceps handle. (*Reproduced by courtesy of W. B. Saunders, Philadelphia*); (b) Negus' modification of Chevalier Jackson's bronchoscopic forceps handle. (*Reproduced by courtesy of The Genito-Urinary Manufacturing Company Ltd.*)

The forceps jaws are screwed on to the stilette and the degree of their closure and the extent of their opening are adjusted by the thumb-nut on the proximal end of the stilette.

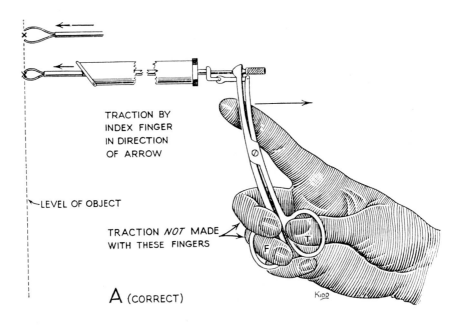

TRACTION BY
INDEX FINGER
IN DIRECTION
OF ARROW

LEVEL OF OBJECT

TRACTION *NOT* MADE
WITH THESE FINGERS

A (CORRECT)

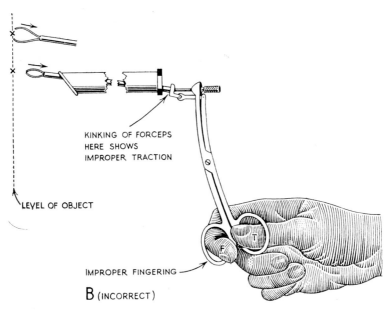

KINKING OF FORCEPS
HERE SHOWS
IMPROPER TRACTION

LEVEL OF OBJECT

IMPROPER FINGERING

B (INCORRECT)

FIG. 109.—(A) Diagram of correct fingering of forceps, manner of closing forceps on object and method of making traction. The thumb and ring finger are inserted into the handle rings. These fingers are used for opening and closing forceps only. All traction is made with index finger, which is placed high on the handle. (B) Diagram showing incorrect method of fingering, closure of forceps and traction whereby object may be missed and forceps kinked.

To close the forceps the handle must be used so that the cannula is forced down on the jaws, causing them to approximate. The handle must not be manipulated so that the jaws are pulled into the cannula as this causes their tips to recede from the target. Fig. 109A illustrates the correct method of closure of the forceps by pushing the cannula on to the jaws. It also illustrates the correct fingering of the handle and the method of making traction for the withdrawal of the forceps with the grasped object. Fig. 109B shows the incorrect method of these manoeuvres by which the object is grasped insecurely and the shaft of the forceps is dragged out of the line of the bronchoscope.

Most of the jaws have been designed by Chevalier Jackson for the removal of foreign bodies or for obtaining specimens of tissue, and the more frequently used types are illustrated in Fig. 110. They have either straight ends or side-curved ends; the latter are of more general use. Each forceps should have its own handle and the set-screws should be on the right side in order to be out of sight.

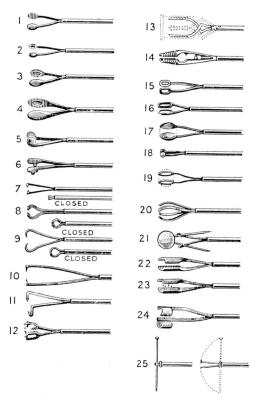

FIG. 110.—Chevalier Jackson's forceps ends. 1–4, Straight grasping forceps; 5, side-curved forceps; 6, Tucker forceps; 7, standard rotation forceps; 8, dangling rotation forceps; 9, sister-hook forceps; 10, long-jaw rotation forceps; 11, side-curved rotation forceps; 12, double-claw forceps; 13 and 14, expansile forceps; 15 and 16, fenestrated forceps; 17 and 18, ball forceps; 19, double-ring forceps; 20, Gordon bead forceps; 21, approximation forceps; 22, cylindrical forceps; 23, cylindrical forceps with teeth; 24, wire-bending forceps; 25, pin-bending forceps. (*Reproduced by courtesy of W. B. Saunders, Philadelphia.*)

Protection of the operator's eyes

Negus has designed a revolving glass disc which is carried on a head-band (Fig. 111) for the protection of the operator's eyes.

The glass disc is wiped over with alcohol after being warmed, and is therefore made aseptic and is prevented from becoming fogged by expired air. If the part of the shield in front of the observer's eyes becomes clouded or soiled by secretion or blood, the disc can be turned with the hand so as to bring a clear area into use. The advantages of the shield over spectacles are that it protects the whole of the face, and that it does not require to be changed when soiled.

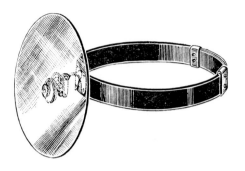

Fig. 111.—Negus' revolving eye shield. (*Reproduced by courtesy of The Genito-Urinary Manufacturing Company Ltd.*)

Anaesthesia

In bronchoscopy, as in laryngoscopy, general anaesthesia is replacing local analgesia but when repeated bronchoscopies are needed and when the examination may take rather longer than usual local analgesia is still preferable.

Local analgesia

This is carried out in the same way as for direct laryngoscopy with the addition that, besides dropping the lignocaine into the interior of the larynx, a further 2 ml. are dropped between the cords into the trachea. This is better than injecting the solution through the cricothyroid membrane.

General anaesthesia

This is also carried out initially as described under direct laryngoscopy. Since a bronchoscope has to be passed, however, an endotracheal anaesthetic tube cannot be used. The anaesthetist, therefore, after inducing with thiopentone and suxamethonium, fully inflates the patient's lungs with oxygen. Alternatively anaesthesia may be maintained through a small-bore catheter. The bronchoscope is then passed and the examination started. The patient is kept apnoeic with intermittent doses of the relaxant and so the anaesthetist must intermittently inflate the lungs with oxygen. This can be effectively done by putting an endotracheal or similar rubber tube firmly into the lumen of the bronchoscope and insufflating the oxygen through it. It may be necessary to repeat the thiopentone injection if the patient shows signs of returning consciousness but the single dose is usually all that is necessary.

A biopsy should not be taken nor the bronchoscope removed until spontaneous respiration is returning.

In young children, deep inhalation anaesthesia with nitrous oxide, oxygen and halothane is sufficient for a short examination and spontaneous respiration is not abolished.

Technique of bronchoscopy

It is unnecessary to state that, except in cases of extreme emergency, all patients before bronchoscopy must have a thorough clinical and radiological investigation, and a routine examination of the nasal fossae, nasopharynx, pharynx and larynx,

274

and they must be prepared in the usual manner either for surface analgesia or for general anaesthesia. Aseptic precautions must be observed during bronchoscopy as in any other major surgical procedure.

Position of the patient

It is customary to carry out bronchoscopic examination while the patient is lying in the dorsally recumbent position. The patient is so placed that the head and shoulders extend beyond the table, the edge of which supports the thorax at about the mid-scapular region; and the head is held by an assistant or a head-rest as the case may be.

As may be seen from Fig. 112, the trachea does not pursue a horizontal course in the thorax, but is directed downwards and backwards. In order to bring the axes of the buccal cavity and pharynx into line with those of the larynx and trachea, therefore, the head and neck must be elevated so that the occiput is about 10 cm. above the level of the table and the head must be extended at the atlanto-occipital joint as shown in Fig. 112. This position is best maintained with the Negus head-rest.

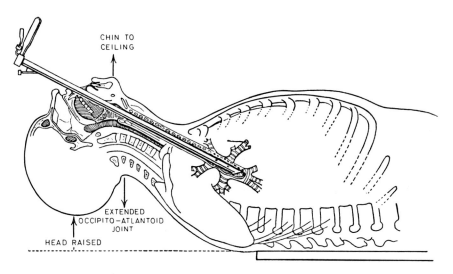

FIG. 112.—Diagram of position of patient's head and neck for bronchoscopy.

Introduction of the bronchoscope

If bronchoscopy is carried out under surface analgesia, it is essential that the procedure and the sensations to be endured shall be explained fully to the patient, so that he may be freed from apprehension and in order that his co-operation may be obtained.

Some laryngologists expose the glottis with a laryngoscope and pass the broncho-scope through this into the trachea; others pass the bronchoscope directly through the glottis into the trachea without the aid of a laryngoscope.

In young children and infants it is always advisable to expose the glottis with a laryngoscope before passing the bronchoscope.

If the bronchoscope is inserted through the laryngoscope after exposure of the glottis, its handle is rotated to the right so that a full view of the left vocal cord is obtained through the bronchoscope (Fig. 113). In this position the tip of the bronchoscope is situated in the long axis of the glottis and it can be inserted gently and easily into the trachea.

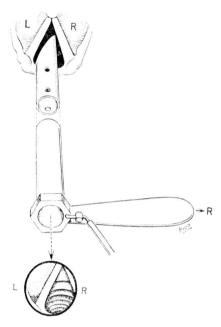

FIG. 113.—Diagram showing method of insertion of bronchoscope through glottis.

When the bronchoscope has been advanced a short distance into the trachea, the handle of the laryngoscope is rotated to the left, its slide is removed and the laryngoscope is then withdrawn.

If the bronchoscope is to be passed directly, without the aid of a laryngoscope, it should be held in the right hand by the shaft—not by the handle—in a pen-like manner, and the patient's upper lip should be retracted by the surgeon's left index finger.

The bronchoscope is inserted to the right of the anterior two-thirds of the tongue and its tip is directed towards the midline when the posterior third is reached. The epiglottis is the first landmark and when this has been identified it is lifted forward on the tip of the bronchoscope to expose the glottis. The bronchoscope is then rotated to the right and so directed that a good view of the left cord is obtained, when the bronchoscope can be inserted gently into the trachea.

When the trachea is entered it is recognized as an open tube with whitish cartilaginous rings, while the expiratory blast is felt and tubular breathing is heard through the bronchoscope.

If a direct-vision bronchoscopic telescope is to be used, it is taken from the vessel of hot water, the lens is dried and it is passed down the bronchoscope until the walls of the trachea are in focus. It is then clipped to the bronchoscope when it can be used with—or as part of—the bronchoscope. It will be necessary to remove the

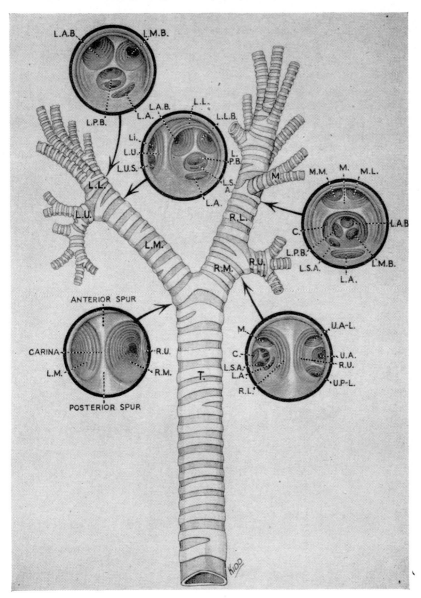

FIG. 114.—Diagram of endoscopic appearances of the bronchial apertures.

T. Trachea.	L.A.B. Lower anterior basal segmental bronchus.
	L.M.B. Lower middle basal segmental bronchus.
Right bronchial tree	L.P.B. Lower posterior basal segmental bronchus.
R.M. Right main bronchus.	
R.U. Right upper lobe bronchus.	*Left bronchial tree*
U.A. Upper apical segmental bronchus.	L.M. Left main bronchus.
U.A-L. Upper anterolateral segmental bronchus.	L.U.S. Left upper lobe bronchus.
U.P-L. Upper posterolateral segmental bronchus.	Li. Lingular lobe bronchus.
R.L. Right lower bronchus.	S.Li. Superior lingular segmental bronchus.
M. Middle lobe bronchus.	I.Li. Inferior lingular segmental bronchus.
M.M. Middle medial segmental bronchus.	U.A-L. Anterolateral segmental bronchus.
M.L. Middle lateral segmental bronchus.	U.A.P. Upper apicoposterior bronchus.
L.A. Lower apical segmental bronchus.	L.U.A. Left upper apical segmental bronchus.
C. Cardiac segmental bronchus.	U.P.A. Upper posterior apical segmental bronchus.
L.S.A. Lower subapical segmental bronchus.	L.L. Left lower lobe bronchus.

277

telescope periodically in order to clean the lens, which must be warmed each time in hot water before re-insertion into the bronchoscope.

The axis of the bronchoscope should be made to correspond as nearly as possible with that of the trachea; any secretion must be removed by aspiration and the walls of the trachea inspected by "weaving" the bronchoscope from side to side or by use of a 90-degree telescope which is self-illuminated.

The carina is recognized as a sharp vertical spur separating the orifices of the two main bronchi. As the carina is situated to the left of the midline the lumen view of the left main bronchus is very incomplete, and in order to view this adequately the tip of the bronchoscope is turned to the left while the patient's head and neck are flexed slightly to the right.

After identification and examination of the carina and of the main bronchial orifices, the main bronchi should be entered in turn, the tip of the bronchoscope being rotated in the direction of the bronchus to be examined and the head and neck flexed to the opposite side.

The bronchial orifices then must be identified seriatim as in Fig. 114.

As a rule, it is impossible to visualize more than a short length of the lumen of any tertiary bronchus through the bronchoscope; and there may be considerable variation of the origins of the tertiary bronchi within "normal" limits.

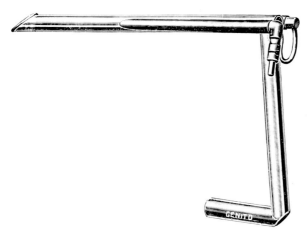

FIG. 115.–Negus tracheoscope. (*Reproduced by courtesy of The Genito-Urinary Manufacturing Company Ltd.*)

The right upper lobe bronchus joins the lateral aspect of the main stem 1 or 2 cm. below the level of the carina at an angle of 90 degrees. This bronchus, though sometimes difficult to find, can always be identified by its vertical spur, and can be examined either directly or indirectly with a retrograde bronchoscopic telescope. Direct examination permits of a very limited lumen view, although it is frequently possible to see the orifice of its anterolateral branch. In order to see into the right upper lobe bronchus, the tip of the bronchoscope is directed to the right and extreme flexure of the head and neck to the left is made.

The right upper lobe bronchus can be viewed more satisfactorily through a retrograde bronchoscopic telescope, and, as a rule, it is possible to view the orifices of its three segmental branches through the telescope.

The right middle lobe bronchus is the only bronchus which joins the right stem bronchus on its anterior aspect, and its almost horizontal spur can be brought into view by directing the lip of the bronchoscope to the right, and dropping the head of the patient until the lip bears strongly on the anterior wall of the right bronchus.

The left upper bronchus, which is about 5 cm. from the carina, can be examined more easily than the right upper lobe bronchus by a similar manoeuvre. The tip of the bronchoscope is directed to the left, the head and neck are flexed strongly to the right and the head is rotated to the right. It is usually possible to visualize the division of the lingular lobe bronchus into its upper and lower segmental bronchi.

The left upper bronchus can also be viewed very satisfactorily through a retrograde bronchoscopic telescope.

Tracheoscopy

The trachea will be inspected during the course of bronchoscopy. If it is desired to inspect the trachea only, the Negus tracheoscope (Fig. 115) is a most useful instrument. It is passed in the same way as a bronchoscope and its shorter length and greater diameter gives a more satisfactory field for inspection.

REFERENCES AND BIBLIOGRAPHY

Baclesse, F. (1938). *Le Diagnostique Radiologique des Tumeurs Malignes du Pharynx et du Larynx.* Paris; Masson.
Holtz, S., Power, S. E., McGavran, M. H., and Ogura, J. (1963). *Amer. J. Roentgenol.*, **89,** 10.
Jackson, C., and Jackson, C. L. (1937). *The Larynx and its Diseases.* Philadelphia; Saunders.
Kleinsasser, D. (1968). *Microlaryngology and Endolaryngeal Surgery.* London; Saunders.
Lewy, R. B. (1953). *Arch. Otolaryng.* **58,** 444.
Negus, V. E. (1947). *Proc. R. Soc. Med.*, **40,** 849.
Thompson, St. Clair, and Negus, V. E. (1955). *Diseases of the Nose and Throat.* London; Cassell.

11

CONGENITAL DISEASES OF THE LARYNX

R. Pracy

DIFFERENCES BETWEEN THE INFANT AND THE ADULT LARYNX

The differences between the infant and the adult larynx are both structural and functional.

Structural differences

The infant larynx is both relatively and absolutely smaller than the adult larynx. It lies higher in the neck and is tucked in under the back of the tongue. This makes the examination of the larynx difficult even if it is carried out under general anaesthesia. The largest diameter of the airway at the level of the glottis in a newborn baby of 3·15 kg. (7 lb.) weight is 6 mm. The diameter of the trachea immediately below the glottis is even smaller—4 mm. The supporting cartilages are very soft and may not provide sufficient substance to act as a rigid frame upon which the intrinsic laryngeal muscles can work. In infants 30–50 per cent of larynges show elongation and narrowing of the supraglottis with "omega shaped" curling of the petiole of the epiglottis, short aryepiglottic folds and a narrow laryngeal introitus. In about 10 per cent of larynges the supraglottis is covered with very lax tissue which may seem to spill over the glottis and to fill the pyriform sinuses. The direction of the airway is straighter in the infant than it is in the adult.

The measurements given above refer to a 3·15 kg. baby and allowance must therefore be made for the size of the child in estimating the possible size of the airway.

Functional differences

In the adult and young child the larynx has a respiratory, an alimentary and a phonatory function. The respiratory function is instinctive, the alimentary function is acquired with relatively little difficulty and at least in part by instinct. Phonatory function is acquired as a result of imitation, experiment and much practice. A hearing child born of deaf parents acquires speech less rapidly than a child born to hearing parents. The newborn child normally exercises its respiratory function instinctively; the vocal cords abduct during inspiration. The alimentary function or protection of the lower airway during swallowing is by no means as perfectly developed and it is a commonplace experience to find the baby choking over both solid and liquid food once it attempts to take food from either a cup or a spoon. There is an abundant and highly sensitive nerve supply to the mucosa of the infant's larynx and once a foreign body stimulates the inner surface of the laryngeal introitus a violent reflex response is initiated. The whole larynx may pass into severe spasm and a period of prolonged breath-holding associated with vivid colour changes in the baby's face may be observed. This is a protective response and the sensitivity of the mucosa is considerably lessened as the child grows into adult life. Since the newborn child has no phonatory ability it has to rely on its cry to attract attention when it is in distress and it is well known that the volume of this cry may at times be out of all proportion to the size of the baby.

SYMPTOMS AND SIGNS OF LARYNGEAL DISEASE IN THE NEWBORN

Stridor

Stridor is a noise made by obstruction of the passage of air into or out of the lower respiratory tract. Where the obstruction lies at the entrance to the tracheo-bronchial tree the noise appears on inspiration and is called inspiratory stridor. The actual sound may vary with the obstructing lesion. The most common form of inspiratory stridor has a musical crowing quality and is traditionally called "croup".

Crying and cough

Obstruction to the airway gives rise to distress and the infant tends to be restless and to cry. In cases where the lesion prevents the complete apposition of the vocal cords the cry may be weak or "wheezy" and on occasion the cry may be absent although the child is making all the other signs of crying such as grimacing and turning its head from side to side and rotating his clenched fists.

Cough frequently accompanies the cry where there is an irritative lesion in the larynx and this cough may have a harsh metallic sound.

Dyspnoea

Many children with laryngeal stridor have no dyspnoea, but where the obstruction narrows the airway by more than 1·5 mm. in a 3·15 kg. baby some degree of difficulty in breathing is always present. Signs of difficult breathing may be sought:

(1) In the face, where the nostrils dilate and the lips may be cyanosed and surrounded by an area of pale skin.

(2) In the neck, where violent inspiratory movements cause the whole larynx and trachea to move downwards towards the mediastinum. This is due to a high negative pressure in the pleural cavity which in effect "sucks" the larynx and trachea into the thorax. This is called "tracheal plunging". When tracheal plunging is very marked it may also be possible to see movements in the muscles of the neck which are used to increase the movements of the thoracic cage.

(3) In the chest, where excessive muscular effort, directed of drawing air through a narrowed glottis, will be accompanied by recession of the intercostal spaces. The earliest place where this is seen is in the lower and lateral part of the chest wall. When the effort becomes more violent the whole sternum may be sucked in towards the spinal column as well as moving up and down with the movements of the thoracic cage.

Feeding difficulties

The young child who has not learned the adult method of feeding usually finds added difficulty if there is any kind of laryngeal lesion. Anything which interferes with the sphincteric action of the supraglottis may lead to stimulation of the sensitive mucosa on the false cords. This will cause not only choking and breath-holding but also overspill into the tracheobronchial tree.

General symptoms and signs

The child who cannot breathe easily and who has difficulty in feeding will not thrive. He will, therefore, tend to be weakly and underweight. However, there are other general effects which are less obvious. Repeated overspill into the tracheo-bronchial tree will lead ultimately to chest infections and toxaemia. Inadequate oxygen intake may result in a high pCO_2 and alterations in the acid–base equilibrium There will also be some measure of cerebral anoxia and to compensate for this the cardiovascular centre will be stimulated leading to a rise in pulse rate. Prolonged severe cerebral hypoxia may lead to brain damage and physical and mental retardation.

Thus, it is extremely important that an assessment of the cause of the obstruction to the child's respiration be made at the earliest possible opportunity. Before a description of the various lesions which may give rise to an obstructed airway is given, the routine assessment of the patient presenting with symptoms of laryngeal obstruction will be described. The assessment may be difficult and time-consuming. It requires patience on the part of the laryngologist and the use of keen clinical observation.

ASSESSMENT

When the symptoms and signs of laryngeal obstruction are manifest the baby should be transferred to hospital and nursed in an incubator with humidity and oxygen supplied. If time permits, that is to say if the patient is not in need of urgent procedures to relieve the obstruction, the history may be obtained from the mother or person who first noticed the symptoms of distress. The surgeon will want to know how long the noise has been present. Is there any abnormality in the baby's cry? Has he a cough? Is there any difficulty in feeding? Has there been any gain in weight since birth? Is the noise louder when the baby is asleep or awake? Does it disappear during sleep or waking periods?

An assessment must be made of the child's general condition. Particular attention should be paid to the general nutrition. The child with a paralysed vocal cord will experience considerable feeding difficulty and will in consequence tend to be under-nourished. The overweight baby obviously does not have a feeding difficulty but may well have a feeding problem. This is the sort of child who develops laryngismus stridulus at about six months of age. Once a general impression of the state of nourishment has been obtained the baby should be examined for signs of dyspnoea. The general colour, pallor, or cyanosis are noted. Abnormal movements of the alae nasi, trachea, larynx and neck muscles or indrawing of the intercostal spaces should be recorded.

If it is at all possible, it is useful to hear the noise which it is claimed that the child is making. The place in the respiratory cycle at which the noise appears is very important. The quality of the noise will help in the making of a diagnosis. It is often helpful to listen at the nares and the mouth to hear if the noise is present. Much can be learned by placing the examining ear on the baby's back and listening to perhaps 30 or 40 respirations. Once the position of the noise in the cycle has been fixed the baby should be placed in various positions. Sometimes a change in position may eliminate the noise altogether. Thus, in Pierre Robin syndrome in which the micrognathia associated with a relatively large tongue causes pressure on the supraglottis, the distress can be relieved at once by placing the baby face down on the surgeon's knee. In less clear cut conditions it can be very profitable to spend perhaps half to three-quarters of an hour turning the baby from side to side and adjusting the position of the head relative to the trunk in order to find in which position the noise is least obtrusive. However, even if the probable diagnosis can be arrived at by such manoeuvres it is imperative that every child with stridor should undergo a direct examination of the larynx in order that the cause may be determined and treatment, if possible, instituted.

Paediatric anaesthesia is now an established specialty in its own right and the good paediatric anaesthetist will make it possible for the surgeon to examine the larynx in a calm and methodical manner. This is absolutely essential if an accurate diagnosis is to be made.

Anaesthesia

The child is anaesthetized with thiopentone and when it is asleep it is saturated with oxygen administered through a face mask. After about 10 minutes a rubber catheter is passed through the nasal cavities into the larynx and is used to supply more oxygen while the examination is being carried out. In this way it is often possible to get a period of 10–15 minutes for laryngoscopy.

Laryngoscopy

Once again method and routine are all important. The most satisfactory instruments for the examination are the Negus infants' laryngoscopes anodized and illuminated by a fibreglass illuminator. An infants' tracheoscope and broncho-scope will also be required (Fig. 116).

The instrument is introduced through the right hand side of the patient's mouth, while the first finger of the operator's left hand is placed between the upper and lower alveolus (Figs. 117–119). When the laryngoscope tip reaches the level of the uvula it is possible to see the catheter and this acts as a reliable guide to the larynx. The first stage in the examination is to pass the beak of the laryngoscope anterior to the epiglottis into the vallecula. In the infant this causes the laryngeal introitus to come into line with the optical axis of the laryngoscope. It allows a good overall view of the larynx and it ensures that in looking for paralysis or paresis of a cord, a false diagnosis of paralysis is avoided because there is no pressure on the aryepiglottic fold. A diagnosis of vocal cord paralysis should only be made when the failure of the cords to move is clearly seen with a laryngoscope in this position (Fig. 120).

The beak should now be used to lift up the epiglottis and in this way the vocal cords, false cords and subglottic regions may be inspected. If, for some reason, subglottic stenosis is suspected the rubber catheter can be removed and an endo-tracheal tube of a size appropriate for the baby's age may be passed. If it fails to pass easily a smaller size should be tried. The operating microscope has made it possible to get a much better view of the larynx. A 275 mm. objective instead of the standard 200 mm. lens enables the surgeon to get a satisfactory view and at the same time to carry out any endoscopic treatment which may be desirable.

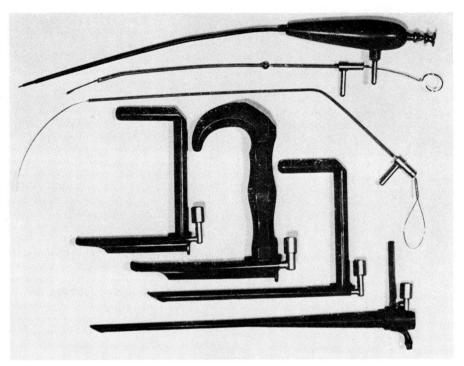

FIG. 116.—Endoscopic equipment for small children and infants.

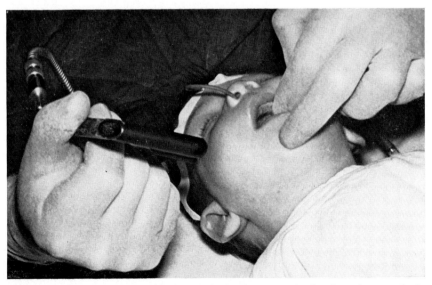

FIG. 117.—Direct laryngoscopy, first stage. (Note the nasotracheal catheter for anaesthetic gases and oxygen.)

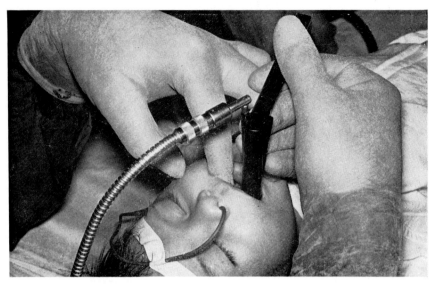

Fig. 118.—Direct laryngoscopy, introduction of laryngoscope. (Note the flexible fibre-optic cable for illumination.)

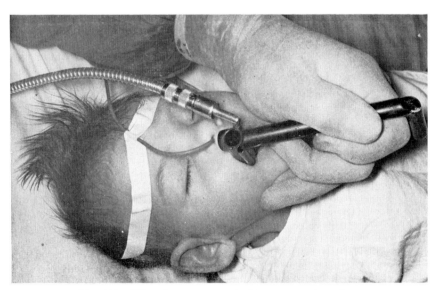

Fig. 119.—Direct laryngoscopy, the larynx comes into view.

If no cause for the symptoms is found as a result of this examination it is necessary to proceed with a tracheoscopy and a bronchoscopy. This will help to determine whether the distress is caused by deficiency of the tracheal rings, by abnormal

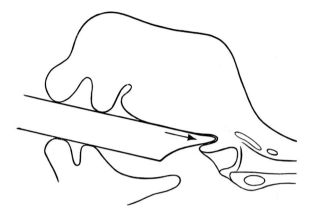

FIG. 120.—The beak of the laryngoscope in the valleculae allows an undistorted view of the vocal cords and their movements.

vessels pressing on the trachea and oesophagus, or whether there is perhaps a tracheo-oesophageal fistula.

MANAGEMENT OF THE NEWBORN CHILD WITH LARYNGEAL OBSTRUCTION

Two main factors have to be considered in planning the management of the patient. These are: (*i*) an adequate supply of correctly humidified air; and (*ii*) adequate nourishment.

Many babies with stridor do not need assistance with their airway unless they develop some form of respiratory infection. However, about one-third of these babies will experience some feeding difficulty in the early months of life. They will be slow feeders and show a marked tendency to cough and splutter as the milk goes the wrong way. It has been found that such babies often progress more rapidly if they are introduced to a solid weaning diet at an earlier age (4–5 weeks) than is usual.

If some artificial assistance with the airway is necessary two possibilities are open to the surgeon. Which he chooses will depend upon how long it will have to be maintained. For the short term case the most satisfactory form of airway, if it can be introduced, is the indwelling endotracheal tube. If this is made from a "non-reacting" plastic (e.g. "Portex") it may be left *in situ* for at least three days in the newborn. It is doubtful if it should remain for longer than four days because of the possibility of frictional trauma to the subglottic region and subsequent stenosis of the trachea and subglottic areas. For all other cases the method of choice is a tracheostomy. A formal tracheostomy is carried out through the second and third tracheal rings and a No. 14 or 16 tracheostomy tube introduced. These tubes are made in plastic and in the more traditional silver. Recent experience has shown that the plastic tube of Aberdeen suffers from the same disadvantage as the Portex endotracheal tube. For this reason the traditional silver tube is to be preferred for long term intubation. The better known adult tracheostomy tubes, made in silver, all suffer from the disadvantage of ending in a plate which fits over the opening in the skin and it is found that in the baby this can lead to obstruction of the mouth of the tube if, as is usually the case, the baby has a short neck and a tendency to a "double chin". For this reason when a silver tube is to be used an Alder Hey Pattern tube (Fig. 121) is to be preferred. In this pattern the inner

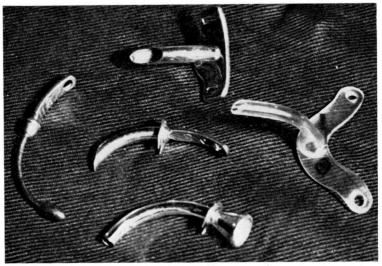

FIG. 121.—The Alder Hey and Aberdeen tracheostomy tubes, in silver and plastic. Note the extended inner tube (*see text*).

tube has an extension which reaches out beyond the neck plate which ensures that it cannot be blocked by overhanging skin. Two additional advantages of this tube are:

(1) A hole is cut in the convexity of the shoulder of the tube. This enables an expiratory tide of air to be directed out through the glottis if the surgeon feels that this is necessary.

(2) The tube is provided with a "blocker" to assist in decannulation.

Decannulation in the small infant presents problems. The usual procedure followed in adults has not been found to be satisfactory in babies. In many conditions occurring in children the surgeon has to keep in mind the concept of the continuing development of the patient undergoing treatment. This may have considerable bearing on immediate treatment and on the prognosis. Thus it is that in the question of tracheostomy in infancy it is necessary to appreciate that the larynx cannot simply be "short circuited" and subsequently expected to function normally. Many of the difficulties encountered in decannulation in the past arose because the larynx was forced suddenly to assume its normal respiratory pattern of function, when it had done so, perhaps ineffectively, for only a few hours after birth. For this reason it has been found that at an early stage in the management of the tracheostomized infant it is essential to introduce a more physiological "expiratory tide" in the trachea. This is achieved by the use of an expiratory valve on the inner tube. Thus the expiratory flow of air is mainly through the glottis and the flow of mucus in the trachea is upwards, towards the glottis. The abolition of this "dead space" is a valuable first measure in the establishment of a normal airway.

Whatever form of artificial airway is decided upon it is imperative that the air supplied to the baby should be properly humidified. Adequate cold humidification greatly reduces the problems of crusting and of cleaning the tubes. This can be supplied by one of several forms of ultrasonic atomizer which delivers a fine mist (Figs. 122 and 123) of particles of less than 3μm. in diameter. If this is done,

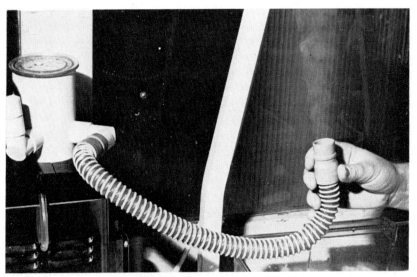

FIG. 122.—Humidifier delivers a fine mist.

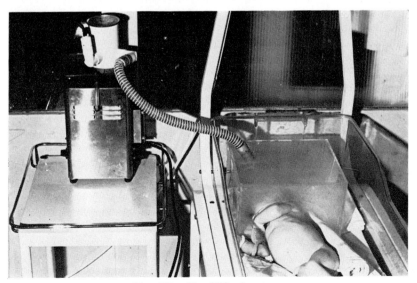

FIG. 123.—Humidifier in use.

289

and aspiration of excessive secretions using a "no touch" technique with disposable sterile gloves is followed, there are very few difficulties in maintaining a small baby's tracheostomy in the short term. In the long term, however, humidification in an incubator cannot be maintained because of the water-logging effect it has upon the baby's skin. Once the cause of the obstruction has been treated and decannulation is possible, the cannula may be removed. If it has been present for some months it is often helpful to pass an endotracheal tube for 12 hours. This allows the original respiratory channel to reform.

Complications which may attend the establishment of an artificial airway

Long-term endotracheal intubation

When this method was introduced by the paediatric anaesthetists there were high hopes that the end had been seen of the complications encountered in the establishment of long-term tracheostomies in small children. There appeared to be good prospects of an end to tracheal strictures and decannulation problems. Initially tubes were left *in situ* for as long as 35 days when this appeared to be necessary, and before long the surgeon was faced with the virtually insoluble problem of strictures running from the lower surface of the vocal cords and for perhaps three or four centimetres down the lumen of the trachea. The reaction to the Portex involved the loss of superficial mucosa and the development of solid rings of fibrous tissue underneath the squamous epithelium which replaced the mucous membrane which had sloughed away. The clearance of mucus from the lungs and bronchial tree became virtually impossible and ultimately the patient died of bronchopneumonia. The period of intubation which was allowed was, therefore, considerably curtailed and experience has proved that it is not safe to leave an endotracheal tube *in situ* for more than seven days. It is probably wiser to make a tracheostomy if after five days there seems to be little possibility of ending the artificial airway in a week. Of the first 180 patients treated at Alder Hey Children's Hospital intensive care unit, only 60 survived and of these 60, 28 were intubated for longer than a week. Of these 28, 6 had residual long term scarring. The scarred areas were found in two sites above the vocal cords posteriorly and below the vocal cords laterally and anteriorly. None of the 60 survivors had severe residual symptoms.

The complications of tracheostomy in children

The immediate complications of tracheostomy are haemorrhage from the wound and sepsis in the track spreading to the tissues of the neck and mediastinum. Both can be prevented by care at the time of the operation. Haemostasis and aseptic technique should be very strictly observed. Long-term complications include the development of granulations in the track which have to be removed and stenosis of the trachea due to the contraction of scar tissue once the tube has been removed. The stricture may have to be dilated many times before the child's airway is satisfactory.

CONGENITAL DISEASES OF THE LARYNX

For many years there was no satisfactory classification of the causes of stridor in infancy. Confusion existed about nomenclature and it was not until 1952 that the first satisfactory classification was published by Wilson. This was a most valuable classification of a difficult area of disease and has certainly not been superseded. It will, therefore, be used here (Table I).

TABLE I

Congenital anatomical abnormalities	Tumours and cysts	Inflammatory conditions	Neurological abnormalities	Trauma	Foreign body
Laryngomalacia (congenital laryngeal stridor)	Benign neoplasms	Acute laryngitis	Tetany (laryngismus stridulus)	Birth injury	Vegetable foreign body
Bifid epiglottis	Cysts of the larynx	Acute laryngo-tracheo-bronchitis	Neonatal tetany	Postnatal injury, e.g. injury caused by intubation	Non-vegetable foreign body
Congenital stenosis of the larynx (webs of the larynx)		Diphtheria Post diphtheritic stenosis	Recurrent paralysis		
		The exanthemata (measles, whooping-cough).			
		Tuberculosis			

Disorders of structure

Laryngomalacia (congenital laryngeal stridor)

Wilson, in his *Diseases of the Ear, Nose and Throat in Children*, regards this condition as an entity. However, experience shows that although there may be no difference to be distinguished in the history or clinical examination of the child there are considerable differences in the laryngoscopic appearances.

Classically the child with congenital laryngeal stridor makes a crowing noise on inspiration because the superstructure of the larynx is driven in by the incoming inspiratory tide of air and when the two sides of the larynx meet vibration occurs (Fig. 124). The classical description of congenital laryngeal stridor attributed to Lambert, Lack, Brown Kelly and Paterson is still seen.

The epiglottis is much elongated, folded on itself and has suspended from it thin and generally short aryepiglottic folds which leave a very small entrance to the larynx. It may be difficult to introduce an endotracheal tube. It must, however, be stressed that not all children with this anatomical state have stridor. There must be an attendant abnormality for this to occur. A second category may be distinguished and to this it would seem appropriate to give the name of laryngomalacia. Here the entrance to the glottis can be clearly seen but the whole laryngeal superstructure is soft and appears to be oedematous. The glottis will admit a normal endotracheal tube for the size of the child. When the baby is relaxed the whole laryngeal superstructure vibrates and produces a crowing stridor.

291

Clinical picture.—Babies with these abnormalities are brought for advice for two reasons. Firstly because they make a loud crowing noise on inspiration when they are asleep. They may also make it when they are awake. Secondly, babies with this abnormality experience feeding difficulties and they fail to thrive. Wilson stated that the condition is essentially benign and disappears by the age of two

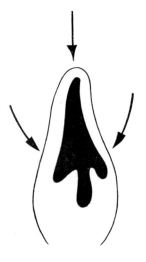

Fig. 124.—Laryngeal superstructure in congenital laryngeal stridor.

and a half years. Very few of these children ever die of their abnormalities but experience shows that the noise may persist up to five years of age. The child may be slow to gain weight and suffer many chest infections on the way through childhood. No treatment has been found to be effective and such empirical and radical procedures as amputating the epiglottis have no place in modern laryngology. As with all cases of stridor the parents should be instructed to bring the child to hospital immediately if the child's respiratory distress increases.

Bifid epiglottis

This is an extremely rare condition. From the accounts which are available it would seem that the symptoms are more acute in onset, and more severe in effect than congenital laryngeal stridor. Cases have been described in which one or other half of the epiglottis becomes impacted in the glottis causing severe laryngeal obstruction. Amputation of the epiglottis after a preliminary tracheostomy is said to cure the condition.

Laryngeal webs and atresia

Some degree of reduction of the normal size of the glottis, due either to webs or atresia is not very uncommon. The condition probably has received more prominence than is warranted in earlier textbooks because in the direct examination carried out without anaesthesia, the lesion was picked up easily. Unless the web is large it rarely requires treatment. The majority cause fusion of the anterior one-sixth of the vocal cords. When the web extends further posteriorly, it is found in practice to be of much greater depth anteriorly.

Symptoms and signs.—When a laryngeal web is large enough to produce symptoms, the infant will be brought for advice because of stridor. The stridor will increase in severity during attempts at crying and coughing, and it will be accompanied by a marked reduction in the volume of the voice. Dyspnoea may be extreme and may be associated with cyanosis and a high pCO_2 in the blood.

On direct laryngoscopy the usual finding is that the anterior one-sixth of the glottis is absent due to the joining of the true cords by a fibrous web. In more severe cases the curved posterior margin of the web stretches between the posterior thirds of the cords and anteriorly the fusion may pass downwards as far as the upper margin of the cricoid ring.

Prognosis.—Small anterior webs which cause symptoms must be treated but in the vast majority of cases the symptoms lessen and eventually disappear as the larynx enlarges. The larger webs with gross anterior thickening cannot be treated at birth and, after safeguarding the airway by tracheostomy, must be left until the child is old enough and the larynx large enough to permit a definitive plastic procedure.

Treatment.—Small anterior webs should be treated by the passage of bougies which will cause the web to split or stretch. Either result leads to an improvement in the airway.

Larger webs will have to be treated by excision and grafting through a vertical midline thyrotomy. This is a difficult procedure and it should be carried out using the operating microscope when the child reaches about four years of age. Until the time of operation the child will have a permanent tracheostomy and should wear an expiratory valve in order to direct the expiratory tide of air through the physiological channel and to encourage the upward flow of mucus from the tracheobronchial tree.

Subglottic stenosis

Subglottic stenosis is a condition which has attracted more attention in recent years. This is probably due to the introduction of direct laryngoscopy under general anaesthesia. This condition is not uncommon and, if the degree of stenosis is severe, will give rise to a severe harsh barking kind of stridor and dyspnoea.

The lesion (Fig. 125) is an area of narrowing of the lower airway about 1cm. below the glottis. The narrowing is due to great thickening of the cartilage of the cricoid and the abnormal cartilage extends round the whole circumference of the airway. It is not uncommon for subglottic stenosis to be associated with other congenital abnormalities such as tracheo-oesophageal fistula. This increases the difficulties which the child has to contend with. The outcome in these cases is usually fatal. Minor degrees of subglottic stenosis may be tolerated reasonably well but constant vigilance is necessary in order to treat the increased dyspnoea which may occur when the airway is further narrowed by inflammation.

Symptoms and signs.—Children with subglottic stenosis are not usually seen at birth unless the abnormality is accompanied by other conditions such as tracheo-oesophageal fistula. In this event the diagnosis will have to be made by the anaesthetist trying to intubate the child for the repair of the fistula. More usually the child is brought for advice at two or three months of age when perhaps after respiratory infection, the characteristic brassy two-way stridor becomes more pronounced and the infection is slow to clear.

The diagnosis is made by the anaesthetist and the laryngologist together after the larynx has been inspected, The glottis is found to be of normal dimensions and the vocal cords mobile. An attempt is made to pass an endotracheal tube with a diameter appropriate to the size of the child. This will be held up at the site of the obstruction about 1 cm. below the glottis. It is then withdrawn and an attempt made to pass a smaller tube. The size of the largest tube to pass the obstruction is taken to be the diameter of the airway at that point.

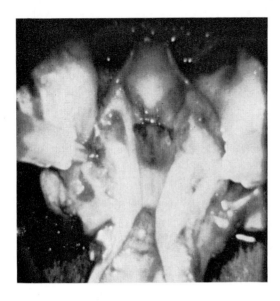

Fig. 125.—Congenital subglottic stenosis.

Prognosis.—The child who has managed to survive the first two or three months of life with subglottic stenosis can be expected to survive into adult life unless some overwhelming infection like acute laryngotracheobronchitis overtakes him. Extra care must be taken when respiratory inflammations occur and it is probably wiser to nurse the baby in hospital where oxygen and added humidity are at hand. Cases should be followed up in the out-patient department until all symptoms have completely disappeared.

Treatment.—Because the narrowing is due to cartilage rather than fibrous tissue, there is little to be gained from procedures such as dilatation with bougies. Indeed these may do positive harm by damage to the mucous membrane of the trachea. If the obstruction is severe and the airway inadequate, the correct treatment is the establishment of a permanent tracheostomy below the stenosis. The tracheostomy tube should be equipped with an expiratory valve. The development of the lower airway must be kept under constant review by routine direct laryngoscopy and measurement of the lumen of the obstruction. It seems possible that in a severe case it might be necessary in later childhood to resect the cartilage submucosally.

Disorders of function

Paralysis of the vocal cords

Some degree of weakness of one or of both vocal cords is one of the more common congenital lesions of the larynx. About 25 per cent of all cases of stridor in infancy which are examined are found to have vocal cord weakness. Unilateral vocal cord weakness is much commoner than bilateral weakness. Unilateral vocal cord weakness appears to be associated with difficult labour and birth and may perhaps be associated with the use of instruments. The right and left vocal cords are affected to about the same extent. Bilateral vocal cord paresis is usually not complete and is therefore an abductor paresis. It is seen most commonly in cases of hydrocephalus. Examination of the vagus nerve in a child who died with hydrocephalus associated with bilateral abductor paresis showed that the nerve had become stretched over the anterior margin of the foramen magnum as the result of the brain stem being forced downwards through the foramen by the raised intracranial pressure. This seemed to offer a reasonable explanation of how the vocal cord weakness occurred.

Symptoms and signs.—The child whose stridor is due to vocal cord paresis frequently is stridulous only when making some physical effort. If the paresis is unilateral therefore the noise will become obvious on crying, coughing or straining at stool and he will sleep quietly. Babies with bilateral paresis on the other hand are in more or less constant distress. All children with laryngeal paralysis have feeding difficulties. This is due to the liquid diet coming into contact with the unrelaxed cricopharyngeus and being regurgitated back over the larynx with consequent overspill into the tracheobronchial tree. For this reason recurrent chest infections are common in these babies and they are both weak and fail to gain weight. Direct laryngoscopy will confirm the diagnosis. There are, however, pitfalls for the inexperienced laryngologist. Holinger has drawn attention to the restriction of movement of the right hemilarynx which may be caused by the introduction of the laryngoscope through the right side of the mouth and posterior to the epiglottis. Wilson has recommended that the laryngoscope beak should be introduced into the vallecula anterior to the epiglottis. Slight pressure in a caudal direction will cause the axis of the glottis to straighten out at right angles to the optical axis of the laryngoscope and will not hinder the movement of either cord. The diagnosis of paresis should therefore be made only with the laryngoscope in this position. Bilateral vocal cord paresis is confirmed by passing an endotracheal tube between the vocal cords when the symptoms will be completely relieved.

Prognosis and treatment.—Unilateral vocal cord paresis seems to recover in about 50 per cent of cases. The larynx is observed at regular intervals up to 18 months. It is possible that the other 50 per cent form the hard core of the so-called idiopathic vocal cord paresis seen in adult life. However, the baby has a stormy infancy, with repeated respiratory infections and poor gain of weight. Since the swallowing of liquids presents such difficulties for these children an improvement in the general condition can often be brought about by the introduction of a semi-solid "weaning" diet at a much earlier age than is usual.

Bilateral paresis has a more serious prognosis. The majority of cases of bilateral paresis are associated with hydrocephalus. When the intracranial pressure has risen to such a degree that stretching of the vagus occurs, the prognosis is grave and the child is unlikely to survive.

When there is no associated hydrocephalus the laryngologist is faced with a most difficult problem. It may not be necessary to carry out a tracheostomy in early infancy when the infant is relatively inactive and yet the occurrence of respiratory inflammation which is to be anticipated as part of the normal development of the child may precipitate a crisis which will call for immediate relief of obstruction. Furthermore, the establishment of a permanent tracheostomy in a small baby imposes great difficulties of management on the mother and the child may have to spend its early life in hospital. This is certainly not the ideal environment for an otherwise healthy baby. The number of cases in this category are small and it is not possible to offer any dogmatic opinion about the course to be followed in every case. However, it has proved possible to steer such cases through the expected respiratory inflammations of infancy and childhood without finding it necessary to establish an artificial airway. If at any time it did become necessary to pass an indwelling endotracheal tube or to carry out a tracheostomy it would be necessary to make a permanent tracheostomy because decannulation would not be possible. Plastic procedures directed towards the improvement of the airway such as arytenoidectomy should be deferred until the age of 14–16 years when the surgeon can count upon the confidence and co-operation of his patient which are so essential to success.

Tumours and cysts

In the course of development the tissues of the larynx and its surrounding structures pass through many complicated phases and foldings and it is not surprising therefore that abnormalities occur when these processes are not completed with the precision normally encountered in embryology. Three varieties of cyst may occur.

(1) Defects of formation of lymph vessels may result in cystic hygroma (lymphangioma) in the region of the floor of the mouth and larynx.

(2) Dermoid cysts which occur in the aryepiglottic folds.

(3) Branchial cysts which are seen in the false cords and may extend laterally.

Congenital cysts of the larynx are rare but a small number of cases can be found in every clinic. Their presence is made known in a very dramatic way, in that the newly-born baby has great difficulty in breathing and intubation is called for urgently in the labour ward.

Clinical picture.—The newborn infant makes violent efforts to breathe. These are unavailing and the standard procedures of the midwife are not effective in clearing the airway. The child's colour and pulse deteriorate rapidly and the anaesthetist is called to pass a tube. On examination of the larynx the normal anatomy will be completely obscured by a rounded swelling which passes over the midline completely obscuring any view of the glottis. An experienced anaesthetist usually has no difficulty in intubating the baby. After intubation the colour and pulse immediately improve and the child should then be transferred to the laryngologist.

Treatment.—Since the endotracheal tube cannot be removed until the cyst has been evacuated treatment must be carried out in the first hours of the child's life. It is not necessary to make a tracheostomy and, if possible, because of the difficulties of decannulation in small infants, tracheostomies should be avoided. Temporary improvement may be effected by removing the top of the cyst with forceps and evacuating the fluid. The disadvantage of this procedure is that the cyst rapidly fills up and it becomes necessary to repeat the procedure. The infant's larynx is so small and sensitive that repeated instrumentation is to be avoided if possible. A modified diathermy needle has been developed for use in these cases. A suction tube is covered with an insulating coat and fitted with a terminal for a diathermy lead. The stilette of the sucker is replaced with a sharpened trocar. The cyst is punctured by means of the trocar and the contents are aspirated by the application of suction when the trocar has been withdrawn. As the fluid is aspirated the superstructure of the cyst falls in and adheres to the mouth of the sucker. This redundant mucosa can then be destroyed by the application of a weak diathermy current.

Larger laryngeal cysts may be too big to be dealt with endoscopically. When the cyst fills the pyriform fossa and extends over the midline of the glottis it is preferable to excise it through an external horizontally placed incision using the approach described by Trotter for lateral pharyngotomy. The cyst can be separated easily, from the lax laryngeal submucosal tissues by blunt dissection. The airway is protected for 24 hours by an indwelling endotracheal tube. Remarkably, little post-operative oedema follows this procedure.

Tumours

Congenital tumours of the larynx are rare. The larynx is composed of a variety of ectodermal and mesodermal derivatives and any of these may give rise to benign tumour formation causing symptoms which are present at birth. These tumours may be divided into two categories.

(1) Pedunculated; these include lipoma, fibroma and leiomyoma. They arise from the posterior surface of the larynx and aryepiglottic folds.

(2) Sessile; in this group chondroma and haemangioma are to be found. They arise from the cartilages and blood vessels of the larynx.

Clinical picture.—Tumours of the larynx may present with dysphagia, dyspnoea or stridor, or with a combination of all three symptoms. Pedunculated tumours fall back into the hypopharynx and only give rise to serious difficulty when the child attempts to swallow. The tumour is then squeezed upwards and comes to lie over the entrance of the larynx causing the baby to choke. Once the tumour has been removed the symptoms are cured.

Chondroma and haemangioma present with stridor and dyspnoea. Chondroma can only be diagnosed by direct laryngoscopy.

Haemangioma may be suspected if the baby is seen to have multiple cavernous haemangiomata on the skin of the head and neck (Fig. 126). Direct laryngoscopy may show that there is a single large lesion of one false cord which is interfering with the movement of the true cord and giving rise to symptoms. The more usual appearance however is of multiple haemangiomata arising over the whole supra-glottis (Fig. 127) and also in the subglotic regions immediately below the true cords. Haemangiomata of this type may be associated with abnormal lymph vessel development. Thus a baby born with multiple congenital cavernous haemangiomata may have minimal symptoms at birth but as development takes place the symptoms may become much more severe as the lymphangiomatous element increases in size. There appears to be a tendency for haemangioma to regress at about 12 months.

Treatment.—Pedunculated tumours are removed most satisfactorily by a snare. Chondroma is best treated when the larynx has enlarged somewhat. Therefore, if the dyspnoea is considerable a permanent tracheostomy must be made, an expiratory valve fitted and the child left to develop for perhaps two or three years before any attempt is made to excise it.

Treatment of haemangioma.—If the haemangioma is causing respiratory distress at birth a tracheostomy must be made because the distress will certainly increase in the first months of life.

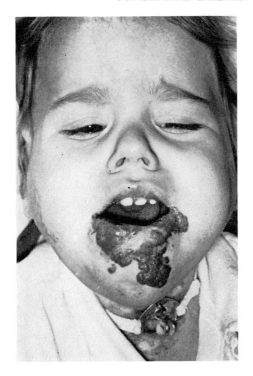

FIG. 126.—Congenital haemangioma of larynx and face.

FIG. 127.—Congenital haemangioma. Direct laryngoscopy revealing large swelling of left false cord.

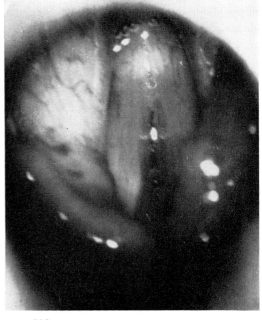

Since the natural history of the condition is that regression may take place at about 12 months of age it may be possible to leave the child with a tracheostomy and expiratory valve and to observe the progress of the lesion. Recent work has indicated that steroids may be helpful in bringing about a regression of the lesion, but experience has not confirmed this finding. Three forms of treatment are available.

(1) *Radiotherapy*. Experience has not shown this to be of much help and the surgeon must bear in mind that a percentage of the children so treated may have a disturbance of growth of the area irradiated and may even develop a carcinoma in that site at a later date.

(2) *Sclerosing agents*. Hypertonic saline and sodium morrhuate have been used. However, the distribution of the sclerosing agent in the subcutaneous tissues is difficult to control and there may be severe post-operative laryngeal stenosis.

(3) *Diathermy and cryoprobes*. Both agents have been applied locally to the tumours—small areas being treated at frequent sessions. This appears to offer the best hope in the treatment of the supraglottic lesion. It may be possible to treat the subglottic lesion by cryosurgery through a thyrotomy at about the age of three years.

REFERENCES

Holinger, P. H. (1948). *Ann. Otol., etc., St. Louis*, **57**, 808.
— (1950). *Ann. Otol., etc., St. Louis*, **59**, 837.
Montreuil, F. (1949). *Laryngoscope*, **59**, 194.
Pracy, R. (1964). *Proc. R. Soc. Med.*, **58**, 268.
— (1970). *J. Laryng.* **84**, 37.
Rees, G. J. (1966). *Brit. J. Anaesth.*, **38**, 901.
Wilson, T. G. (1962). *Diseases of the Ear, Nose and Throat in Children* (2nd ed., p. 249). London; Heinemann.

12

TRAUMA AND STENOSIS OF THE LARYNX

DOUGLAS RANGER

TRAUMA

The shape of the neck, with the mandible projecting forwards above and the clavicles and sternum below, serves to protect the larynx from injury in a number of accidents such as falls and blows. The lateral mobility of the larynx also reduces the effects of compression injuries. The cartilaginous framework provides protection to the contained soft tissues, but once this framework is fractured or dislocated the injuries inside may be accentuated because of the adherence of the soft tissues to the cartilage. Despite these protective factors the larynx may be involved in open wounds and closed injuries, foreign bodies may lodge in the larynx and damage may result from burning.

Open wounds

Gunshot wounds may injure the larynx. Wounds with knives and razors and other sharp weapons may open the larynx and this may sometimes occur with self-inflicted neck incisions.

Diagnosis

Open wounds of the larynx will often prove fatal before the patient can obtain any medical treatment. In those patients who survive, laryngeal involvement will usually be obvious because of bubbling of blood due to air passing in and out of the wound during respiration.

Treatment

Treatment is usually required urgently to establish a free airway and prevent more blood from entering the bronchial tree. Under these circumstances an emergency tracheostomy is required and this will be rendered more difficult if there is extensive haematoma formation. In a few patients it may be possible as an emergency measure to pass a tube into the larynx through the opening resulting from the wound.

Once a tracheostomy has been established the wound of the larynx can be dealt with on general principles; foreign bodies must be removed, devitalized tissue excised and the mucosa sutured. No raw surfaces must be left uncovered but the skin edges must never be sutured under tension. Where a large amount of skin from the neck has been destroyed it may be necessary to advance or re-arrange flaps.

An antibiotic will be required and prophylaxis against tetanus is advisable. Oedema persists for several days and the tracheostomy must be maintained until there is a clear airway through the larynx and there is no longer any risk of laryngeal swelling from tissue reaction to the trauma or from secondary infection. Difficulty in swallowing will usually necessitate the use of a nasogastric tube for feeding purposes for several days post-operatively.

Closed injuries

The larynx may be damaged as a result of the moving neck coming into sudden contact with a rigid structure; such an injury is liable to occur in falls on to objects projecting transversely, such as a railing or the back of a chair. This also happens in the whiplash injuries of road accidents when the larynx strikes the steering wheel or windscreen in the case of front-seat passengers, or the back of the seat in the case of rear-seat passengers and those in coaches or buses.

Moving objects may strike the neck and injure the larynx. This occurs as a result of accidental or deliberate blows from the edge of the hand, the fist, or the elbow or even from a kick with the foot in the case of people lying on the ground. Injuries are also liable to occur as a result of the impact of inanimate objects such as a swing seat, hockey stick, cricket ball, rake handle and many others.

Compression injuries result from strangulation either manually or by rope.

One unusual injury which occurred to a patient seen by the author was caused by pressure from a collar stud under a tight collar. During an episode of shouting the base of the stud was forced inwards between the cricoid and thyroid cartilages. This produced a haematoma and considerable hoarseness.

Pathology

Haematoma formation is the most common lesion occurring as a result of closed laryngeal injuries. It may be localized to a small area of the larynx such as one vocal cord or extend diffusely throughout the larynx and beyond it into the trachea, pharynx and oesophagus. Bruising also occurs in the muscles surrounding the larynx and in the subcutaneous tissues. The hyoid bone and the thyroid cartilage may be fractured and, more rarely still, the cricoid cartilage. Even fracture of the epiglottis has been reported by Chadwick (1960) in a patient with multiple injuries. In that case death occurred suddenly from asphyxia some hours after the injury. Rarely the cricothyroid and crico-arytenoid joints may be dislocated. The recurrent laryngeal nerves may be torn across, especially with dislocations of the crico-thyroid joint, or laryngeal paralysis may occur as a result of involvement of the nerve in haematoma or oedema. In the absence of any paralysis a vocal cord becomes fixed as a result of post-traumatic fibrosis occurring in the cord itself or outside it, or in the crico-arytenoid joint. Laceration of the mucosa can occur and this may give rise to haemoptysis and also to surgical emphysema.

Symptoms and signs

In severe crush injuries of the larynx the most prominent feature is the obstruction of the airway requiring immediate alleviation by tracheostomy. If the mucosa has been torn there will be bleeding into the airway and surgical emphysema which may be extensive over the chest and face as well as the neck and may involve the mediastinum. Cough may be a troublesome feature and will add to the emphysema. There is nearly always great difficulty in swallowing.

In less severe injuries which do not immediately jeopardize the airway pain or discomfort is usually present especially on coughing, speaking or swallowing. Hoarseness is common but the presence of a normal or near normal voice in the early stages does not necessarily indicate that the injury is only slight. The subsequent development of scar tissue in the damaged larynx may lead to obstruction of the airway if treatment is not undertaken early.

Injuries to other parts of the body such as the chest and the face may also occur at the same time and require treatment.

Diagnosis

In most patients the damage to the larynx and adjacent tissues is the only injury sustained and attention is automatically directed to the region. However, in patients with multiple injuries, and especially in those rendered unconscious, the laryngeal lesions may well be overlooked and this sometimes leads to sudden unexpected death from asphyxia.

All recent laryngeal injuries must be regarded seriously and steps should be taken to assess the full extent of the damage so that the risk of a sudden respiratory obstruction can be avoided and so that injuries which might give rise to severe symptoms later are not overlooked.

Examination of the neck may reveal little abnormality apart from some tenderness. Indirect laryngeal and pharyngeal examination will reveal any swelling and also indicate whether the recurrent laryngeal nerve has been involved. Tomograms give an assessment of the extent and exact site of any swelling or obstruction. In late cases laryngograms may be of particular value. Open operation gives the most accurate assessment of the degree of damage.

Treatment

The treatment of closed laryngeal injuries will depend on the extent of the injuries and also on the time that has elapsed since the trauma. A few patients are seen on account of voice changes which date from a comparatively minor laryngeal injury which occurred several days or weeks earlier. Such patients will not be at risk on account of complications and they require voice rest in the early stages and graduated speech therapy later.

All patients who require a tracheostomy on account of respiratory obstruction or bleeding will also require open operation on the larynx to reduce dislocated or fractured cartilage, suture lacerations of the mucosa and splint the larynx if necessary. In addition open operation should be undertaken in patients who have had a laryngeal injury and in whom there is evidence of dislocation or fracture of cartilage as shown by tomography or by displacement of the arytenoid on laryngoscopy. Under these circumstances if operation is delayed until the voice is severely affected or there is evidence of significant obstruction of the airway the amount of scar tissue which has formed may prevent a satisfactory ultimate result being achieved.

At exploration, after a preliminary tracheostomy, cartilage which is fractured and displaced should be repositioned and will be retained in position by an internal mould of non-reactive plastic such as polyvinyl introduced at the end of the operation. Fragments of cartilage should not be removed unless they are extensively damaged and loose and likely to act as a future focus of infection. However, if the arytenoid cartilage has been disarticulated from the joint surface of the cricoid then a better result will be obtained by excising it than by leaving it to become ankylosed in scar tissue. The larynx is opened by laryngofissure and lacerations of the mucosa are sutured carefully. A polyvinyl mould of suitable size is then inserted to splint the larynx and retained in position for one month by means of an anchoring stitch or wire.

In very severe laryngeal injuries there may be gross fracturing of the cricoid cartilage as well as the thyroid carilage and Conley (1953) has reported excision of the cricoid cartilage with end-to-end anastomosis. Careful attention has to be paid to the recurrent laryngeal nerves.

The treatment of stenosis of the larynx resulting from the late effects of laryngeal trauma is discussed on p. 308.

Burns and scalds

The laryngeal mucosa may be damaged by the inhalation of burning gases or of very hot air from a fire, by the inhalation of steam or irritant gases, and also by the swallowing of corrosive liquids. In all these injuries there is likely to be associated damage to the mucosa of the mouth and pharynx and often to the trachea as well. The effects are erythema and oedema and also necrosis of the mucosa and, perhaps, of the underlying tissues as well.

Treatment

Unfortunately, many of these injuries prove rapidly fatal, either as a result of the laryngeal lesions alone or of the extent of burns in other areas also. In those who survive, any degree of dyspnoea is an indication for tracheostomy as it is almost certain that the oedema will increase, possibly very rapidly, and respiratory obstruction should be avoided rather than awaited. In all except the most minor burns steroids should be administered and in the initial stages the most satisfactory method of administration will usually be the injection of hydrocortisone intravenously or intramuscularly. In all patients requiring steroids an antibiotic will also be needed.

Pain is usually a distressing feature, and powerful analgesics and sedatives such as morphine or one of its derivatives will often be required for many days. Associated dysphagia will usually necessitate feeding the patient through a nasogastric tube.

Foreign bodies

Foreign bodies which are inhaled into the air passages seldom become impacted in the larynx but pass through it into the trachea and bronchi. Impaction in the larynx is more liable to occur in children than in adults. Coins and other similar objects may lodge in the larynx and care must be exercised in prescribing tablets or capsules for children. These have been known to be inhaled rather than swallowed and have, on occasion, become wedged in the larynx between the true and false cords with fatal consequences. In adults, food—particularly a piece of poorly masticated meat—may enter the larynx and be held there due to spasm of the muscles. Also bizarre foreign bodies occasionally become impacted in the larynx. The museum of one institute contains the pharynx and larynx of an edentulous man with a billiard ball stuck in the laryngeal inlet. The author has removed a piece of glass 8 cm. × 1·5 cm. whose pointed end was impaled in the under surface of the left vocal cord with the remainder of the glass lying free in the lumen of the larynx and trachea.

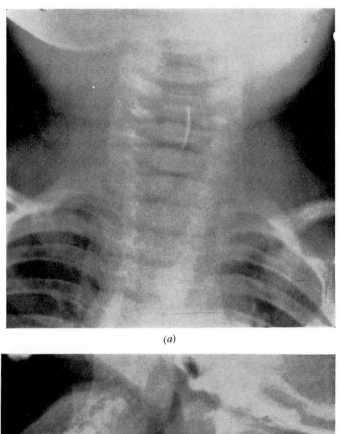

(a)

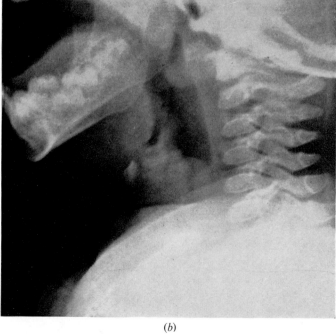

(b)

FIG. 128.—Radiographs of piece of eggshell in the larynx of a child: (a) anteroposteral view showing eggshell seen "end-on"; (b) lateral view— eggshell not visible.

305

Symptoms and diagnosis

Foreign bodies which impact in the larynx are liable to produce sudden and often complete asphyxia but occasionally the dyspnoea develops gradually as a result of increasing oedema due to the presence of a small sharp foreign body. When the symptoms are slow in onset it is difficult to decide in children whether the foreign body is lodged in the larynx itself or in the pharynx with consequent oedema of the arytenoids. The length of time elapsing between the "swallowing" of the foreign body and the onset of symptoms gives some guidance but the most reliable help before endoscopy is likely to be obtained from an x-ray. Flat foreign bodies in the pharynx tend to lie transversely, those in the larynx anteroposteriorly in the long axis of the larynx (Fig. 128).

Treatment

The urgent relief of asphyxia from the impaction of a large foreign body has usually to be undertaken without any facilities for tracheostomy or laryngoscopy. Fortunately, if children are raised by the legs and slapped hard on the back the foreign body will often be dislodged. Also in both adults and children it is often possible to extract the foreign body by a finger passed through the mouth.

In patients without urgent dyspnoea the foreign body should be removed as soon as possible by direct laryngoscopy. The presence of oedema will indicate the need for a tracheostomy.

STENOSIS

Narrowing of the lumen of the larynx with obstruction of the airway occurs in a wide variety of conditions. Many of these are considered in detail in other chapters of this book but an attempt will be made to list here the main causes of stenosis and review the general management of chronic stenosis of the larynx.

Causes of laryngeal stenosis

Congenital abnormalities

    (1) Atresia.
    (2) Web.
    (3) Bifid epiglottis.
    (4) "Congenital laryngeal stridor".
    (5) Congenital cysts and tumours.
These are discussed in Chapter 11.

Traumatic conditions

    (1) Impaction of a foreign body.
    (2) Haematoma formation from injury.
    (3) Acute oedema from foreign body or injury.
    (4) Fibrosis as a late result of injury.
    (5) Stenosis as a late result of a very high tracheostomy.
    (1)–(4) are discussed on pp. 301–304; (5) is discussed in Chapter 19.

Inflammatory conditions
  (1) Acute:
    (*a*) acute (non-specific) laryngitis;
    (*b*) acute epiglottitis;
    (*c*) laryngotracheobronchitis;
    (*d*) diphtheria and other acute specific fevers.
  These are discussed in Chapter 13.

  (2) Chronic:
    (*a*) tuberculosis;
    (*b*) scleroma;
    (*c*) syphilis;
    (*d*) leprosy;
    (*e*) glanders.
  These are discussed in Chapter 14.

Vasomotor and allergic conditions
  (1) Angioneurotic oedema.
  (2) Drug sensitivity.
  These are discussed in Chapter 13.

Impaired abduction of vocal cords
  (1) Recurrent laryngeal paralysis.
  (2) Spasm of the adductor muscles.
  (3) Laryngismus stridulus (laryngeal tetany).
  (4) Arthritis of the crico-arytenoid joint.
  (5) Fibrosis around the crico-arytenoid joint.
  (1)–(3) are discussed in Chapter 20; (4) and (5) in Chapter 14.

Cysts and neoplasms
  (1) Benign.
  (2) Malignant.
  These are discussed in Chapter 15.

The management of chronic stenosis of the larynx

It is now proposed to discuss in general terms the management of a fibrotic stenosis of the larynx, without attempting to deal with any specific therapy for a particular type.

Initial assessment

Before attempting any treatment it is necessary to determine precisely the nature and severity of the patient's symptoms and also the exact level and extent of the stenosis. In addition, when the stenosis is a late result of an inflammatory or neoplastic condition, any residual activity of the disease must be excluded. The general state of the patient and the presence or absence of any chest disease must be determined.

The site and extent of the stenosis must be assessed accurately by indirect and direct laryngoscopy. Tomograms and laryngograms may be useful in demonstrating the stenosis, the latter being obtained by using a radio-opaque medium instilled into the larynx either through the mouth or through a tracheostome.

Patients with a laryngeal stenosis have a respiratory obstruction and usually a hoarse voice as well, unless the stenosis is confined to an area low in the subglottic region. It is unlikely that any operative treatment will produce much improvement in the voice and treatment should be undertaken solely in an attempt to relieve the laryngeal obstruction. If the stenosis is so extensive that it seems probable that even after treatment a tracheostomy will still be necessary, or if it appears likely that operation may seriously damage the voice, no operation should be undertaken.

Treatment

Treatment of stenosis of the larynx may be palliative or curative. As a palliative measure the laryngeal obstruction can be overcome by means of a tracheostomy. Most patients will have a sufficient lumen to allow expiration through the larynx and can wear an inspiratory valve in the tracheostomy tube. In this way the inspiratory obstruction is overcome but the patient retains the same voice as before.

Congenital laryngeal webs may be so thin that they can be treated by simple division via a laryngoscope and a few patients with stenosis from other causes can be treated in a similar way. In the vast majority, however, curative treatment will require an open operation with excision of the stenotic area and grafting of the residual raw surfaces.

In these patients a tracheostomy will usually have been performed previously. If not, a tracheostomy should be established and the patient allowed to become accustomed to it before the stenosis is dealt with. The larynx is opened via a laryngofissure approach to allow a thorough inspection of the interior of the larynx and to permit complete excision of the stenosed area which may be of considerable length. Meticulous attention must be paid to securing haemostasis and a support is then prepared to fit the cavity so that it is ready to use after the graft has been applied to the raw area.

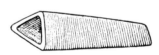

FIG. 129.—Triangular mould of plastic material around which the skin graft is wrapped. This is made in six different sizes by Portland Plastics Ltd., after the Negus design.

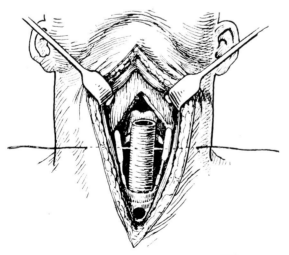

FIG. 130.—The larynx has been opened and a tube inserted after excision of scar tissue. The tube is held in position by a transfixing silver wire suture.

Supporting materials of a wide variety of types have been used by different surgeons and have usually succeeded in keeping the graft in position. They may be solid pre-formed moulds or hollow tubes (Fig. 129). They may also be fashioned individually for each patient from rigid materials like wax or stent or from elastic materials such as sponge rubber or sponge nylon. If a rigid substance is used it should be somewhat larger than the normal lumen of the larynx to allow for subsequent contraction of the graft. This should be of thin split-thickness skin obtained from a smooth hairless area such as the inner aspect of the arm.

The piece of skin must be sufficiently large to cover the raw area completely. The graft is wrapped round the prepared mould and then both are kept in position by wire stitches transfixing the alae of the thyroid cartilage, mould and skin graft as advocated by Schmiegelow (1938) (Fig. 130). Firm fixation of this type is desirable to prevent movement of the graft during coughing. The laryngeal and skin incisions are then closed and this provides further support and fixation for the graft. Opinions differ on the length of time during which the mould should be retained in position and vary from ten days to as long as six months. Kilner (1954), with extensive experience of plastic surgery in this region, advises that the mould should be retained for six weeks, but that periodic observation of the patient is required for six months as contraction in the grafted area may continue during that period. The tracheostomy should be maintained until it is clear that the laryngeal lumen is adequate and that further contraction will not occur.

REFERENCES

Chadwick, D. L. (1960). *J. Laryng.*, **74**, 306.
Conley, John J., (1953). *Ann. Otol., etc, St. Louis.*, **62**, 477.
Jackson, C., and Jackson, C. L. (1937). *The Larynx and its Diseases.* Philadelphia; Saunders.
Kilner, T. P. (1954). In *Modern Trends in Diseases of the Ear, Nose and Throat* (Ed. by Maxwell Ellis). London; Butterworths.
Martin, J. A. M. (1963). *J. Laryng.*, **77**, 290.
Montreuil, F. (1949). *Laryngoscope*, **59**, 194.
Schmiegelow, E. (1938). *J. Laryng.*, **53**, 1.
Thomson, J., and Turner, A. L. (1900). *Brit. med. J.*, **2**, 1561.
Wilson, T. G. (1952). *Proc. R. Soc. Med.*, **45**, 355.

13

ACUTE LARYNGITIS

MAXWELL ELLIS

INTRODUCTION

The usual form of this condition occurs as part of the common cold and is due to an acute inflammatory process in the laryngeal mucosa. It is variously called a cold in the throat, simple laryngitis or acute catarrhal laryngitis.

Aetiology

The disease is usually associated with, and secondary to, an acute inflammation of the nasal cavities, accessory sinuses and pharynx, and in the same way as these conditions are infectious, it too may be contagious. At times acute upper respiratory tract infections are epidemic and then usually one or other part of the tract seems to bear the brunt of the infection. Thus acute laryngitis is sometimes sufficiently ubiquitous to suggest an epidemic. It is a droplet or air-borne infection and in the initial stages the infective agent is usually one of the viruses of the common cold, but later secondary invasion by other organisms nearly always occurs. For the most part these organisms are normally present in the upper air passages and seem to be activated to pathogenicity in a manner as yet undetermined. They are commonly the haemolytic streptococcus, haemolytic staphylococcus, pneumococcus, *Micrococcus catarrhalis,* and the influenza baccillus. Others are occasionally responsible, such as the virus of influenza, measles, whooping-cough or smallpox, and bacilli of the enteric group. Exposure to cold, damp, dust and irritating vapours including tobacco, are predisposing conditions, as is a lowered general resistance, particularly a deficiency of vitamins. Vocal abuse and chronic infection in the upper air passages, accessory sinuses or lymphoid tissue, are important contributory factors. Finally there is the idiosyncrasy whereby certain individuals recurrently contract the condition for no obvious reason.

Pathology

This is identical with acute inflammation anywhere else in the body. Initially there is a dilatation of the peripheral vessels in the mucous membrane with resulting exudation of fluid into the cellular tissue together with diapedesis of granulocytes and some lymphocytes (Fig. 131). The infecting agent breaches the surface sheet of mucus, where present, and penetrates the epithelial layer to the submucosa where the vascular and lymphatic plexuses are situated. It is in this layer that the invading organisms usually travel from above to involve the larynx. The inflammatory reaction later involves the whole thickness of the mucous membrane as well as the intrinsic muscles and occasionally the crico-arytenoid joints. Areas of epithelium may be destroyed and exfoliated and the oedema may cause respiratory

311

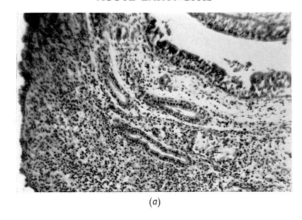

(a)

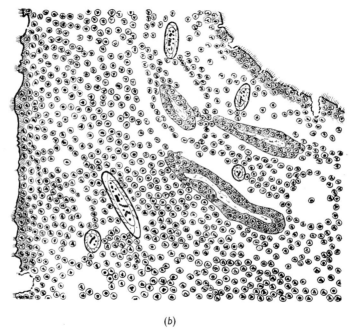

(b)

FIG. 131.—(a) Photomicrograph of a section through the mucous membrane of the larynx of a child aged 5 who died 12 hours after the onset of an acute respiratory tract infection. There is a heavy infiltration of neutrophils and lymphocytes together with vascular congestion and oedema. Areas of the epithelium have been destroyed and have desquamated: (b) a diagram of the photomicrograph in (a).

embarrassment. Excessive secretion is not a feature of the condition, indeed much of its peculiar discomfort is due to dryness. When the infection has been overcome, the waste products are removed both by leucocytes into the blood stream and by cough and expectoration. Complete resolution is the rule, but the condition may persist in a subacute form, especially if untreated or in unfavourable circumstances. A round-cell infiltration of the tissues then takes place, gradually progressing to fibrosis. This change is irreversible, occurring not uncommonly in the mucous membrane and probably also in the intrinsic muscles. Permanent crico-arytenoid arthritis is rare however. Different parts of the larynx seem to be affected disproportionately and often, in patients subject to recurrent attacks, the same part recurrently suffers.

Vocal cord paralysis

Occasionally a paralysis of one or other vocal cord occurs (it is rarely bilateral) and is possibly due to a peripheral neuritis of the vagus or of the recurrent laryngeal nerve. The condition may be more frequent than is usually supposed, as hoarseness with a cold is accepted as a more or less normal symptom and laryngologists rarely get an opportunity of examining these patients. A sufficient number of cases have been seen to identify the condition and also to record that the paralysis usually recovers spontaneously.

Symptoms

These are chiefly hoarseness, discomfort or pain in the larynx and an irritant, paroxysmal cough, and they are generally preceded by the symptoms of the ante-cedent infection higher up in the respiratory tract. The voice becomes rough and varies in pitch and strength. It is never completely lost although it may be reduced to a husky whisper. Oedema of the mucous membrane of the vocal cords and vocal processes together with sticky secretion in the glottic chink are partly responsible, but some of the dysfunction is due to infiltration of the intrinsic muscles. The cough often lasts after the voice has recovered. It is spasmodic and distressing and, in the early stages, unproductive. It frequently has a most trying nocturnal persistence. The pain is felt in the larynx itself and occurs at the outset. The sensation is one of rawness, heat and dryness, and has a peculiarly disagreeable quality. Fortunately, it rarely lasts more than a day or two. The symptoms diminish about the fifth to the seventh day, but an associated tracheitis may delay their departure and especially prolong the duration of the cough. General disturbance is usually slight and pyrexia of any magnitude or duration is uncommon.

If part of the hoarseness is due to paralysis of one or other vocal cord, the rough timbre disappears as usual, but the voice may remain a little weak or breathy for some weeks, until the palsy recovers.

Physical signs

Examination of the nasal cavities and pharynx is necessary to reveal any exciting cause. The larynx on indirect laryngoscopy will reveal mucosal redness and swelling, ecchymosis and occasional superficial ulceration. The vocal cords and arytenoids are usually most affected, but the epiglottis, ventricular bands or subglottic tissues occasionally bear the brunt (*see* Plate II). The vocal cords are generally last to assume the characteristic dull red colour and to become noticeably oedema-tous owing to the tight attachment of the mucous membrane to the vocal ligament. They are also late in showing the changes of resolution. Sticky secretion is nearly always visible on the cords or in the anterior commissure. In severe cases the vocal cords move sluggishly, and perhaps asymmetrically, and paralysis, usually unilateral, may sometimes be seen. The disease is self-limiting and physical signs have usually disappeared by the tenth to the fourteenth day.

Diagnosis

The lack of correlation between the sudden onset of somewhat alarming symp-toms and the general fitness of the patient is almost diagnostic. Tuberculosis may occasionally be responsible for acute symptoms of a similar nature, but other features will readily identify the condition (*see* p. 336). Diphtheria can sometimes be simulated when there is much exudate, but it is rare in adults. In a suspected case the diagnosis is made by means of a culture from the secretions—preferably before the stage of membrane formation.

Complications and sequelae

These are rare, but the most serious is oedema sufficient to cause respiratory obstruction. It is a function of virulence and perhaps poor resistance and depends upon a time factor, the rate of fluid exudation into the tissues, and also an anatomical one, the looseness of these tissues. Severe oedema thus usually occurs in debilitated children, where the conditions are ripe. Tracheitis commonly accompanies laryngitis. Very infrequently abscess formation and even cartilage necrosis may occur. In inadequately treated cases and those subject to idiosyncratic recurrence, permanent changes in the tissue may result, producing a chronic laryngitis.

Treatment

Prophylaxis

Prevention is naturally the best treatment and could be achieved by segregation and prophylaxis. The desirable ideal is to immure every sufferer from the common cold until his infectivity is past, but this pitch of social perfection has yet to be attained. The initial invasion can be due to so many different viruses that specific passive or active immunization is not practicable. The most that can be done in prevention is the avoidance of crowded and ill-ventilated assemblies and the maintenance of resistance by a good mixed diet and hygiene. Fresh air and sunlight undoubtedly help to improve resistance, and the regular use of the ultra-violet lamp can be useful. As a corollary, cold and damp lower the resistance and predispose towards infection.

Local susceptibility in the nasopharyngeal mucosa is increased by chronic irritation. In industry the avoidance of exposure to noxious vapours or dust must be secured or at least attempted. This applies also to tobacco. However, so much of the epidemiology is inherent in modern urban living conditions that precautionary measures are largely unavailing.

Remedial measures

Complete voice rest is the most important measure, preferably from the earliest stages of the infection, and greatly reduces the duration of the disability and its later discomforts. Unfortunately, even if the patient presents early, which is unusual, the constitutional disturbance is so slight that he will rarely follow this advice. Ideally he should be put to bed and forbidden to speak or even whisper. The room must be well ventilated, although not necessarily cold, and a reasonable degree of humidity procured. The measures usually adopted in acute infections are applicable—mild purgation and diaphoresis together with a plentiful supply of bland fluid. The traditional drugs used are calomel followed by a saline next morning; Dover's powder, 300 or 600 mg., three times a day, or a similar dose of aspirin, are suitable diaphoretics. Fruit juice drinks, sweetened or not by personal inclination, and preferably of lime or lemon are not only pleasant to take but help to clear away secretions in the hypopharynx. The diet need not be of any special character providing only that it is readily digestible, and the patient's own wishes can usually be humoured; alcohol and tobacco should be avoided. If there is much general disturbance or any fever over 37·8°C, a sulphonamide compound or antibiotics, preferably penicillin, should be given in appropriate dosage. To ease the discomfort and cough, medicated steam inhalations every two or three hours are useful. Pine or eucalyptus are perhaps the most fragrant and soothing, although some patients object to the latter. The irritant cough is best relieved by a linctus. Linctus Gee can be taken in doses of one or two teaspoonfuls every three or four hours, and where the cough is very troublesome codeine or diamorphine can advantageously be included in the linctus. The illness is brief and the risk of habit formation therefore theoretical. The sleep and rest procured by relief of the cough will more than compensate for the slight risk. If the patient remains ambulatory, very little except local alleviative measures are possible, but he will generally be able to manage a few inhalations during the day. Should his occupation demand much talking warm alkaline throat sprays are helpful in temporarily clearing away viscid secretion. The local application (by spraying or swabbing) of astringent or vasoconstrictor substances is distinctly harmful, as it interferes with the normal body mechanism of inflammation and repair. However, in an emergency, singers may be treated with a solution of 0·1 per cent adrenaline, or public speakers with 0·5 per cent ephedrine and 0·5 per cent phenol in liquid paraffin, sprayed directly on the vocal cords.

Prognosis

Unless the infection is of uncommon virulence the symptoms will usually subside in a few days or a week if treated energetically, and in an uncomplicated case will rarely last as long as a fortnight. In patients who attempt to lead a normal life, the condition may persist for a great deal longer and may even become chronic.

ACUTE LARYNGITIS IN CHILDREN

This is usually associated with an acute infection of the upper respiratory tract but may also occur as part of an acute lower respiratory tract infection which will be more fully discussed in the section on acute laryngotracheobronchitis. The disease has been called pseudocroup or laryngitis stridulosa.

Aetiology and pathology

The bacteriology and epidemiology are identical with that of the disease in adults. It is of less frequent incidence as most of the irritant factors in causation do not apply. On the other hand, it is generally more serious, partly owing to a child's undeveloped immunity to upper respiratory tract infection and partly for anatomical reasons. The opening of the glottis is relatively small and is encroached upon by the curled-in *omega* shape of the infantile epiglottis. The epithelium is separated from the cartilage by an abundance of loose areolar tissue containing rich vascular and lymphatic plexuses, permitting the maximum of oedema and the ready spread of infection. Obstruction thus occurs easily, resulting in cyanosis and spasm which in turn increase the vascular engorgement. In addition, a child is less able to expel by coughing the sticky secretion which forms in the larynx.

Clinical picture

During the course of a bad cold or acute bronchitis, or perhaps both, a cough of a croupy nature develops and dominates the illness. In severe cases the cough and associated spasm can become almost suffocating. The larynx must then be inspected. With patience and coercion mirror laryngoscopy may be possible in older children. Direct laryngoscopy is preferable in a young child or infant, restrained by wrapping it tightly in a sheet or blanket. The intense mucosal redness and swelling will then be revealed. If the subglottic tissues are particularly affected, red semi-elliptic brawny bands are visible immediately below the cords, narrowing the airway.

Diagnosis

In mild cases the diagnosis can be made by inference, without necessarily examining the larynx, but if the symptoms worsen laryngoscopy is essential. In diphtheria the child is generally more ill, but less febrile, and some evidence of membrane should be visible. Cultures must be taken if there is the slightest suspicion. Very young children may inhale a foreign body into the larynx with resulting suffocating attacks, but the absence of any general disturbance or infection should indicate the possibility and examination should reveal it.

Treatment

As effective control can be exercised over the movements of children, the treatment already described as ideal for adults is possible. Penicillin by injection is the mainstay of treatment. It is important to obtain a high level in the blood stream as soon as possible and injections of a soluble preparation should be given every six hours for the first two days, followed by a daily or twice daily injection of a less soluble one. Where the causative organism is insensitive to penicillin, one of the tetracyclines made up as an elixir is usually effective. If the child is too young to use a steam inhalation, a tent is erected over the cot with sheets and medicated steam is introduced under it. Secretions can be loosened in a severe case by the administration of ipecacuanha syrup, 2g. every half hour until the child vomits. Occasionally the obstruction and dyspnoea are so severe that energetic measures to restore the airway may become necessary. The choice lies between blind intubation, intubation by direct laryngoscopy (using a Magill anaesthetic tube or a rubber catheter cut across obliquely at the end) or tracheostomy. Antibiotics and the oxygen tent have undoubtedly reduced the frequently of active intervention; increased oxygenation results in a lessenging of dyspnoea which in turn reduces both the muscle spasm due to vascular engorgement and that due to fright. The infection tends to last longer in children than in adults and is subject to the same complications.

ACUTE EPIGLOTTITIS

This condition is a special form of acute laryngitis and is the name given to a particularly clearly demarcated pathological and clinical entity. It arises in the same ways, but the brunt of the disease falls upon the loosely attached mucous membrane on the anterior surface of the epiglottis, with very little reaction in the surrounding tissues. The resulting localized oedema may obstruct the airway in children, where the amount of loose mucosa is great and the glottic aperture relatively small and additionally encroached upon by the *omega*-shaped epiglottis. In adults, the greater size of the larynx, the lesser amount of loose mucosa and the more spatulate shape of the epiglottis diminish the effects on the airway, but the enlarged, rigid and less mobile epiglottis may affect swallowing.

Clinical picture

Children

When the condition occurs in children, progressive respiratory obstruction may become alarming and even urgent enough to demand tracheostomy. Deaths have occurred from a failure to recognize the potential danger. The condition is unusual, but it should be considered in any child developing increasing dyspnoea for no very obvious reason, and in some way the larynx must be inspected.

Adults

The symptoms are more pharyngeal than laryngeal. Deglutition is painful, leading to an accumulation of viscid saliva in the mouth. The tongue feels stiff and swollen and some degree of trismus increases the misery of the patient. The picture is similar to that presented by a case of quinsy. The oedema may sometimes be considerable enough to cause respiratory difficulty, but this is unusual. The condition is readily diagnosed by indirect laryngoscopy.

Treatment

The general lines of treatment have already been discussed, and sulphonamides and antibiotics are the most important measures in the relief of this rather odd and sometimes dangerous condition.

ACUTE LARYNGOTRACHEOBRONCHITIS

Aetiology

This condition usually occurs in infants or small children, is rarely seen after the age of seven or eight years, and may be due to any of the pathogenic organisms of airborne disease, predominantly the haemolytic streptococcus. It is a severe disease for the anatomical reasons given on page 315 and, in addition, as the trachea and bronchi are also involved in the infection, the dyspnoea and cyanosis are considerably increased. It has occasionally been a consistent complication of certain influenza epidemics and in this way has acquired an epidemic incidence.

Pathology

The process of acute inflammation of mucous membrane already described occurs here throughout the bronchial tree from the subglottic tissues to the alveoli. A characteristic feature is the production of a tenacious exudate and crusting composed of all the products of an acute inflammatory process together with desquamated surface epithelium embedded in fibrin. This tough and adherent deposit may not be large, but it encroaches on a child's air spaces with disproportionate effect. In addition, it is removed only with great difficulty by his own inco-ordinated and inexperienced coughing efforts. It is present chiefly in the trachea and bronchi and may occlude the latter, resulting in atelectasis and collapse of areas of lung. When it is wiped away no ulceration is seen and little bleeding occurs, affording a ready distinction from diphtheria. In the larynx oedema is the usual feature with semi-elliptic "mounding" of the subglottic tissues. Sometimes the mucosa appears dull red, dry and glazed throughout, and secretions are absent.

Symptoms and physical signs

The disease may take a fulminant course with high fever, perhaps up to 41°C, and toxaemia initiated by convulsions and vomiting, rapidly followed by laryngeal obstruction with cyanosis, and finally prostration and death from cardiac failure. More usually the onset and course are gradual. Following a cold or influenza the child develops a hard, dry, croupy cough with hoarseness. There is a fever of 38·9°–40°C, restlessness and a marked ashy-grey colour. With increasing laryngeal obstruction stridulous breathing develops until finally the child struggles for breath with "tugging" in the supraclavicular spaces, suprasternal notch and lower chest. The mucous membranes appear blue-tinged and careful examination of the chest reveals scattered areas of pulmonary collapse. At this stage, on broncho-scopy, the subglottic tissues would be found to be oedematous, "mounding", the mucosa red and velvety with oozing points of blood, and tenacious secretion would be seen throughout the trachea and bronchial tree, sometimes occluding the smaller branch bronchi-by plug-like accretions or by crusting. The child can take nourishment only with difficulty and rapidly becomes dehydrated and weak. Death may occur because of prolonged fatigue with eventual circulatory failure. Throughout the illness examination of the blood rarely reveals more than a moderate granulocytosis.

Differential diagnosis

Simple laryngitis is nothing like so severe a disease and is not accompanied by the peculiar secretions. The most important differentiation must be made from true diphtheria and membranous laryngitis, and from both of these diseases it is diag-nosed positively by bacteriological examination of the laryngeal secretions. Clinic-ally, this distinction can be made earlier by the trained observer on direct laryngo-scopy when the velvety nature of the mucosa together with the absence of membrane is revealed. Bronchopneumonia may run a similar course in some ways, but it is not usually accompanied by bronchial exudation and crusting. Bronchial obstruc-tion by foreign bodies, especially vegetable ones, and more rare conditions like abscess or tumour must be excluded.

Prognosis

This is a function of obstruction and complications. The degree and duration of dyspnoea with its attendant anoxia govern the production of exhaustion and the onset of cardiac failure. The supervention of toxaemia, bacteraemia, broncho-pneumonia, pericarditis, endocarditis or nephritis is usually fatal. The younger the child the worse the outlook, and the disease is distinctly dangerous in infants under three years of age. The mortality was as high as 70 or 80 per cent, but it has been reduced to 10 or 15 per cent by earlier recognition and early treatment with modern antibiotic drugs.

Treatment

It is extremely important in this disease to identify the causative organism as soon as possible and to test its sensitivity to antibiotics. Meanwhile, penicillin and a soluble sulphonamide should be given in full doses. If the organisms prove insensitive to these drugs as judged by the clinical course of the case, tetracyclines should be substituted even before the results of bacteriological examination.

The room atmosphere must be kept warm, about 21°C, and also rather humid, about 80 per cent. If this is impracticable a tent can be erected over the cot or bed and a steam kettle used. The child's strength must be conserved by good nursing and the minimum of disturbance. Sleep is a problem and careful use of opiates is justifiable to ensure rest. Some authorities strongly oppose this and any other measure which may depress the respiratory centre and inhibit cough. However, in any serious illness, especially a self-limiting one such as this, in which ultimate survival may depend upon vitality and physical strength, a compromise may be necessary to conserve energy as opposed to risking something else. A child's cough reflex is not well developed as a protective mechanism and, in addition, the membrane in the bronchial tree is often too adherent and tough to be removed in this way. Coughing efforts may thus merely weaken the child to no purpose. There are other ways of securing an adequate respiratory exchange and removing obstruction. Each case must therefore be treated on its own merits and if rest is needed it must be ensured. Syrup of chloral in doses of one teaspoonful or even two is an effective sedative, as is a drop or two of Nepenthe. Dehydration must be avoided and the child given plenty to drink. Except in the last stages of exhaustion the child will rarely become too weak to swallow, but saline solution and glucose must then be administered by continuous intravenous drip. Protein concentrates can be given in the drinks, but as the disease seldom lasts longer than two weeks food is less important than fluid. Blood transfusions are valuable for toxaemia or debility and should be given before much general deterioration becomes manifest.

Maintenance of an airway

The mucosal swelling together with the tough membranous exudate combine to produce the most serious aspect of the disease—the asphyxia from anoxia and resulting exhaustion from exaggerated respiratory efforts. Minor degrees of this condition are best treated by placing the child in an oxygen tent in which, if necessary, he can be kept throughout the illness. The obstruction, of course, is unaffected as is the carbon dioxide concentration in the blood, but the anoxia is relieved with a consequent improvement in cerebral nutrition and thus in the general condition of the patient. The dyspnoea gradually lessens as the frequency of respiratory movements diminishes and their amplitude increases. The physical strain of the illness is thus to some extent eased and the cardiac embarrassment consequent upon exertion mitigated. However, some attempt must be made to loosen the membrane and facilitate its expulsion. Steam inhalations of pine or benzoin should be tried and may be successful in less severe cases. If the membrane is massive and extensive, severe obstruction and cyanosis may supervene in spite of these measures. Active steps to secure an airway are then necessary and should not be delayed. The choice lies between repeated bronchoscopic removal and aspiration, intubation of the larynx or tracheostomy. Although the first of these measures is mechanically effective, it involves considerable disturbance of the child, however well organized and however skilful the technique, and may prove too exhausting. The choice between intubation and tracheostomy largely depends upon the skill with which the former can be performed as well as the readiness with which the tube can be replaced if coughed up. Intubation can be indirectly achieved with O'Dwyer's instruments—a method that has stood the test of half a century—or a tube such as is used by anaesthetists can be inserted under direct vision through a laryngoscope. Practice will determine the choice of method, as will the availability of the different instruments and of technical assistance, but in either case a suction tube cannot easily be introduced into the trachea, and this is a most important part of the subsequent treatment. For these reasons tracheostomy is generally preferable. The opening must be made as low as possible, through or below the second ring of the trachea, and the operation is more easily performed if a bronchoscope is first inserted and kept in position. A nurse must subsequently pass a soft rubber catheter connected with a source of suction through the tracheostomy cannula and clear the brochial tree at frequent intervals. If the secretions become too crusted or viscid for removal in this way, it is a comparatively simple matter to pass a bronchoscope through the tracheostomy opening and remove the obstruction under direct vision with the sucker or forceps. Crusting can be lessened by moisture, and a few drops of warm saline solution should be introduced through the tracheostomy tube from time to time as necessary and followed by suction. It helps to tie a layer or two of damp muslin round the neck to hang over the opening of the tube. This phase of the illness may last a week or more and demands the most meticulous and intelligent nursing as well as shrewd medical judgment. It is particularly important to delay decannulation or closure of the tracheostomy until it is certain that the infection has resolved. Complications are usually serious and adversely affect the prognosis, but they do not as a rule demand any deviation, other than the purely symptomatic, from the treatment described.

OEDEMA OF THE LARYNX

This is a wide term applied to a condition of oedematous infiltration in the loose corium of the larynx and may be due to local or general causes.

Aetiology

In marked and dangerous degree the condition is uncommon, but the lesser manifestations are fairly frequent. Two groups can be recognized, the infective and non-infective. The former is by a long way the larger group and can itself be subdivided into primary or secondary infections of the larynx. However, as already described, there is no clear line of demarcation since acute laryngitis usually occurs during the natural history of a host of acute upper respiratory tract infections and is only sometimes an entity. In every such case oedema is present to some extent although rarely of clinical significance. Oedema of the larynx is thus occasionally a complication of acute laryngitis. The various responsible predisposing conditions have been discussed, but there are, in addition, certain others such as quinsy, Ludwig's angina and retropharyngeal abscess and, in children, acute zymotic disease and influenza. Acute pyogenic invasion may occur in granulomatous, neoplastic or other ulcerations of the larynx, and tuberculosis occasionally assumes a subacute oedematous form. In this category can also be included the oedema secondary to the perichondritis of syphilis or irradiation, or to irradiation alone. The second group includes angioneurotic oedema, constitutional diseases with fluid exudation such as nephritis and cardiac failure, and reactions occasionally caused by iodides and acetylsalicylates. Direct wounding of the larynx may be responsible as may the indirect trauma of ingested irritants, caustics, hot fluids or alcohol, the inhalation of noxious gases or fumes, vocal abuse or excessive tobacco, operations in the neighbourhood of the larynx or on unerupted molars, or the nearby lodgment of foreign bodies.

PLATE II

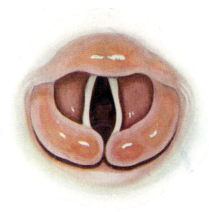

(a)

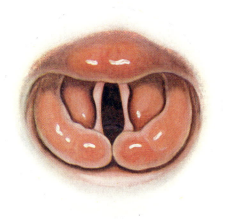

(b)

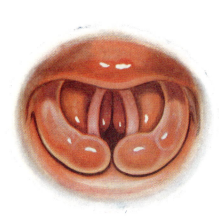

(c)

Acute laryngitis: (a) an early stage showing hyperaemia of the aryepiglottic folds, arytenoids, epiglottis and ventricular bands; (b) a later stage with deepening congestion and swelling of the structures in (a) and noticeable hyperaemia of the vocal cords; (c) a severe and very late stage, the whole larynx is uniformly dusky red and the subglottic tissues are also congested and oedematous—so-called "mounding".

PLATE III

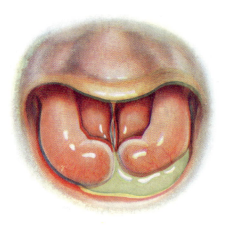

Radio-necrosis and perichondritis with abscess formation. The inflammatory infiltration and oedema almost occluded the airway and a tracheotomy was necessary.

Pathology

The essential change is an effusion of fluid into the loose tissues of the corium and submucosa chiefly affecting those areas where the mucosa is most loosely attached to the underlying cartilages or membranes, namely, the aryepiglottic folds, vestibule and, occasionally, the subglottic tissues. Where infection or trauma is responsible, the onset of this oedema takes an appreciable time, perhaps even days, and can be predicted and faced with awareness. In cases of angioneurotic oedema the onset may be of dramatic, even fatal, rapidity. Angioneurotic oedema is sometimes herediatry but, although it is probably an allergic or hypersensitivity reaction, other allergic manifestations are uncommon. It is similar to urticaria, but the reaction is more delayed and occurs in more deeply seated tissues. In all cases crusting or secretion may encroach upon and further restrict the airway.

Symptoms

Although the oedema may be due to a chronic cause the onset of symptoms is usually sudden as the constriction attains a certain threshold value of size. Hoarseness amounting to aphonia and rapidly increasing stridor and dyspnoea then supervene. Cough and pain are usually absent. If the oedema is largely vestibular or supraglottic, the breathing is stertorous; in glottic or subglottic obstruction it is more muffled and high pitched. Associated with the dyspnoea the patient is at first ashy-grey and later cyanotic. The respiratory embarrassment is otherwise evident by indrawing at the suprasternal notch, epigastrium, intercostal spaces and around the clavicles. In allergic cases there may be subcutaneous swellings on the hands, feet and face, or other manifestations in the gastro-intestinal tract.

Physical signs

On mirror examination the oedema is readily seen. When the cause is inflammatory and acute, the surface of the mucous membrane is reddened and congested. Non-inflammatory oedema is characterized by a pale, grey, shiny, sodden mucosa, and one side of the larynx may be more affected than the other. During this examination an estimate must be formed of the size of the glottic chink and the further degree of obstruction of the lumen still likely or possible, since it is on such a judgment that energetic treatment will largely depend.

Prognosis

The immediate outlook depends on the amount of obstruction and the promptness with which it is relieved. The onset of cyanosis, indicating a late stage of asphyxia, is a grave sign. More remotely the prognosis rests upon the cause of the oedema and it is clearly poor if there is an underlying serious constitutional disease.

Treatment

Relief of the obstruction is essential and may be achieved by the treatment of the primary cause or by measures applied locally to the larynx. On the first count the assistance of a physician will often be helpful to decide both the diagnosis and the appropriate measures. In other cases the timely evacuation of a neighbouring collection of pus or the removal of a foreign body may be indicated.

If allergy is the cause, a hypodermic injection of adrenaline may abort or reduce the swelling, while resolution may be assisted by antihistamine drugs, Phenergan or Thephorin, or ephedrine by mouth. Local treatment may be useful whether or not the primary cause is determined or treatable. To a large extent it follows the same lines as that for acute laryngotracheitis but, in addition, the laryngeal obstruction may be relieved by a spray of 1·0 or 2·0 per cent cocaine mixed with an equal quantity of 0·1 per cent adrenaline, and in this strength the spary may be repeated every four hours. The oxygen tent is an almost essential part of treatment when there is even the slightest stridor. The dyspnoea may be so urgent that the immediate re-establishment of an airway is essential, and the choice between intubation and tracheostomy must then be made. The factors governing this choice have already been discussed and require no further amplification except a renewed insistence upon the dangers of vacillation and delay. Once the patient has reached the stage of even slight cyanosis his expectation of life may be counted in hours and few even of those. It is justifiable and even desirable to place him in an oxygen tent while preparing for intubation or tracheostomy, but emphasis cannot be too strongly laid upon the disasters awaiting indecision.

ACUTE PERICHONDRITIS OF THE LARYNX

The space between the enveloping perichondrial membrane of the larynx and the cartilages is occasionally the site of infection. This condition is difficult, if not impossible, to separate from that due to infection of the cartilage itself, and both are usually present together. Very rarely the invasion is acute and primary, and is then usually due to a streptococcal infection. Most cases, however, are secondary; a few occur acutely, often with abscess formation, as a complication of an acute exanthem, but most are chronic and arise insidiously during the course of a pyogenic or granulomatous infection or of a neoplasm. The chronic form sometimes follows irradiation, "high tracheostomy" performed through the cricoid cartilage, or direct external trauma to the larynx with or without fracture of the cartilages.

The primary form

The primary form generally arises suddenly as a severe pain in the larynx which may be worse on swallowing, The temperature is raised to 37·8°C or more, and the patient is ill. In addition, he has a strained look, partly due to the pain but also because of his anxiety over his breathing. The cervical tissues superficial to the larynx are oedematous and deep palpation is extremely painful. The framework of the larynx becomes so hard and rigid that respiratory movements set up a vibration which can be felt on light palpation. After some hours the clinical picture changes as the infection develops either to a diffuse or circumscribed variety.

Diffuse infection

The diffuse variety is very rare and nearly always fatal from the combined toxaemia and respiratory obstruction. It is characterized by apparently complete and rapid disappearance of the thyroid cartilage before any localization and pus formation can occur. The local pain becomes more and more severe, especially on swallowing, and the patient passes through the stages of increasing toxaemia—sweating, dehydration, tachycardia and high fever, and also increasing asphyxia, and anoxaemia followed by deepening cyanosis and exhaustion. The cervical tissues over the larynx become oedematous, reddened and adherent, and indirect laryngoscopy, if practicable, shows similar mucosal changes. Tracheostomy is followed by descending infection and mediastinitis and thus cannot be performed to relieve the respiratory obstruction.

Treatment.—The treatment consists in early recognition of the imminent grave danger and the exhibition of massive doses of both penicillin and sulphonamide drugs, the latter preferably in a soluble form intravenously. As swallowing is difficult, if not impossible, a saline infusion must be given and maintained. The rationale is to induce localization of the infection, meanwhile maintaining the patient's strength, and with advances in chemotherapy the prognosis has undoubtedly improved.

Circumscribed infection

The circumscribed variety is much less severe than the former, and is rarely fatal. The infection usually involves the thyroid cartilage, although sometimes the cricoid cartilage is affected. The temperature usually falls and the laryngeal pain localizes to the area attacked. The patient's general condition may improve a little as compared with that in the invasive stage, and both swallowing and breathing may become easier. An irritating and exhausting cough frequently develops, and the voice has a muffled or croaking sound. A tender and often red swelling develops in the neck, localized to the area of cartilage involved and, in addition to the generalized redness and oedema, a similar intralaryngeal swelling may be visible on indirect laryngoscopy. The symptoms and signs may all gradually subside as the infection resolves, and this likelihood is increased by chemotherapy. A localized residual abscess may form.

Treatment.—The treatment is exactly the same as for the diffuse type of infection until abscess formation occurs. Subsequent measures are discussed in the section "Abscess of the Larynx" (*see* below).

The secondary form

Chronic infection in the perichondrial membrane may follow an acute infection, but it is usually secondary to chronic disease inside the larynx, and is rarely an isolated event. The precursory diseases have been enumerated above, and in the relevant articles dealing with these diseases an account is given of the clinical features and the approrpriate treatment in each type of case.

ABSCESS OF THE LARYNX

Aetiology

This is a comparatively rare condition compared with the extreme frequency of non-suppurative inflammations. The most usual cause at one time was typhoid fever, but this disease is now rather uncommon. Other causes are the acute exanthems, erysipelas, pyogenic infection following influenza, and, rarely, agranulocytosis and mononucleosis. An abscess may form in more chronic conditions for instance, tuberculosis, syphilis or gonorrhoea, especially if there is a super-added pyogenic infection. The most frequent of all chronic precursors is perichondritis (rarely chondritis) due to one of the above infections, malignant disease or radiotherapy. Occasionally in elderly patients, in whom ossification in the thyroid or cricoid cartilage is not infrequent, osteomyelitis may occur complicated by abscess formation. Other causes are secondary infection following direct trauma from without, or injury resulting from an ingested or inhaled foreign body. Infection reaches the larynx either by direct extension from neighbouring structures or by the blood stream.

Pathology

Whatever the underlying cause, the formation of an abscess in the larynx involves the same pathological processes as elsewhere in the body. The collection of pus begins either in the submucosa where the vascular and lymphatic plexuses are situated, or under the perichondrium, depending upon the aetiology. Swellings may therefore occur anywhere inside the larynx or sometimes on the external surface of the thyroid cartilage. There is always some measure of oedema of the surrounding tissues and this may occasionally result in respiratory difficulty. After evacuation and drainage of the pus resolution may be complete, but if the infection has involved cartilage portions slough away as sequestra, leaving various residual deformities. Among the more serious of these is laryngeal stenosis and ankylosis of the crico-arytenoid joint. The cricoid cartilage is only rarely affected.

Symptoms and signs

Apart from the symptoms of the exciting causes those due to the abscess itself are pain and respiratory difficulties. During the stage of formation of an acute abscess pain is marked and usually well localized. There is often a referred earache. If the lesion is in the posterior portion of the larynx there is pain on deglutition and perhaps dysphagia, or at least a sensation of a lump or a "tickle in the throat" which cannot be removed by swallowing. As a result, a thick mucoid salivation may be a prominent feature. The space occupied by the abscess itself and the accompanying oedema result in some measure of respiratory obstruction which may amount to asphyxia. Cough is almost invariably due to the presence of the lump and also to the sticky intralaryngeal secretion. Hoarseness of some degree is a constant feature for the same reasons. The local condition seldom causes much constitutional disturbance or fever although some of the more acute precursory events may be accompanied by a great deal of both. If the abscess is large and involves neighbouring structures, trismus or spasm of various cervical muscle groups occurs. The larynx is usually tender on palpation even with an intralaryngeal abscess; with a perilaryngeal involvement induration or sometimes a fluctuating external swelling is present. There is usually some enlargement of the deep cervical glands.

Laryngoscopy

On indirect laryngoscopy the site of the abscess may be revealed by a localized area of more intense redness even before an actual swelling is visible. This congested area becomes progressively more boggy and orange-coloured. Abscesses formed in association with the thyroid cartilage are the most common and are usually present in the pyriform fossae, often beginning as a swelling of the lateral wall of the fossa but sometimes of the floor. Exceptionally, however, such abscesses may point in the anterior commissure, on a ventricular band or below the cords. When the cricoid cartilage is involved the abscess appears behind the interarytenoid space (*see* Plate III). These collections of pus and the surrounding oedema may cause grotesque abnormalities of vocal cord movements. An oozing, ulcerated area indicates the site of spontaneous evacuation of the abscess. When doubt exists even after a careful mirror examination, direct laryngoscopy is necessary. Oedematous tissues can then be pressed aside and a more careful search made.

Differential diagnosis

The chief confusing conditions are retropharyngeal abscess, laryngeal cyst or new growth. Abscesses presenting externally must be differentiated from suppurative cervical adenitis or infection in a thyroglossal cyst. Although there is some superficial similarity none of these conditions should really present any distinguishing difficulty if a careful appraisal of the history and physical signs is made—providing the possibility of a laryngeal abscess is remembered.

Treatment

Apart from the treatment of the cause the condition itself may require special measures in certain circumstances. If there is any danger of asphyxia tracheostomy is necessary independently of any attempt to evacuate the abscess. Incision of an intralaryngeal abscess can be performed indirectly with the laryngeal mirror using a curved laryngeal scalpel after anaesthetizing the larynx with applications of 5–10 per cent cocaine. A more precise operation is possible by direct laryngoscopy under magnification and the use of a long straight knife and suction. This is the procedure of choice, with local cocaine anaesthesia or intravenous sodium thiopentone muscle relaxant, and intubation. Abscesses of any extent involving cartilage, even if not pointing externally, are best treated by external incision and free removal of necrotic cartilage. An abscess lying deep to the thyroid cartilage and not easily drained by direct laryngoscopy should be treated by an external approach and the removal of a window of overlying cartilage. In the special case of multiple abscesses with cartilage necrosis following irradiation, total laryngectomy may become necessary. This operation then presents unusual difficulties and dangers due to the combined devitalizing effect of the irradiation and the infection. The author has found in these cases that no pre-laryngeal tissue should be left since it invariably dies, and further that a deliberate pharyngostome should be created to facilitate subsequent plastic closure.

Prognosis

If the condition is recognized and treated there should be no danger to life, but subsequent fibrosis, especially when there has been necrosis of cartilage, may result in stenosis. This may also occur from infection of the crico-arytenoid joint with resulting ankylosis.

HERPES OF THE LARYNX

This is a very rare condition and is usually accompanied by a similar involvement of the buccal cavity, pharynx and sometimes lips, presumably due to the same virus. The symptoms begin with an unpleasant pricking sensation in the throat which soon becomes a real pain in the larynx more marked on swallowing. There may be slight hoarseness and perhaps a little fever. Mirror examination will reveal a number of small vesicles with a surrounding zone of congestion. They are at first discrete but later become confluent. The surface of the vesicles then sloughs away leaving a shallow, irregularly shaped ulcer. The epiglottis, arytenoids, aryepiglottic folds and posterior wall of the vestibule of the larynx are the usual sites.

Differential diagnosis

The differential diagnosis from smallpox or chicken-pox is readily made on the more general character of these diseases. Pemphigus occasionally occurs in the pharynx, but the vesiculation is more widespread and on a larger scale. The monilia sometimes cause blisters but are recognizable on microscopic examination.

Treatment

No specific treatment is known so that therapy must be symptomatic to relieve pain along lines already fully described. The disease always resolves and owing to the superficial character of the lesion there is no residual scarring.

MEMBRANOUS LARYNGITIS

This, too, is a rare condition and consists of an acute inflammation of the larynx accompanied by membrane formation. It is also known as croup or pseudo-membranous croup. It is not due to the Klebs–Loeffler bacillus but to the streptococcus, pneumococcus, *Bacillus pyocyaneus* or Vincent's organisms. Occasionally it results from chemical (gaseous) irritation with secondary infection. The disease occurs in infancy or early childhood often as a complication of zymotic disease, and exposure to cold and damp are important factors.

Pathology

The membrane consists of a yellowish surface epithelium set on a layer of fibrous tissue, and it is only loosely attached to the laryngeal mucosa. When removed no bleeding occurs and no ulceration remains. It is presumably formed by the desquamation of a rapidly proliferating epithelium. It occurs on the aryepiglottic folds and in the vestibule—less frequently on the vocal cords. It can spread from above as part of a Vincent's infection of the pharynx, but most commonly it is confined to the larynx and is accompanied by a generalized congestion of the hypopharynx.

Symptoms

The onset suggests acute laryngitis. There is usually some febrile constitutional disturbance with anorexia and also thirst. The skin is dry and hot and the temperature may reach 38·9° or 39·4°C. Swallowing is painful. Cough is always a marked feature and is later followed by laryngeal spasm and dyspnoea due to the expulsive efforts to get rid of the obstructing membrane. It is then that the inspiratory croup is manifest. If the condition progresses asphyxia may supervene. The physical signs have already been indicated in the discussion of the pathology and are clearly seen in the laryngeal mirror or on direct laryngoscopy.

Differential diagnosis

The disease must chiefly be differentiated from diphtheria which it often markedly resembles. Laryngoscopy and the removal of a piece of membrane are essential. The histological examination of this may be sufficient, but a bacteriological investigation should always be made and will almost invariably establish the diagnosis. Clinical examination revealing the presence of membrane suffices to distinguish the disease from all forms of acute laryngitis and other causes of stridor.

Treatment

As the organisms responsible are usually sensitive to the sulphonamides and penicillin, these drugs should be given in adequate doses. If the organism proves resistant, tetracyclines or, rarely, chloramphenicol must be substituted, preferably on the results of bacteriological examination of sensitivity. The treatment otherwise is the same as for laryngotracheobronchitis.

Prognosis

Modern chemotherapy has altered the outlook considerably. The younger the child the worse the outlook because of the increased likelihood of asphyxia. At one time the disease was fatal in nearly 50 per cent of cases, but death should now be exceptional if the condition is recognized reasonably early in its course.

DIPHTHERIA OF THE LARYNX

This is a special form of acute laryngitis due to the *Corynebacterium diphtheriae* or Klebs–Loeffler bacillus and characterized by the formation of a membrane on the affected areas. It usually spreads from the pharynx, but it may be the sole lesion. It is an ancient disease and probably formed the bulk of the cases known as "croup".

Aetiology

The disease is endemic with epidemic phases. Local outbreaks often occur unassociated with any general increase in incidence. A seasonal increase occurs during the autumn and winter. Children under 15 years are chiefly affected, the ages between 1 and 5 years bearing the brunt, and the mortality diminishes with increasing age. During the past few years there has been an enormous decrease in the number of cases and a decline in the severity of the infection. It is nowadays a rare disease in the United Kingdom.

Bacteriology

The disease is due to a bacillus. The body of the organism contains a varying number of granules which stain differently from the rest of the organism with Neisser's methylene. When cultured from smears the bacilli grow in a curious arrangement suggesting Chinese characters. Other and non-pathogenic corynebacteria, the diphtheroids, are frequently found in the upper respiratory tract and have a very similar, sometimes indistinguishable, morphology. Further tests are then required. These are the fermentation reactions with sugars, the behaviour of colonies of growth on selective tellurite media and the biological estimation of virulence. The second of these methods can also be extended to yield information concerning the type of diphtheria organism itself, for the varying appearance of colonies on tellurite media corresponds closely to strains known as gravis, intermedius and mitis. The gravis strain is further differentiated from the other two by fermenting starch. Upon the strain or organism involved largely depends the severity of the case of diphtheria, although the individual's own resistance plays some part. It is important to know the strain chiefly responsible in an outbreak before arranging the necessary combative measures. The virulence of any organism is finally determined biologically by the injection of suspensions of the bacteria mixed with

327

antitoxin into the skin of a guinea-pig's abdomen. Toxigenic strains can also be recognized by a gel-precipitin test in which diphtheria toxin interacts with its homologous antitoxin to form a precipitate. The incubation period varies from two to four days, but may be as little as 24 hours or as much as six days. The disease is spread by air-borne droplets or by fomites. There can be direct contact from a patient by the reception of his discharges into a vulnerable part of the body, or indirect contact to remote persons by contamination of food or from infected domestic animals. However, the most usual source of infection is from carriers who are of two types—the convalescent carrier and the contact carrier. The former individual is actually convalescent from a known attack of the disease, but continues to harbour the C. *diphtheriae* at or near the site of the infection 12 weeks after the condition has subsided clinically (this time is arbitrarily chosen and serves as a convenient epidemiological standard). The latter individual may again be of two types—a Schick "positive", that is susceptible, or Schick "negative", immune person. The former acquires a latent and transient infection, never becoming clinically apparent and lasting only a few hours or days. He does not usually constitute a source of infection to others. The latter may carry the organism for months or years and is exceedingly difficult to detect. He is the chief source of infection and, especially if he carries the gravis strain, tends to be a persistent one. The organisms for the most part are carried in the nose or throat or both places, usually in lymphoid tissue which is involved either in bulk, as in the tonsils or adenoids, or diffusely throughout its distribution in the corium, whence bacilli are extruded into the normal mucus secretions. This is why they are occasionally present in aural discharges.

Diagnosis and treatment of carriers

Carriers are diagnosed by the presence of virulent organisms in an apparently normal person, and the chief aim is to detect and treat the Schick-negative chronic persistent type. The detection consists in routine bacteriological examination as already discussed. In treatment, when discrete lymphoid tissue (the tonsil particularly) is affected, surgical eradication is easy and the results excellent. Adenoidectomy is not quite so successful; and when the nasal or sinus mucosa harbours the bacilli both surgical and conservative measures become more difficult and relapse is common. There is, however, a case for the routine removal of tonsils and adenoids from all recovered cases of diphtheria.

Pathology

After alighting on the mucosa the bacilli multiply on the surface while their exotoxins diffuse more deeply. The body repair mechanism responds with its usual hyperaemia and exudation which therefore occur chiefly in the more superficial layers of the mucosa. This process results in the formation of a membrane consisting of fibrin and leucocytes in which the organisms are trapped. If the infection involves stratified squamous epithelium the superficial, cornified layers necrose and, with engorged capillaries, are caught up in the membrane which can then only be detached with some difficulty, leaving a bleeding surface. Membrane soon reforms on this area. Over ciliated epithelium the attachment is loose. Detachment is easy and not accompanied by bleeding. In the larynx, therefore, membrane can be of both varieties, but the loosely attached variety is more usually responsible for obstruction and cough and is hence called croupous. The membrane is greyish-white in appearance, but may be brown or even black if there has been haemorrhage into it. The consistency also varies somewhat and although usually tough may be friable. Occasionally, because of underlying thrombophlebitis, it sloughs away together with portions of the mucous membrane giving rise to so-called "gangrenous diphtheria".

The toxin produced by the organisms is absorbed into the lymphatic and vascular systems. The degree of toxaemia depends partly on the strain of bacillus responsible and partly on the site of infection. Absorption is a direct function of the amount of membrane and its adherence, and since this latter depends on the type of mucosa involved it follows that toxaemia from pharyngeal lesions is usually greater than that from laryngeal ones. The toxin is rapidly disseminated, and equally rapidly and irreversibly taken up by the tissues. They are all damaged by it, but cardiac muscle and nervous structures are markedly susceptible. The myocarditis, consisting of cellular degeneration of an acute type with hyaline and fatty changes and oedema, has no specific features. Nerves exhibit the changes of a toxic peripheral invasion with rapid fatty demyelinization, and those chiefly involved are associated with the site of the lesion, especially the ninth and tenth cranial nerves. The interference with general metabolism occasioned by the tissue damage is measurable by sugar tolerance tests and others which thus serve as a laboratory index of the severity of the attack.

Symptoms

In general, the clinical course of the disease, especially the tonsillar and pharyngeal type, is roughly divisible into three stages—an initial stage of general toxaemia and a local lesion lasting about a week; a week of circulatory disorders; and an uncertain period up to seven weeks in which paralyses may appear. In mild attacks nothing but the first stage may occur, whereas in more severe cases all three stages supervene although the time relations may show considerable variation. Often either the second or third stage is inconspicuous or absent; for example, after an apparently quite mild attack with a brief first stage, paralyses may appear in the fifth or sixth week. However, such variations are uncommon, and in general the frequency of remote manifestations varies with the severity of the first stage.

In pure laryngeal involvement toxaemia is not great and the second and third stages are therefore not clearly marked and may not even occur at all. The local lesion is of paramount importance, and the clinical picture is of an acute upper respiratory tract infection which rapidly seems to settle down in the larynx. The chief symptoms are pyrexia and malaise with some hoarseness and an irritant cough. Membrane formation then begins, and as it accumulates, together with vascular congestion and muscle spasm, the hoarseness increases sometimes to the point of aphonia, while the cough becomes dry and short as well as paroxysmal and exhausting. Respiration is wheezy and an inspiratory whistle or stridor develops. The respiratory difficulty is shown by recession of the supraclavicular fossae and epigastrium. As anoxaemia progresses cyanosis and restlessness appear. All these symptoms occur in bouts. The final stages are characterized by briefer intervals between the paroxysms, which themselves become more violent, with deepening cyanosis until at last the child dies of cardiac failure either already unconscious and stuporose or during a convulsion. In very severe cases the disease extends into the trachea, and even into the bronchi, with consequent exaggeration of the respiratory embarrassment.

Diagnosis and differential diagnosis

In any case of acute laryngitis several features may lead to a suspicion that one is really confronted with laryngeal diphtheria, notably the presence of membrane in the pharynx or nose, a foetor peculiar to this infection, or paroxysms of asphyxia. As the patient is usually a small child or infant direct laryngoscopy is necessary, although this may reveal no membrane but only the changes of a severe acute infection. However, the examination by smear and culture of aspirated secretions should reveal the true state of affairs even in the absence of membrane, while similar investigation of this latter is usually conclusive. It is the presence of membrane with consequent exaggeration of obstructive signs that differentiates laryngeal diphtheria from other forms of acute laryngitis.

In both membranous laryngitis and acute laryngotracheobronchitis there are certain similarities, but the bacteriological findings are diagnostic. When laryngeal diphtheria is an extension of a pharyngeal involvement a distinction must be made from acute follicular tonsillitis, quinsy, Vincent's angina, leukaemia and agranulocytosis, and again a bacteriological examination is imperative and diagnostic.

Treatment

As in all acute infections the first and essential step is to neutralize the toxin which is still not yet anchored to the cells susceptible to its action. It is the circulating toxin which here causes the damage and, as already explained, it reaches and combines with the tissues extremely rapidly. Specific treatment must thus be begun as early as possible and consists of intramuscular or intravenous administration of the antitoxin. The benefit conferred by the first dose far outweighs that of subsequent injections. It is better therefore to err on the generous side with this dose and ensure an effective blood concentration as swiftly as possible. As a working rule, using refined serum, up to 10,000 units should be given to mild cases, from 15,000 to 30,000 units to moderate cases, and as much as 100,000 units to severe cases. When large doses—20,000 units and upwards—are given the intravenous route is preferable. In grading cases it must be remembered that delay in coming under observation increases the hazards—any case presenting after the third day is late. Also the more severe the case the less time is available for serum therapy: in bad cases there may be no longer than 24 hours in which successfully to make the diagnosis and give antitoxin. It may sometimes be impossible to determine the precise bacteriological diagnosis in time, and in this event the clinical condition must be the guide to the giving of antitoxin. With modern enzyme-digested serum sensitization reactions are rare and the administration of antitoxin on suspicion need not be withheld for fear of such reactions. Strains of C. diphtheriae, especially of the mitis type, are usually sensitive to penicillin, which should always be given.

As has already been described laryngeal diphtheria is not characterized by toxaemia so much as by the local obstruction. Although the treatment of the latter is usually more pressing than that of the general symptoms, they must not be neglected. The child is generally best nursed flat or with one pillow and only gradually allowed a more upright position. Glucose and fluids should be pushed, and complications, which are chiefly cardiac and nervous, treated symptomatically. The most important preliminary measure in local treatment is a direct laryngoscopy both to establish the diagnosis with certainty and to clear the airway by aspiration. No anaesthetic is necessary in skilled hands and the discomfort should be slight. That part of the obstruction due to muscle spasm may be relieved by a steam kettle or by belladonna, and restlessness by sedatives such as chloral or bromides.

If it becomes clear that the airway is failing and must be re-established, several alternative measures are available in addition to aspiration by direct laryngoscopy. These measures have already been mentioned and their techniques and several merits discussed (*see* p. 319, and in Chapter 19). They are intubation, either by direct laryngoscopy or blindly, and tracheostomy. The latter is the more certain method, but the former is widely used particularly in the United States of America. It is immaterial which technique is employed provided only that the procedure is not delayed until obvious exhaustion and cardiac weakness have occurred.

Prophylaxis

The disease is preventable. Energetic measures of active immunization of the child population have in many places reduced the incidence enormously and together with early diagnosis and antitoxin treatment have removed the disease from its high place as a frequent and serious, often fatal, infection of childhood.

Prognosis

Laryngeal diphtheria, when it occurs, has a definite mortality, especially in early childhood. However, with prompt and efficient treatment recovery should be the rule.

14

CHRONIC LARYNGITIS

MAXWELL ELLIS

TUBERCULOSIS OF THE LARYNX

Aetiology

Tuberculosis of the larynx may be secondary to tuberculous lesions elsewhere in the body or a primary affection from inhaled tubercle bacilli. Most authorities are agreed that the former is the usual method and that the latter is very rare. The source of infection is nearly always pulmonary although it need not be an open lesion.

Incidence

There has unquestionably been an immense decline in the incidence of the affection during the past few years, not only in Great Britain but all over the world. Whereas 40 years ago laryngeal tuberculosis was found in 25–30 per cent of cases of pulmonary tuberculosis, in 1941 the percentage was 3–6, and it is now rare. This is probably the result of the earlier diagnosis and the more efficient methods of treatment of pulmonary tuberculosis, as well as of its diminishing incidence. In addition, the laryngological examination of any case presenting symptoms indicative of involvement is now an almost universal routine technique in the management of cases of tuberculosis. Catarrhal laryngeal lesions which might otherwise have progressed to tuberculous ones are thus discovered early and treated.

Sex

There is no special sex incidence. At one time males were rather more prone to the disease than females, possibly because of their more active and exposed lives, but this social distinction and its pathological counterpart are disappearing.

Age

The disease is most common between the ages of 20 and 40 years, perhaps because pulmonary tuberculosis then has its heaviest incidence. It was thought to be rare in children, but more frequent and careful examinations have shown this to be an error.

Occupation

It cannot be said that any special occupations predispose towards laryngeal tuberculosis. Undoubtedly exposure to certain dusts as well as to weather may lead to pulmonary lesions, but not markedly to laryngeal ones; this also applies to environment and social and economic factors, as well as to race, upper respiratory tract disease and indulgence in alcohol and tobacco.

Pregnancy

Undoubtedly, however, pregnancy has the same accelerating effect on the extension of the laryngeal lesion as it has on the pulmonary lesion.

Pathology

This is best considered under the headings of: (1) pathways of infection; (2) histology; and (3) topography.

Pathways of infection

It has already been noted that the infection reaches the larynx from a pulmonary lesion—usually an active one. The actual pathway of invasion is a matter of some doubt. The possible routes are: (*a*) contact of sputum containing tubercle bacilli; (*b*) blood-borne or lymph-borne bacilli deposited locally; and (*c*) hypersensitivity, that is, an allergic tissue reaction.

Contact of sputum containing tubercle bacilli.—When sputum is coughed up it tends to remain in contact with certain parts of the larynx. In the interarytenoid region and the ventricles the mucosa is thrown up into folds and sputum is easily caught and retained in the crevices, until removed by swallowing or expelled by coughing. The supine position to some extent intensifies stagnation. Tubercle bacilli in the secretion can gain the depths of the mucosa through unbroken surface epithelium, but may do so more easily if abrasions are present. This mechanism does not entirely explain why tuberculous lesions are rare in the bronchi and trachea or why they occur in the larynx in the absence of sputum. Conversely, the larynx is often unaffected in cases in which sputum is copious, indicating that some further and as yet unknown factor is necessary.

Blood-borne or lymph-borne bacilli deposited locally.—The cases in which tuberculous laryngitis occurs in the absence of sputum are explicable on the assumption that the tubercle bacilli are carried in the submucous lymphatic or vascular networks from the site of the pulmonary infection. They leave these channels and are deposited in the submucosa of the larynx.

Hypersensitivity.—It has been shown by Koch (Pagel and colleagues, 1964) that certain tuberculous lesions are allergic reactions, that is, the reaction of hypersensitive tissue to the introduction of an antigen. The usual antigen is a sudden multiplication of tubercle bacilli which may result from the non-specific stimulus of constitutional diseases, like diabetes mellitus, or of endocrine changes, as in puberty, pregnancy and the puerperium. Tuberculous lesions tend to progress rapidly in these conditions, and pathologically the deterioration is due to the rapid liquefaction of the infected tissues which is a tuberculous allergic reaction. Certain of the oedematous lesions in the larynx may be of this type.

Histology

In whatever way the infection reaches the larynx it begins in the subepithelial cellular tissues with exudation followed by a round-cell infiltration and slight peripheral hyperaemia. This progresses to the formation of a tubercle consisting of a nodule of necrotic or caseous tissue surrounded by small lymphocytes and larger endothelial cells (some of which may coalesce into giant cells) and encompassed by a noticeable but not intense hyperaemic reaction. When a number of these tubercles are present, the mucosa presents a lumpy appearance and a varying degree of vascularity and oedema which is known as the stage of infiltration (*see* Plate IV*a*).

Confluence of these tubercles eventually leads to the death of the overlying epithelium from occlusion of blood vessels. This surface sloughing produces the stage of ulceration. The ulcers have thin ragged and undermined edges, often slightly congested, and the base is sloughy and contains foci of caseation; secondary infection then occurs. As a rule the ulcers are shallow, but they may extend more deeply and involve the cartilage or invade the crico-arytenoid joints. The perichondritis which thus occurs is usually confined to the epiglottis and arytenoids.

Tuberculosis is to some extent self-limiting and heals by fibrosis (*see* Plate IV*b*), and in lesions of slow growth the processes of invasion and resolution may be occurring simultaneously, leading, in rare cases, to the formation of a tumour-like nodule called a tuberculoma. Such a nodule may be sessile or pedunculated, more often the latter, and is generally found arising from the posterior portions of the larynx or from one or other of the vocal cords. In this slowly evolving type of invasion there sometimes occurs a pachydermatous tissue reaction in the inter-arytenoid region which may be confused clinically with the non-specific variety (*see* pp. 359–364). In any healed case much fibrosis is present, and the scarring may even lead to a degree of stenosis.

Slight oedema is part of a typical tuberculous reaction, but it is not usually a noticeable feature. Sometimes, however, the lesions are intensely oedematous and rapidly progressive, and are then perhaps allergic reactions as described above, due to the antigen of a rapid increase in the number of tubercle bacilli. As such an increase indicates a failing resistance, the appearance of the lesions augurs a bad prognosis, and they are often seen as terminal events.

In those cases in which the general disease has become widespread, miliary tubercles may be deposited anywhere in the larynx.

In general, apart from the obvious lesions, the laryngeal and also the pharyngeal and palatal mucosae are said to exhibit a characteristic pallor, but this is probably only the case in the absence of secondary infection. It is perhaps due to the combined effect of general anaemia and the obliteration of blood vessels in the corium by the spread of tuberculous granulation tissue in this layer.

Topography

This has been given a disproportionate importance in the literature. Minute descriptions of the percentage incidence of lesions in the different parts of the larynx really add nothing to the clinical picture of the disease and have relatively little place in the prognosis and treatment. In general terms it can be said that the evidences of tuberculous invasion are frequent and marked in those areas of the larynx equipped with stratified squamous epithelium, that is, the posterior portion, the vocal cords and the epiglottis. Lesions may appear in several different sites, and in any one case any of the various stages may be visibly in progress. Where there is a lax corium in which tuberculous granulation tissue can spread the lesion is apt to be bulky and ulceration relatively late. Such areas are the aryepiglottic folds and the ventricular bands. Where the epithelium is more tightly attached to the underlying membranes or cartilage, as on the vocal cords, arytenoid cartilages and epiglottis, ulceration occurs earlier.

Thus, thickening or an oedema-like appearance in the posterior part of the larynx, especially the interarytenoid space or over the arytenoids, should immediately arouse the suspicion of tuberculosis.

Symptoms

In the early stages of involvement a slight irritation low down in the throat may be felt together with some dryness which may give rise to an irritating clearing cough. Slight hoarseness then occurs, often only in the later part of the day. It may be independent of any visible lesion on the cords and is due to muscular weakness from infiltration and anaemia. Cough is usual for one reason or another; it is generally pulmonary in origin and also generally productive. There may also be some discomfort on swallowing, especially of solid food, if the aryepiglottic folds, arytenoids or epiglottis are involved. Localized pain together with referred earache are common symptoms.

These symptoms increase in severity as the lesions progress until in late stages the voice becomes a harsh whisper and there is an incessant, hard, productive cough due to the stasis of secretion in the larynx; pain in the larynx and hypopharynx and also shooting into the ear are prominent, and the dysphagia almost unbearable. If oedematous lesions are present, dyspnoea may be an additional misery. It must be stated, however, that in most parts of the world nowadays few cases reach this degree of severity.

Physical signs

Pallor of the soft palate, fauces and posterior pharyngeal wall is often a noticeable feature and is due to general anaemia.

One of the earliest recognizable features in the larynx is some interarytenoid thickening or enlargement of the posterior end of one aryepiglottic fold. Sometimes the epiglottis is attacked early and is seen to be turban-shaped. All these infiltrations are pale and soft and are accompanied by secretion. In known cases of tuberculosis undergoing routine laryngeal examinations the earliest sign may be slight congestion or discoloration of one vocal cord, a loss of tension or a weakness of adduction.

Various indirect laryngoscopic appearances have been described as "infiltro-oedematous", "fibro-ulcerative" or "ulcero-oedematous", but no special significance is conveyed by such a descriptive nomenclature, except as a means of focusing attention on the extent of the ulceration and the degree of oedema.

When the epiglottis is thickened and overhangs the glottis, direct laryngoscopy may be necessary to ascertain the presence or absence of further lesions. This should be performed in any doubtful case.

Diagnosis

In general, the pallor of the surrounding mucosa, the soft, greyish infiltrations, the shallow ulcers with thin undermined edges, and the distribution of the lesions are characteristic. In most cases clinical and radiological examination of the chest will reveal the primary source of the infection, and examination of the sputum, or of a laryngeal smear, will disclose tubercle bacilli.

Differential diagnosis

Infiltrative phases of the disease must be differentiated from the various types of chronic non-specific laryngitis and from scleroma, and the ulcerative forms may be confused with lupus vulgaris, syphilis or carcinoma. The points to observe are the relative vascularity and symmetrical appearance of chronic non-specific laryngeal lesions compared with tuberculous ones. The ulceration of syphilis or carcinoma is

PLATE IV

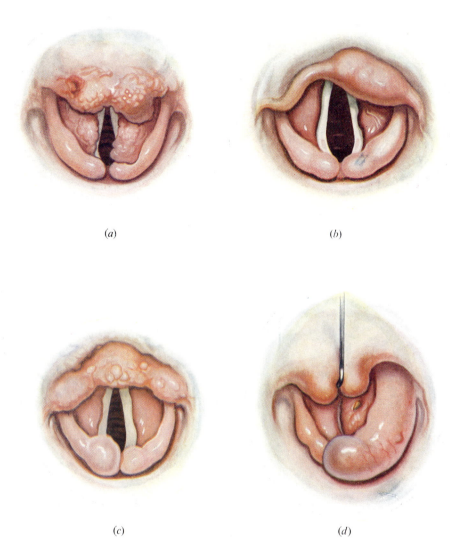

(a)

(b)

(c)

(d)

(a) Shows massive tuberculous infiltration of the epiglottis and ventricular bands with some destruction of the former. (b) Healed tuberculosis with massive fibrosis resulting in deformity, pallor and atrophy. (c) Lupus showing the fibrosis of healing over the arytenoids and aryepiglottic folds and persisting activity over the surface of the epiglottis. (d) Syphilis. A gummatous involvement of the whole of the left side of the larynx. The massive oedema of the arytenoid and aryepiglottic fold probably indicates subjacent perichondritis.

PLATE V

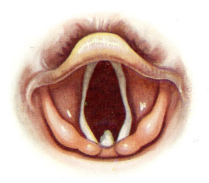

(*a*) Chronic localized hyperplastic laryngitis. Interarytenoid mass, paler than usual, and as it is not spreading to the vocal processes probably best classified as chronic localized hyperplasia.

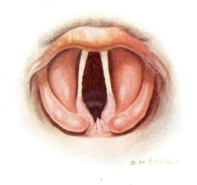

(*b*) Interarytenoid pachydermia. Pachydermatous proliferation in the interarytenoid region and spreading along both vocal processes. The membranous portions of the cords are slightly nodular on the upper surfaces, and the ventricular bands are somewhat thickened.

of a quite different nature, and the latter is rarely situated posteriorly except in advanced lesions. Lupus vulgaris is usually painless, and the lesions are not oedematous. The most important factor is the presence of a pulmonary lesion. When the diagnosis is still in doubt a biopsy is necessary.

Treatment

Throughout this description of laryngeal tuberculosis the connection between it and its pulmonary precursory condition has been reiterated. It must again be emphasized that the most important aspect of the treatment is that of the lungs. In addition, local measures may be needed both to assist healing and to relieve symptoms. Until recently these consisted of strict voice rest, cleansing sprays or soothing inhalations or local applications, and a number of more active procedures, to be mentioned later. The introduction of streptomycin (Feldman and Hinshaw, 1948) has, however, quite revolutionized this regimen and has made almost unnecessary nearly all the local measures which were at one time used in laryngeal tuberculosis.

Streptomycin

The tubercle bacillus is markedly sensitive to streptomycin, especially when combined with para-aminosalicylic acid. The former is given intramuscularly in doses of 0·5–1·0 g. and the latter orally in doses of 12·0 g. daily, continued for 60 days or even longer. Laryngeal pain when present rapidly disappears, and few lesions fail to resolve with this treatment.

Streptomycin in larger doses than those recommended (and in some patients even with these smaller doses) can have a toxic action on the vestibular portion of the inner ear or the vestibular nuclei. If a patient complains of the slightest sensation of giddiness, the drug must be discontinued at once. Longer administration may result in permanent damage, causing unsteadiness or vertiginous attacks when making even slight movements which may be extremely disabling. Cortical compensation usually occurs in time, but persisting ataxy is not uncommon. Fortunately, this toxic action can usually be noticed in time and the dosage reduced.

Naturally enough, biochemists have produced many drugs similar to streptomycin hoping to improve on its action and also to avoid its side-effects. One of these compounds, *dihydrostreptomycin*, unfortunately enjoyed a considerable vogue before it was discovered that it had a lethal action on the auditory portion of the inner ear. It is still made, but should never be prescribed.

Voice rest

The next most important measure is voice rest, and in any bad case this means absolute silence. The patient is provided with a pad and pencil and forbidden even to whisper. In less severe cases he is allowed to speak at certain times of the day.

Local applications

Numerous local applications have been advocated at different times, have enjoyed a vogue and then disappeared. The irritation and cough of a catarrhal exudate can be relieved by laryngeal sprays of alkaline solutions or of mineral oils containing chloretone or balsams, as in chronic laryngitis. Chaulmoogra oil has been used in this way for its analgesic action. With all oils the danger of lipoid pneumonia must be remembered. Lozenges and linctuses may also be helpful. Steam inhalations

337

containing pine preparations are soothing, but dry inhalations used with a Burney-Yeo inhaler are easier to handle and equally efficacious; spirits of cinnamon can be recommended.

The surface of ulcers can be painted with medicaments applied on a bent probe tipped with cotton-wool and introduced by indirect laryngoscopy. Among the drugs advocated are formaldehyde solutions, 0·5 per cent increasing to 10 per cent, and lactic acid, from 5 per cent to 30 per cent. Various cauterizing drugs such as chromic acid may be used in the same way after cocainization.

If pain and dysphagia are troublesome, equal parts of Orthoform and benzocaine powder can be insufflated into the larynx with a Leduc tube. The local anaesthesia so produced may last for a day, but the method is often unsuccessful. Lozenges containing cocaine or other analgesics, or direct spraying with these drugs, can be used in bad or advanced cases, but the effect soon disappears, even with increasing dosage, and their general action on the body is harmful.

When ulcerating areas become necrotic and secondarily infected the removal of fungating tissue may afford considerable relief. Under a local anaesthetic and preferably by direct laryngoscopy such tissue can be excised cleanly with punch forceps or gently curetted away. A tuberculoma causing any respiratory difficulty can be removed and a grossly diseased epiglottis amputated by the same techniques.

Galvanocautery

Infiltrated areas or small ulcers can be treated with the galvanocautery. Long bent applicators with distal cautery points turned in different directions are used under local anaesthesia; they are introduced by indirect laryngoscopy. The point is brought to white heat while held in the lumen of the larynx and then inserted into the area selected; if at white heat it is easily withdrawn again. It is introduced until an increase in resistance indicates healthy tissue. Several areas may be treated at a sitting. The intent is to limit spread of the disease and assist its healing by provoking fibrosis. The method is most successful in cases that seem at a standstill and appear to need something more to start them on the road to recovery, and it should not be used in acute cases or where the lesions are oedematous. The regions of the cricoarytenoid joints must be avoided because of the subsequent danger of cord fixation. Treatments can be repeated at monthly intervals.

Heliotherapy

Heliotherapy by the various carbon or quartz lamps, Finsen light and even the sun itself (reflected by an alloy material absorbing the heat rays) has had advocates, but the results have been indifferent.

Nerve injection or resection

When pain or dysphagia is intractable the superior laryngeal nerve can be injected with 80 per cent alcohol or 2 per cent Novocaine, or resected. If the head is extended to put the neck on the stretch, the nerve is almost subcutaneous where it passes into the thyrohyoid membrane between the great cornu of the hyoid bone and the superior cornu of the thyroid cartilage. A fine needle inserted into this area will reach the nerve at about 0·5–1·0 cm. from the skin. The location is determined by the patient who complains of pain shooting into the ear. The injection is performed with a local anaesthetic in the skin and with the index finger of the other hand behind the point of insertion of the needle to protect the vascular sheath. A few drops of alcohol are first injected to be sure that the needle point has not entered the larynx, and, if no coughing occurs, 1–2 ml. are slowly given. If the patient coughs the needle is withdrawn slightly and another trial made. The nerves on both sides may be treated at one sitting, but this should be avoided if possible. The anaesthesia lasts for several weeks and may be repeated. By using a short straight needle on a curved shaft and a laryngeal mirror, the nerve can also be injected in its course through the lateral wall of the pyriform sinus where it lies immediately under the mucous membrane. Section of the nerve offers no real advantage over a successful injection, as cases in which the procedure is needed at all are of poor prognosis. Section is performed under a local anaesthetic, such as infiltration with Novocaine, through an incision 2·5 cm. long, parallel to the hyoid bone and just below it and centred over the anterior border of the sternomastoid muscle. After the platysma and fascia are divided, the sternomastoid muscle and carotid sheath are retracted laterally and the omohyoid and sternohyoid muscles are retracted medially; the nerve then becomes visible on the lateral portion of the thyrohyoid membrane. It is here accompanied by a branch of the superior laryngeal artery from which it must be separated before being divided.

Referred earache may be treated by cocainizing the sphenopalatine ganglion.

Paralysis of the recurrent laryngeal nerve

There have been advocates of paralysing the recurrent laryngeal nerve in cases of strictly unilateral lesions in order to put this half of the larynx completely at rest. This procedure could scarcely be justified in early cases, and more advanced ones are rarely unilateral. The indications, if any are considered acceptable, must therefore be most uncommonly encountered. The nerve can be exposed in the neck after retracting the lateral lobe of the thyroid gland forward, and it is then divided, frozen with ethyl chloride or injected with 80 per cent alcohol. It can also be reached by blind injection alongside the first tracheal ring until the vertebral column is reached and then withdrawing the point of the needle 1–1·5 cm.

Operative measures

As final desperate measures gastrostomy for intractable dysphagia and tracheostomy for severe dyspnoea are available, but when the disease has reached this degree of severity the patient must have lost all resistance to the disease and be mortally ill from its ravages in other organs. When these operations have been performed, the results, as might be expected, have been almost uniformly bad.

General management

The management of cases of tuberculous laryngitis has in the past called for considerable experience and judgment in the use of the various forms of treatment available which have been briefly described above. However, the greatly lessened incidence of the disease and its earlier diagnosis, together with the administration of modern antibiotics has, within the last few years, completely altered the clinical picture and considerably reduced the active role of the laryngologist.

Prognosis

The outlook has nowadays been entirely transformed by the use of streptomycin, but even in the immediate few years before its introduction the earlier diagnosis of the lesion, and of the disease in general, together with the improvement in treatment of the pulmonary condition, had greatly improved matters. The prognosis is always dependent on the degree of pulmonary involvement, but, in addition, extensive ulceration or considerable oedema are of bad import. Other factors of adverse influence are copious sputum laden with tubercle bacilli, pregnancy, local complications such as perichondritis, or other extrapulmonary tuberculous lesions.

LUPUS VULGARIS OF THE LARYNX

This is a rare disease and, like tuberculosis of the larynx, is becoming even more rare. It is nearly always accompanied by active lesions in the nose or pharynx, but sometimes appears after such lesions have healed. It probably never occurs as a primary infection.

Pathology

The disease is probably an attenuated form of tuberculosis and the histological picture is very similar. However, the tissue reaction is less acute and oedema and hyperaemia are absent, but, on the other hand, the round-cell reaction is intense. These factors lead to superficial necrosis or ulceration, and also much fibrosis. To the naked eye the lesions are therefore grey in colour, ulceration is widespread but in small, discrete patches, the base of the ulcers is covered with scanty and viscid secretion, and much cicatrization is visible both in and around the areas of active disease (*see* Plate IV*c*).

The epiglottis is the most common site of invasion, but lesions are also found on the aryepiglottic folds, over the arytenoids and, sometimes, on the ventricular bands. The epiglottis is occasionally partly or wholly destroyed, but the other cartilages are almost never involved.

Symptoms and physical signs

The progress of the disease is so slow and painless that it may have occurred and healed spontaneously without having given rise to any noticeable symptoms, but usually some degree of hoarseness or cough or local discomfort is present. The disease is never painful and, indeed, local anaesthesia may occur even to the point of causing swallowing difficulties. The evidences of past or present lupus may be visible in the nose or pharynx, and in the larynx the superficial, grey, irregular lesions, the nibbled-away appearance of the epiglottis and the irregular scarring can be seen on mirror laryngoscopy.

The general health is often surprisingly unaffected, and there may be no demonstrable pulmonary or other tuberculous lesions.

Diagnosis

This condition can only be confused with tuberculosis, but from the description given the differences are sufficiently clear-cut except in certain cases of fibrogranuloma. Here the distinction may be so difficult that such cases have been labelled lupoid tuberculosis. A precise diagnosis is often only reached after a period of expectant treatment and exhaustive general investigations.

Treatment

Spontaneous healing is almost the natural tendency in the larynx, and indeed cases are occasionally encountered where routine examination of the larynx reveals destruction and scarring, almost certainly due to healed lupus, but with no laryngeal history. Cauterization of the edges of the lesions as described on page 338 assists resolution and is a valuable measure.

The patient should also be ordered the full benefits of fresh air, a full diet and such tonics as may seem to be indicated. In this connection the administration of calciferol (vitamin D_2) has been shown (Dowling, 1946) to have an almost specific effect on lupus. It is given in doses up to 150,000 International Units per day and may be continued for some months. However, calciferol in large doses acts as a decalcifying agent, and patients must take, in addition, at least two pints of milk a day. Even so, toxic effects, especially renal damage, are not unusual and a strict clinical and laboratory control must be exercised (Anning and colleagues, 1948).

Prognosis

As already indicated, the prognosis is good, as quite apart from any treatment the condition may heal spontaneously. Even severe lesions may be expected to heal with the administration of calciferol if the condition of the patient is otherwise favourable.

SYPHILIS OF THE LARYNX

This disease, at one time relatively common, has now become a rarity in the United Kingdom. Congenital lesions may occur, usually tertiary, about the time of puberty. In the primary and secondary stages of the disease, syphilis of the larynx is rarely diagnosed. There has been a progressive decline in all tertiary syphilitic manifestations for some years owing to the earlier diagnosis and to treatment with arsenical and bismuth compounds and, more recently, with penicillin. The disease is most common in middle or early adult life and males are more often affected than females.

Pathology

In the secondary stage, which occurs shortly after birth in congenital cases, mucous patches and condylomas may form on the laryngeal mucosa.

Tertiary syphilitic granulation tissue invades the mucous membrane by a peri-arteriolar infiltration. It occurs at first as a discrete nodule, the specific granuloma, consisting of a centre of amorphous, necrotic tissue surrounded by an exudate of plasma cells and lymphocytes with sometimes a few eosinophils and giant cells. At a later stage a fibrous reaction is prominent. These processes occurring in relation to the peripheral arteries result in an obliterative endarteritis with secondary necrosis of tissue. An accumulation of granulomas often forms a distinct mass which is known as a gumma.

These histological processes are visible in the larynx as gummatous swelling on the epiglottis or in the aryepiglottic folds, or more commonly as a diffuse infiltration which sooner or later ulcerates. The lesions have a slight predilection for the epiglottis and anterior portions of the larynx. When ulceration occurs it is nearly always deeply seated. The base of the ulcer contains a tenacious, yellow, necrotic slough (*see* Plate IV*d*), the margins are deeply punched out with sharply defined and somewhat hyperaemic edges. Considerable destruction may thus be caused, the epiglottis usually bearing the brunt.

The depth of the infiltration is such that the perichondrium may be reached and the resulting perichondritis can be most destructive. The perichondrium may occasionally be the primary site of the granulomatous process. In either case secondary infection usually occurs and adds to the destruction. The deep penetration may also involve the crico-arytenoid joints directly, or later restrict their movements by fibrosis.

In some cases a very slowly progressive hypertrophic tissue reaction resembling pachydermia occurs in the interarytenoid region, and rarely this may spread throughout the larynx.

The final stage of healing is accomplished by dense fibrosis and the resulting scarring after much destruction gives rise to the most bizarre appearances and deformities.

Symptoms

Any or all of the usual symptoms of laryngeal disease may occur, depending entirely on the site and extent of the lesions. Generally the voice becomes hoarse or raucous, and, as the epiglottis is so frequently involved, some degree of dysphagia occurs. Deep ulceration into the valleculae or lateral pharyngeal wall increases the severity of this symptom. Pain is not a noticeable feature unless rapid destruction is taking place. Cough is also uncommon, as the disease rarely assumes a catarrhal form, but it may be troublesome in later stages when ulceration and secondary infection have occurred and it is then accompanied by a foul sputum. Some degree of dyspnoea is usual as the glottic space is often encroached upon, and it may become severe in cases with oedema, perichondritis and abscess formation. It is also a frequent late phenomenon, coming on insidiously, as cicatricial stenosis develops in healing.

Physical signs and diagnosis

In the secondary stage the mucous patches are also present in the pharynx, from which indeed the laryngeal invasion has spread. A slight confusion with an acute or subacute laryngitis could arise, but only if the lesions were casually studied and no careful history taken.

The various tertiary appearances when seen in the laryngeal mirror may sometimes be sufficiently characteristic for immediate diagnosis, but usually the whole gamut of investigation is necessary to distinguish between these lesions and those due to tuberculosis or cancer—clinical and radiological examination of the chest, serological and sputum examinations and perhaps even a biopsy. It must always be remembered that these diseases may occur together and that the presence of one does not exclude either of the others. Potassium iodide can be given as a therapeutic test in any case unaccompanied by oedema, as it has a noticeable and rapid healing power in syphilitic lesions. A clinical diagnosis must be based on the history, the character and situation of the lesions, the kind of ulcer and the nature of its base and margins, the degree of hyperaemia or the amount of scarring.

Treatment

A course of penicillin injections must be started at once and continued for as long as seems necessary. It is a mistake to discontinue the drug unless complete healing has occurred.

Potassium iodide may be administered at the same time, especially in treating late tertiary lesions, as it apparently has some power of removing gummatous tissue. The initial dose should be 300 mg. three times a day and can be increased to as much as 13,000 mg./day where gummatous involvement is severe. The depression sometimes caused by large doses of the drug may be relieved by including sal volatile in the prescription, and plenty of water must be taken with each dose to assist its absorption. The catarrhal exudate produced by the drug may be dangerous when oedema already exists, and the patient must be carefully watched, especially in the early stages of administration.

In addition, and particularly in any acute case, both voice rest and rest in bed are necessary together with abolition of all irritants such as tobacco and alcohol. Cartilage erosion and sequestration following perichondritis may require direct laryngoscopy and either incision of an abcess or removal of fragments. Occasionally, if dyspnoea is severe, a tracheostomy must be performed.

Prognosis

The condition usually resolves with treatment, but the residual cicatrization can so impair the airway that a permanent tracheostomy may be necessary. The voice may always remain hoarse.

MYCOSES OF THE LARYNX

These are all very rare diseases due to various forms of fungus.

Actinomycosis

This condition probably never occurs as an isolated laryngeal affection. It gives rise to a yellowish, tumorous, granulomatous infiltration which soon breaks down into a suppurating mass. Lymphadenitis is an early feature. The suppurating areas burrow deeply and destructively and small yellow masses containing the ray fungus of actinomyces are extruded with the purulent discharge. Metastatic deposits are frequent, especially in the lungs. Hoarseness and cough with a foetid sputum are constant features together with increasing cachexia. The diagnosis can be made with certainty only by a microscopic examination of the pus or from the result of its inoculation into a guinea-pig. The administration of massive doses of potassium iodide together with penicillin or tetracyclines may, in early cases, effect a cure but, in addition, surgery of a most radical nature may be necessary.

Leptothricosis

Even more rare, this disease is said to be due to the so-called *Leptothrix buccalis*. It is almost never primary in the larynx but secondary to pharyngeal or lingual lesions and appears as small white areas in a relatively normal mucosa, bearing a slight resemblance to leucoplakia. Hoarseness may occur or the disease may be symptomless. The fungus does not thrive in an alkaline medium, and treatment therefore consists of tablets of sodium bicarbonate to suck and of large doses of potassium iodide.

Blastomycosis

Blastomycosis, although also rare, is the most common of these diseases and may be a primary affection of the larynx. It occurs almost entirely in South America among grain workers and is due to a number of species of yeast fungus.

343

The larynx and lung are involved more often than the pharynx, and the histological picture is that of a chronic granuloma. There is a proliferation of round cells, a formation of giant cells resembling those of tuberculosis, and, later, minute areas of necrosis or small abscesses followed by ulceration. The base of the ulcers is soft and granular and the edges are irregular and undermined, but a purulent discharge is constantly thrown off which tends to crust. A red, sometimes almost purple, areola surrounds the ulcer.

It is said that the organism cannot be found in the sputum unless there is a pulmonary involvement, and that as mycelium is often absent the ovoid or globular organism must be looked for and is more easily identified in unstained smears. In biopsy specimens the organism may be found in the giant cells, but again unstained sections must be used. The fungus can be grown, although slowly, on Sabouraud's medium. Blastomyces vaccine may give a positive intradermal reaction.

Hoarseness and cough are early symptoms, and dyspnoea and dysphagia are later ones and are accompanied by increasing debility. Although the disease is only slowly progressive it is fatal if untreated.

The lesions as seen on indirect laryngoscopy must be differentiated from those of tuberculosis, syphilis and cancer. The ultimate diagnosis can be made by careful microscopical examination of the sputum or tissue, or by culture, and by a positive skin reaction.

The administration of large doses of potassium iodide is the only efficacious treatment so far known. It may need to be given for months and continued in smaller doses for a year or more after the lesions have apparently healed. Irradiation with x-rays is said to be helpful and may be used in addition to iodides.

The effects of streptomycin on all these mycotic infections await trial and report since they are all so rare, but its administration seems well worth while on empiric grounds.

SCLEROMA (RHINOSCLEROMA)

This is an unusual disease endemic in Poland, from which country it is slowly spreading over Europe in a southerly and south-easterly direction, to Egypt and India. Sporadic cases occur everywhere. It consists of a submucous infiltration chiefly in the nose and in the oral cavity round the lips, extending gradually backwards into the pharynx and larynx. It is sometimes seen first of all in the larynx. Dense fibrosis resembling a keloid follows, and there is no tendency to suppuration or ulceration.

Pathology

The mucous membrane is first of all infiltrated with small round cells and plasma cells. Almost no other evidence of an inflammatory reaction occurs. Fibrosis gradually follows and the cicatricial tissue assumes a characteristic density and induration which has been likened to cartilage. In this granulation tissue are found the eosin-staining hyaline bodies of Russell and large vacuolated cells that resist staining, described by Mikulicz. From this tissue can be cultured the diplo-bacillus of Frisch which may be identical with Friedländer's bacillus. Specific agglutination reactions of the serum can be obtained with filtrates of cultures of bacilli isolated from the tissues or secretions. There is, in addition, a specific complement fixation test of the Bordet-Gengou type between the serum and filtrates. The overlying epithelium after undergoing some hyperplasia atrophies.

The disease usually begins in the subglottic region of the larynx and may be unilateral or bilateral. The fibrous tissue is laid down in crescentic bands or in mound-like deposits. The affected areas are covered with crusts.

Symptoms

The laryngeal involvement produces increasing hoarseness. At a late stage breathlessness and an irritating cough, with the expectoration of crusts, may occur. On indirect laryngoscopy the typical subglottic encroachment becomes visible.

Diagnosis

The chief diseases to be differentiated are syphilis, carcinoma and the subglottic form of chronic laryngitis. The absence of ulceration distinguishes it from the first two and its induration from the last. The complement fixation test is diagnostic in over 90 per cent of cases, but biopsy will be necessary to establish the diagnosis beyond doubt unless, as is usual, the nose and lips are also involved (Ellis, 1951).

Treatment

Streptomycin is often extremely successful in arresting the disease and is almost a specific remedy. Unfortunately, some cases are resistant but may heal with tetracyclines. Chemotherapy is only of value in the active invasive stage of the disease, when cortisone may also be helpful in preventing the deposition of fibrous tissue.

When the deposits of fibrous tissue have formed, little can be achieved except the removal of obstructive adhesions. On two occasions the author has by laryngofissure under general anaesthesia (with a tracheostomy) performed a submucous dissection of obstructing subglottic mounds of scleromatous tissue. The recurrent laryngeal nerves must be avoided and it is prudent to administer streptomycin and cortisone for a month or so afterwards. The reaction usually takes this length of time to subside, and the tracheostomy can then be closed.

CHRONIC NON-SPECIFIC LARYNGITIS

Chronic non-specific laryngitis is a condition chiefly affecting the superficial portion of the mucous membrane, especially the epithelium, but often extending more deeply. It rarely reaches to the underlying cartilage. The disease may be fairly diffusely spread throughout the larynx or certain areas may bear the brunt. In the same way the changes may be variously distributed in the thickness of the mucosa. Thus certain fairly clear-cut varieties of the condition can be distinguished although the common and characteristic symptom is persisting hoarseness.

Aetiology

There are a number of ways in which the disease may arise, as follows.

Susceptibility

Certain individuals are susceptible to recurrent attacks of acute catarrhal laryngitis. Although these infections generally resolve rapidly they occasionally linger in a subacute form throughout the winter. Yearly repetitions of this process may result in permanent changes in the mucosa.

Physical abnormalities

In addition to constitutional reasons predisposing to recurrent catarrhal attacks there may be a persisting abnormality in the nose or throat responsible for them, and from which infection also spreads directly to the larynx. Among the most important are infection in tonsils (and also adenoids in children) or teeth.

The irritant postnasal discharge of chronic sinusitis is often directly responsible.

Anatomical nasal abnormalities such as gross septal deviation or enlargement of turbinals may cause mouth breathing. Air which has thus not been properly cleansed, warmed and moistened by passage through the nasal cavities is inhaled directly into the larynx, and it would be surprising if this chronic irritation did not occasionally produce mucosal reactions there.

Finally, chronic irritation from a disease process in the neighbourhood, such as one of the granulomata or carcinoma, may cause the condition.

Occupational factors

There are other forms of irritation, apart from those due to abnormalities in the upper respiratory tract, for example, occupational exposure to climatic inclemency or extreme, as in chauffeurs or costermongers on the one hand and bakers and stokers on the other. Exposure to dusty atmospheres in mines or metal shops or the repeated inhalation of irritant chemical vapours is attended by the same risk. Tobacco is undoubtedly irritating to the mucosa and workers in smoky, unhygienic atmospheres, such as cinemas, may suffer equally with the heavy addict.

Alcohol

Alcohol is a chronic pharyngeal irritant, especially in the more concentrated form of spirits, and in hard drinkers there is frequently an associated laryngeal involvement.

Trauma

Long continued trauma is a not infrequent cause of chronic hyperplastic changes. It is exemplified by persistent crying, screaming or shouting in children, or by vocal mismanagement in singers or persons whose occupation demands much speaking. Proper voice production is an uncommon natural blessing, but it is surprising how often professional voice users, such as actors, clergymen or lawyers, have poor and untrained voices. Their lack of vocal training is readily apparent when they are confronted with unfavourable conditions, and the forcible efforts to make the voice "carry" sometimes induce actual physical damage to the vocal apparatus. If suitable periods of rest are possible, the voice may recover completely, but when this is impracticable, or when the unfavourable circumstances recur frequently, the condition may become fully developed. In certain occupations, those of the course bookmaker and costermonger, for instance, it is apparently desirable to make as much noise as possible, and with such ill-use an almost characteristic voice is developed, hoarse and raucous, from the resulting chronic changes in the larynx. In all these cases there may be in addition any of the factors already discussed, particularly exposure to weather and smoky atmospheres, as well as the necessity to be heard over noise. There are numerous other forms of vocal abuse which will be recognized easily when encountered.

Other disorders

In cardiac, renal and various gastro-intestinal conditions, as well as in gout, rheumatism, diabetes mellitus and asthma, permanent changes often occur. They result possibly from vasomotor disorders and secondary vascular abnormalities.

Incidence

Males are more often affected than females, and adults than children. The incidence is likely to be heaviest between the ages of 30 and 50 years, which are the average person's most active period of life, and in damp and cold climatic conditions.

General pathology

Various clinical types of the disease are fairly readily distinguished, and correspond on the whole to specific pathological changes. However, certain general changes are common to all types and are really the processes of inflammation and repair occuring simultaneously in different parts of the mucosa. There is a generalized hyperaemia of the mucous membrane leading to over-activity of the mucus-secreting cells in the ciliated portions of the epithelium, namely, most of the vestibule including the posterior surface of the epiglottis, the ventricular bands and ventricles. The anterior surface and free margins of the epiglottis, the upper border of the aryepiglottic folds, the interarytenoid space and the true vocal cords are covered with stratified squamous epithelium, and here a lymphocytic infiltration of the deeper layers occurs. As the disease progresses the infiltration spreads to the submucosa and even to the intrinsic muscles. It is uncommon for the perichondrium or cartilage to be involved, but this may occur together with invasion of the crico-arytenoid joint. The stimulation of hyperaemia is in time followed by hyperplasia of the mucus-secreting glands in the corium. These changes result in some thickening of the mucosa, but complete resolution is still possible at this stage. If for any reason the condition persists for an undue length of time, or recurs frequently, the cellular infiltration is followed by fibrosis with consequent glandular atrophy and ultimately metaplasia of the ciliated epithelium to a stratified squamous epithelium. This squamous epithelium usually becomes hyperplastic and often hyperkeratotic in localized areas, producing certain well defined clinical pictures. During the course of the changes the mucosa is first bulky, dusky red and covered with viscid secretion. It gradually becomes more slaty in colour while still remaining thickened, and the secretion lessens. In long-standing cases the colour is often pale and there may be considerable residual thickening localized to certain areas. The intrinsic muscles may undergo similar changes and, in addition, often hypertrophy under the stimulus of over-action to correct the speech defects and then gradually atrophy as a result of interstitial fibrosis and deficient nutrition. Terminal changes of the same kind may involve the crico-arytenoid joints and sometimes result in fibrous ankylosis.

Classification of clinical types

The clinical types of chronic non-specific laryngitis may be classified as follows:

(1) Chronic diffuse (or hyperaemic) hyperplastic.

(2) Chronic localized hyperplastic:

    (*a*) supraglottic: (*i*) dysphonia plicae ventricularis of Jackson (1935), (*ii*) prolapse or eversion of the ventricle of Morgagni, (*iii*) cystic protrusion from the ventricle.

(b) glottic

(c) subglottic.

(3) Pachydermia:

    (a) red: (i) simple pachydermia of the vocal cords, (ii) granular laryngitis, (iii) posterior hypertrophic pachydermia (or "contact ulcer" of Jackson (1928)), (iv) interarytenoid pachydermia

    (b) white: (i) vocal nodules (or chorditis nodosa), (ii) leucoplakia.

(4) Chronic laryngitis of childhood.

(5) Chronic hyperaemic laryngitis in systemic disease.

Microlaryngoscopy

The closer study of laryngeal lesions made possible by the use of the Zeiss operating microscope has tended to confirm the above classification, formulated by the author 20 years ago. Kleinsasser (1969) by microlaryngoscopy has arrived at a closely similar description of laryngeal hyperplasias, superbly illustrated in colour. This method of examination has enormously improved the ability of the laryngologist in diagnosing non-malignant conditions where slight visual changes may mark important differences between one type of lesion and another. The method has also immeasurably assisted the techniques of precise and delicate excision when this is necessary. In any case not readily diagnosed by indirect laryngoscopy, direct laryngoscopy with magnification (under a general anaesthetic) is nowadays imperative.

Chronic diffuse hyperplastic laryngitis

Aetiology

Of all the factors already enumerated in the general discussion the ones responsible here are those likely to exert a uniform effect throughout the larynx. The most important are: (a) chronic suppuration in the nose or throat, especially in the sinuses, tonsils or teeth; (b) mouth breathing; (c) over-use of the voice by professional voice users; (d) irritation by tobacco or alcohol; and (e) occupational chemical or physical irritants.

Pathology

The pathology conforms with the description given above. There is a generalized hyperaemia of the whole laryngeal mucosa and diffuse thickening due to hyperplasia of glandular elements, interstitial cellular infiltration and fibrosis. Where vocal abuse is mainly responsible, the membranous portions of the vocal cords are more congested than the remainder of the larynx and this engorgement may even cause partial obstruction of the airway. The colour of the vocal cords depends upon the amount of hyperaemia and varies from dusky red to grey through all shades of pink and brown, but occasionally they may appear fairly normal. The rest of the laryngeal mucous membrane shows a similar variation in colour changes for the same reason. Excessive viscid secretion is nearly always produced in the ventricles and appears on the upper surfaces of the cords. It is often adherent and difficult to expel, and when it reaches the free margins the voice may almost disappear, or a slight "apologetic" cough occurs which may amount to a tic. In long-standing cases there may be actual deformity of the epiglottis, ventricular bands and vocal cords from fibrosis, and at this stage the mucosa is pale and covered with a fine network of vessels, and secretion is scanty. Occasionally the interarytenoid region is thickened and prevents apposition of the vocal processes. Finally, atrophy of the intrinsic muscles, especially the thyro-arytenoideus, may occur.

Symptoms

Hoarseness is the essential feature of this condition and may persist for weeks or years. It is generally the continuance of this symptom which causes the patient to seek advice. Characteristically it is unaccompanied by pain or by any general disturbance, but the patient often complains of other local sensations such as a pricking, smarting or tickling and dryness. The accumulation of these subjective sensations together with the excessive efforts of the laryngeal muscles to produce an intelligible voice often result in local irritability and spasmodic cough. Another cause of cough is the presence of sticky secretion on the free margins of the cords which also gives rise to the well-known "frog in the throat" feeling and often sudden aphonia.

Laryngeal vertigo.—Cough, however produced, may occasionally occur in violent attacks associated with a glottic spasm in a manner resembling pertussis. On rare occasions, during such an attack, the patient may fall to the ground unconscious. Charcot (1876) applied the name laryngeal vertigo (ictus laryngé) to this sequence of events believing it to be analogous to aural vertigo or Menière's disease. However, there is no confirmatory evidence for this belief. It may be due to either forced expiratory or inspiratory efforts against a closed glottis. In the former case a positive pressure is exerted on the great vessels in the thorax leading to cardiac embarrassment, and in the latter the increased negative pressure induced in the thorax leads to accumulation of blood on the right side of the heart. Cerebral vascular disturbances sufficient to produce a momentary loss of consciousness may occur whichever mechanism is responsible.

Another possible mechanism may be cerebral anaemia induced by movements of the head and neck during spells of severe coughing if there is atheromatous narrowing of the vertebral or basilar arteries. The arterial insufficiency may not need to be great to result in momentary loss of consciousness.

Recovery is usually rapid and complete although some mental confusion may persist for a short time. There is no loss of sphincter control. The features may be congested, but are sometimes pale, and haemorrhages are occasionally found locally in the larynx and elsewhere as a result of suffusion. The attacks are unpredictable in onset and frequency, and usually occur in middle-aged or elderly males. The irritation of tobacco and alcohol has been specifically blamed, and rheumatism and gout as well as a psychoneurotic tendency are predisposing factors (Baker, 1949).

In singers the speaking voice may be relatively good and the hoarseness only revealed while singing in a certain range when the voice suddenly roughens or "breaks". If secretion is at all excessive the voice may have a "flat" and somewhat rough tone throughout which can be overcome in the early stages by good technique, but later it becomes permanently lowered in register and harsh in timbre. The increasing efforts necessary to produce a clear tone result in more and more rapid fatigue with shorter periods of clarity, and finally, in permanent hoarseness. All these events are more sharply accentuated in singers and professional voice-users whereas in others the early stages are apt to pass without recognition. The usual history here is hoarseness on awakening in the morning which gradually passes off during the day, but returns by evening. The period of remission becomes shorter until an almost permanant condition of hoarseness is reached, although even in quite severe cases the voice rarely disappears altogether. Secretion accumulates overnight, is partly responsible for the severity of the symptoms in the morning, and, after being cleared away by coughing and hawking, gradually re-accumulates during the day. It is this collection of mucus, as well as laryngeal muscular fatigue, which causes the evening exacerbation. It also produces the frequent "clearing" cough which is a characteristic feature of the condition, frequently annoying the sufferer's associates. The hoarseness becomes permanent when structual changes develop in the larynx.

Physical signs

The physical signs are entirely confined to the larynx and are readily distinguished by indirect laryngoscopy. At an early stage, when the symptoms are chiefly restricted to the morning and evening, the usual finding is a generalized dusky red colour of the mucosa throughout the larynx. The surface has a leathery and crinkly appearance, and may be covered with sticky secretion. The ventricular bands, arytenoids and interarytenoid region, and occasionally the epiglottis, are swollen, often disproportionately. The vocal cords are at first injected and thickened and later this thickening may even cause some respiratory difficulty. The edges lose their sharp demarcation and appear rounded. At a later stage still the cords acquire the dusky red colour of the remainder of the larynx. In long-standing cases the mucosa appears pale and a fine vascular arborization may be visible throughout the larynx. The epiglottis may be thickened and deformed and similar changes may be evident in the ventricular bands and interarytenoid region. Movements of the vocal cords, at first limited by inflammatory deposits and oedema, are ultimately affected by muscular atrophy and peri-articular fibrosis or arthritis of the crico-arytenoid joints. The cords themselves then appear pale and somewhat enlarged, with irregular free margins, but occasionally they are thin and atrophied and almost transparent in appearance. There is no ulceration at any stage.

Differential diagnosis

The most important disease which may closely resemble this condition is tuberculosis, although syphilis and the early stages of carcinoma can be confused. All these diseases occur in the larynx in a variety of different ways and there are numerous superficial points of physical similarity which can usually be resolved by direct microlaryngoscopy. In any extremely doubtful case biopsy and microscopic examination may be needed and are diagnostic, but clinical examination should usually suffice.

Both the secondary and tertiary stages of syphilis may involve the larynx diffusely, but there is nearly always ulceration; manifestations elsewhere in the body, together with serological examination, should reveal the true state of affairs.

It is rare for carcinoma to appear in the posterior part of the larynx except in the later stages, when its neoplastic character should scarcely be in doubt. In the early stages, however, the lesion is markedly unilateral and may be confused with other types of chronic laryngitis to be described later.

Tuberculosis does occasionally appear as a diffuse and oedematous infiltration, but is then an acute condition and almost invariably associated with an active pulmonary infection. The symptoms are usually of comparatively short duration and, in addition, the mucosa is markedly pale and quite unlike the dusky redness of chronic laryngitis. In those cases where no active lung lesion is present there will nearly always be some history or radiological evidence of previous pulmonary involvement. Wegener's granuloma is rare and may cause difficulty in diagnosis *see* Volume 3.

The association of unconsciousness occurring during coughing attacks with diffuse chronic laryngitis is sufficiently uncommon to suggest laryngeal vertigo (q.v.), but psychoneurosis, epilepsy and tabes dorsalis must first be excluded.

Treatment

To a very large extent treatment is governed by the cause, since the disease is usually a secondary effect of a preventable or curable condition. Certain measures are therefore automatic. All foci of sepsis in the upper respiratory tract must be eradicated as far as possible; thus infected lymphoid tissue and teeth should be removed, and sinusitis treated in any appropriate fashion. Causes of nasal obstruction must be remedied and the possibility of systemic disease investigated. All this demands nothing active of the patient except his consent, but there is unfortunately another aspect of treatment which will tax his patience and assiduity and perhaps also necessitate the cessation of his long-standing and pleasure-giving habits. In addition, where vocal abuse or misuse is present, his immediate livelihood or occupation may be involved in such treatment, making him even more unwilling to follow the advice. It is this attitude which will prove the greatest obstacle to efficacious treatment, and herein lies a possible explanation of the indifferent results usually obtained.

Patients can be divided into two groups; cases largely secondary to infection, and others secondary to irritation.

The chief method of handling the first group has already been considered prophylactically, and therapeutically follows the lines laid down in the treatment of acute laryngitis.

The second group includes, on the one hand, professional voice-users and persons exposed to irritant atmospheres and, on the other hand, persons who indulge more freely than they should in alcohol and tobacco. It is also unfortunately true that those in the former category can often be included with equal propriety in the latter. All sufferers must be strongly advised against any indulgence in tobacco or alcohol, and if anything is to be conceded alcohol in moderation should be given the preference over tobacco. Industrial exposure to irritant vapours scarcely comes within the range of the average laryngologist as the Factory Acts and official inspection provide against undue normal risk, but here too avoidable extra irritation must be governed.

This elimination leaves those patients whose laryngeal condition is occupational or is due to improper use. The cardinal maxim here is strict silence if it is possible to exact it, failing which voice rest, or avoiding use of the voice in ill-ventilated places, must serve. After an adequate period, assuming recovery or a substantial measure of it to have occurred, efficient re-education and training are essential for singers or public speakers with faulty voice production. Naturally enough, the older the patient and the more advanced in his career, the less is either of these aims likely to be fulfilled, and this disappointing reaction must be expected by the laryngologist who should have ready some appropriate counter-persuasion. It is of great help to know of several good teachers of singing and elocution in order that advice may be couched in concrete terms and leave less open to evasion.

Steam inhalations.—Local applications in the larynx are of little fundamental value, but occasionally they may give some symptomatic relief. The most useful are steam inhalations containing volatile oils; those mainly employed are eucalyptus and pine either made up in suspension in water with light magnesium carbonate or dissolved in industrial spirit. To some extent inhalations act like hot fomentations and assist the bodily processes of repair. These same oils made up in liquid paraffin may be employed as a soothing laryngeal spray, but cautiously and infrequently owing to the possibility of lipoid pneumonia.

Alkaline sprays.—Alkaline sprays sometimes help the expectoration of tenacious secretion.

Penicillin.—Penicillin aerosol has been used and to the extent that it dilutes secretion is of value, but it is difficult to see what other direct effect it could exert.

Astringent sprays.—Astringent sprays have also been used in an attempt to shrink up some of the excessive tissue in very chronic cases. Silver nitrate, tannic acid in glycerin, zinc sulphate or Protargol, each in strength up to 10·0 per cent, and sometimes even stronger, have been used in this way or directly painted on a particular part. In order to avoid laryngeal spasm, 5·0 per cent solution of cocaine containing a few drops of 0·1 per cent adrenaline should first be sprayed into the larynx. The painting can then be easily achieved using a suitable bent applicator or brush and a laryngeal mirror while the patient grasps and holds out his tongue with his thumb and forefinger. On the whole, this method of treatment can hardly be recommended on rational grounds of pathology, as a condition primarily due to irritation is hardly likely to subside if treated with irritants.

Expectorants.—Mild expectorant mixtures containing ammonium carbonate, squills or ipecacuanha are of some value in thinning secretion, but potassium iodide should be avoided as it sometimes produces oedema.

Change of climate.—In addition to the advice regarding voice rest and training discussed above, a change of climate can often be helpful for those who can afford it. A warm, moist climate is ideal for this condition and a holiday in some Mediterranean region may work wonders. The régime at many watering places may be beneficial and certain resorts cater for such cases, notably Cauterets and Allevard. The benefits at these resorts are supposedly the sulphurated or carbonated waters, but there is no doubt that the strict and healthy general regimen of existence imposed on the patient is probably more important.

Local massage.—Where muscular weakness or atrophy has occurred in very old cases, local neck massage may be helpful and a strychnine tonic should be tried.

Special measures.—Laryngeal vertigo occasionally demands special measures if the attacks are violent. A little chloroform may relieve the spasm, as may the inhalation of amyl nitrite or octyl nitrite. If the patient is convulsive he must be prevented from injuring himself by padding his head with rugs or clothing and by introducing a rolled-up handkerchief or a piece of wood between his jaws to protect his tongue.

Prognosis

In cases due to a specific, exciting, infective or irritant factor which can be evaluated, complete recovery can be expected provided the local changes are not already too far advanced and the patient is amenable to whatever the treatment entails. If vocal mismanagement is the underlying trouble the outlook is doubtful, as the patient's livelihood is often inextricably involved. In all cases, once the pathological changes have passed the point where complete resolution is possible, a permanent residual disability is inevitable. It is also unfortunate that whenever a condition of hoarseness exists the automatic remedial efforts made by other parts of the larynx nearly always result ultimately in intensifying it, unless exceptionally good vocal re-education and training are available. It must be remembered that the higher registers in singing and the speaking voice in women may be permanently affected by apparently trivial laryngeal changes, and this should always be considered when giving an opinion based on the physical appearance of the larynx.

Chronic localized hyperplastic laryngitis

Localized areas of the larynx often exhibit changes which are remarkably uniform from case to case. Although the pathological processes already described are distinguishable as the fundamental ones, the physical appearances are sufficiently specific to suggest distinct entities.

The causes of these conditions are largely those already given for chronic diffuse laryngitis. In this group the emphasis falls more on vocal misuse and chronic irritation than on infection. Shouting and screaming, stuffy atmospheres, tobacco and alcohol are probably the chief aetiological factors.

Supraglottic

The ventricular bands are the main structures affected and, very uncommonly, the laryngeal ventricles. The epiglottis and aryepiglottic folds do not exhibit any uniformly recurring localized changes. The two specific clinical conditions which thus result are dysphonia plicae ventricularis and prolapse or eversion of the ventricle of Morgagni.

Dysphonia plicae ventricularis.—The condition was first described under this title by Jackson and Jackson in 1935, but enlargement of the ventricular bands had been noted as a physical sign for many years previously. Anatomically these bands are composed of muscle and connective tissue, chiefly elastic fibres, enveloped by a thick fold of mucous membrane which contains many acinous glands and is surmounted by a columnar ciliated epithelium. The muscle fibres are derived from the thyro-arytenoideus. The bands assist in closing the airway as well as in producing the voice and, therefore, any lesion of the true vocal cords inhibiting their function is likely to be accompanied by a compensatory over-activity and hypertrophy of the false cords. The usual lesions are tumour, removal by operation, congenital abnormality, atrophy or sluggishness following infection, or impairment of mobility from arthritis in the crico-arytenoid joints or lesions of the recurrent laryngeal nerves. True muscular hypertrophy, however, is uncommon compared with the incidence of inflammatory hyperplasia. This selective infiltration is possibly the result of several factors. First, as already described, when the function of the true vocal cords is at all hindered, the activity of the false cords becomes correspondingly greater, and constant use of an inflamed part tends to prolong the duration of the inflammation and to impede its resolution. Secondly, permanent and hyperplastic changes are easily produced in the loose and glandular corium. Thirdly, the conditions chiefly responsible are those most likely to endure since they are so frequently occupational.

Symptoms and physical signs include the characteristic roughness and harshness of the voice, which is low in pitch and often "breaks"; sometimes two tones are

353

produced simultaneously. A sensation of vocal fatigue may occur and is a most unpleasant symptom. On indirect laryngoscopy the ventricular bands are seen to be reddened and thickened, and they almost hide the vocal cords even during quiet breathing. On phonation they come together in the midline and obscure the view of the cords. The enlargement of the bands is fairly uniform, and it is unusual to find any other abnormality elsewhere in the larynx. The diagnosis is thus relatively straightforward.

Treatment, for reasons already mentioned, is apt to be disappointing, as an essential part of it is voice rest. In addition, of course, all irritants should be removed, and astringents thus have no place in the treatment. Vocal re-education is important and the patient must be taught by proper breath control to speak in a low-pitched tone. It is possible to determine when the bands begin to move in phonation and by suitably devised exercises to correct this tendency. In stubborn cases a small piece from the centre of the free margin of each band can be punched away with suitable forceps. However, by the time the patient comes under treatment so much permanent structural change has occurred that symptomatic relief and arrest of progress are about as much as can be expected.

Prolapse or eversion of the ventricle of Morgagni.—This is probably a misnomer. The case reports exhaustively investigated by Moore up to 1922 reveal no more than two or three that could claim this title. In these few the mucous membrane of the sacculus laryngis, perhaps owing to the negative intralaryngeal pressure of a severe coughing attack, had undoubtedly become everted, and had herniated into the ventricle itself and thence into the main laryngeal lumen. In all the remaining cases either the mucosa of the saccule or ventricle, or both, had become infiltrated and hyperplastic and had perforce burgeoned into the larynx proper, or the normal mucosa had been pushed or dragged into this position by the growth of an underlying tumour or by the traction of a superficial one. A chronic, non-specific, inflammatory thickening in the corium of the ventricle itself is the most common of these causes. The redundant mucosa is forced out of this confined space and comes to lie on the upper surface of the vocal cord. The mass may eventually cover the whole length of the cord from end to end and also from side to side, even reaching beyond the midline, and, if bilateral, respiratory obstruction may be produced. The weight of the mass impedes the free movement of the vocal cord. The covering epithelium may undergo metaplasia and become stratified and squamous, but it does not ulcerate. By the time the condition has become recognizable spontaneous regression is probably impossible.

Symptoms and physical signs again include some degree of hoarseness as the predominant, almost the only, symptom, due to the damping action of the weight of tissue lying on the vocal cord. A slight irritant cough is sometimes present and, rarely, respiratory obstruction. Indirect laryngoscopy reveals a dusky-red, almost violet, mass partly or completely obscuring the cord. The spatial relationships of the ventricular bands, the protruding mass and the vocal cords are usually distinguished on phonation. Occasionally, however, the ventricular band cannot be identified with certainty. The whole area should then be painted with 5 per cent cocaine and 0·1 per cent adrenaline in equal parts, which will cause the inflammatory mass to shrink up, withdrawing partly or wholly into the ventricle, and thus clarifying the position. The relationships may also be determined by palpation with a blunt probe. These manoeuvres are best performed under magnification. A protrusion over the anterior portion of the cord is due to eversion of the sacculus alone.

Diagnosis is made on the physical appearance, which is generally sufficiently characteristic, but tuberculosis may occasionally present a similar picture. The presence of ulceration, a careful search for lesions elsewhere in the larynx together with an examination of the chest and sputum (or laryngeal secretion) will define the position. Syphilis very rarely gives rise to this appearance alone—there is nearly always some neighbouring involvement of the ventricular band or arytenoid cartilages—and necrosis and ulceration are almost invariable. Tumours, both innocent and malignant, are readily distinguished on inspection. In any difficult case a biopsy will establish the diagnosis.

Treatment consists in puncturing the mass in several places with a galvanocautery to promote fibrosis and shrinkage, or pieces may be removed with a suitable punch. Both forms of treatment may be combined. They can be performed under cocaine anaesthesia by indirect laryngoscopy or under general anaesthesia by direct laryngoscopy, using the microscope. Apart from such efforts to reduce the weight and size of the protruding mass, the usual general measures already discussed can be used, largely in the attempt to prevent recurrence.

Cystic protrusion from the ventricle.—This is a rather more common condition and is probably due to circumstances similar to those producing eversion. The proliferating subepithelial deposits interfere with drainage from the ducts of the mucous glands in the deeper layers of the mucosa and retention cysts form. They are sometimes large enough to overlap the vocal cord and prevent clean adduction in phonation, and occasionally they are multilobed.

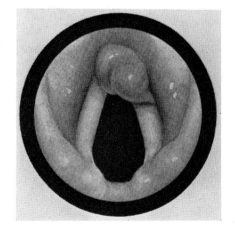

Fig.132.—Lobulated cystic mass arising from the right ventricle and overlying the anterior end of the vocal cord and glottis.

The symptom is hoarseness, at first most marked with vocal fatigue and gradually becoming permanent if the cyst reaches the free margin of the vocal cord. On indirect laryngoscopy the cyst will usually be seen as an obvious circumscribed gelatinous mass coming from the opening of the ventricle and lying on the upper surface of the cord (Fig. 132).

Diagnosis is relatively straightforward on the physical appearance of the cyst, even more apparent seen with the microscope, when the origin from the ventricle will be in no doubt.

Treatment is by excision, preferably under magnification. The ventricular band is pushed aside and the origin of the cyst dissected out. Occasionally a further lobe will be found burrowing upwards under the loose epithelium and it must be enucleated with the main mass.

Glottic

In this variety some of the more marked forms of local hypertrophy are found. Deposits of inflammatory products chiefly in the corium and only to a lesser extent in the epithelium organize into swellings which may closely resemble neoplasms. The hyperplastic tissue consists of exudate and cellular elements of which one or other may predominate in the ultimate reaction at any site. Thus the following distinct clinical forms are distinguishable, especially with microlaryngoscopy:

(1) A bilateral oedematous hyperplasia of the membranous vocal cords, usually bilateral, due to a proliferative process in Reinke's space, sometimes called Reinke's oedema.

(2) A gelatinous mass, so-called "mucous polypus", arising from a localized area on the under surface or free margin of the anterior half of a vocal cord. It is sometimes bilobed or multilobed.

(3) Tumorous masses in the interarytenoid region.

Which form will occur in any given case is unpredictable, but the basic underlying pathological changes are identical, presumably the result of similar conditions and of these the irritative are again believed to be more important than the infactive.

Symptoms and physical signs.—As before, hoarseness is the outstanding symptom, but in this group the hoarseness is apt to be intermittent, and phases of an almost normal speaking voice lasting weeks at a time may alternate with similar phases of hoarseness. The voice is also apt to deteriorate during the day from a relatively normal one in the morning to a muffled croak in the evening. This phasic and diurnal incidence is probably related to fatigue and may indicate the fleeting appearance of a syndrome already described, namely dysphonia plicae ventricularis (*see* pp. 353, 354). Secretion is not a prominent feature and thus cough is infrequent. However, a "clearing" cough is sometimes present. There is no interference with respiration as the hypertrophic masses rarely become sufficiently large. In general the disability is slight for a long time and perhaps noticed in the early stages only by singers or professional voice users, but the hoarseness is almost invariably progressive.

The physical signs vary with the form of pathological change but are readily identified on indirect laryngoscopy.

(1) The membranous portions of the vocal cords have a rounded spindle-shaped appearance due to gelatinous masses which apparently form on the upper surfaces of the cords and drop flabbily into the glottic space. One usually overlaps the other (Fig. 133). Occasionally the masses become large enough to cover the vocal processes, but they do not arise from the mucosa in that region. The appearance is unmistakable on indirect laryngoscopy. In a fully developed case the voice is permanently muffled and non-resonant, as the masses by their weight interfere with the movements of the cords and by their size obtrude between them. The remainder of the larynx usually appears normal.

(2) A smooth globular mass projects into the glottic space from one or both cords. It may be stalked or sessile. It is usually white and gelatinous in appearance

(Fig. 134), but sometimes, if vocal trauma with localized haemorrhage was the precursor, the mass may be red or pink. The polypus is usually in the anterior portion of the larynx and the unaffected part of the vocal cord looks normal. These polypi are usually stalked although the pedicle may be short and widely based.

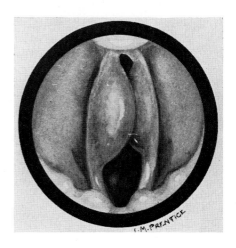

FIG. 133.—Massive spindle-shaped cystic masses arising from the whole length of the vocal cords and overlapping one another.

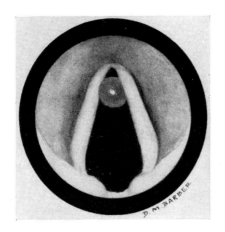

FIG. 134.—Polypus arising from the under-surface of the anterior end of the right vocal cord.

(3) Firm deposits may be seen in the interarytenoid region (Plate V*a*). Here the tissue is thrown up into a central mound or several small hillocks because of the constant movements of the arytenoid cartilages, and may reach a size sufficient to prevent proper approximation of these cartilages. The surface of the mass is generally a duskier red than the normal mucosa of this area, and is often covered with sticky secretion. Except when large, the swelling usually interferes very little with vocal cord movements.

Unless the physical appearance is completely obvious in the mirror, a direct laryngoscopy, preferably with magnification, should always be performed in order to leave nothing to chance. These conditions sometimes closely resemble more serious ones, and a satisfyingly careful examination of every portion of the swelling and surrounding larynx must be made.

Diagnosis.—These lesions with the possible exception of (3) bear little resemblance to malignant conditions or to tuberculosis, syphilis or scleroma. Biopsy will differentiate type (3) from these other diseases.

Treatment.—The usual general and local measures already discussed may serve to relieve the symptoms and perhaps to prevent recurrence or progress, especially of the oedematous varieties of the disease. The fully formed lesions will probably need more active local treatment such as galvanopuncture to obtain shrinkage by fibrosis, electrocoagulation to reduce the mass of the swellings or, preferably, excision by direct microlaryngoscopy. Localized lesions of types (2) and (3) are removed by careful incision of the epithelial layer only round the base of the tumour followed by scissors dissection of this layer and its contained tumour. The cases of type (1), Reinke's oedema, are best treated by excising an oval strip of epithelium along the length of the swelling on one cord only, the other side being similarly treated three or four weeks later.

Subglottic

A chronic inflammatory hyperplasia more or less uniformly diffused through the loose corium of the subglottic mucosa and symmetrically situated on either side of the midline is a rare finding, and one which has aroused some controversy. There is no doubt that the tissue involved is one in which such a change could occur. Why it should do so without involving the superjacent and more vulnerable parts of the larynx may be inexplicable, but it is not impossible. However, although uncommon, a sufficient number of such cases have been observed to confirm the existence of the condition. It seems to follow the acute laryngitis of certain severe infections, chiefly typhus, typhoid fever and erysipelas, and also repeated attacks of simple acute laryngitis. In children it may gradually form in repeated attacks of laryngismus stridulus.

Symptoms and physical signs.—A hoarse and harsh voice of low pitch is associated with slight dyspnoea and stridor. An irritant cough is present which is often brassy in note, but may be croupous. On indirect laryngoscopy the subglottic tissues are seen to be swollen and are visible on either side below each vocal cord as smooth, pale-rose cushions. Very rarely there may be a similar enlargement posteriorly. These swellings are said never to reach the size of granulomatous infiltrations in this area, but they are sometimes large enough to arrest the cords in the cadaveric position. They are soft and never ulcerate.

Diagnosis.—The rarity of this condition compared with somewhat similar appearances occurring more frequently in syphilis, tuberculosis and especially cancer, demands that the diagnosis be made by a process of exclusion. Thus, unless the case has been observed throughout from the acute phase, direct laryngoscopy must be performed and the swellings actually moved with instruments in order to estimate their consistency and to detect any ulceration. All the usual investigations for the presence of tuberculosis or syphilis must be made, and if doubt still remains there should be no hesitation in performing a biopsy. Scleroma occasionally appears in this region unaccompanied by lesions in the pharynx or nose, but this disease is rare even in the limited geographical areas to which it is confined. The best means of diagnosis is the microscopic examination of a piece of tissue. As a practical measure it is advisable to perform a biopsy in every case to avoid the disaster of missing a subglottic cancer.

Treatment.—Once the condition is well established there is little to be done but to assist resolution by the conservative measures already described, and to organize the patient's existence in an endeavour to prevent recurrence. Some measure of thickening nearly always persists, but does not require active treatment unless it causes respiratory obstruction. Tracheostomy may then be necessary. If the disease is still in an active phase the tube must be retained until no sign of activity remains, when it can be removed providing the airway is adequate. In forming this estimate the possibility of oedema from further acute attacks of laryngitis must be remembered. Fortunately, such an end result is exceedingly rare. Unless the disease process is defunct radical attempt at cure by excision of the hyperplastic tissue and skin grafting is unlikely to be successful.

Pachydermia

Pachydermia is the clinical term given to a localized hyperplastic condition, possibly another form of those described in the previous sections, but distinguished by the characteristic pathological change of hyperkeratosis. The symptoms are identical. The subject was first investigated and to some extent defined by Virchow in 1887, after the historical case of the Emperor Frederick III, and he called it "pachydermia verrucosa laryngis". Two varieties are recognizable, the red and white, and each is divisible into several others.

Red

In the red variety of pachydermia the epithelium is excessively thickened and cornified in those areas where it is stratified and squamous, and elsewhere first undergoes metaplasia followed by hyperkeratosis. The papillae enlarge projecting downwards into the corium in which hyperplasia of the connective tissue elements occurs. The basement membrane remains intact (Fig. 135). Occasionally the reaction becomes more vigorous and rapidly dividing cells spread along the superficial surface of the basement membrane, carcinoma *in situ*, or even break through the basement membrane to form a true invasive squamous cell carcinoma. Thus the condition can sometimes be pre-cancerous.

Chronic irritation is believed to be the major causative factor. The deposits occur in certain sites in the larynx with sufficient peculiar characteristics restricted to each to warrant their being described separately.

Simple pachydermia of the vocal cords.—This occurs as a bilateral, but sometimes unilateral, diffuse infiltration throughout the membranous portions of the cords, which then appear as reddened, smooth, cylindrical bands. The colour is less vivid than in acute laryngitis, but movements are more restricted. The condition is relatively frequently encountered. It may be the end result of a form of chronic laryngitis already mentioned as occurring almost specifically in singers and professional voice-users where the secretion has become scanty and the epithelium in particular has undergone hypertrophy.

Its symmetrical appearance, the mobility of the cords and the normal appearance of surrounding structures, make the diagnosis relatively straightforward. Acute oedematous tuberculous laryngitis may resemble it locally, but there will be other signs and symptoms of extralaryngeal involvement.

No specific treatment is known, but tobacco and alcohol should be forbidden and the other general measures applied which have been described. A change of climate, especially a stay at a spa with its strict routine, are said to be particularly helpful.

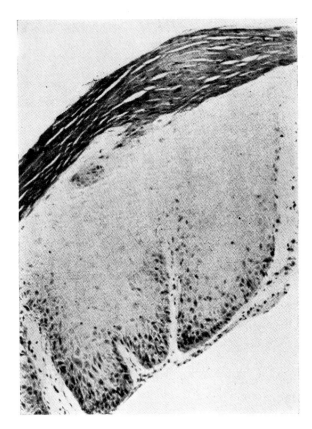

FIG. 135.—Red pachydermia. Photomicrograph showing excessive proliferation of epithelium and papillary downgrowth.

Granular laryngitis.—This is possibly a final stage of chronic diffuse hyperplastic laryngitis. The upper surfaces of the vocal cords become studded with small reddish granulations which are most numerous on the membranous portions (Fig. 136), and which to some extent resemble the swollen lymphoid nodules occasionally occurring on the posterior pharyngeal wall. Where it can be seen between the granulations the surface of the vocal cord itself is pink, and the condition in this stage is called *cordite en îlots.* The granulations occasionally become confluent and the whole cord then has a warty or lumpy appearance. The sinuous edge may give the illusion of ulceration, but a careful examination will reveal that the surface epithelium, although irregularly and grossly thickened, is intact. The condition is the typical "pachydermia verrucosa" and has also been called "chorditis tuberosa". Granulations are occasionally found on the epiglottis and on the ventricular bands. The disease is often unilateral. Curiously enough, women are a great deal more affected than men, and children are sometimes sufferers.

Hoarseness, as can well be imagined, is very severe in the advanced cases and is always troublesome. On the other hand, cough and symptoms associated with the irritation of secretion are relatively slight.

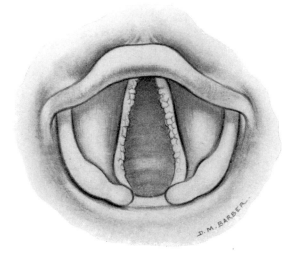

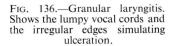
FIG. 136.—Granular laryngitis. Shows the lumpy vocal cords and the irregular edges simulating ulceration.

The diagnosis from tuberculosis and syphilis is chiefly made on the lack of ulceration, but the latter disease often gives rise to cases bearing a close resemblance. The usual general investigations will clarify the position. Cancer may be difficult to exclude, especially in a unilateral case, and biopsy will then be necessary.

The condition is treated on exactly the same lines as is glottic localized hyperplastic laryngitis (*see* p. 356).

Posterior hypertrophic pachydermia.—This variety is distinguished by localized deposits occurring on the vocal processes exclusively, leaving the membranous portions of the cords clear. The hyperplastic tissue usually takes the form of an oval mound, with its long axis horizontal, mainly on the inner surface of the vocal process but extending also on to its upper surface. On phonation these mounds come into apposition and prevent full adduction of the cords. Perhaps as a result of this constantly recurring trauma, crater-like depressions form in the mounds, one usually much larger than the other, but they may be due to the closer attachment of the mucosa to the tip of the vocal process than elsewhere. Into the larger crater the whole mound of the opposite side may seem to fit when the vocal processes are opposed, and so deep and rough is this depression that it frequently simulates an ulcer (Fig. 137). Jackson (1928) believed that trauma is always responsible and described this condition as an entity without reference to pachydermia, calling it "contact ulcer" (*see* p. 352). He stated that the depression is an actual ulceration and that necrotic cartilage of the tip of the vocal process is often present in the depths. It seems more likely that the condition is a true pachydermia and that ulceration, when it occurs, is due to persistence of the causative factors and to lack of treatment.

The mound-like elevations are roughened and extend from the tip of the vocal process spreading sometimes on to its upper and lower surfaces, to the body of the arytenoid cartilage. The periphery of the swelling is reddened and becomes paler and more grey in appearance until the crater is reached. This is often white or yellow. Ulceration or superficial erosion, if present, may be difficult to detect, even after careful drying of the surface with cotton wool on suitable applicators and inspection with a magnifying lens. The vocal cords are generally smooth and normal in outline and either uniformly pink or injected. They both move well although full adduction is hindered by the mounds. On phonation the characteristic cup and ball fitting of the mounds is seen.

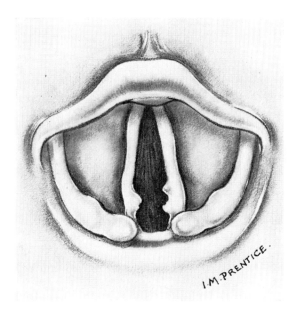

Fig. 137.—Posterior hypertrophic pachydermia ("contact ulcer"). Shows the typical masses, one larger than the other, with apparent central ulceration over each vocal process.

Hoarseness is the chief symptom and in this type of case is extremely intractable and unpleasant. It is constant and causes rapid and often painful vocal fatigue. There is usually some excessive secretion with its resulting irritation and cough. Men are the chief sufferers and the lesions may be caused by an attempt to speak in a deep and "manly" voice, a "belly-voice" so-called. This causes a squeezing together of the posterior portions of the vocal cords, creating by friction a corn-like condition at the tip of each vocal process.

Diagnosis is readily made on the characteristic position and shape of the epidermal masses, and there is no other disease which bears much resemblance. However, biopsy is always available in case of doubt.

Treatment is generally disappointing. The patient can rarely be persuaded out of his speaking habit or the usually accompanying alcohol and drinking habits. Clean local excision under magnification may often be possible, but the lesions have a strong tendency to re-form.

Interarytenoid pachydermia.—One form of glottic chronic localized laryngitis has already been seen to affect the loose interarytenoid tissues, and these same tissues are also vulnerable to pachydermia, but this latter condition rarely remains so localized and generally spreads on to the vocal processes and over the arytenoids

(Plate V*b*). The excessive tissue between the cartilages is thrown up into prominent rugae separated by clefts which give the impression of ulceration. However, although some superficial erosion of the hyperplastic cornified layers may occur, ulceration is unusual. The general colour of the tissue is greyish and the whole mass has a velvety appearance.

Although it is said that the diffuse simple type of pachydermia is of most common occurrence, there can be no doubt that it is the interarytenoid form which is most commonly seen and diagnosed. It is more frequent in males and is considered to be largely the result of chronic irritation.

The symptoms resemble those of posterior hypertrophic pachydermia, and the hoarseness is severe and distressing.

The physical appearance of the hypertrophic masses is fairly characteristic, and the criteria of differential diagnosis are the same as those above, but microscopic examination may be necessary to establish the diagnosis from the similar form of chronic localized laryngitis.

In treatment, removal of the superfluous tissue under magnification is relatively successful, and although it will probably re-form, the intervening period of relief can be used to correct the causal conditions. On rare occasions thyrotomy has been necessary to remove firm masses of tissue which could not be adequately treated by direct laryngoscopy.

White

This form of pachydermia is characterized by hyperkeratosis as well as hyperplasia of the epithelium which dips long papilliform processes into hyperplastic and hyperaemic corium. A well-defined layer of lymphocytic infiltration surrounds the affected areas. The tissue so formed is firm in consistency and white or yellow in colour, as the thickened epithelium conceals the blood vessels in the corium. It is thus pathologically a leucoplakia, similar to that occurring on the tongue or in the pharynx, and it may be pre-cancerous. There are two varieties.

Vocal nodules (*chorditis nodosa*).—This is largely a disease of professional voice-users, chiefly singers in the higher range, e.g. sopranos and tenors (*see* also p. 551). It is simple hyperkeratotic reaction in a specific part of the vocal cord and is due to trauma, chiefly bad voice production, but additional irritative factors are tobacco, alcohol and dusty and stale atmospheres. In speaking, and especially in singing, the cords do not vibrate as a whole but in segments depending on the pitch of the note. The anterior portion of the cord is active while the posterior portion is inert; the active portion lengthens posteriorly as the pitch is lowered. This can be well seen with the stroboscope.

Where singers are producing high notes in a faulty manner, often because of singing beyond their natural range or using certain methods such as the *coup de glotte*, the cords come together in an abnormally violent manner. If other unfavourable circumstances are present, or if this vocal abuse is too frequently repeated, small nodules develop, usually on the free margins of the cords opposite each other at or near the junction of the anterior and middle thirds (*see* Plate X*c*). These nodules consist of hyperkeratotic epithelium and some underlying fibrosis and round-celled infiltration, and are thus a leucoplakic condition. It is also held that the predisposing conditions described above may result in submucous haemorrhage and that the nodule may be started by the fibrosis consequent on the organizing of

363

such a haematoma. The fact that the nodules are nearly always bilateral is somewhat against this contention.

The early symptoms are slight roughness of the voice, usually in the higher frequencies, and sometimes whenever a note of a certain pitch is reached. This can be overcome by conscious laryngeal effort which in turn induces vocal fatigue. As the condition progresses the roughness extends to notes in the lower registers and cannot be eliminated by compensatory efforts. The speaking voice then thickens and a more or less continuous hoarseness follows. A slight irritant cough often occurs.

On examination, in the early stages, on the anterior portion of the cords a little sticky secretion will be fairly constantly seen which draws out on phonation into a thin band between the cords at the level of the junction of the anterior and middle thirds. Later, a tiny elevation will be noticed on the free margin of one cord at first, but very soon afterwards on the other, and eventually definite nodules develop at these sites. They never attain any great size, but their almost exact apposition prevents complete adduction of the parts of the vocal cords which produce sound. The nodules therefore give rise to a degree of hoarseness entirely disproportionate to their bulk. They are dead white or greyish-white in colour. The vocal cords themselves are nearly normal in appearance, although perhaps not quite the characteristic pearly-white colour. Other hyperplastic chronic or acute changes are not often seen, unless, of course, the patient, in addition to vocal abuse, is exposed to the sort of conditions which produce them. The cords move normally except for their inability to come into complete apposition. The nodules are rarely ulcerated in spite of the trauma to which they are subjected.

The diagnosis is made on the history, the symmetrical position of the nodules and on lack of evidence of other disease, but tuberculosis and syphilis may need to be excluded by the usual general investigations. Cancer is never bilateral, but in cases where the vocal nodule is unilateral confusion may arise which must be settled by biopsy.

Treatment consists entirely of rest, and to obtain resolution even of small nodules months of silence may be necessary, Despite this, however, the growths may persist and surgical removal may become indicated. The operation is a delicate and responsible one, as the patients are nearly always professional voice-users and often singers. It should be performed by direct laryngoscopy under general anaesthesia and magnification and the nodule on one cord is delicately cut away with a sickle knife or scissors without injuring the underlying membrane. The other cord is treated similarly about a month later. Even when the nodules have been successfully removed, months may elapse before healing and resolution and restoration of muscle tone are complete and the singing voice returns.

In addition to this treatment it is most important that the patient should not be exposed subsequently to unfavourable surroundings, and, more important still, that he should undergo a period of vocal re-education and training; a relapse is otherwise certain. Unfortunately, in any case, there is a great tendency to recurrence.

Leucoplakia.—Leucoplakia is a condition in which hyperkeratosis develops on the upper surface of one or both cords. It sometimes takes the form of a number of discrete white or pale yellow horns projecting from the cord, and at other times consists of one or more flat plaques of similar colour. These nodules are often loosely attached and can be wiped away, although they soon re-form. The underlying vocal cord is generally, although not invariably, hyperplastic to some extent

(Fig. 138), but the movements are rarely hindered. There is considerable evidence that malignant changes may occur here as in leucoplakia elsewhere (Fig. 139), and that irritation is a possible exciting factor; treatment with caustics or astringents should therefore be avoided. There are no constant findings to indicate that such a change is imminent or is in progress, and, moreover, as it begins in a localized part of the lesion it may not necessarily be revealed by biopsy. Close observation of all such cases is thus of great importance.

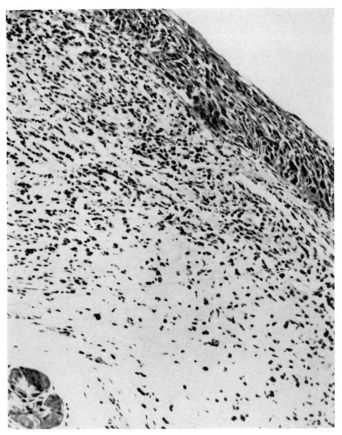

FIG. 138.—Leucoplakia. Photomicrograph of a section of a vocal cord showing excessive cornification with subjacent hyperplasia.

Hoarseness is the only symptom and is often not very marked. However, as the condition is slowly progressive the hoarseness gradually increases. Indirect laryngoscopy reveals the changes already described and these must be differentiated chiefly from those of syphilis and carcinoma. The diagnosis may be impossible without a biopsy and even this may not be conclusive. Repeated careful examinations over a period are then essential. There is very little resemblance to any form of tuberculosis.

In the treatment avoidance of caustics has already been noted. From the practical point of view the local lesion itself should be ignored and conservative general measures adopted, chiefly those designed to prevent irritation. The larynx must be inspected at regular intervals and if progressive changes induce any uneasiness a biopsy should be performed. This may not clarify the position, and, should the local appearance continue to deteriorate, it is far better not to wait until definite evidence of malignancy appears and not to perform small localized excisions. With careful technique under magnification the lesion can sometimes be stripped completely off the vocal cord without damaging the vocal ligament. This may be impossible because of deeper infiltration, and the whole cord is then best removed by laryngofissure (Ellis, 1957).

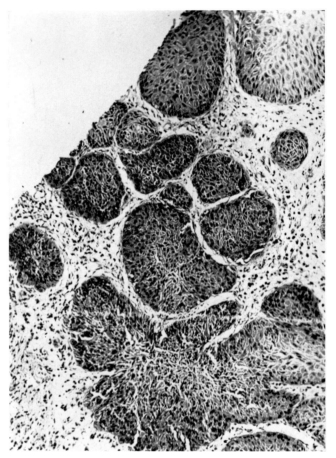

FIG. 139.—Leucoplakia. Photomicrograph of another section through a different portion of the same vocal cord as Fig. 138, showing papillary downgrowth and commencing malignant infiltration.

Although the possibility of malignant change has been stressed because of its disastrous import, it is not common, and, in general, the prognosis to life and health is good. The lesion, however, may persist indefinitely.

Chronic laryngitis of childhood

Aetiology

A raucous voice occasionally develops in children usually between the ages of five and ten. All the various causes that have been enumerated in the section on chronic diffuse hyperplastic laryngitis are applicable except those specifically encountered in adult or industrial life. Infection and vocal abuse are the chief factors, and of the former the acute specific fevers are the most important. Severe laryngitis with mucosal erosion and sometimes ulceration very occasionally complicates measles, and a similar condition may occur in scarlet fever, the enteric fevers, influenza, pneumonia and diphtheria. This laryngitis usually resolves, but persistence may be induced by other abnormalities such as mouth breathing, sinusitis and infected tonsils. Many children seem incapable of speech or conversation or enjoyment in general except at the tops of their voices, particularly in city life where the level of background noise is high. Other children sing in choirs in an unnatural range. Benign growths, particularly papillomas, sometimes occur in children and provoke undue effort in an endeavour to produce a clear voice. All these types of vocal abuse may induce chronic changes in the larynx.

Finally, a condition of hereditary hoarseness is known in which the vocal cords may seem normal on inspection, although atrophy and scarring have both been recorded.

Pathology

The pathology is exactly as in chronic laryngitis in adults.

Symptoms and physical signs

Hoarseness is the only symptom and the voice has an unpleasant harsh and raucous timbre which is constant. Examination of the larynx with a mirror is often possible, with patience and persuasion, but when the child is unco-operative direct laryngoscopy must be performed with or without an anaesthetic, depending on the technique used in the particular clinic. Garel (1921) has described the following three distinct laryngeal changes.

First, nodules are symmetrically placed on the cords identical with the condition of vocal nodules in adults.

Secondly, the whole anterior two-thirds of each vocal cord is slightly hyperaemic and uniformly swollen and rounded into a semi-elliptical shape with the convexity along the free margin, so that on apposition a small space remains between the vocal processes (Fig. 140).

Thirdly, the portion of the cord adjacent to the free margin atrophies and a line or groove of demarcation running the whole, or almost the whole, length of one or other cord, or both, appears.

Garel gave the names *laryngite à type nodulaire, laryngite à grains d'orge* and *laryngite à sillons atrophiques* to these respective appearances, and, in addition, maintained that the last-named occurs only in children, and if seen in an adult is pathognomonic of such affection in childhood. It is due to atrophy of the thyroarytenoid muscle and is usually a late change seen in older children. This atrophy may extend to the interarytenoid muscles.

Diagnosis

Tuberculous laryngitis is rare in children, as is nowadays hereditary syphilis. For practical purposes it remains only to differentiate the condition from a benign growth, readily achieved by an examination of the larynx which will also disclose the type of laryngitis present.

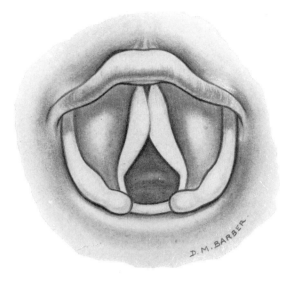

FIG. 140.—Chronic laryngitis. This drawing was made from the larynx of an adult, but shows the precise change more commonly occurring in children.

Treatment

Absolute silence is desirable, but this is almost impossible in a child. However, he can perhaps be prevented from singing, shouting or speaking in anything more than a quiet voice. All foci of sepsis must, of course, be eliminated. The results are frequently disappointing and the child may carry his raucous voice with him throughout life, especially if muscular wasting has occurred. On the other hand the appearance *à grains d'orge* is rarely seen in adults, which suggests that in a number of cases resolution does occur. It may not be possible to persuade the child of the importance of treatment until he grows older and more self-conscious, when willing co-operation often quite suddenly occurs, and a condition of some years' standing may clear up in a comparatively short time.

Chronic laryngitis in systemic disease

This is not a common finding, but occurs from time to time in any general systemic condition involving vasomotor changes or vascular congestion. The evolution of chronic changes depends upon the persistence of such vascular abnormalities. Myxoedema, nephritis, diabetes mellitus, gout, chronic bronchitis, chronic rheumatism, intestinal disorders and various blood dyscrasias are diseases in which it has been found, as well as in obesity, and at the menopause. Rarely, Wegener's granulomatosis affects the larynx, and biopsy will be necessary for diagnosis.

Pathology

The mucous membrane alone is affected and never the underlying cartilage. The changes are those of submucous hyperplasia already described diffusely spread throughout the larynx and usually also involving the pharynx. The pathology of Wegener's granuloma is described fully in Volume 3.

Symptoms and physical signs

The symptoms are identical with, although rarely as severe as, those already described in the section on chronic diffuse laryngitis, of which it is in reality one variety. Cough is often more troublesome than hoarseness, as secretion is usually produced in excess. The larynx is diffusely wine-coloured, almost violet, but the hyperaemia may be dusky and punctate. The neighbouring pharynx generally has a similar appearance. Movements of the vocal cords depend upon the degree of infiltration. In addition to these local signs will be those of the systemic condition.

Diagnosis

The differential diagnosis of the laryngeal appearances has been discussed (*see* p. 350), and the precise systemic illness is a matter for the general physician.

Treatment

The underlying cause is usually a more serious matter than the laryngeal involvement, and is the primary concern of treatment. However, both hoarseness and cough, especially the latter, are often disturbing. The appropriate conservative measures have already been fully described (*see* pp. 351, 352). Obstruction necessitating tracheostomy can occur in cases of Wegener's granuloma of the larynx.

ATROPHIC LARYNGITIS

This disease is also called "laryngitis sicca" and "ozaenatous laryngitis". It is characterized by discomfort in the throat, hoarseness, a spasmodic cough and the formation of crusts in the larynx, and is nowadays uncommon.

Aetiology

The condition is generally considered to be secondary to diseases in the nose or throat. The most important and usual of these is atrophic rhinitis, but it is also seen in cases of suppurative sinusitis, especially posterior ethmoiditis and sphenoiditis. However, it may arise as a primary disease in the larynx, since it is found only in adults, whereas atrophic rhinitis and suppurative sinusitis may well be developed at puberty or adolescence. Syphilis can be an associated factor. In whichever way the disease originates exposure to dusty or smoke-laden atmospheres is undoubtedly deleterious. No specific organism has been isolated.

Pathology

The basic change is fibrosis in the corium of the mucosa leading to anaemia and glandular atrophy. Where the overlying epithelium is ciliated and columnar, metaplasia occurs to the stratified squamous variety. The anaemia also leads to atrophy of other mucosal elements and of the intrinsic muscles, especially the thyro-arytenoideus. The result of these changes is the extrusion of a scanty, thick secretion in which epithelial debris and pus cells are present. Owing to the absence of cilia and because of its own high viscosity, this secretion moves very slowly and is dried by the currents of air moving to and fro over it in respiration. Crusts are thus formed in various parts of the larynx, most frequently in the interarytenoid region and also over the vocal processes and on the cords. Where these crusts overlie ciliated epithelium their pressure eventually causes atrophy and further metaplasia.

369

When the secretion and crusts are rubbed away, the underlying mucous surface is generally pale and glazed, but it may be dull red and thrown up into folds, especially in the interarytenoid region, suggesting hypertrophy or pachydermia, and in the fissures of this type of mucosa superficial erosion or even ulceration may occur. All these changes may extend distally into the trachea and also be traceable proximally through the hypopharynx to the nasopharynx and nasal cavities.

Symptoms and physical signs

The most worrying and important symptom is the constant irritable cough which gradually wears down the patient's strength. It is sometimes accompanied by glottic spasm which has been of such severity as to necessitate tracheostomy. The cough is associated with the expectoration of crusts and secretion occasionally streaked with blood. Rarely, haemoptyses of measureable amount occur.

Hoarseness is, of course, a constant but less urgent symptom. It is worse on awakening in the morning, because of the nocturnal accumulation of crusts, and improves after the patient has got rid of them by coughing and expectoration. It then gradually re-appears or worsens during the day, as the crusts re-accumulate and the poorly vascularized muscles become fatigued.

There is nearly always a pricking or burning sensation in the larynx accompanying the constant feeling of dryness, and this may amount to actual pain. A foetid odour is said to occur sometimes, but it may emanate from the nose rather than the larynx.

The outstanding and often the only physical sign is the collection of blackish-grey or green crusts in the larynx, readily seen on indirect laryngoscopy. In early cases the crusts chiefly gather in the posterior portion of the larynx and only to a slight extent on the vocal cords, but later they may completely obscure the cords. Crusting may also be seen in the subglottic region and even in the trachea. Slight ulceration or erosion may be present. Movements of the vocal cords are generally normal until the disease has reached an advanced stage, when the muscular atrophy may be noticeable in the slightly flaccid outline of the membranous portions and in the lack of full adduction. Apart from the local laryngeal appearances, examination of the nose and throat may reveal an atrophic rhinitis (most commonly) or sometimes a posterior sinusitis or chronic tonsillitis.

Diagnosis

The diagnosis is hardly in doubt as no other disease gives rise to such widespread crusting. An examination of the nasal cavities may reveal the source of the condition.

Treatment

This is naturally divisible into the treatment of any primary cause on the one hand and symptomatic treatment on the other. The former scarcely falls within the range of this discussion and is described in various sections elsewhere. In the latter, stimulation of secretion and the removal of crusts are the desiderata. Secretion can be encouraged by the administration of small doses of iodides or ammonium chloride or ammonium carbonate. Mucus so formed is less viscid than that normally present in the disease and this, together with the increase in bulk, facilitates cough and expectoration. To some extent, therefore, the irritant cough can be relieved medicinally. The glands can also be stimulated by the local application of Mandl's paint. The most important part of treatment is the removal of crusts by spraying the larynx with an alkaline or sulphurated solution. An excellent device is to use a spray nozzle on a rubber tube connected to a soda-water syphon; the effervescent alkaline solution is most effective as well as refreshing. Where crusts are present in the nose and pharynx similar cleansing of these regions is necessary. After the mucosa has been cleared of crusts and secretion, erosions or ulceration may be revealed and can be painted with 10 per cent zinc chloride solution, a similar strength of silver nitrate or compound tincture of benzoin. Simple lubrication is soothing and can be obtained by spraying the larynx with a 5 per cent solution of chloretone or a 1 or 2 per cent solution of one of the aromatic oils in liquid paraffin. Occasionally steam inhalations containing an aromatic oil will be found useful both in the stimulation of secretion and in the loosening of crusts.

If there is any appreciable haemorrhage from the ulcerated areas the best treatment is careful forceps or sucker removal of crusts by direct laryngoscopy, followed by the application of 5 per cent tannic acid or ferric perchloride solution to the surface of any ulcers thus revealed.

In a general way lozenges containing either ammonium chloride or phenol with mucilage are comforting to suck at intervals during the day.

All irritant habits such as indulgence in alcohol and tobacco should be abandoned, and dusty and ill-ventilated places avoided. A warm and moist climate is ideal for these patients; it will not cure the condition, but the symptoms will be greatly relieved.

Prognosis

Where the condition is secondary to a suppurative focus elsewhere, the outlook is good if this focus is treated and eradicated before extensive metaplastic changes have occurred in the larynx, for it must be remembered that stratified squamous epithelium is an irreversible end result of epithelial metaplasia, and that the symptoms are proportional to the extent of its occurrence. The cases occurring together with atrophic rhinitis are probably slowly progressive. There is no evidence that the condition is prejudicial to life in a direct way, but the tendency to bronchitis and pulmonary infection is probably increased.

SUBMUCOUS HAEMORRHAGE

An extravasation of blood into the mucosa of the vocal cords can occur (*see also* p. 551). It has been called "haemorrhagic laryngitis", but this term is more properly applied to and should be restricted to those severe cases of acute laryngitis in which the haemorrhage occurs as a result of the inflammatory process. In this condition the bleeding follows the vocal trauma of sudden shouting or screaming (Fig. 141). It is possible that vocal nodules in singers may occasionally originate as small haematomas produced in this way. Larger localized collections may organize to fibromas or granulomas of some size and are only histologically distinguishable from true benign neoplasms.

Symptoms and physical signs

Immediately following the trauma slight pain occurs in the larynx and the voice becomes hoarse and easily tired. Rarely a little frothy blood may be coughed up or expectorated. On indirect laryngoscopy the haemorrhage will be visible on one vocal cord (rarely both), either in a small localized area, often on the free margin, or more diffusely along the length of the cord. If the blood has broken through the epithelium it will be seen streaking the glottis. The haematoma is normally absorbed and can then be observed exhibiting the usual colour changes. Complete resolution is the rule when the extravasation is small, but when larger it may organize to a permanent fibrotic nodule or a soft granuloma.

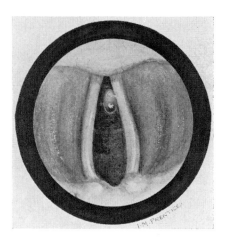

FIG. 141.—Localized polypoidal haematoma on right vocal cord caused by shouting at a football match. (View at direct laryngoscopy.)

Treatment

There is no specific treatment. Voice rest is all-important. If, despite this, nodules or permanent tumours form, they must be removed by direct laryngoscopy under magnification. With strict management complete healing is to be expected.

LARYNGEAL ARTHRITIS

Laryngeal arthritis is always secondary to or part of some other disease. It may occur as a complication of inflammatory conditions in the larynx or pharynx; it may be secondary to various acute infections such as typhoid fever and influenza or to more chronic ones like syphilis or tuberculosis; it may be due to a focal metastatic infection; it may be part of a gouty or rheumatic invasion; it may result from external trauma; and, finally, it occurs in the crico-arytenoid joint in any fairly long-standing case of recurrent laryngeal paralysis. Some of these conditions are so serious in themselves as to absorb all the attention, and the arthritic condition may only later become noticeable. In others, while the joint involvement is observed or suspected during the course of the underlying disease, it again takes a subsidiary place. The crico-arytenoid joint is much more often affected than is the cricothyroid joint, since from its anatomical position it is vulnerable to intralaryngeal pyogenic or granulomatous infection. The involvement may be unilateral or bilateral. It may resolve completely or may leave a residual fibrous ankylosis leading to bizarre positions of the vocal cords.

Symptoms and physical signs

The symptoms of cricothyroid joint disease are similar to but less marked than those of infection of the crico-arytenoid joint. Ignoring all symptoms due to the various aetiological diseases, localized pain and hoarseness are chiefly complained of by the patient. He can frequently, with his forefinger, press deeply on the neck near the lower end of the posterior border of the thyroid cartilage indicating this as the region of pain. It is said that crepitation may occasionally be felt here due to friction between surfaces of inflamed synovial membrane. In the absence of actual pain in the larynx there is often a sensation of pricking, heat or tension. Sometimes dysphagia is present. The hoarseness is most marked if the affection is bilateral.

On indirect laryngoscopy the arytenoid region is seen to be red and swollen in acute cases, but this is less marked in more chronic ones. The vocal cord may move slightly or not at all and may be fixed in any position varying from complete adduction to complete abduction. In chronic cases this immobility and variable fixation may be the only physical signs, giving rise to confusion with recurrent laryngeal nerve paralysis. The distinction is best made by direct laryngoscopy and palpation of the arytenoid cartilage with a forceps or other instrument to disclose the presence or absence of ankylosis. However, repeated careful examination by indirect laryngoscopy will generally be sufficient.

Treatment

Naturally the causative disease must be treated in the appropriate fashion. If the joint is acutely inflamed absolute silence is desirable and certainly voice rest. Cold packs to the neck are comforting and may assist absorption of fluid. If ankylosis occurs bilaterally in a manner leading to respiratory obstruction and to stridor, tracheostomy may be necessary. In favourable cases this need not be permanent, as an arthroplasty and fixation in abduction can be performed, as advocated by Woodman (1946) for bilateral recurrent laryngeal nerve paralysis (*see* p. 535).

REFERENCES AND BIBLIOGRAPHY

Anning, S. T., Dawson, J., Dolby, D. E., and Ingram, J. T. (1948). *Quart. J. Med.*, **41**, 203.
Baker, C. (1949). *Guy's Hosp. Rep.*, **98**, 95.
Charcot, J. M. (1876). *Gaz. méd. Paris*, Série IV, **3**, 588, 602.
Dowling, G. B. (1946). *Brit. J. Derm.*, **58**, 45.
Ellis, M. (1951). "Rhinoscleroma". In *British Encyclopaedia of Medical Practice* (Vol. 10, 2nd ed.). London; Butterworths.
— (1957). *J. Laryng.*, **71**, 379.
Feldman, W. H., and Hinshaw, H. C. (1948). *Brit. med. J.*, **1**, 88.
Garel, J. (1921). *Monogr. oto-rhino-laryng. int.* No. 4. Paris.
Jackson, C. (1928). *Ann. Otol., etc., St. Louis*, **37**, 227.
— and Jackson, C. L. (1935). *Arch. Otolaryng., Chicago*, **21**, 157.
— — (1942). *Diseases and Injuries of the Larynx*. New York; Macmillan.
Kleinsasser, O. (1969). *Microlaryngoscopy and Endolaryngeal Microsurgery*. London; Saunders.
Moore, I. (1922). *J. Laryng.*, **37**, 263, 333, 381.
Pagel, W., Simmonds, F. A. H., Donald, N., and Nassau, E. (1964). *Pulmonary Tuberculosis* (4th ed.). Ed. by W. Pagel. London; Oxford University Press.
Woodman, De G. (1946). *Arch. Otolaryng., Chicago*, **43**, 63.

15

TUMOURS OF THE LARYNX

Henry Shaw

BENIGN TUMOURS

Simple laryngeal tumours are not uncommon, occurring in an approximate ratio of 2:3 with malignant lesions in adult males, while in women the ratio is reversed. It is, however, important to realize that the great majority of cordal benign "tumours" are non-neoplastic, thus emphasizing the comparative rarity of true benign neoplasms of the cords (Table I).

TABLE I

Benign Tumours of the Larynx Seen at the Royal National Throat, Nose and Ear Hospital, 1948–56

Non-neoplastic		Neoplastic	
Polyps and nodes	283	Papilloma	34
Cysts	23	Fibroma	8
Non-specific granuloma of		Angioma	4
vocal process:		Chondroma	3
(a) Intubation granuloma	12	Adenoma	2
(b) Contact ulcer granuloma	14	Myoblastoma	2
Papillary keratosis	18		
Laryngocoele	3		
Primary amyloidosis	1		
Total:	354 (87%)	Total:	53 (13%)

In the larynx simple tumours exhibit certain anomalous features which must be carefully noted. There is often difficulty in deciding clinically whether a swelling is neoplastic or of an inflammatory, degenerate or traumatic nature, and even histological appearances may frequently be confusing.

A swelling which appears clinically to be a simple fibroma, may, on histological examination, prove to be a tuberculoma, whilst a cordal haematoma due to abuse of the voice as in shouting at a football match, may organize and develop into a tumour that appears to be a fibro-angioma.

Following the use of endotracheal anaesthetic tubes, especially after a prolonged operation, small granulomas may sometimes occur on the vocal processes of the arytenoids. If they are not removed at an early stage they may later resemble closely a typical fibroma.

Again the common bilateral condition of "singer's nodules" is certainly due to

375

misuse of the voice and may disappear with complete rest of the voice, but histological appearances may range from simple polypoid degeneration of the cordal margin through vascular fibrous tissue to what is impossible to differentiate from a true fibroma.

SYMPTOMS

The location and size of the tumour will mainly determine the presence and type of symptoms. Small swellings or even those of some size in areas such as the outer side of the aryepiglottic folds or around the epiglottis, may produce no symptoms and may only be discovered accidently on routine inspection of the larynx.

Tumours large enough to displace muscle fibres may cause a feeling of discomfort in the throat, especially on speaking or swallowing, and also variable alterations in the timbre of the voice.

Since the majority of simple tumours are found on the vocal cords, hoarseness will be an early symptom in many cases. Quite a small tumour in the anterior commissure or a small sessile swelling on the cordal margin may cause marked dysphonia, whereas a larger but pedunculated tumour on the upper or lower cord surfaces may be displaced upward or downward on phonation and may produce little more than slight fatigue or tiredness of the voice.

Pain as opposed to discomfort is a rare symptom, as also is dysphagia. An irritating or paroxysmal cough sometimes occurs with pedunculated tumours. Dyspnoea and stridor are predominant symptoms in the more bulky benign tumours, especially in multiple papillomas of childhood and more rarely with large chondromas or adenomas in the adult.

DIAGNOSIS

After consideration of the history this can usually be made by inspection with a laryngeal mirror. However, confirmation of the diagnosis by histological examination must be sought whenever possible.

Direct laryngoscopy

This technique remains the essential means of performing any intralaryngeal operation, especially where tissue must be removed for biopsy (*see* Chapter 10). Although often performed under local anaesthesia, the rapid development of safer general anaesthetics and relaxants, has now made direct laryngoscopy under general anaesthesia the method of choice in most centres. Much greater accuracy for inspection and biopsy is achieved at little risk and with greater comfort to the patient. Certainly much of the increased value of direct laryngoscopy today is also due to the use of fibre-optic lighting systems giving better and more reliable illumination.

In young children where mirror examination of the larynx would be impossible, there should be no hesitation in proceeding to direct laryngoscopy under general

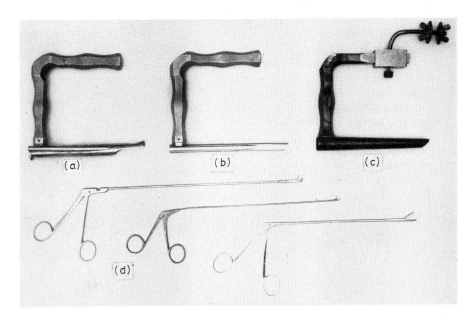

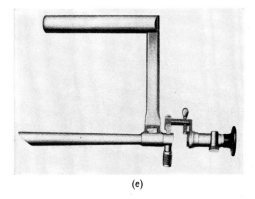

FIG. 142.—Jackson laryngoscopes using twin proximal fibre-optic lighting; (*a*) general inspection type; (*b*) anterior commissure type; (*c*) modified larger calibre with suspension bracket for microlaryngoscopy; (*d*) three types of biopsy forceps; (*e*) Broyles' pattern anterior commissure laryngoscope with distal fibre-optic lighting and built-in × 6 magnification system.

anaesthesia, both for establishing a diagnosis and very often for regular treatment of multiple papillomas.

Microlaryngoscopy

During the past three years the technique of direct inspection under general anaesthesia has been taken a stage further in the interests of greater accuracy of observation and surgical precision. Kleinsasser (1965) adapted the Zeiss operating microscope, fitted with a 400 mm. objective lens to work with wide calibre tapered laryngoscopes of his own design and held in place by a suspension system supported on the patient's anterior chest wall (*see* Fig. 102, p. 265). General anaesthesia with relaxants and a small calibre endotracheal tube are employed.

The method has proved extremely successful, being also particularly useful for endoscopic photography and accurate surgical manipulations within the larynx.

Both hands of the surgeon are free to work with the special set of small instruments designed for use under magnification (Fig. 142).

Earlier investigators have also given thought to developments of this kind and it was Broyles of Baltimore (1941) who first linked a fibre-optic lighting system with built-in (x6) magnification to an anterior commissure pattern laryngoscope (Fig. 142e).

Both of these refinements of the basic technique of direct laryngoscopy have a valuable application and also some limitations. In certain aspects they are complementary, the Kleinsasser method being invaluable for photography and operative intervention but having problems in application to the "anatomically

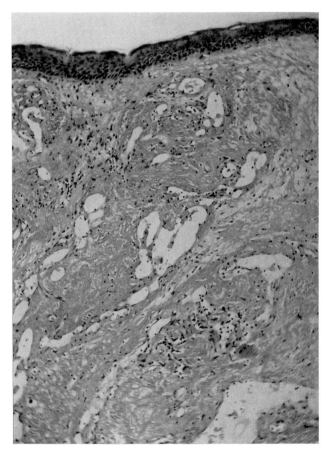

FIG. 143.—Vocal nodule showing marked vascularity and fibrinoid change. (× 120, reduced to three-quarters on reproduction.)

difficult" throat, whereas the Broyles' instrument is ideal for inspection of the "difficult" throat, but less suitable for surgical intervention other than simple biopsy.

It should be emphasized that these techniques are additional to but do not replace the traditional methods and instruments used for routine direct laryngoscopy.

PAPILLOMAS

These are the most common true benign neoplasms in the larynx; even so they are relatively infrequent. In the large Mayo Clinic series of benign laryngeal tumours in 1938 (New and Erich) they formed approximately 25 per cent of the total; whereas Winston and Epstein (1958) give their incidence as roughly 10 per cent (Table I). They may be single or multiple. The solitary types are more common in adults and the multiple more frequent in children. Of 39 cases reported by the latter authors 31 were single and in adults (Plate VId, e and f), and 8 were multiple and in children (Plate VIIa).

Solitary papillomas

These usually grow from the edge of the vocal cord in its anterior two-thirds, but they may also arise from the ventricular band or subglottic region. They are twice as common in males and are most frequent in the 30–50 age group.

Sites of occurrence

When pedunculated and growing from the edge of the vocal cord, papillomas may be difficult to see on quiet respiration because they hang down into the subglottic region. However, on phonation they are immediately displaced upward and may then appear to lie on the upper surface of the cord (Plate VIe and f).

They occasionally arise in the anterior commissure but are very rarely found growing from the posterior part of the larynx. They range from pink to deep red in colour with a warty or papilliferous surface and vary in size from a millet seed to a walnut (Fig. 144). In the condition called pachydermia of the larynx there may be multiple areas of hypertrophy of the posterior part of the cord and the inter-arytenoid region. These areas of papillary keratosis are very similar in appearance to papillomas and often most difficult to distinguish histologically.

Treatment

If small, removal is easily accomplished by using sharp cup forceps through direct laryngoscopy. The use of microlaryngoscopy can be most helpful in dealing with many of these small tumours. The occasional large papilloma may require careful excision via the laryngofissure approach.

Danger of recurrence

If removal is incomplete, a small proportion of solitary papillomas will recur. A further and more serious feature is a definite tendency for a small number, probably not more than 3 or 4 per cent of these tumours, to undergo eventual malignant change (Jackson and Jackson, 1942). Winston and Epstein (1958) found definite carcinoma in only one of the 31 adult papillomas they described, but gradations of cell atypia in several others may well be significant. All tissue removed from the cords must therefore be subjected to microscopic scrutiny.

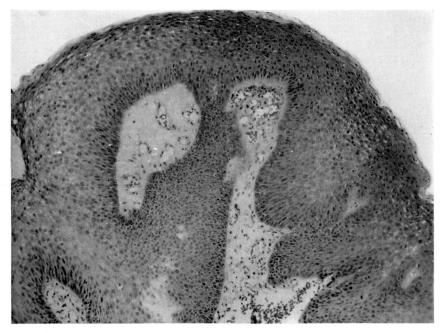

FIG. 144.—Massive but regular squamous cell proliferation in a papiloma with intact basement membrane. (× 160, reduced to three-quarters on reproduction.)

Multiple papillomas

These interesting tumours, by reason of their multiplicity, tendency to spontaneous regression and alleged response to the tetracyclines (Holinger, Johnson and Anison, 1950; Zaprzewski and Sobocynski, 1957) have, by analogy with the common infective wart, a suspected viral aetiology. Bjork and Weber (1956) claim to have produced clinical evidence of this, and also of a possibly significant amino acid dietary deficiency in their patients. Inclusion bodies have also been demonstrated in juvenile papillomas. The tumours appear in childhood chiefly between the ages of 5 and 15 but may commence in infancy. Their frequency is about equal in the sexes and there is generally a tendency to regression at puberty. However, the evidence for this is tenuous (Winston and Epstein, 1958) (Plate VIIa; Fig. 145).

Their multiple nature may cause dyspnoea in young children and a low tracheostomy may be required for months or even several years.

Danger of recurrence

Unfortunately these tumours show a tendency to recur with spread to almost any site in the larynx, pharynx or trachea. Sometimes they may even reach an external tracheostomy orifice. Histologically, unlike adult papillomas they normally show no tendency to become malignant, however frequently removed. Even so, Capps (1957) quotes three cases of malignant change in adults who had suffered recurrent papillomas in childhood. However, all had had irradiation to their larynges in childhood with subsequent malignant change 18–20 years later.

380

They show further resemblance to skin warts in that after recurring for years, they may suddenly disappear for no apparent reason. Since this may happen about puberty and because of the ultimate natural limitation of the disease, it is very desirable to damage the mucosa as little as possible by surgical intervention.

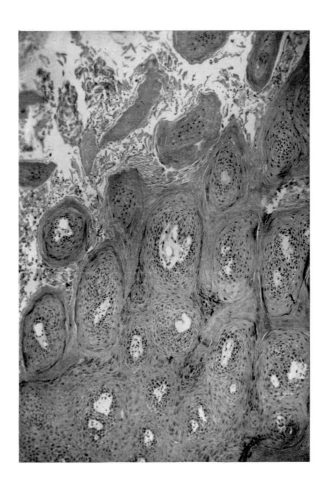

FIG. 145.—Papilloma of childhood showing papillary processes surrounded by whorls of desquamating keratin. (× 125, reduced to three-quarters on reproduction.)

Treatment

The principal method of treatment is by repeated accurate surgical removal by "scalping", using the side of a sharp cup forceps for each individual tumour, or by the use of diathermy. Such intervention should always be conservative, often requiring repeated sessions at appropriate intervals. Microlaryngoscopic techniques are most helpful (Pracy, 1970). Medical treatment using tetracyclines (Holinger, Johnson and Anison, 1950), systemic hormones, bovine wart vaccine (Moffitt, 1959) and autogenous vaccine therapy, particularly the latter, have been useful in a number of cases (Holinger and colleagues, 1962). A further report by Holinger, Schild and Maurizi (1968) states that some success has been achieved using antimetabolites such as Methotrexate intravenously and also with some of the alkylating agents.

Tracheostomy must be carried out without hesitation if indicated. It should always be placed well below the cricoid cartilage to avoid subsequent stenosis, and be as far as possible from the papillomas. An inner tube may also be used which can be fitted with a speaking valve. A decision to decannulate should not be made until some months have elapsed after the last recurrence has been successfully removed.

Irradiation is mentioned only to be condemned as being completely unjustified in this disease (Capps, 1957). These tumours are seldom radio-sensitive and frequent disasters have occurred. Majoros, Devine and Parkhill (1963) have recently reported that 14 per cent of children receiving external irradiation for this complaint developed squamous carcinoma of the larynx at a later date.

Cryosurgery.—Crysosurgical destruction of multiple papillomata is currently under trial.

Local applications.—Caustics such as silver nitrate or podophyllin are alleged to have been helpful in many cases (Holinger, Johnson and Anison, 1950; Pinsker and Proud, 1958). Some evidence has also been given to support the use of painting the tumour sites with oestrogens after removal (Broyles, 1941; Zalin, 1948). The application of ultrasound has been described by Birck and Manhart (1962).

FIBROMAS

The true neoplasm, as distinct from a fibrous polyp or node, is a rare tumour. Stewart (1957) found only nine over a twelve-year period at the Royal Infirmary, Edinburgh. In a recent nine-year survey at the Royal National Throat, Nose and Ear Hospital, London (Table I) only eight were reported. It may occur in any age group, but mainly in adults between the ages of 30 and 50, and most commonly on the edge of the vocal cord at the junction of the middle and anterior thirds (Plate VI*b*). However, they may also occur at any other laryngeal site. Off the cords they may well go undetected owing to their small size and the absence of symptoms.

Treatment

They are usually round, firm, smooth and sessile and their treatment is by complete endoscopic removal with suitable forceps under general anaesthesia.

CYSTS

Those cysts that have origin within the larynx may be usefully divided into:

(1) True cysts, having a secretory lining epithelium of columnar or cubical cells interspersed with goblet cells, as in congenital cysts and the retention cysts of seromucinous glands.

(2) Pseudocysts, due to degeneration of simple tumours such as polypi or fibromas, and those due to trauma such as lymph or blood cysts (El-Mofty, 1959).

Congenital cysts

Congenital cysts are very rare. New and Erich (1938) reported only one out of 35 laryngeal cysts of all types. They conclude that these cysts originate from a sequestration of embryonic cells in the saccule or appendix of the laryngeal ventricle. It is also possible that some of these cysts are of branchiogenic origin from the third branchial pouch (Wilson, 1955; Taylor, 1965). Among laryngeal tumours they are relatively rare, being most likely to be encountered in early infancy. Asherson (1957) refers to the congenital cyst as "a benign lesion which belies its deadly nature". They are most commonly diagnosed post-mortem and their sinister repute gives emphasis to the importance of early endoscopic examination in all cases of infantile stridor. These cysts are found even less frequently in adults, and by this time they tend to be larger, sometimes extending through the thyrohyoid membrane into the anterior triangle of the neck (El-Mofty, 1959) (*see* Chapter 11).

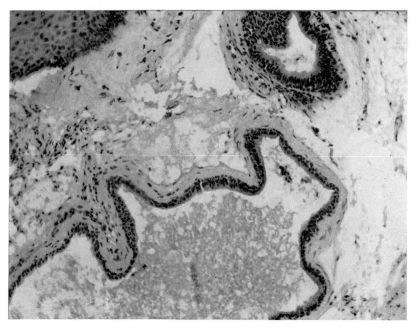

Fig. 146.—Retention cyst of the larynx lined by columnar epithelium with occasional goblet cells. (× 160, reduced to three-quarters on reproduction.)

Retention cysts

Retention cysts of seromucinous glands are easily the most common. They form the great majority of all adult cysts and at least 50 per cent are located on or adjacent to the epiglottis, although they are sometimes found in the ventricles and on the ventricular bands or aryepiglottic folds (Plates VI*c* and VII*f*). They are typically lined by columnar epithelium, and are more thin-walled, smooth, sub-mucous, translucent grey swellings compared with congenital cysts which are deeper, have thicker walls and are therefore less easy to identify (Fig. 146). In young children they can also be extremely dangerous, although perhaps less so than the congenital variety.

Pseudocysts

Pseudocysts, whether due to simple tumour degeneration or traumatic inplantation, and blood or lymph cysts are also rare. They may occur in any part of the larynx, although the vocal cords and immediately adjacent areas are the more frequent sites. They are usually small and their differential diagnosis presents little difficulty if there is an accurate history.

Symptoms and signs usually point to airway obstruction of variable degree in childhood, often with added huskiness or stridorous "cry". In adults interference with the airway may well be apparent but hoarseness and a fluctuant swelling in the anterior triangle of the neck may also be found.

Diagnosis and treatment should always be prompt owing to their great potential danger. Endoscopic inspection and diagnosis followed by marsupialization, using diathermy, or removal by snare excision, may be effective in children. External removal via pharyngotomy or thyrotomy are sometimes required in adults.

ANGIOMAS

Three different conditions are described under this name and must be carefully distinguished.

Pseudo-angiomas or vascular polyps

Such lesions are produced by trauma to the vocal cords causing subepithelial rupture of a small blood vessel. The resulting haematoma soon becomes converted into vascular reparative tissue with distended blood spaces, and then takes on an angiomatous appearance both clinically and histologically. As previously mentioned these tumours are simply a variety of cordal polyp. Any collection of blood occurring as a result of voice strain should ideally be evacuated rather than allowed to form a submucous haematoma (*see also* p. 371).

Congenital telangiectasia (Osler-Rendu disease)

These small swellings are usually multiple, occurring diffusely on the skin and in mucous membranes. They are familial in nature. The face, neck and fingers are common sites on the skin; while the mucosa of the lips, nose, tongue, cheeks, palate, epiglottis and interior of the larynx may be variously involved (Plate VII*c*). Hoarseness is not a usual symptom, but bleeding may occur on very slight trauma and this is one of the causes of haemoptysis for which the help of the laryngologist may be sought. If bleeding is persistent it may be necessary to cauterize the bleeding point electrically.

True angiomas

These are rare tumours compared with the pseudo-angiomas. In the well known series of 722 benign laryngeal tumours reported by New and Erich in 1938, there were only 25 true angiomas and one lymphangioma. The capillary cavernous variant may be represented separately or combined in any haemangioma. Two definite varieties are recognized, the infantile and the adult. The former usually presents in the first three months of life and both sexes seem equally affected. It tends to grow rapidly after birth, is usually subglottic, may be associated with dermal angiomas and causes afebrile episodic laryngeal obstruction. Diagnosis

PLATE VI

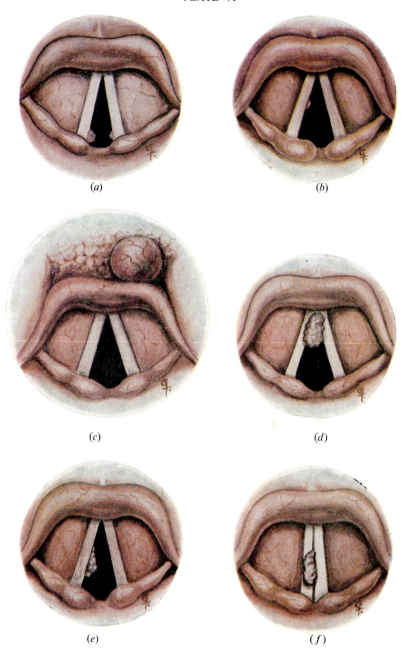

(a) Intubation granulomas on the vocal processes of the arytenoids. (b) Fibroma growing from the edge of the right vocal cord. (c) Retention cyst of the left vallecula. (d) Pedunculated papilloma growing from the anterior commissure. (e) Single papilloma of right vocal cord on quiet respiration. (f) Effect of phonation on papilloma shown in (e).

PLATE VII

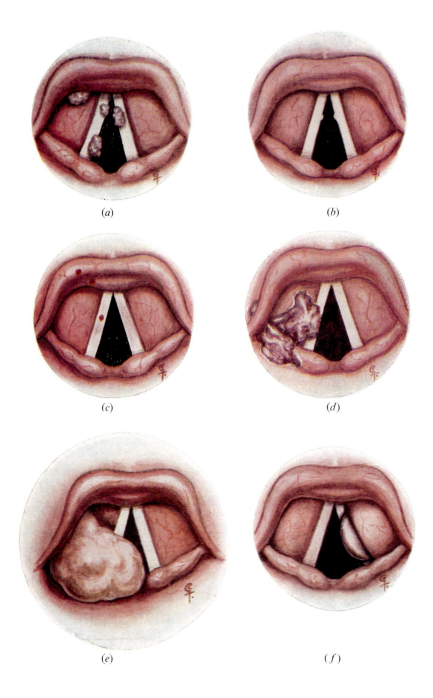

(a) Multiple papillomas in the larynx. (b) Bilateral vocal nodules in the typical position. (c) Multiple congenital telangiectases in the larynx (Osler–Rendu disease). (d) Large angioma of the right ventricular band and aryepiglottic fold. (e) Chondroma growing from the right arytenoid. (f) Retention cyst of left laryngeal ventricle projecting into the larynx between the left vocal cord and ventricular band.

PLATE VIII

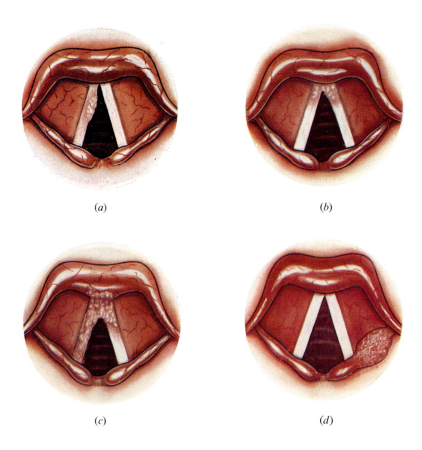

(*a*) (*b*)

(*c*) (*d*)

(*a*) Stage 1 carcinoma limited to the membranous right vocal cord. Irradiation is the treatment of choice. (*b*) Carcinoma involving the anterior commissure and anterior thirds of both vocal cords (Stage 2). Irradiation preferable to partial laryngectomy. (*c*) Stage 3 glottic carcinoma involving the anterior third of the left cord, the anterior commissure, the base of the epiglottis and the whole length of the right vocal cord to include the arytenoid. Some reduced mobility of the right cord. Total laryngectomy would be the treatment of choice. (*d*) Early (Stage 1) carcinoma of left aryepiglottic fold. Treatment by irradiation or partial laryngectomy (*continued overleaf*).

PLATE VIII (*continued*)

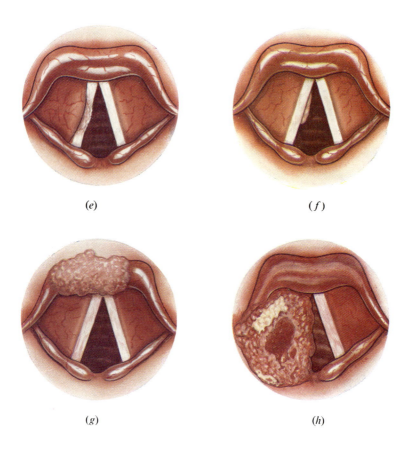

(*e*)   (*f*)

(*g*)   (*h*)

(*e*) Stage 2 carcinoma of right ventricle involving the middle third of the right vocal cord. Treatment by irradiation or total laryngectomy. (*f*) Subglottic (Stage 1) carcinoma beneath mobile right vocal cord. No posterior extension. Irradiation is the treatment of choice. (*g*) Extensive epiglottic carcinoma (Stage 2). Treatment by total laryngectomy. (*h*) Massive carcinoma involving the whole fixed right hemilarynx with subglottic extension and two mobile palpable homolateral neck nodes (Stage 3). Treatment by total laryngectomy with right radical block dissection in continuity.

may be difficult owing to the depth of the tumour beneath normal mucosa, and biopsy confirmation is certainly dangerous. Despite possible risk of later carcinoma, the only effective treatment is by small doses (200–500 r) of x-radiation. This is only justified by the high mortality of the untreated condition. Holborow (1958) and Mawson (1961) give good descriptions of the hazards involved.

Adult haemangiomas appear as rather large sessile purplish tumours usually in the supraglottic region and often extending submucosally into the laryngopharynx (Plate VII*d*). They do not project into the lumen, do not grow and as a rule there are no symptoms. If possible they should be left alone.

CHONDROMAS

Chondromas are also rare tumours. Little more than 100 have so far been reported in the literature. They chiefly affect men in the 40–60 age group. They are slow-growing, smooth, hard, sessile and generally subglottic, often growing from the posterior plate of the cricoid cartilage. They may also arise from other laryngeal cartilages, for example the arytenoid, as described by Salmon (1957) (Plate VII*e*). They vary from the size of a cherry to that of an orange. The smaller variety are

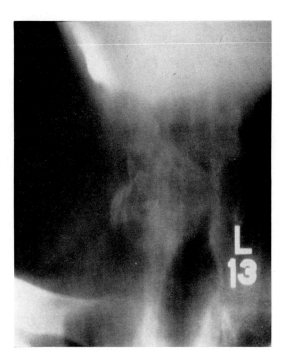

FIG. 147.—Tomogram to show position of a massive chondroma of the cricoid cartilage causing gross obstruction of the airway and distortion of the whole larynx.

the most numerous and consist equally of enchondromas and ecchondromas; the larger are usually mixed (Capps, 1957). They can grow to a large size and, by causing dyspnoea, may necessitate tracheostomy (Fig. 147). Bronchopneumonia and asphyxia are the less common complications which may endanger life. In some cases calcification and myxomatous degeneration may occur. Sarcomatous degeneration has also been described but this appears extremely rare.

Treatment

Treatment is by laryngofissure and local removal of the tumour if not too large. At times the whole larynx may become so involved that total laryngectomy will be required but surgery should be as conservative as possible.

AMYLOIDOSIS

The classical description of homogeneous intercellular amyloid material states it to be a well known secondary manifestation in generalized chronic toxaemia. In the primary disease without any apparent precipitating condition, there is maximal diffuse involvement of the heart and striated muscles with less striking abdominal involvement (Bayliss, 1957). Many cases of a third type in which local "amyloid tumours" occur typically in the upper air passages or bladder may sometimes be found at post-mortem to have more widespread primary disease. Nevertheless, in a large number of such cases the local deposit is quite solitary.

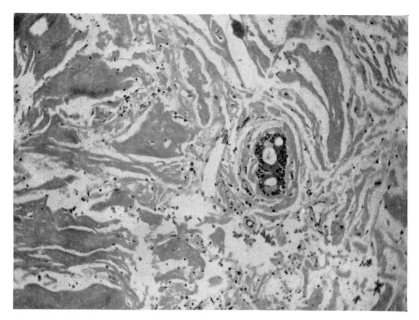

Fig. 148.—Hyaline intercellular amyloid material surrounding mucous gland ducts.
(× 160, reduced to three-quarters on reproduction.)

These local amyloid tumours are most often found in the larynx and trachea, but may also occur in the tongue, nose, pharynx and elsewhere in the respiratory tract (Payling Wright, 1958; McAlpine, Radcliffe and Friedmann, 1963). The sex incidence is about equal, although with a slight male preponderance, and they are found usually in adults in the 40–70 age range. The vocal cords are the most common site, although any intralaryngeal structure may be involved. Appearances are variable, but two types are recognized, the localized swelling or subepithelial deposit seen as a slightly raised smooth pink nodule or plaque, and the diffuse infiltrative variety (Falbe-Hansen, 1955) (Fig. 148).

The aetiology of primary localized amyloidosis is obscure. Experimental studies have suggested that the formation of amyloid is a perverted phase of protein synthesis, the initiation of which is still hypothetical. Chronic local infection or irritation is a suspected but unproven cause (Holinger, Johnson and Delgado, 1959).

Symptoms

Symptoms arise entirely from the mechanical effects of the lesions depending upon their precise situation in the larynx. Hoarseness, irritation and dry cough are therefore usual.

Treatment

Treatment of the localized variety is by simple endoscopic removal; if complete, recurrence is rare. The diffuse type requires more consideration since medical measures and irradiation are ineffective, despite some claims for corticosteroid therapy (Creston, 1961). It would seem that simple excision of as much affected tissue as possible via a laryngofissure approach with free skin grafts to the raw surface is the most effective. However, such treatment should be reserved only for those cases in which the airway is embarrassed. No case of malignant change has yet been reported.

ADENOMAS

These tumours are very rare, few having been described since Moore's description of 13 cases in 1920. Stewart (1960) stated that only about 20 cases had been reported in the English literature in the past 30 years, and the recent large series referred to in Table I lists only two cases (Epstein and colleagues, 1957).

They are found occasionally throughout the mucosa of the respiratory tract, more commonly below the larynx, Willis (1953) stating that they account for about 5 per cent of bronchial tumours. In the larynx they usually arise in the supraglottic region, frequently in the ventricles where mucous gland aggregates are most numerous. Growth is slow and symptoms are those of mechnical interference. They are mostly sessile, with well defined margins, covered with an intact epithelium, and having a congested, smooth or mammillary appearance. They have a slight preponderance in men and vary greatly in size from a millet seed to a hen's egg.

Pathology

Histologically, they are a distinct entity arising from the mucus-secreting glands of the air passages. There is thus no need to invoke the presence of ectopic salivary tissue. They range from the typically solid variety resembling a benign mixed salivary tumour to an extremely cystic tumour akin to the adenolymphoma of Warthin, the main distinction being the usual absence of lymphoid tissue in the laryngeal tumour (Fig. 149) (Lennox and colleagues, 1968). A further variant is an eosinophilic glandular cell cystadenoma (Heath, 1961).

Treatment

Treatment is by surgical removal via an external approach where the tumour is of any size, since excision must be complete if recurrence is to be avoided. Prognosis remains excellent if removal has been adequate.

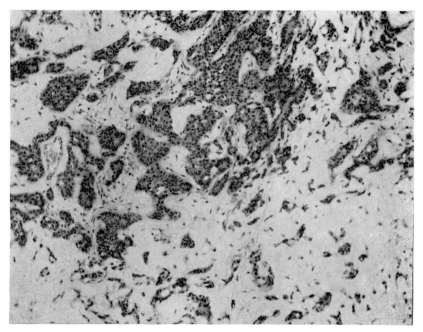

FIG. 149.—Laryngeal adenoma showing epithelial cells and tubule formation lying in a soft fibrous stroma.

MYOBLASTOMA

This unique and rare tumour was first described on the vocal cord by Abri-kossoff in 1931, although it had been described quite frequently in the tongue, also in skeletal muscle and a few subcutaneous sites, some years before. At least 25 cases have now been described in the larynx. MacNaughton and Fraser (1954) reviewed 14 adult laryngeal cases and one in a child of nine years. The sexes are almost equally affected and the fourth decade has furnished the highest frequency. They appear as small flat or nodular submucous plaques, pink or yellow in colour, with a poorly defined margin. They tend to arise in the posterior half of the larynx and are of slow growth. Symptoms again result entirely from their size and situation.

Pathology

The aetiology of these tumours is not known with certainty. Willis (1953) regarded lingual myoblastomas as degenerative lesions of muscle fibres and not true neoplasms. Others have considered them to be a type of neurofibroma, since there is alleged evidence of a possible neural origin (Fust and Custer, 1949).

Histologically, the most important feature is the marked pseudo-epitheliomatous hyperplasia of the overlying squamous epithelium. Not infrequently this results in a mistaken diagnosis of squamous carcinoma. However, no true case of malignant change has yet been reported (Fig. 150).

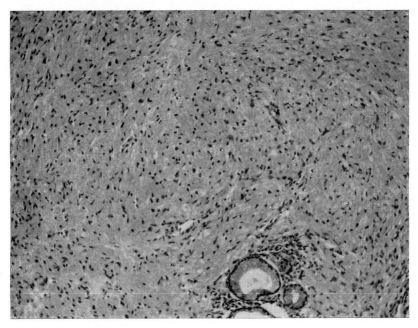

FIG. 150.—Granular cell myoblastoma of the larynx, showing typical fibrillar streaming pattern and incorporating mucous glands. (× 160, reduced to three-quarters on reproduction.)

Treatment

Treatment is by endoscopic removal for the majority of small tumours. Larger lesions or recurrences may require excision via laryngofissure. Prognosis is excellent although the tendency to recurrence through poor clearance of margins imposes a necessity for prolonged follow-up.

Neurofibromas, lipomas, rhabdomyomas, plasmacytomas, xanthomas and thyroid gland rests occur so rarely in the larynx as to need no detailed discussion here, except to state the rarity of their appearance. Cummings, Montgomery and Balogh (1969) give a good account of neurofibroma, noting that 15 per cent of cases reported were associated with Von Recklinghausen's disease.

MALIGNANT TUMOURS

CLASSIFICATION

Cancer of the larynx accounts for about 2 per cent of all reported cases of malignant disease, but there is still some difficulty in assessing its relative frequency because full accord has not yet been reached on terminology and classification. Nevertheless, in recent years a greater appreciation of the natural history and surgical pathology of laryngeal cancer has resulted in growing agreement. This has been much helped since 1954 by the work of the International Union Against Cancer, which then accepted the task of drafting a precise classification for cancer of the breast, cervix uteri and the larynx. A further scheme of classification was then added to include the buccal cavity, pharynx and bladder (U.I.C.C. Report, 1962). Since then the latest U.I.C.C. Report (1968) offers full classification for 27 main anatomical sites, which in the head and neck include the buccal cavity (including lip and oropharynx), nasopharynx, hypopharynx and larynx.

The earliest and most important attempts at classification were made by Isambert (1876) and Krishaber (1879) who separated tumours into two main groups—intrinsic and extrinsic—although Isambert also suggested that subglottic growths should constitute a distinct subdivision. Many years later, Thomson suggested four main subdivisions: (1) intrinsic; (2) subglottic; (3) extrinsic; and (4) mixed (Thomson and Colledge, 1930).

From pathological and therapeutic viewpoints there is basic soundness in Krishaber's original division into intrinsic and extrinsic lesions, in view of the very different behaviour of growths arising within the larynx, especially on the vocal cords, and those arising outside. However, there was much dispute as to the precise topographical limits of these areas, intrinsic often being held to include the true cord, ventricle and ventricular band, and extrinsic to include those growths arising in the laryngopharynx. Consequently these terms are now in decline and today the distinction survives in some measure as cordal and non-cordal laryngeal cancer.

The scheme of classification of the larynx shown in Table II has been fully discussed by the various responsible committees since 1958 and after being recommended for a five year trial period from January 1st 1963 this has been extended by the U.I.C.C. for a further five years until 1972. It would seem to meet all reasonable requirements by dividing the larynx into anatomical regions and sites (Figs. 151–153).

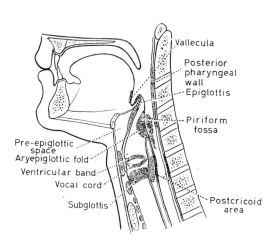

FIG. 151.—Sagittal section to show common sites of origin of laryngeal and laryngopharyngeal carcinoma.

In the United States a report of the Sub-Committee on the Larynx of the American Joint Committee on Cancer Staging and End Results Reporting recommended in 1961 the adoption of a similar scheme, with the exception that marginal zone sites be included with the laryngeal supraglottic sites (Norris, 1963).

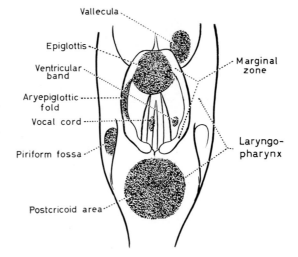

FIG. 152.—Posterior view to show common sites of tumour origin; also the marginal zone between the larynx and laryngopharynx.

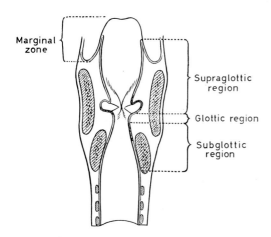

FIG. 153.—Coronal section to show the division into laryngeal regions and marginal zone.

TABLE II

Regions	Sites
Larynx Supraglottic	Posterior surface of the epiglottis (infrahyoid)
	Ventricular bands
	Ventricles
	Arytenoids
Glottic	Vocal cords
	Anterior and posterior commissures
Subglottic	Walls of the subglottis
Marginal zone	Tip of epiglottis (suprahyoid)
	Aryepoglottic folds
Laryngopharynx (hypopharynx)	Pyriform fossae
	Postcricoid area
	Posterior pharyngeal wall

In 1954 the Committee on Clinical Classification and Applied Statistics of the International Union Against Cancer also proposed the "T.N.M." system as a universal method of classification for each anatomical site. This defines the extent of the disease in terms of its three main components: T = extent of primary tumour; N = condition of regional lymph nodes; M = distant metastases.

Variation or degrees of local extension, fully described, are designated by numbers (for example, T_1, T_2 as below). The same procedure may then be used for the clinical condition of the regional lymph nodes (N) and distant metastases (M).

Having been under trial for a number of years a wide measure of agreement through international discussion has now been reached for these U.I.C.C. proposals. However, it is felt that more time is required and, in the case of the larynx, a final decision is not intended until 1972. The descriptive details are set out below in Table III.

TABLE III

Supraglottic	Glottic	Subglottic
T. Primary tumour		
T_1S. Pre-invasive carcinoma, so-called carcinoma *in situ*		
T_1. Tumour confined to one anatomical site within the larynx		
Tumour confined to laryngeal surface of epiglottis, or to an aryepiglottic fold or to a ventricular cavity or a ventricular band	Tumour confined to one vocal cord and mobility of cord remains normal	Tumour limited to one side of the subglottic region, exclusive of the under-surface of cord
T_2. Tumour confined to one anatomical region within the larynx		
Tumour involving the epiglottis, extending to the ventricular cavities or bands	Tumour involving both cords with normal mobility; or one or both cords with fixation of cords	Tumour extending to two sides of subglottic region, exclusive of the under-surface of the cords
T_3. Tumour extending beyond one anatomical region but confined to the larynx		
Tumour of the epiglottis and/or ventricles or ventricular bands, and extending onto the cords	Tumour extending from cord either to subglottic region or to supraglottic region, that is, to ventricular bands or ventricles	Tumour involving the subglottic region and extending onto the cords
T_4. Tumour extending beyond the larynx		
Tumour as in T_1, T_2 or T_3, but with direct extension to pyriform sinus, postcricoid region, vallecula, or base of tongue	Tumour as in T_1, T_2 or T_3, but with direct extension through cartilage to skin, to the piriform sinus, or to the postcricoid region	Tumour as in T_1, T_2 or T_3, but with direct extension to trachea, skin or postcricoid region

N. Lymph nodes
    N_0. No lymph nodes palpable
    N_1. Homolateral movable lymph nodes
    N_1 a. Nodes not considered to contain growth
    N_1 b. Nodes considered to contain growth
    N_2. Bilateral or contralateral movable lymph nodes
    N_2 a. Nodes not considered to contain growth
    N_2 b. Nodes considered to contain growth
    N_3 Homolateral or bilateral fixed lymph nodes

M. Metastases
    M_0. No evidence of distant metastases
    M_1. Distant metastases

The American Joint Committee has given approval to this scheme, but has recognized the practical day-to-day need for a simpler plan of malignant "staging" than the unwieldy use of all the individual combinations of the T, N and M categories. It has therefore proposed the summary of stage groupings shown in Table IV.

TABLE IV

Stage I:	T_1, N_0, M_0	Stage IV:	T_4, N_1, M_0
Stage II:	T_2, N_0, M_0		$T_1, N_{2/3}, M_0$
	T_3, N_0, M_0		$T_2, N_{2/3}, M_0$
	T_4, N_0, M_0		$T_3, N_{2/3}, M_0$
			$T_4, N_{2/3}, M_0$
Stage III:	T_1, N_1, M_0		T_{1-4}, M_1
	T_2, N_1, M_0		
	T_3, N_1, M_0		

The four stages as indicated may then apply to lesions arising in each of the three laryngeal regions, giving a total of twelve major groups. The Committee on Clinical Classification of the U.I.C.C. do not at present recommend any stage grouping.

Although a number of alternative methods of classification have been proposed in recent years by other authorities, it is not proposed to list them here since the above schemes are at present under wide international trial and, it seems, are likely to be adopted, either as set out or with slight modifications.

General features

There is some evidence of a slow increase in the incidence of the disease in recent years in the United States, although apparently not in the United Kingdom (Curwen and Kennaway, 1954). In a recent analysis Wynder, Bross and Day (1956) have stated that laryngeal cancer occurs in about 3–4 individuals per 100,000 U.S. citizens. Shumrick (1969) gives some evidence that the frequency rate of laryngeal cancer may be increasing to as much as 4 per cent in the U.S. By far the highest rates are among Asian races, particularly Indians, in whom the incidence is more than double that of Western races.

No definite causes are yet known for the disease although it is likely that chronic mucosal irritation by heavy smoking, excessive intake of alcohol, particularly spirits, and the chewing of tobacco or aromatic nuts in Asian countries play a definite rôle in its aetiology. The U.S. Surgeon-General's Report on Smoking and Health (1964) specifically finds a definite correlation between heavy smoking and laryngeal cancer. Auerbach, Hammond and Garfinkel (1970) have now shown that metaplasia and malignant change in human laryngeal epithelium develops in proportion to the tobacco smoke exposure, especially with cigarettes, and that the changes may be reversed by abstention. Very prolonged vocal strain with severe chronic laryngitis and previous irradiation of the neck may also be contributory causes, although it may be doubted whether chronic upper respiratory infection alone plays any real part (Siirala and Siirala, 1966).

Throughout the larynx and pharynx the disease predominantly affects men in the ratio of 8:1, with the sole exception of the postcricoid type of tumour. This ratio is reversed in tumours of the postcricoid region, being associated with the pre-cancerous mucosal changes of the Paterson–Kelly syndrome of women. Laryngeal cancer may occur at any age, although rare in young people under 30.

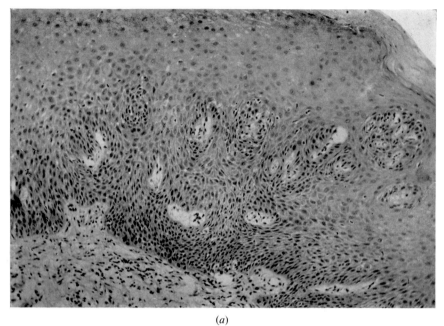

(a)

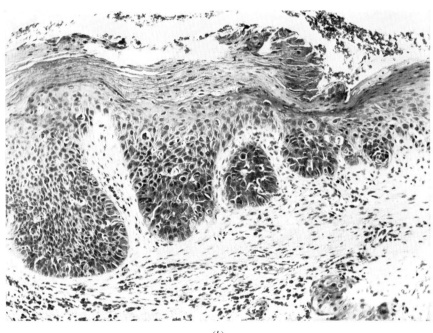

(b)

Fig. 154.—(a) Hyperkeratosis of a vocal cord showing acanthosis in deeper layers but intact basement membrane; (b) keratotic epithelium with *in situ* carcinoma changes in deeper layers but no penetration of basement membrane. (× 160, reduced to three-quarters on reproduction.)

The youngest case reported was in a boy of 10 (Crookes, 1953). In males the sixth and seventh decades are most affected, whereas in females the peak age groups are often one decade younger.

Histopathology

By far the most common variety of tumour is the squamous cell carcinoma. It is usually well differentiated, but in this respect there is a difference according to the main region affected. Cordal tumours show a relatively high degree of differentiation, 80 per cent in a recent series, whereas in a parallel non-cordal and laryngo-pharyngeal series there was only a 55 per cent proportion of well differentiated tumours (Shaw, 1965) (Figs. 155–157).

In any large series it is generally found that 96–98 per cent are squamous cell carcinomas with the occasional transitional cell carcinoma of the epiglottis (Fig. 159). Adenocarcinoma of mucous glands (Fig. 158), and basal cell carcinoma also occur.

Cady, Rippey and Frazell (1968) reported a series of 31 cases of non-epidermoid cancer of the larynx out of a total 2,500 cases of laryngeal cancer seen at Memorial Center, New York. Of these, 17 were adenocarcinomas. Eleven cases of laryngeal cancer other than squamous carcinoma were seen at the Royal Marsden Hospital 1948–1967 inclusive, out of a total of 1,516 new patients, and are listed as follows:

Adenocarcinoma	5
Malignant lymphoma	2
Fibrosarcoma	1
Chondrosarcoma	1
Plasmacytoma	1
Malignant melanoma	1

Seven cases of pseudosarcoma (Fig. 161) were seen in this period. Although the stromal cells of this lesion have a sarcomatous appearance, the tumour is epithelial in origin and contains inconspicuous and often intramucosal elements of squamous carcinoma. It must be treated as such. True sarcomas are very rare and those reported have usually been an occasional fibrosarcoma (Fig. 160), rhabdosarcoma or reticulosarcoma. Malignant melanoma has also been found in the larynx, but must be regarded as extremely rare (Welsh and Welsh, 1961); only about 12 cases have been reported.

Since Broders proposed his scheme for histological grading of squamous carcinomas of the lip in 1920, it has been customary to use the system of four grades applied to the larynx as indicated in Table V.

TABLE V

Grades	Percentage of cells undifferentiated
1	0–25
2	25–50
3	50–75
4	75–100

However, in this country during the past 35 years Broders' grading has increasingly been used in the modified form of three categories: "well", "moderately" and "poorly" differentiated—expressions that are descriptively adequate providing

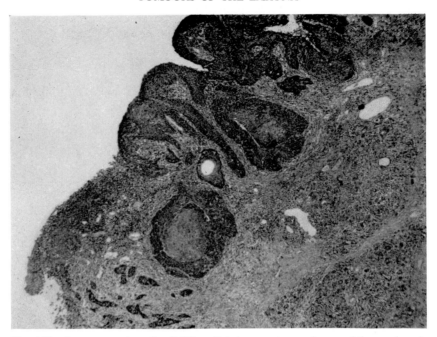

FIG. 155.—Low power view of well differentiated squamous carcinoma of the vocal cord, showing general features, cell nest formation and invasion of the stroma. (×50, reduced to three-quarters on reproduction.)

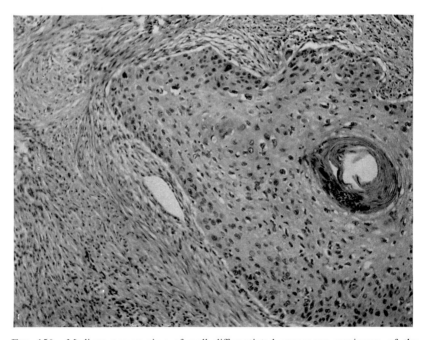

FIG. 156.—Medium power view of well differentiated squamous carcinoma of the supraglottic region, showing nuclear irregularity, cell mitosis and pearl formation. (× 160, reduced to three-quarters on reproduction.)

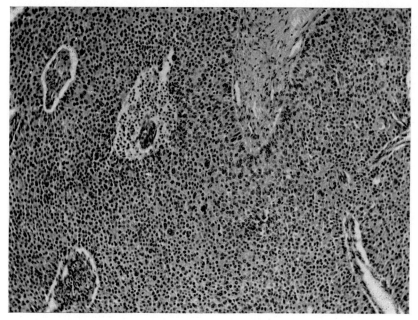

Fig. 157.—Undifferentiated laryngeal carcinoma, showing nuclear pleomorphism and hyperchromasia. (× 160, reduced to three-quarters on reproduction.)

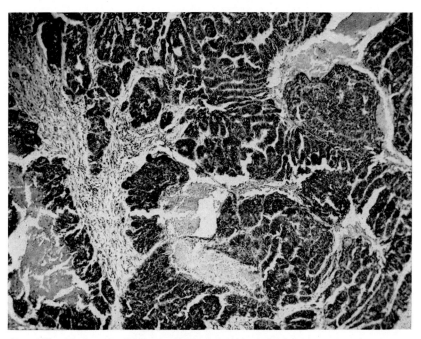

Fig. 158.—Moderately differentiated adenocarcinoma of the larynx showing invasion of stroma by hyperchromatic masses of columnar epithelium. (× 85, reduced to three-quarters on reproduction.)

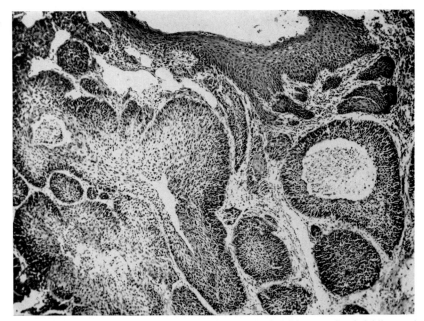

Fig. 159.—Transitional cell carcinoma of the epiglottis with extensive infolding and cystic pseudonecrosis.

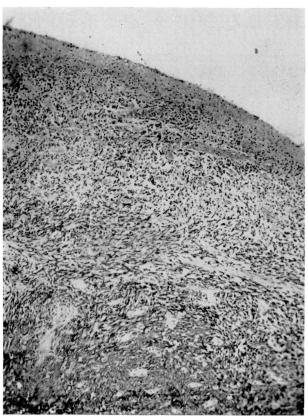

Fig.160.—Fibrosarcoma of larynx, showing spindle cell patterns. Post-radiation changes are present.

precise statements are included regarding *"in situ"* or *"invasive"* characteristics of each tumour (Figs. 154 and 161). The description *"in situ"* carcinoma is now generally known to mean intra-epithelial malignant change without penetration of the basement membrane (Fig. 161). Added clinical significance also lies in the fact

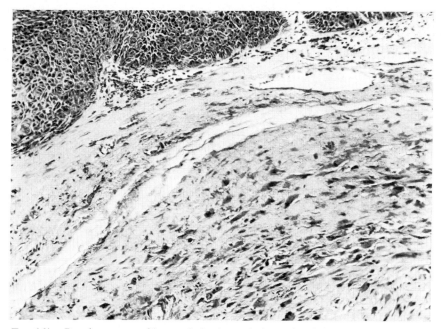

FIG. 161.—Pseudosarcoma of larynx. Lying beneath the surface layer of *in situ* carcinoma is the so called pseudosarcomatous stroma. (× 160, reduced to three-quarters on reproduction.)

that its natural history is not necessarily progressive. As with simple keratosis it may regress and disappear, although progress to an invasive carcinoma occurs in a high proportion of cases.

GLOTTIC REGION

Glottic cancer is by far the most common type of laryngeal neoplasm in the adult. It is also the most frequent variety of laryngeal cancer, estimates varying from 50 to 85 per cent being quoted by Negus (1955). This is fortunate since its diagnosis is quicker, its treatment usually simpler and prognosis infinitely better than that of cancer in other regions of the larynx or of most other sites in the head and neck.

It generally arises on the free margin or upper surface of the true vocal cord in its middle or anterior third—the area of maximal work-load (Plate VIIIa). Local spread along the cord in both directions is slow, owing to the dense layers of elastic and fibrous tissue present, and metastasis to cervical lymph nodes is uncommon owing to the absence of any lymphatics in Reinke's subepithelial connective tissue layer. Ten cases only out of a total of 306 consecutive cases of glottic cancer seen at the Royal National Throat, Nose and Ear Hospital during the years 1947–56, were found to have clinically positive neck nodes on first attendance (Shaw, 1965).

Tumours arising in the anterior commissure are rare and also treacherous (Plate VIII*b*), only five being encountered in the above series. Growths in the posterior commissure are almost unknown.

SUBGLOTTIC REGION

Although this area is frequently involved to some degree by tumours spreading downwards from the true cords—at least one-fifth of the above series having had some evidence of this type of spread—it is uncommon for cancer to arise *de novo* in the subglottic region. When it does, it is usually in the anterior half of the sub-glottis, it often spreads anteriorly across the mid-line, and may be difficult to detect clinically (Plate VIII*b*). It differs significantly from cordal lesions in that it gains early access to lymphatics draining directly into the prelaryngeal, paratracheal and lower deep cervical chains of nodes. A further danger is of direct spread through the cricothyroid membrane into the thyroid gland or deep fascia and strap muscles. Diagnosis and treatment are always correspondingly more difficult and prognosis must always be guarded.

SUPRAGLOTTIC REGION

Ventricles and ventricular bands

These are uncommon sites of origin for laryngeal cancer (Martin, 1947). They are most often involved by tumours spreading upward from the true cords. Disease is generally extensive by the time the diagnosis is made owing to lack of early symptoms. The laryngeal ventricle has a bad reputation as it may conceal early lesions and often leads to delayed diagnosis (Plate VIII*e*).

Infrahyoid epiglottis

This is the most frequently involved area of the epiglottis and was found to give 12 per cent of a large series of laryngeal tumours at all sites (Shaw, 1959). Even so, this is a low incidence compared with reports from Continental and U.S. authorities. Early diagnosis is again difficult owing to the "silent" nature of small lesions, which may be hypertrophic and proliferative in type, or more often may form a slow but deeply penetrating ulcer just above the petiolus. On a backward curling epiglottis they are easily missed at mirror examination.

These tumours have a particularly sinister repute owing to their mid-line position, easy access to bilateral deep cervical lymphatics and tendency to early invasion of the pre-epiglottic space (Plate VIII*g* and Fig. 151).

MARGINAL ZONE

Suprahyoid epiglottis

The projecting or free part of the epiglottis is a much less common site for the origin of laryngeal cancer, although it is often involved by spread from neigh-bouring areas. It generally appears as a slowly growing superficial ulcer associated with gradual erosion of the tip and with minimal symptoms. Alternatively a proliferative granular lesion is sometimes found. Owing to the presence of fewer lymphatics in the area and its comparative isolation, a tumour confined to this site is more amenable to treatment and has a better prognosis than on the infrahyoid epiglottis.

Aryepiglottic folds

These tumours are usually large when diagnosed because there are few early symptoms. In the relative frequency of primary tumours of this region, they occupy a position midway between the ventricular bands and epiglottis. However, the area is commonly involved by tumours that have spread from the vallecula or epiglottis and from the lateral pharyngeal wall or pyriform fossa, or even from the upward extension of an advanced cordal tumour (Plate VIII*d* and *h*). In appearance they are usually nodular and proliferative, and although accessible to treatment they generally carry a poor prognosis due to their extent and the frequent invasion of the rich lymphatic field.

SPREAD OF MALIGNANT DISEASE

The spread of malignant disease in this area is exactly the same as in other parts of the body: (*a*) by direct extension; (*b*) lymphatic spread; and (*c*) blood stream metastases.

Direct extension

Inside the larynx extension occurs for the most part along the surface of the mucosa or by submucous infiltration. The presence of the surrounding cartilage seems definitely to limit its spread beyond these borders in most cases.

On the vocal cord the general direction of spread is anteroposteriorly; there is little tendency to invade the false cord but spread readily occurs backwards to the tip of the arytenoid and forwards to the commissure, and from there along the opposite cord. In the case of subglottic tumours, the spead may be downwards into the trachea or horizontally around the anterior wall, affecting the subglottic region of the opposite side before there is any invasion of the edge of the cord. This is a bad point in the prognosis of such tumours, which frequently prove to be quite extensive before any symptoms of hoarseness are apparent.

Occasionally a subglottic tumour will spread through the cricothyroid membrane and a glottic lesion may penetrate the thyroid cartilage, but this is unusual—especially the latter unless it arises in the anterior commissure. Similarly, a tumour commencing on one surface of the epiglottis may spread around the tip and invade the other surface before it invades the epiglottic cartilage. Reference has already been made to the tendency for epiglottic cancer to invade the pre-epiglottic space.

Tumours in the region of the anterior commissure, however, may invade the epiglottis in the neighbourhood of the petiolus as well as the thyroid cartilage and there may be deep burrowing ulceration in this area at an unexpectedly early stage. Tumours of the aryepiglottic fold and edge of the epiglottis often spread along the fold very rapidly and also spread along the pharyngo-epiglottic fold to the lateral wall of the pharynx.

401

Direct invasion of small veins or nerve sheaths passing through the thyrohyoid or cricothyroid membranes may sometimes take place; this causes rapid permeation of these minute channels leading to separate involvement of structures well outside the larynx.

Lymphatic spread

The lymphatic spread is of great importance from the point of view of treatment and prognosis. There are practically no lymph vessels in the true vocal cord and, while a tumour is limited to the cord, there is very little tendency to involvement of lymph nodes. It is because of this feature that it is possible to remove an early neoplasm of the vocal cord by a limited local excision, with a very good prospect of cure. This fact, combined with the early onset of symptoms of hoarseness in carcinoma of the vocal cord, makes the prognosis of such lesions more favourable than anywhere else in the body cavities. Below the vocal cord, in the subglottic region, the lymphatic supply is again not very free. The lymph vessels drain into the cricothyroid, pretracheal and paratracheal nodes. Unfortunately the prognosis is not as good as in carcinoma of the vocal cord because symptoms occur later and therefore cases may not come under observation until the tumour has already become extensive. In addition, involvement of the paratracheal lymphatics may be bilateral and may pass undetected until the disease has reached the mediastinum.

The lymphatics of the ventricle drain upwards through the thyrohyoid membrane with those of the supraglottic region to the lymph nodes of the upper and middle deep cervical groups. Neoplasms of the epiglottis metastasize into the same group of nodes but also occasionally affect the submaxillary and submental nodes. This is particularly the case with the papilliferous types of tumour. Of particular importance in a midline area such as the epiglottis is the likelihood of bilateral lymphatic involvement.

The work of Pressman and Simon (1961) has indicated that the vocal cords may be considered almost a "lymphatic divide", there being virtually no transglottic lymph channels. This is of great importance when considering the theoretical basis of supraglottic partial laryngectomy. Nevertheless, transglottic tumours are not infrequent, but since they are usually extensive it would seem likely that direct growth in two directions from the cord is responsible.

Metastatic spread

Metastatic spread by the blood stream is not common, but cases have been reported with deposits in the lungs, liver and bones, sometimes three or four years after operations on the larynx and when there has been no evidence of local recurrence. In patients dead from uncontrolled laryngeal cancer the incidence of distant metastasis was reported as low as 16 per cent (Ormerod and Shaw, 1956). The disease, as a rule, remains localized to the head and neck throughout its course, and upon this are based the concepts of early radical treatment.

SYMPTOMS

Hoarseness is the main early symptom of malignant disease of the larynx. This will occur with very early lesions of the vocal cord but usually occurs at a late stage with supraglottic tumours, and will probably be absent or slight in those of the marginal zone of the laryngopharynx. There are no early symptoms of any constancy in tumours in these last two situations.

Other symptoms of laryngeal cancer are vague discomfort in the throat, some increased expectoration, a thickness rather than huskiness of the voice and occasionally an irritable cough, but the disease is usually already well established before such symptoms appear.

It might be expected that cough would be an early symptom of glottic carcinoma of the larynx but this is not the case. It is, in fact, more common as a symptom of marginal zone tumours.

Alteration of the voice and possibly some dyspnoea on exertion may be two of the early symptoms to become evident in subglottic disease. This is due to infiltration of the vocal cord from below and limitation of its movement before the tumour becomes evident on mirror examination.

Discussion of late symptoms is of no great value; they naturally include dyspnoea, dysphagia, loss of appetite, cachexia, foetor of the breath, haemorrhage and earache, and will depend on the situation of the tumour, its direction of spread and such complications as it may cause.

DIAGNOSIS

Diagnosis of malignant disease will be made after consideration of: (1) the history; (2) examination of the pharynx and larynx by both indirect and direct methods; (3) examination of the neck; (4) general examination of the patient, which may include examination of blood and sputum for bacteriology and cytology; (5) radiological examination of the chest, neck and larynx; and (6) histological examination of a portion of suspected tissue.

History

The symptoms have already been considered and nothing more need be said than that practically any other disease affecting the larynx may exhibit symptoms compatible with malignant disease; the converse is also true. Again, malignant disease may co-exist with other diseases such as tuberculosis or syphilis, and a condition such as leucoplakia of the larynx may undergo malignant change without any apparent change in the symptoms.

Examination of the larynx and pharynx

The appearance of the lesion will, of course, vary with the site but may also vary considerably in any one situation on the vocal cord. It is very rare for a growth to arise on the arytenoids or in the interarytenoid region. A typical raised nodule may be seen with a flat rather rough surface, or a hypertrophic papillary growth; in other cases there may be a local thickening of one vocal cord or sometimes a typical epitheliomatous ulcer (Fig. 162a). If there is much keratinization of the surface the appearance will be pale or white; in other cases it may be pink or red, particularly if there is associated inflammation.

A tumour originating at the anterior commissure may appear as a small bud of granulation tissue, whereas in the subglottic region a lesion may be quite extensive and yet not be seen on indirect laryngoscopy because it is hidden by the overlying edge of the vocal cord (Fig. 164). A tumour in the commissure, or one arising just above the commissure on the epiglottis, may fail to be seen by mirror examination because it is hidden by the tubercle of the epiglottis or by overhang of its tip.

Impaired mobility of the vocal cord is not an early sign of malignant disease since it is usually due to invasion of the thyro-arytenoid muscle and often the

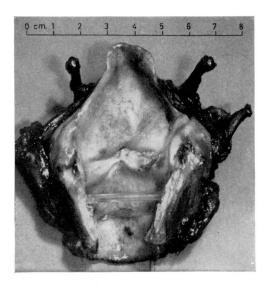

(a)

Fig. 162.—Surgical specimens of two larynges split open posteriorly to show: (a) carcinoma involving the whole right vocal cord with fixation; (b) extensive transglottic carcinoma of the right side of the larynx.

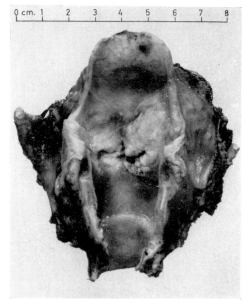

(b)

adjacent cartilages; nevertheless it is unfortunately present in many cases when first sent for examination and is therefore an important sign in the differential diagnosis. It is particularly important in the case of a subglottic lesion as this may not produce any symptoms in the early stages and will only cause some alteration in the voice when it begins to infiltrate the submucous tissues and produces limitation of cord movement. This impaired mobility is mostly a limitation of full abduction together with some sluggishness in adduction.

Fig. 163.—(a) Specimen opened posteriorly to show massive carcinoma invading the base of the epiglottis and anterior commissure with some transglottic spread; (b) specimen of larynx split sagittally to show gross penetration by tumour through thyroid cartilage into the pre-epiglottic space, and soft tissues of the neck.

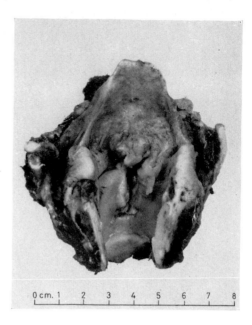

(a)

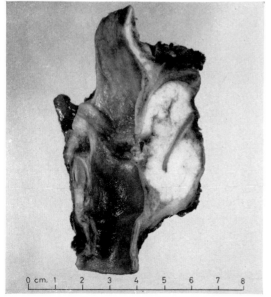

(b)

When a tumour commences in the ventricle the only indication of its presence in the early stage may be a slight fullness of the ventricular band on that side, and later, an appearance suggesting some oedema or prolapse of the mucosa of the ventricle. If the ventricular band is then pushed outwards it may be seen to be hiding a comparatively large tumour.

In all cases of doubt it is wise to pass a direct laryngoscope and the subglottic region must always be inspected. In such cases microlaryngoscopy and the use of a right-angled telescope are of value.

In the aryepiglottic region the appearance is usually that of a localized swelling of the fold with ulceration—generally of the outer or upper surface (Plate VIII*d*). Occasionally one sees a small indurated ulcer, without much swelling—in this case most commonly on the posterolateral aspect of the arytenoid—and rarely a pedunculated tumour which may obscure the whole field of view and cause doubt as to the true site of origin. Such a lesion may sometimes be removed with biopsy forceps completely while being examined by direct laryngoscopy. This can also occur with very small tumours on the vocal cords.

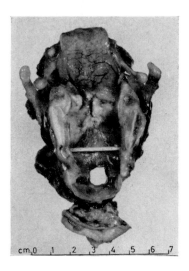

FIG. 164.—Extensive subglottic infiltration by carcinoma of both vocal cords, especially left, with bilateral midline fixation, in female aged 72 years. Tumour found microscopically in strap muscles on specimen. Tracheostomy fistula completely excised.

Similar variations occur on the epiglottis; the most common type is a nodular ulcerating tumour arising more frequently from one edge than from the tip, or as a secondary extension from a carcinoma of the vallecula. Less commonly is seen a cauliflower type of tumour completely hiding the vocal cords and arytenoids and yet rather surprisingly causing very little dyspnoea. Rarely one sees a deeply infiltrating tumour of the petiolus; this does not cause symptoms early and may be missed on examination for reasons already given.

Examination of the neck

As already mentioned, involvement of the internal jugular chain of lymph nodes occurs rarely with carcinoma of the vocal cords and seldom occurs early with subglottic tumours. If nodes are affected it is frequently the small prelaryngeal node on the cricothyroid membrane in cordal tumours, and in subglottic growths the pretracheal and paratracheal nodes, that are first involved.

There may be some swelling of the larynx which can be felt on palpation. This is due either to associated perichondritis, when the cartilage will be tender on pressure; or to a mass of tumour directly infiltrating through the cricothyroid membrane. This occurs only at a late stage and with extensive lesions.

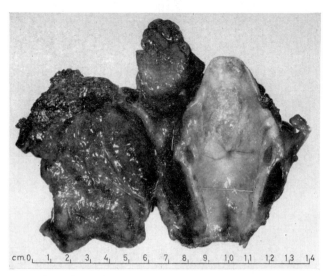

FIG. 165.—Advanced Stage 3 carcinoma of epiglottis, left ventricular band and aryepiglottic fold. Specimen showing combined total laryngectomy and left radical neck dissection.

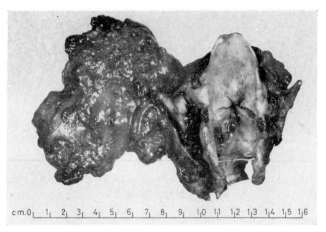

FIG. 166.—Massive Stage 3 carcinoma involving left subglottic region with fixation of left vocal cord. Specimen to show combined total laryngectomy and elective left radical neck dissection.

Occasionally an aggressive tumour of the anterior commissure invading thyroid cartilage or with some subglottic spread will produce a midline indurated swelling beneath the skin over the lower border of the thyroid cartilage at the junction with the cricothyroid membrane.

With supraglottic and marginal tumours the nodes most frequently affected are the homolateral upper and middle deep cervical groups. In tumours of the epiglottis similar deep cervical node groups may be affected, often bilaterally, and spread may occasionally take place to the submaxillary or submental nodes of either side.

Where there is doubt about the palpable presence or otherwise of any lymph node, it should be assumed to be involved until proved otherwise.

General examination

General physical examination of any patient suspected of malignant disease of the larynx or laryngopharynx should be carried out as a routine measure. It is essential to perform serological tests for syphilis, and the sputum should be examined for tubercle bacilli. Also, a haemoglobin estimation and white cell count with blood urea and electrocardiogram are minimal requirements. The co-existence of diabetes mellitus, renal, chronic pulmonary or cardiovascular disease may well modify the line of treatment to be advised.

Radiological examination

The chest should be examined radiologically before treatment is undertaken (a) to eliminate or verify the co-existence of a tuberculous infection or other lesion, (b) to note the presence of any retrosternal mass of nodes in the mediastinum or pulmonary hilum, and (c) to detect any metastatic disease in the lung fields themselves.

Radiological examination of the neck is of considerable value, partly as an aid to diagnosis but more especially in assessing the extent of a tumour which can only be seen from above, before planning radiotherapeutic treatment. Lateral and postero-anterior plain films of the larynx will often demonstrate the presence of a tumour of the epiglottis with possible invasion of the pre-epiglottic space, the extent of the tumour mass in a postcricoid carcinoma or the presence of a subglottic neoplasm growing in the anterior or lateral part of that region.

Modern tomographic techniques are of much value in certain situations, particularly for suspected tumours in the ventricular and subglottic regions. Positive contrast laryngography and pharyngography using Dionosil and local anaesthesia can also be of the greatest value, especially in determining the lower extent of supraglottic tumours and the integrity of the ventricles, subglottic region and pyriform fossae (Brindle and Stell, 1968; Howell, Gildersleeve, and King 1968). However, it must be remembered that the use of these techniques should be selective and that none of them is reliable in evaluating the post-irradiation larynx (Figs. 172–175).

Histological examination

Histological examination of any tumour or ulcer is essential before treatment can be considered. Nowadays the removal of a sample of tissue for microscopical examination will almost invariably be done by direct laryngoscopy, using the pattern of laryngoscope that seems most suitable for the particular case. It has been suggested that the removal of a specimen for histological examination was undesirable (a) because it made metastatic dissemination of the growth probable, although this is not borne out by practical experience, and (b) because a diagnosis could rarely be made from the material removed. This objection may sometimes have applied in the days of removal of tissue by indirect laryngoscopy, but has ceased to be true if adequate portions of tissue are removed by direct laryngoscopy. It

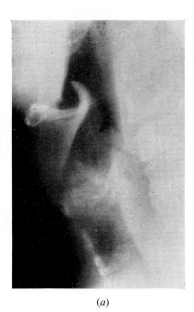 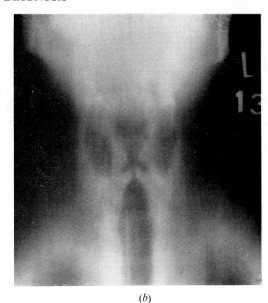

(a)   (b)

FIG. 167.—(a) Normal soft tissue lateral radiograph of larynx showing calcification in laryngeal cartilages and tracheal rings; (b) normal tomograph of larynx showing vocal cords, ventricular bands, ventricles and pyriform fossae.

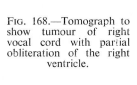 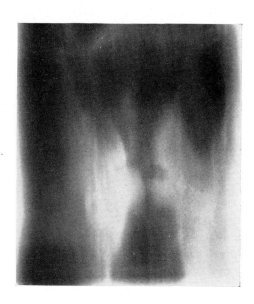

FIG. 168.—Tomograph to show tumour of right vocal cord with partial obliteration of the right ventricle.

is generally agreed by most surgeons that histological examination is essential for the following reasons.

For the purpose of diagnosis

Even the most experienced of laryngologists has been guilty of diagnosing a tuberculous laryngitis as carcinoma, and a carcinoma of the cord may occur in a

409

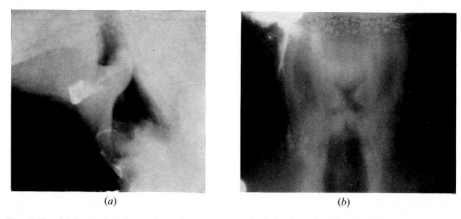

(a) (b)

FIG. 169.—(a) Lateral radiograph to show tumour of epiglottis and vallecula with invasion of the
pre-epiglottic space; (b) tomograph of similar epiglottic tumour.

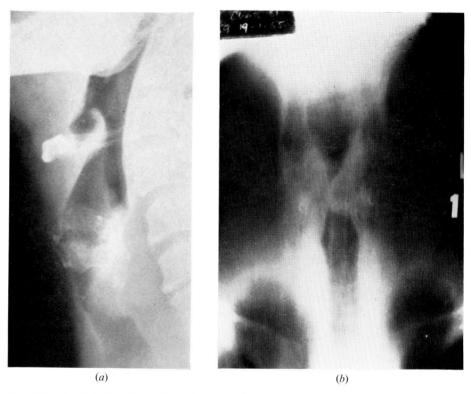

(a) (b)

FIG. 170.—(a) Lateral radiograph to show growth on posterior wall of subglottic region; (b)
fibrosarcoma of left hemilarynx.

patient with obvious signs of pulmonary tuberculosis. Again, it may be impossible to be certain that a case of leucoplakia has not undergone malignant changes without microscopic examination, and to what extent such changes may show invasive disease or be confined to carcinoma *in situ*.

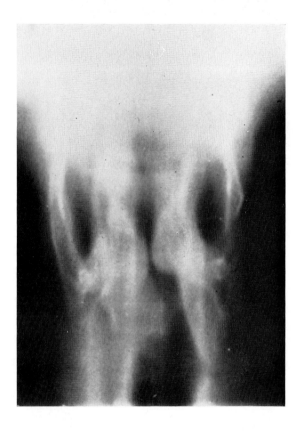

FIG. 171.—Tomograph to show extensive right subglottic tumour.

For the purpose of selecting treatment

In well differentiated tumours it may be reasonable to advise conservative surgery in a borderline case, whereas in cases with poor differentiation and active mitosis conservative surgery should not be attempted in any other than very favourable circumstances and the alternative line of treatment by radical surgery or radiotherapy would be advised.

Multiple primary tumours

The incidence of multiple primary carcinoma in the air and upper food passages is slowly increasing with the rising cure rates of cancer and the rising age of the population. At present it is about 5 per cent of all patients who have been success-fully treated for any one lesion in this area. Especially significant is the high incidence of 19 per cent bronchial carcinoma associated with preceding primary cancer in the upper air and food passages (Epstein and Shaw, 1958). This reflects a tendency to widespread mucosal degenerative changes throughout the air passages

411

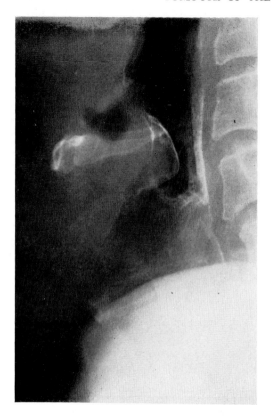

FIG. 172.—Laryngogram to outline large tumour of laryngeal surface of the epiglottis. Probable involvement of pre-epiglottic space but not reaching anterior commissure.

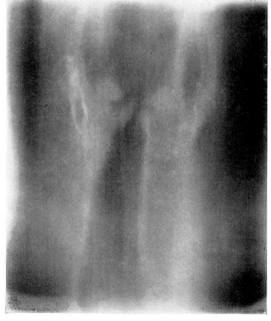

FIG. 173.—Tomograph to show tumour involving left vocal cord, left subglottic region and possibly left tracheal wall.

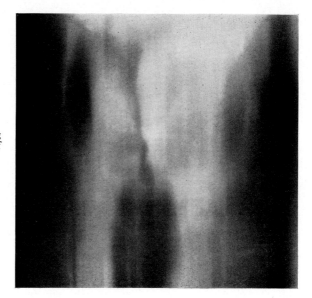

FIG. 174.—Tomograph showing massive transglottic tumour of left hemilarynx.

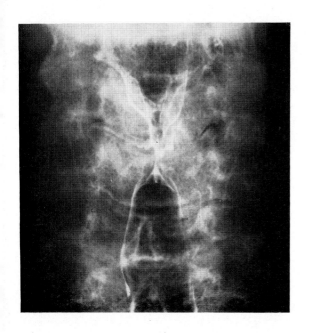

FIG. 175.—Laryngogram during phonation to reveal crater of small recurrent tumour on left ventricular band.

in particular (Wynder, Bross and Day, 1956; Auerbach, 1956). The occurrence of mucosal field changes and multiple tumours within the larynx itself has also been noted (Rabbett, 1962; Shaw, 1964).

It is also interesting to find that there is now evidence for an increased frequency of carcinoma of the larynx in patients successfully treated for bronchial carcinoma (Lavelle, 1969).

These findings emphasize the necessity for prolonged follow-up of all successfully treated patients, if possible throughout their natural life.

DIFFERENTIAL DIAGNOSIS

Confusion with malignant tumours can arise mainly from four conditions affecting the larynx. These are chronic laryngitis, benign tumours, tuberculosis and syphilis.

Less frequently the chronic benign lesions of pachydermia and leucoplakia may give rise to doubt, and more rarely still such conditions as scleroma, inflammation of the crico-arytenoid joint, or prolapse of a ventricle may cause difficulty. When a well established lesion is present on first examination a tentative diagnosis will be made by consideration of the history, by routine examination, by examination of the neck, by examination of the nose and pharynx and by indirect laryngoscopy.

Final diagnosis will be made by histological examination of a sample of tissue removed at direct laryngoscopy. Other investigations may exclude or confirm associated conditions and will be undertaken at the discretion of the physician. In cases of doubt it may be wise to keep a patient under observation for a few weeks. It is necessary to forbid tobacco and alcohol during such a period and also to put the patient on strict silence. A course of wide-spectrum systemic antibiotics may also be desirable.

A more difficult question by far is to decide if and when a previously non-malignant lesion has become malignant. The question arises most commonly in cases of cordal carcinoma supervening on leucoplakia. The leucoplakic condition may have been present for some years and the patient probably kept under quarterly observation (Fig. 154). The change to malignancy is insidious and may occur in only one part of the leucoplakic area. A single biopsy may be misleading, especially if the specimen is taken from a non-malignant part while another area, from which no specimen is removed, is undergoing malignant degeneration.

In this situation it is necessary to examine the patient at more frequent intervals, remove specimens whenever it might be thought necessary and to treat the condition as malignant if the reports are at all equivocal. Leucoplakic areas which become malignant do not always respond favourably to irradiation.

Persistent and asymmetric oedema in the larynx or localized perichondritis may give rise to some doubt as to whether residual disease is present or not in cases following treatment by irradiation. However, where the larynx has returned to normal as a result of this treatment, and some months later persistent hoarseness supervenes with further oedematous swelling of the arytenoid region or of the false cord, there are much greater grounds for suspicion of recurrent cancer. Prompt imposition of absolute voice rest and the use of antibiotics may alter the picture favourably within a few days, but if it does not respond within two or three weeks resort must be made to careful biopsy under antibiotic cover. In these difficult cases one negative biopsy alone is insufficient evidence since residual tumour is often deeply buried in oedematous tissues.

Nevertheless, it is also well recognized that such oedema may persist for six months or more following irradiation, the larynx eventually returning to normal without recurrent disease.

CURATIVE TREATMENT

There are still only two methods of curative treatment in use today: surgery and irradiation. They have complementary rôles in the treatment of laryngeal cancer. In the last 30 years considerable changes have occurred involving both indications for, and the application of, these methods.

From 1920 to 1935, following the introduction of Coutard's technique of fractionated external irradiation, the larger tumours were treated by this method and the smaller Stage 1 and 2 lesions by surgery. A phase of disillusionment then set in, and shortly after World War II, with its rapid development of newer surgical aids, it was realized that irradiation with preservation of function was more effective in the smaller tumours, whereas the safer use of radical surgery could give greatly improved results in the more extensive tumours. This trend continues and the more recent developments are towards greater safety with preservation of function in the application of both methods.

Surgery

Resection of primary tumour

The operation of vocal cord excision by partial lateral laryngectomy via the laryngofissure approach has had much popularity over the years and continues to give excellent results, although at the price of permanent voice impairment (Thomson and Colledge, 1930; Jackson, 1940). The main indications for this operation are that the tumour shall be superficial and limited to one vocal cord. It should not have spread to any other site or region, nor shall it have infiltrated the cordal muscles to produce limitation of movement. Extension to the cordal extremities may render this operation inadvisable, especially in poorly differentiated tumours. However, various modifications or extensions of this procedure, for example, frontolateral resection, may also be used when the tumour extends to the anterior commissure or even onto the opposite cord. These are based upon the concept of Hautant's original hemilaryngectomy and are well described by Leroux-Robert (1956) and others (Alonso, 1957; Norris, 1958; Ogura, Saltzstein and Spjut, 1961; Ogura and colleagues, 1969).

For tumours causing fixation of one vocal cord, marked subglottic or transglottic spread, wide extension to the opposite cord, or involvement of the arytenoid or posterior commissure total laryngectomy is the only safe alternative. However, in the latter regions, where the tumour is confined above the cords, supraglottic partial laryngectomy may be carried out with preservation of the vocal cords, via a transverse or lateral pharyngotomy approach (Norris, 1962; Ogura and colleagues, 1969). The simplest and most successful example of this technique is amputation of the free part of the epiglottis for a tumour confined to its tip (Martin, 1957).

These conservative operations are often difficult, suitable cases are few and must be selected with care. Restoration of the normal swallow may give much anxiety.

There is also the added danger that preservation of vocal function may obscure the main objective—to give a patient the best initial chance of a cure by complete resection of the tumour. All these hazards are increased after irradiation. Nevertheless, partial resections are still possible.

The disadvantages of total laryngectomy are that it involves the loss of the laryngeal voice, interruption of the natural airways with substitution of a permanent tracheal stoma in the neck, and definite limitations on some forms of physical activity such as swimming and heavy manual work. Nevertheless, a reasonable oesophageal voice can be developed after operation in about two-thirds of patients, while the remainder today can be fitted with effective speech aids. The operation itself is not technically difficult. It now has a low mortality rate of 1–3 per cent, equivalent to other major head and neck operations, and healing is usually rapid.

Neck dissection

The place of radical block dissection of the neck in laryngeal cancer has been much debated in recent years. Where palpable evidence of metastatic disease to one or both sides of the neck exists in the absence of distant metastases, there is no doubt that dissection of one or both sides in continuity with excision of the primary disease is mandatory if a cure is to be obtained. There is also evidence that courses of pre-operative irradiation for palpable and resectable cervical metastases will give some improvement in cure rates (Strong and colleagues, 1969; Lindberg and Jesse, 1968).

In the past this was the only indication for neck dissection, but the detailed work of Ogura (1951), Kuhn, Devine and McDonald (1957), Pietrantoni and Fior (1958), McGavran, Bauer and Ogura (1961) and others in the past 15 years has demonstrated the existence of a high percentage of impalpable metastatic deposits in the cervical lymphatics of patients with supraglottic, marginal and laryngopharyngeal cancer. As a result, the concept of elective block dissection of the neck has evolved. Accordingly, it is felt that elective in-continuity neck dissection should today be carried out with all extensive well lateralized primary carcinomas at these sites (Figs. 186 and 188).

A modification of the original Crile radical neck dissection may also be made by preservation of the spinal accessory nerve in many elective dissections. This imposes little extra risk of failure and functionally gives a better result.

Where bilateral neck dissection is required it is better carried out with an interval of three to four weeks between operations. Nevertheless, if necessary, bilateral simultaneous dissection with sacrifice of both internal jugular veins involves no increased operative risk to life, although morbidity may be prolonged in some cases (Ewing and Martin, 1962). In selected cases one vein may be spared.

If neck dissection is required on one or both sides without surgery to the larynx, but where the larynx or neck has been previously irradiated, a temporary tracheostomy must always be performed.

Irradiation

The greatest single benefit of recent developments in radiotherapy is the increasing ability to direct high cancer-lethal dosage into the tumour while causing minimal damage to the surrounding normal tissues. In the last few years the achievement of even greater accuracy by the introduction of the linear accelerator, giving energy output up to 35 MeV or more, does not yet appear to have produced much better results than with the more modest supervoltage techniques (Lederman, 1958).

Because modern irradiation can achieve a high percentage of cures in limited laryngeal cancer there is a tendency to justify its initial application to all cases in the cause of preserving function; the subsequent argument being that all failures have a "second chance" of cure by radical surgery. Although beguiling, this is an oversimplification for the following reasons: (1) The true extent of the tumour cannot always be accurately established. (2) It may progress locally and undetected during treatment. (3) It may metastasize during treatment. (4) Deceptive appearance at follow-up leads to (5) delay in surgery after failed irradiation. (6) Inability of the patient to attend for regular follow-up. (7) Increased chance of post-operative healing problems and other complications. Moreover, it has been shown that adequate surgery gives the best overall cure rate in laryngeal cancer, and it is a long established principle that the most effective initial treatment gives the best chance of a permanent cure. It is therefore essential that treatment must be highly selective in every case.

Although opinions differ in detail, there is also today some evidence that pre-operative irradiation to the primary lesion and appropriate neck fields up to a total of 3,000–4,000 rad. can give a slightly increased cure rate for more extensive laryngeal and pharyngeal carcinomas. This applies particularly to large growths of the supraglottis, subglottis, pyriform fossa and postcricoid area (Biller and colleagues, 1969). It is essential, however, that treatment of such lesions is based on radical surgery about three weeks after the preliminary irradiation. The patient and relatives must be told that his condition requires an operation for cure and that irradiation is a preparatory tactic to give greater assurance.

Choice of treatment

The initial method of treatment will depend principally on the facilities available, the site and stage of the tumour and upon its histology. In addition the physiological age, general fitness, psychology and personal factors pertaining to each patient must be weighed. Calendar age itself is no bar to surgery and physicians or anaesthetists should not be asked whether a patient is fit or unfit for surgery. They should be requested to aid in achieving optimum fitness. Where there is doubt as to the most suitable method a report of poor histological differentiation should weigh in favour of irradiation in view of the bad prognosis in such cases whatever the treatment.

With these factors in mind it can then be said that external irradiation should be used for the common small Stage 1 tumours confined to the vocal cord or anterior commissure and also for the uncommon Stage 1 tumours at other laryngeal sites. For early Stage 2 tumours without fixation of the cord, especially in professional voice-users, irradiation may still be used providing a regular follow-up is feasible. In some centres these two types of tumour are treated initially, as already discussed, by various methods of partial laryngectomy (Leroux-Robert, 1956; Alonso, 1957; Norris, 1958; Ogura and colleagues, 1969). In other centres such conservative operations may sometimes be used successfully after full courses of irradiation (Lewis, 1961; Shaw, 1966), but in most of these cases total laryngectomy is advisable.

For the later Stage 2 tumours of all sites with or without mobile palpable neck nodes or cord fixation, and the majority of Stage 3 tumours, radical surgery correctly performed is the best initial method of treatment often with a preliminary short course of irradiation (4000 rad.). This will frequently involve a wide-field total laryngectomy combined with radical neck dissection performed as a monobloc resection on the same side.

The majority of Stage 4 growths are suitable only for palliation, although it is possible sometimes to salvage occasional cases by radical surgery alone or combined with precedent irradiation or chemotherapy.

It is also felt that an elective neck dissection should be combined with ablation of the primary tumour in all supraglottic and marginal late Stage 2, Stage 3 and operable Stage 4 cases.

Further effective support for the above clinical indications for partial or total laryngectomy is given by the serial section of resected larynges (Kirschner, 1969). In particular this author shows that cord fixation is usually a result of muscular infiltration by tumour, and that many larger tumours responding poorly to irradiation, especially in the subglottic area, also show invasion of cartilage.

If initial surgery is carried out without preliminary irradiation, but some reasonable doubt exists that all disease was removed from the primary region or neck, then it is essential that a full course of irradiation be given to such areas, to start as soon as healing is complete. Any "wait and see" policy is perilous since post-operative irradiation is usually ineffective in the presence of palpable recurrence. This applies especially to Stage 2 and 3 subglottic carcinoma, where at least the paratracheal and superior mediastinal lymphatics should be irradiated routinely after surgery.

In summary, all small Stage 1 tumours confined to their anatomic site of origin and with no sign of metastases are today best treated by external irradiation and regular follow-up. With very few exceptions, all more extensive tumours of the larynx, producing cord fixation, marked supra- or subglottic extension or palpable metastases are better treated by wide resection, combined with radical neck dissection in a high proportion, and often preceded by a shortened course of irradiation.

PALLIATIVE TREATMENT

Surgery

If there is any reasonable possibility of surgically removing an ulcerated tumour in the throat with immediate healing and re-establishment of the natural swallow in an otherwise fit individual this should be done, providing any untreatable metastases are small and symptomless. In this way the worst terminal sufferings of the patient may be avoided. Otherwise surgery is generally limited to timely tracheostomy or gastrostomy.

Chemotherapy

The use of cytotoxic drugs, such as alkylating agents or the anti-metabolites, has greatly increased since Bierman and Klopp independently noted in 1950 that the intra-arterial administration of nitrogen mustard produced profound local effects on a variety of tumours.

Although there have been only a few useful additions to the number of drugs effective against squamous carcinoma in the last 20 years, we do know more about the uses and limitations of the few which are of value. The main indication for their use is pain, or other severe and unrelieved distress. For this they can be effective for limited periods and preferably given on an out-patient basis by oral or intra-venous routes. The most reliable and least generally toxic are considered to be

Cyclophosphamide and Methotrexate. These agents are described in more detail in Chapter 18.

Irradiation

Short, well-spaced courses of 250 kV grid x-ray therapy or occasionally even supervoltage irradiation, and the carefully planned insertion of gold grain or radium needle implants can often produce marked regression of inoperable growths, even in a previously irradiated field. Probably the most useful effect of irradiation in these cases lies in the reduction of pain and prevention of fungation.

Symptomatic relief

Dyspnoea

This can be very disturbing, and if a tracheostomy must be performed it is better that it should be done before the stage of urgency is reached. It is usually carried out under local anaesthesia and should be as low as is convenient, especially when there is likelihood of any subglottic spread.

Dysphagia

All efforts must be directed to preserving the natural swallow by judicious variation in the pattern of diet. But in terminal cases where tube feeding becomes inevitable, an effective early gastrostomy avoids the unpleasant features of the continuous use of a naso-oesophageal feeding tube.

Infection

This will tend to aggravate both of the preceding conditions and will also cause increased pain. Careful attention to local hygiene, especially in the mouth, is desirable. The use of oral antiseptic sprays and mouth-washes with short courses of systemic wide-spectrum antibiotics can do much to diminish the extent of secondary infection.

Salivation

Increased salivation is not uncommon in uncontrolled cancer of the larynx or pharynx, but if the patient has had irradiation the secretions are more likely to be highly viscid and distressing. Mouth-washes of 1 per cent bicarbonate of soda or potassium chlorate and phenol, with plenty of watery or milky drinks and simple-flavoured glycerin lozenges can be helpful. In excessive secretion small doses of belladonna or Pro-Banthine are useful.

Pain

Most commonly this is a referred otalgia or pain in the side of the neck. It can be extremely severe, especially in growths with involvement of the internal laryngeal or glossopharyngeal nerves. It is seldom possible to divide the internal laryngeal nerve surgically as it is usually involved in the tumour masses, but a well placed nerve block infiltration can sometimes be most helpful. Occasionally it may be justifiable to perform a prefrontal leucotomy for really severe and poorly controlled pain. In general, however, reliance must be placed first on the aspirin group of drugs often combined with a tranquillizer, such as Sparine or Librium, before proceeding to pethidine and eventually to chlorpromazine and the morphine group, of which heroin is by far the most effective drug in terminal cases. A standard mixture of aspirin and Nepenthe can be most effective. Other useful substitutes are methadone (Physeptone), levorphanol (Dromoran), dextromoramide (Palfium) and pentazocine (Fortral).

The use of anaesthetic powders and local anaesthetic lozenges, emulsions or sprays may help especially if used before meals, but generally they tend to be disappointing owing to the involvement of nerve trunks. A patient should be allowed to decide for himself whether he takes alcohol or tobacco in reasonable quantity. For ensuring sleep, alcohol is the best choice at night for many elderly people once pain has been controlled. Glutethimide (Doriden) or chloral compounds are to be preferred to the barbiturates. Combinations of Nepenthe and cocaine with additives such as gin and honey often give the best results. Severe secondary haemorrhage in these patients is better dealt with by sedation than by active interference. When simple drug relief of pain seems ineffective consideration should be given to cytotoxic chemotherapy.

TREATMENT BY IRRADIATION

Those who treat laryngeal cancer by this method must have considerable technical knowledge and experience with facility in clinical examination of the larynx. Only in this way can a radiotherapist achieve the best results and, in view of the comparative infrequency of the disease, there is much to be gained by treating these patients in large centres. Close co-operation with a laryngologist is essential and regular joint clinics should be established.

As soon as the diagnosis has been confirmed histologically, further investigations may be required to ascertain as accurately as possible the site of origin within the larynx and the extent of the growth. A clear idea of the extent of the disease is important in planning irradiation not only to include the whole tumour within the treated area but also to minimize the amount of normal tissue irradiated.

Selection of cases

This is discussed in Chapter 18. Apart from the indications for irradiation discussed therein, it may also be used in the presence of co-existing disease which makes surgery too hazardous; when operation is refused; or when surgical resection of the primary tumour is technically impossible, or non-resectable nodes are present. In some cases a good response to irradiation may make a successful resection possible.

Irradiation should also be considered: (a) whenever biopsy shows the tumour to be poorly differentiated; (b) after surgical resection if there is good reason to suspect that removal of disease has been incomplete or (c) in overt and inoperable recurrence following radical surgery. In the latter case it is unlikely to be curative.

Irradiation is generally contra-indicated: (a) where there is fixation of one vocal cord by tumour; (b) where the thyroid cartilage is infiltrated; and (c) when established perichondritis is present.

Methods of treatment

Irradiation to the larynx may be given as follows.

External irradiation

The many varieties of apparatus which are now available to the radiotherapist, together with the more important advantages and disadvantages of each, are described in Chapter 18.

In cancer of the larynx, there is much to be said for using a convenient means of gamma-radiation in the medium supervoltage range, such as the small telecurie therapy unit especially designed for treatment of head and neck tumours. Radio-active cobalt-60 and caesium-137 are highly satisfactory and relatively cheap sources of energy for these units. Two or three fields are planned to give a homo-geneous dose to the whole volume of tissue possibly invaded. A dose of 300 r is usually given through one field per day for 5–6 days per week, the total tumour dose varying from 5,500 r to 8,000 r in 6–8 weeks (Fig. 176). It must be emphasized that the patient's best chance of cure is proportional to the skill and practical experience of the radiotherapist in day-to-day observation of the clinical response to treatment. Adjustments to the fields and decisions regarding total dosage can thus be made according to local and general progress.

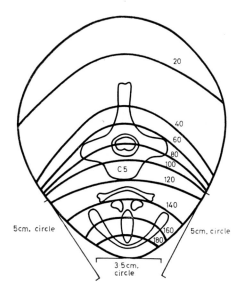

FIG. 176.—Cross-section through the neck at the level of the vocal cords with a radiation distribution superimposed. The 150 curie Cobalt-60 unit is applied through three portals at a source-to-skin distance of 8 cm.

Interstitial irradiation

The Finzi–Harmer operation.—This is mentioned mainly because of its historical importance, since it is now little used. By exposing the thyroid cartilage, partially resecting the ala adjacent to the tumour, and inserting a palisade of radium needles for a period of 6–8 days, it is possible to deliver a high dose of about 10,000 r to the tumour without damaging the skin. It was suitable only for limited Stage 1 cordal growths before the advent of efficient external telecurie therapy, and was an excellent, often better, substitute for 250 kV x-radiation. In skilled hands it gave equal results to partial laryngectomy without impairment of the voice. A possible application today is in the treatment of poor-risk elderly patients in situations where skilled supervoltage therapy is not available or might prove too arduous for them.

Radio-active gold grain implants.—Using a special type of "gun" these tiny pellets can be inserted in any suitable pattern into a metastatic tumour mass in the neck. If planned and inserted with surgical exposure under direct vision they can deliver a depth dose of up to 10,000 r at 1 cm. distance without excessive skin damage, despite a previous full course of external irradiation. For this reason they are particularly valuable in the palliation of tumour masses considered to be unresectable. Occasionally they can even be curative.

Reactions and complications

The degree of morbidity after external irradiation is very variable. It depends upon the relative biological sensitivity of the tumour and host tissues, the total dosage and the total area of tissue irradiated: for example, whether large neck fields are included; and upon the individual tolerance of the patient. Very few patients require hospitalization during, or as a result of, their treatment, and those in poor general health or whose daily attendance involves much travel are boarded as hostel patients from the start.

In the third or fourth week of treatment some erythema of the skin and oedema of the laryngeal tissues will appear which may cause enough pain, dysphagia and difficulty with speech to require full hospitalization for the last one or two weeks of treatment and for about a similar period after its termination.

True perichondritis is today very uncommon during irradiation and generally occurs in advanced disease with cartilage invasion or due to an error in dosage. It may well indicate the need for a change to surgical treatment but, if slight, it is often feasible to continue irradiation under an antibiotic cover and with a modified dosage. A mild subacute perichondritis is occasionally encountered as evidenced by localized tenderness, earache and laryngeal oedema. It occurs towards the end of treatment or shortly afterwards and usually responds well to voice rest and antibiotics which may be required for several weeks. This type of perichondritis may also occur some years after irradiation and is often associated with respiratory infections.

Persistent localized laryngeal oedema, often with some degree of cervical subcutaneous oedema, is occasionally seen when high dosage has been given. The presence of residual disease is especially difficult to rule out in these cases as already discussed (p. 414).

Tracheostomy for radiation-induced oedema is now a rare event and, if it occurs, may be due to faulty radiotherapy technique. With large and infected tumours, nevertheless, laryngeal oedema is often difficult to avoid, however much care is taken. Post-radiation tracheostomy is usually a result of failure to control the disease.

Moist skin desquamation is unusual today but may occur in patients with especially sensitive skins. Other forms of tissue necrosis are now rare and would indicate errors or failure in treatment.

Among minor sequelae, dryness of the mouth and throat with bizarre aberrations of taste may cause discomfort for some months, but they nearly always resolve in time. By the fourth week dry desquamation of the skin with some atrophy and tanning are usually present, but marked telangiectasia and subcutaneous fibrosis should be encountered.

General symptoms such as malaise, insomnia, anorexia and some loss of weight by dehydration and dysphagia are much less frequent today, but may occur if large cervical fields are used. Dietary measures to increase the fluid intake to six pints daily and to adjust the semi-solid nature of food intake may be required towards the end of treatment. The use of an aspirin or benzocaine emulsion before swallowing is often very useful in these patients. Breathing exercises, mouth hygiene and the maximum possible movement are important, especially in older patients in whom bronchopneumonia is always a risk.

A patient undergoing modern irradiation for laryngeal cancer may therefore expect a mild local and general reaction to therapy which is transient and which usually allows a return to work about six weeks after completing treatment. He must, however, take great care of the voice, no shouting or excessive strains—and ideally no smoking—are permitted for at least three months after the end of treatment.

SURGICAL TECHNIQUES

Many different techniques for surgical treatment of laryngeal cancer have been devised since Gordon Buck in 1851 first performed a successful partial laryngectomy by laryngofissure for this disease in the United States; and Billroth of Vienna carried out the first total laryngectomy for cancer in 1873. All the subsequent techniques, however, have derived from the work of these early pioneers, and later modifications have concerned mainly such details as anaesthesia, skin incisions, succession of stages and methods of closure.

In the early years of the present century although these operations were increasingly used, serious complications were the rule and operative mortality due to haemorrhage, wound infection and bronchopneumonia was at times as high as 25 per cent for the smaller procedures and even 50 per cent or more after complete removal of the larynx.

From about 1910 onward this toll was gradually reduced through the work of pioneers such as Gluck (1914), MacKenty (1925), St. Clair Thomson and Colledge (1930). Their achievements were obtained not merely by technical skill, but by a realization of the importance of adequate preparation of the patient before surgery and careful post-operative nursing to combat the dangers of infection.

After 1940, with the advent of surgical aids such as antibiotics, safer anaesthetics and efficient blood transfusion, the whole scene has changed. There are now few definite contra-indications to laryngeal surgery and serious complications are rare. Operative mortality for major laryngeal operations is no more than 2–3 per cent.

Today the following types of procedure are employed;

(1) By laryngotomy

    (*a*) Lateral partial laryngectomy ("laryngofissure").

    (*b*) Frontolateral partial laryngectomy.

    (*c*) Extended frontolateral partial laryngectomy.

(2) By pharyngotomy

    (*a*) Epiglottectomy.

    (*b*) Supraglottic partial laryngectomy.

    (*c*) Glottosupraglottic partial laryngectomy.

(3) By wide field dissection

    (*a*) Total laryngectomy alone.

    (*b*) Total laryngectomy with partial pharyngectomy and/or partial glossectomy.

    (*c*) Total laryngo-pharyngo-oesophagectomy.

The operation of radical block dissection of cervical lymphatics on one or both sides may need to be combined with any of these procedures (Figs. 186 and 188). It is seldom required in the first two owing to the absence of lymphatics on the true cords and therefore the improbability of metastatic cervical disease. In addition, partial or total thyroidectomy may be obligatory in the major resections.

Lateral partial laryngectomy (Fig. 177a, b), often termed "laryngofissure", is today performed less frequently, owing to the more effective results achieved by teleradiation in suitable cases. However, it still has a very definite place in situations where good radiation is not available, in some cases of irradiation failure and possibly for limited cordal tumours in young adults, where irradiation may be liable to provoke future neoplastic changes; perhaps also in a few older patients unsuitable for prolonged irradiation. It is an essential operation for the removal of many large benign laryngeal tumours, and occasional areas of persistent keratosis on the vocal cord (cordectomy) (Howie, 1957).

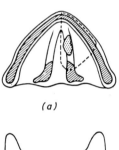

(a)

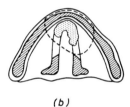

(b)

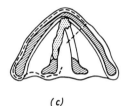

(c)

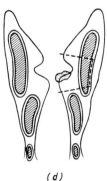

(d)

FIG. 177.—Diagrams of transverse section (*a*) and coronal section (*d*) through the larynx to show the extent of tissue removed by lateral partial laryngectomy (laryngofissure) for Stage I growth of the vocal cord. Diagram (*b*) of transverse section to show extent of tissue removed by frontolateral partial laryngectomy for growth involving the anterior commissure. Diagram (*c*) to show extended frontolateral resection.

Frontolateral partial laryngectomy may be useful where a glottic tumour crosses the anterior commissure to involve the anterior third of the opposite cord and without any reduction of mobility ("horseshoe tumour" (Fig. 177c)) (Som and Silver, 1968).

The older more complete hemilaryngectomy of Hautant (1937) is not now employed, but an extension of the lateral partial laryngectomy technique to include the whole ventricular band and arytenoid cartilage may on occasion be used in highly selected cases, providing there is no evidence of deep infiltration (Ogura and Mallen, 1965).

Pharyngotomy, either by the anterior transverse approach or by the lateral route (Trotter, 1926), provides a satisfactory access to limited Stage 1 or 2 supraglottic tumours. The anterior pharyngotomy approach is also useful in excising small tumours of the tip of the epiglottis and marginal aryepiglottic folds (Martin, 1957) (Fig. 179). The larger operation of supraglottic partial laryngectomy for Stage 1 and 2 lesions of the infrahyoid epiglottis and adnexae is more modern in its concept. Although growing in popularity in some centres (Alonso, 1957; Bocca, Pignatoro and Mosciaro, 1968; Ogura and colleagues, 1969, it is still not widely practised in this country, mainly owing to the success of irradiation in many suitable cases, also to difficulties of case selection and subsequent rehabilitation.

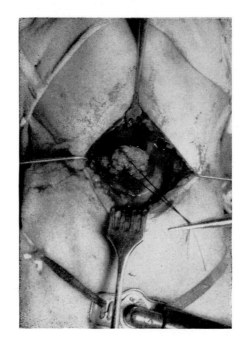

FIG. 178.—Tumour of suprahyoid epiglottis being removed through anterior pharyngotomy.

Consent for total laryngectomy must always be obtained before attempting any type of partial resection. Previous radiotherapy is not necessarily a bar to partial laryngectomy.

LATERAL PARTIAL LARYNGECTOMY (LARYNGOFISSURE)

Using this technique it is possible to remove completely many tumours confined to the vocal cord, with an adequate margin of healthy tissue and without removal of the arytenoid cartilage. The principles involved in operative surgery for malignant disease elsewhere will naturally apply in the case of this operation, with the exception that it is unnecessary to remove the associated cervical lymph nodes for reasons already given.

The tumour must be removed in one piece with as wide a margin of apparently healthy tissue as is practicable. It has been suggested that this margin should be 1 cm., and although this suggestion is of some practical value the tissue removed must be as much as is possible and prudent. Even in the earliest case it should consist of the whole of the side of the larynx anterior to the arytenoid cartilage, including its tip; and from the upper border of the cricoid cartilage below, to the upper border of the thyroid ala above. It may be more than 1 cm. above, but may be less anteriorly if the tumour approaches the commissure, or less posteriorly if it approaches the tip of the arytenoid cartilage.

Naturally, the smaller the margin of healthy tissue removed, the less satisfactory are the results likely to be, and it is only by the judgement of the individual surgeon that a decision can be taken as to whether this method is satisfactory in any particular case.

If, on histological examination of the specimen removed at operation, it would appear that doubt exists as to the complete removal of the lesion with an adequate margin of healthy tissue, a full course of irradiation should at once be given if the larynx has not previously been irradiated. However, in the latter event, vigilant follow-up alone is possible with recourse to total laryngectomy at the first sign of recurrent disease.

Pre-operative care

The most important pre-operative measure in this type of surgery is to ensure as far as possible the cleanliness of the mouth. All carious teeth should be filled or removed and, in particular, attention must be paid to the gums. Gingivitis or pyorrhoea are more important even than caries of the teeth. Operation should not be undertaken until the mouth has completely healed. Nasal sepsis should be eliminated as far as is practicable and it is wise to forbid alcohol and smoking for some days before operation in all but exceptional cases.

From a psychological point of view the surgeon will naturally assess each case individually and will tell the patient as much or as little about the operative procedure as he thinks wise. His attitude will be encouraging, sympathetic and optimistic; and rightly so, for if optimism is not justified it is doubtful if partial laryngectomy is the correct line of treatment. The surgeon should always obtain the patient's permission for total laryngectomy in case it should prove necessary.

Anaesthesia

The operation can be performed under local anaesthesia or a combination of local with general anaesthesia. The choice will depend upon the surgeon's own particular preference, upon the availability of an experienced anaesthetist and upon the suitability or otherwise of the patient for either a local or a general anaesthetic.

Whichever form of anaesthetic is used it is important that the cough reflex shall return immediately after the operation. Pre-operative medication other than atropine or scopolamine may be disadvantageous and morphine should not be used before or after surgery.

For local anaesthesia, Xylocaine 1 per cent with adrenalin 1/200,000 is used for infiltration of the skin and tissues superficial to the larynx, while cocaine 5 per cent is used for intralaryngeal surface application.

For general anaesthesia after induction with thiopentone and relaxant, halothane with nitrous oxide and oxygen via a small calibre cuffed peroral endotracheal tube is satisfactory.

Where the resting airway is seriously reduced by the tumour, there should be no hesitation in carrying out a preliminary tracheostomy under local anaesthesia with insertion of a right-angled cuffed anaesthetic tube. As soon as the trachea is exposed, a few drops of 5 per cent cocaine solution are injected into the lumen before insertion of the cuffed tube and induction of general anaesthesia.

Position of the patient

This should be similar to that used for tracheostomy; the head is extended by placing a sandbag or a flat firm pillow beneath the shoulders. The degree of extension will vary with the individual patient and must not be so great as to cause dyspnoea. It is important that the pillow or sandbag be evenly placed under the two shoulders; if it is not, one shoulder may be higher than the other and the neck will tend to be rotated so that the trachea and larynx will not be accurately in the midline.

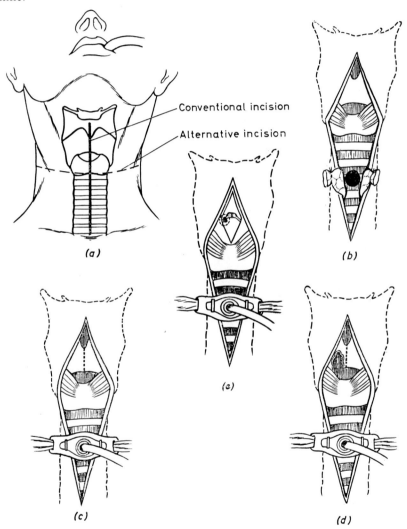

FIG. 179.—Partial lateral laryngectomy (laryngofissure). Diagram to show: (a) the incisions; (b) infrahyoid muscles retracted, larynx exposed, thyroid isthmus divided and trachea opened; (c) tracheostomy tube inserted. Dotted line shows saw cut groove in thyroid cartilage; (d) ala of thyroid cartilage being removed on the side of the tumour, up to the midline groove and back to the area of muscle attachments, prior to incision of cricothyroid membrane and internal perichondrium; (e) larynx opened to expose tumour for excision.

Operative technique (Figs. 177 and 179).

Exposure of the larynx

The classical incision is vertical in the midline and extends from the hyoid bone to a finger's breadth above the sternum. However, adequate exposure can also be obtained through a transverse curved incision centred on the lower border of the cricoid cartilage. The flaps are developed, strap muscles exposed then separated mainly by blunt dissection, and at some point below the cricoid cartilage the isthmus of the thyroid gland will be identified. Up to this stage the only difficulties encountered will be the division of one or two transverse connecting veins, and occasionally some difficulty in deciding the line of separation between the muscles; hence the importance of the head and neck being in the correct position. No endeavour should be made to identify the muscles individually by dissection and there should be no dissection of the neck much to the side of the middle line.

The muscles should be separated in the midline to just below the lower border of the thyroid isthmus. The isthmus is now elevated from the anterior surface of the trachea. It may be necessary to incise the pretracheal fascia immediately above the isthmus for this purpose, but there is no difficulty in separating the gland from the trachea once the dissector can be passed behind it.

The isthmus of the gland is now clamped and is divided between the forceps. Although bleeding is not usually marked, there may be large veins which will cause trouble later and for this reason it is wise to ligate the divided ends of the isthmus by transfixion. The front of the larynx and upper part of the trachea should now be well exposed.

Injection of the larynx and trachea

The next step will be to inject some cocaine into the larynx and also into the trachea, 0·3 ml. of a 5 per cent solution are injected first into the trachea between the second and third rings, and then a similar amount through the cricothyroid membrane.

The object of this is to anaesthetize the mucosa of the trachea and larynx and so avoid any coughing spasms on subsequent opening. As soon as the injections have been made, all remaining ligatures are tied and if a transverse main incision is used, a short vertical limb or separate horizontal incision may be required. The trachea is then opened.

Tracheostomy

The tracheostomy opening is made by excising a circular or elliptical piece of the anterior tracheal wall; the piece removed will be large enough to allow the insertion of a large size cuffed plastic tube and will include part of the third and, if necessary, part of the fourth ring of the trachea.

At this stage the right-angled cuffed tracheostomy tube is inserted as the per-oral tube is withdrawn, and connected to the anaesthetic circuit after inflation of its cuff. If the operation is being performed wholly under local anaesthesia, a large metal tracheostomy tube is passed at this stage and packed off from the larynx with 2·5 cm. ribbon gauze. Ordinarily the tube is retained for 12–24 hours after operation but may then be safely removed in the absence of complications.

Excision of thyroid ala

Formerly it was the practice to divide the thyroid cartilage in the midline together with the subjacent mucous membrane and, after removing the neoplasm by

428

subperichondrial dissection, to leave the thyroid ala on the affected side intact, the perichondrium on the outer surface not being touched. This method leaves the bare inner surface of the cartilage to line the larynx on the side from which the growth has been removed. Healing over such an exposed surface is necessarily slow and some sequestration or necrosis of cartilage is possible, with formation of granulomas and considerable subsequent scar contraction. The present accepted practice is to excise almost the whole ala on the affected side, leaving the larynx to be lined by the external perichondrium. This removal of the thyroid ala is not followed by falling in of the soft parts but healing occurs much more rapidly than if bare cartilage is left exposed. Additional advantages are that the removal of the growth is made much easier and haemorrhage in the deeper part of the larynx after removal of the growth is much more easily dealt with.

The external perichondrium should be separated laterally on the affected side using a blunt elevator as far as possible. The most adherent part, where a sharp dissector may be needed, is at the oblique line where the inferior constrictor, sternothyroid and thyrohyoid muscles are attached, and is the usual limit of this dissection. A sharp elevator is next used to separate the perichondrium of the deeper surface at the upper and lower edges of the ala, care being taken not to separate more than about 0·6 cm. The middle line of the cartilage is next outlined by a small saw. No attempt should be made to divide the whole thickness of the cartilage but merely to make a vertical groove in the midline. The cartilage is now removed piecemeal on the involved side using a small pair of bone nibbling forceps.

After each bite the internal perichondrium is separated for another 0·6 cm., until a column of cartilage has been removed to one side of the saw-cut groove. The internal perichondrium can now be separated quite easily from the cartilage which is then removed as far back as necessary, usually back to the region of the muscular attachments.

The affected side of the larynx is now exposed and if the growth, as previously examined by direct laryngoscopy, approaches the commissure then some of the cartilage on the unaffected side must be similarly removed.

Opening of the larynx

An incision is now made in the cricothyroid membrane in the midline extending from the upper edge of the cricoid cartilage as far as the level of the lower border of the thyroid cartilage.

The incision is now carried upwards. If the growth is of the early type, already described as suitable for this operation, then the incision is made in the midline using a pair of fine, straight, blunt-pointed scissors, and carried upwards for a distance of about 2·5 cm.; the upper end will probably divide the petiolus of the epiglottis.

When the larynx has been opened in this manner the interior can easily be inspected by pulling the edges of the incision apart. A flat type of self-retaining mastoid retractor is most useful at this stage for exposing the interior of the larynx, leaving the assistant free to manage suction and swabs.

Excision of growth

If the growth proves to be more extensive than was first thought, it may be necessary to carry out a total laryngectomy, the patient's consent having previously been obtained.

Careful preliminary examination, especially by tomography or laryngography, should enable such a possibility to be avoided, but it frequently happens that the growth extends further downwards into the subglottic region than had been suspected. In such a case removal of tissue down to the upper edge of the cricoid cartilage may be allowed, and if this seems insufficient it is possible to divide the cricoid cartilage in the middle line anteriorly and remove part of its lateral aspect in the same way as for the thyroid cartilage. In this event very fine judgment is required.

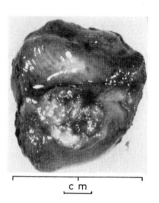

FIG. 180.—Specimen following lateral partial laryngectomy for limited cordal cancer.

c m

After packing normal-saline-moistened 2·5 cm. ribbon gauze down onto the tracheostomy tube the excision of the growth is carried out with scissors. Transverse cuts are first made well above and well below the growth for a sufficient distance posteriorly. The upper cut will always be through the ventricular band and the lower one will be at least 1 cm. below the apparent lower border of the growth. These incisions are best made with short straight scissors.

A troublesome vessel is usually opened at the back of the lower incision and it is wise to secure this before removing the growth. Well-placed suction is extremely useful at this stage of the operation. The specimen posteriorly is best divided with a fairly large pair of scissors curved on the flat. It should be pulled well forwards with forceps and the tip of the vocal process of the arytenoid cartilage must always be included.

Haemostasis and closure

All packing should now be removed and bleeding points carefully controlled. A further proof of haemostasis is to allow the cough reflex to return at this time.

After spraying the raw surface in the larynx with a suitable antibiotic the external perichondrium is sutured vertically with a few stitches of 1/0 chromic catgut and the wound then carefully closed in layers and again sprayed with antibiotic. A drain is not usually required. Simple gauze dressings with a crepe bandage are applied and the tracheostomy tube checked and secured with tapes.

Post-operative care

The main complications to be feared after operation are haemorrhage from the larynx, and chest infections due to aspiration of blood or inability to expectorate blood or mucus. Both these conditions are preventable. If care is taken in ligation of bleeding vessels, particularly subcutaneous veins, and the patient is allowed to cough before the incision is sutured, then there is little likelihood of severe post-operative haemorrhage. If this should occur the most satisfactory procedure is to reopen the wound. Blood clots and free blood are removed by suction and the area from which the bleeding arises is identified. The most common single vessel will be a subcutaneous vein which has been overlooked at operation. Alternatively, there may be free bleeding from the raw intralaryngeal surface and this may give rise to some difficulty. If the bleeding does not yield to diathermy coagulation or the use of adrenaline or thrombin, it may be necessary to pack the larynx, and the tracheostomy must then be retained.

Freedom from chest complications depends upon avoiding aspiration of blood and the preservation of an active cough reflex. This, again, is one of the advantages of tracheostomy as part of the operation, since the trachea can then be packed off from the larynx during surgery. The effect of cocaine in the trachea and larynx will have worn off by the end of the operation and the patient should not be allowed to leave the operating table until his cough reflex has returned. Morphine should be avoided both before and after the operation and, indeed, no analgesic other than aspirin compounds or pethidine should be necessary. The patient must be sat up as soon as possible after return to bed as it is so much easier for him to cough in this position. A further essential is the administration of a systemic antibiotic in full doses, starting if possible the day before surgery. Tetracycline or ampicillin are usually chosen.

The patient should not be left alone during the first five or six hours and should be in an intensive care unit for the first 24 hours after operation. A nurse must be in constant attendance to make sure the tracheostomy tube is in position, and to wipe away or aspirate any mucus or blood that is coughed out. If necessary, the tracheostomy tube can be occluded by the finger to allow the patient to cough occasionally through the larynx and so clear away any bloodstained mucus which may have collected. He should be allowed to have frequent mouth-washes of iced water to keep the mouth moist, but should not at this stage swallow.

The surgeon should visit the patient some five or six hours after operation and the patient should then be given a few sips of water to swallow. Swallowing is usually a little painful and occasionally a drop or two may trickle into the larynx and cause a spasm of coughing, or be coughed out through the tracheostomy. This is only temporary and swallowing should be fairly satisfactory after 24 hours, although somewhat painful for the first day or two.

If the swallow is satisfactory, two or three tablets of codeine compound in solution may be given and may be repeated later during the night if necessary. The patient may have sips of water throughout the night as he desires.

If there is no evidence of glottic oedema, the tracheostomy tube can be removed next morning, but if any doubt exists it should be left in for 24–48 hours. The larynx may be examined with a mirror, but the best test is to put a finger over the tracheostomy tube and see if the patient can breathe comfortably with the tube occluded.

A dry gauze dressing is all that is now required for the wound, which will usually heal without any trouble. If the tracheal fistula is moist it should be dusted with antibiotic powder at each change of dressing.

If he so desires, the patient may be allowed to get up to pass water and should be encouraged to sit out of bed the day after operation. Sepsis is not a likely complica-tion if the operative and post-operative technique has been sound, but if local sepsis does occur it will be treated on conventional lines. Semi-solid food may be given the day after operation and normal diet on the third or fourth day.

The interior of the larynx will take much longer to heal than the outside because of the large area which has to be covered with granulations and epithelium.

It will probably be two months before the interior of the larynx is completely healed. When the operation is performed after irradiation the importance of continuing antibiotic cover up to three weeks after operation should be noted. In such circumstances also healing inside and outside the larynx may well be delayed. Occasionally, a granuloma appears in the region of the commissure or at the site of resection a few weeks after operation. It may grow to a size sufficient to cause some dyspnoea but usually is no larger than a lentil. If left alone it tends to disappear after two or three months, but it is better to remove it in the same way as one would remove a papilloma of the larynx and, needless to say, it should be examined microscopically after removal. It is probably due to a small area of necrosis of the cut edge of the thyroid cartilage.

The patient can usually leave hospital at the end of 7–14 days but must be examined at monthly intervals for the first year after operation and at three-monthly intervals during the second year, with continued regular follow-up there-after.

Late results of operation

That part of the larynx from which tissue has been removed heals by slow fibrosis and epithelialization. This is not excessive and does not result in any stenosis of the larynx, especially if the thyroid ala has been removed. It is usually found, however, that in the region of the vocal cord the scarring is more pronounced and that a fibrous replica of the cord is produced which, after a year, may make a very passable substitute for the true cord. Conley (1961) claims better healing and an improved voice by fashioning a new cord from an inturned flap of cervical skin used to line the raw side of the larynx.

There is no satisfactory movement of this band of scar tissue and, although the voice will be useful, it is rough and cannot be said to approach the normal. Singing is impossible. There is always some stenosis if the anterior part of the second cord has been removed as in the frontolateral operation. In such cases the voice is seldom so good as in those in which the operation has been limited to one cord. The patient must not use his voice during the first week after operation but may use a quiet unstrained voice gradually after the first week.

Local recurrence of growth is uncommon but may take place in the scar, or in that tissue adjacent to the area which has been removed. If a growth occurs on the opposite cord it is often difficult to say whether it is a recurrence or a second primary growth.

Metastasis may become evident in the cervical or mediastinal lymph nodes some years after operation and with no evidence of local recurrence in the larynx.

SUPRAGLOTTIC PARTIAL LARYNGECTOMY

Most of the general aspects of this type of surgery have already been covered in the previous pages relating to lateral partial laryngectomy. It is therefore intended to limit this description to relevant differences of detail and technique.

As regards pre-operative care, anaesthesia and position, there is nothing to add except that general anaesthesia with relaxation is essential for this delicate and precise surgery.

Slight variations in the incisions favoured in the past for anterior or lateral pharyngotomy are usually employed, an essential being that they can be rapidly extended for purposes of neck dissection. It is also preferable that the tracheostomy should be made through a separate transverse incision. The T shaped incision illustrated in Fig. 183a and described by Som (1969) is entirely satisfactory.

Approach to the supraglottis

After elevation of the flaps the strap muscles are exposed and divided close to the hyoid bone. The thyrohyoid membrane should then be exposed and the upper border of the thyroid cartilage identified. The larynx should be gently rotated and the superior laryngeal vascular bundle identified and ligated. The superior cornu and posterior border of the thyroid cartilage can now be defined, displacing the superior thyroid pedicle as necessary. An opportunity is now taken to palpate the jugular chain of lymph nodes and if necessary specimens are sent for cryostat section. If neck dissection is indicated it should be done at this stage.

The external perichondrium on the upper border of the thyroid cartilage must now be incised and stripped downward with its muscle attachments until the upper half of the cartilage can be divided horizontally as shown (Fig. 183b, c), with the

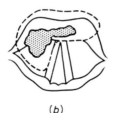

(a)

(b)

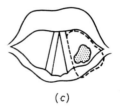

(c)

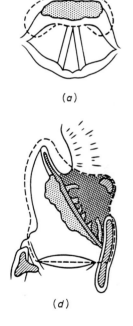

(d)

Fig. 181.—(a), (b), (c). The larynx from above to show approximate lines of resection for supraglottic tumours with sparing of the vocal cords; (d) sagittal section showing resection to include the pre-epiglottic space.

anterior end of the incision crossing the midline on an upward bevel to facilitate closure. The upper half of the cartilage is now dissected away leaving the internal perichondrium intact. At this point it is convenient to carry out a tracheostomy and continue anaesthesia through a cuffed right-angled plastic tube, the peroral tube being withdrawn.

Exposure of the tumour

The pharynx is now entered through a horizontal incision about 1 cm. above the cut margin of the thyroid cartilage. This will pass through the lateral wall of the pyriform fossa and should be continued forwards towards the epiglottis until a good view of the tumour is obtained.

Excision of the tumour

Assuming that a resection of the whole supraglottis including the ventricular bands is required, incisions are now carried posteriorly along the summit of the aryepiglottic folds of both sides, then forwards across the front of the arytenoid cartilages and along the lateral walls of the ventricles to meet just above the anterior commissure of the vocal cords. The anterior end of the original incision opening into the pharynx is then continued slightly upwards dividing the mucosa of the pharyngo-epiglottic fold, across the floor of the vallecula and then joining the incision on the aryepiglottic fold of the opposite side. The supraglottis is now surgically encompassed but it must be removed *en bloc* with the pre-epiglottic space and body of the hyoid bone.

The next and final stage of the resection is therefore division of the hyoid body from its cornua and superior muscle attachments. It is then grasped with a vulsellum and the whole specimen of hyoid body, thyrohyoid membrane, pre-epiglottic tissues and supraglottis bearing the tumour, also with the relevant part of the thyroid internal perichondrium, is removed.

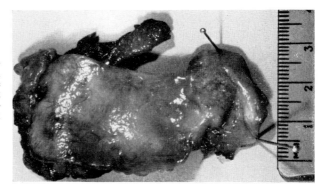

Fig. 182.—Specimen following supraglottic partial laryngectomy to include epiglottis, hyoid bone, left ventricular band, left ventricle and part of left vocal cord.

Cricopharyngeal myotomy

At this stage it is convenient to displace the upper pole of the thyroid gland and expose the lower pharyngeal constrictor muscle. This is facilitated by the vertical limb of the T incision. With one finger in the hypopharynx as a guide, the fibres of the cricopharyngeus are vertically and completely divided down to the submucosa. Following this a No. 12 or 14 F.G. plastic naso-oesophageal feeding tube should be passed.

Closure

After haemostasis is thoroughly assured, with tracheostomy and feeding tube in place, all raw surfaces are sprayed with antibiotic and the sandbag removed from beneath the patient's shoulders. The first step is to eliminate all raw surfaces within the larynx. In most cases this is easily achieved by approximating the cut edge of the mucosa at the top of the medial wall of the pyriform fossae and valleculae to the divided laryngeal mucosa in the walls of the ventricles and in the anterior commissure. Occasionally it is necessary to "borrow" mucosa from the pyriform fossae by simple undermining and advancement or by using local rotation flaps. Interrupted atraumatic sutures of 2/0 chromic catgut are used.

When this is completed, attention is directed to closure of the pharynx. Four or five strong horizontal mattress sutures of 1/0 chromic catgut are then used to approximate, without excess tension, the suprahyoid muscles, pharyngeal mucosa and the cut edge of the thyroid cartilage as composite sutures. This can be further aided by gentle flexion of the head. The flap of thyroid external perichondrium is then brought up as a second layer and tacked down to the suprahyoid muscles with interrupted 2/0 chromic catgut sutures. A third layer of external strap muscle remnants is now carefully secured to the suprahyoid muscles and hyoid cornua. The wound is again sprayed with antibiotic and the flaps approximated and sutured with a small drain of Paul's tubing leading from the posterior limb of the transverse incision. A large gauze, wool and crepe bandage is applied, separate from the tracheostomy dressings and tapes. The nasal feeding catheter is secured and the patient moved to the intensive care unit.

Post-operative care

A similar routine to that following lateral partial laryngectomy is followed at first. The drain is removed in 24 hours and the wound redressed. After 3–4 days the cuffed plastic tracheostomy tube is changed and it is emphasized that during this time the cuff must be deflated for five minutes every 1–2 hours.

Aspiration of tracheal secretions must be regular and thorough as some laryngeal spillover of saliva is almost bound to occur during the first week despite the use of a cuffed tube. All being well small naso-oesophageal tube feeds may be gradually started 24 hours after surgery. However, if regurgitation or coughing occurs it is better to continue intravenous feeding alone for 4–7 days.

The patient should remain in the intensive care unit for about 48 hours or longer if there is any great problem with spillover or managing the tracheostomy. After the first week, skin sutures can be gradually removed and dressings reduced. The tracheostomy tube is changed every 3–4 days. After the second change the cuff can be deflated for longer intervals, and the patient encouraged to clear his larynx and trachea by coughing so as to reduce the need for frequent suction.

Rehabilitation

After 10 days, gradual use of the voice is allowed under the care of a speech therapist, and if spillover is well controlled first attempts at normal swallowing are begun. Ice-cream, jellies, soft-boiled eggs and puréed foods are usually easiest and will be better swallowed if the tracheostomy tube can be plugged during eating. The biggest problem lies in the taking of fluids by mouth. In the early stages drinking with a straw or feeding cup may be helpful, and weeks or months may sometimes be necessary before complete control in this respect is achieved. As soon as there is an adequate fluid intake by mouth the nasal feeding tube can be removed.

Usually the patient will be able to return home in 3–4 weeks although full control of normal swallowing may take longer especially in older patients.

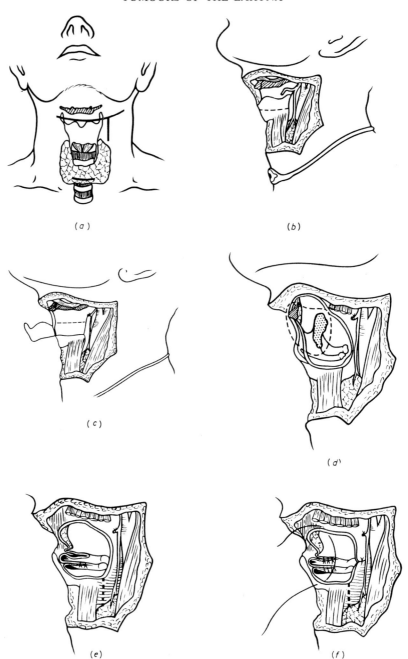

(a)

(b)

(c)

(d)

(e)

(f)

FIG. 183.—Serial diagrams to show steps in supraglottic partial laryngectomy: (a) incisions, easily adaptable to include radical neck dissection; (b) and (c) exposure of larynx and excision of the upper part of thyroid cartilage; (d) opening pharynx, exposure of tumour with extent of excision; (e) covering of raw surfaces by suturing of laryngeal mucosa; (f) first stage closure. The dotted line indicates the site of pharyngeal myotomy.

436

Contra-indications

Any established transglottic disease or gross extension of tumour into the anterior commissure; any major involvement of arytenoid or posterior commissure mucosa; any marked extension into the pyriform fossa. In other words, the tumour must be confined to the supraglottis and/or vallecula.

In addition to the usual general medical and surgical contra-indications, it is felt with experience that this type of operation should not be carried out on patients who have reduced pulmonary function or who are over the age of 65.

TOTAL LARYNGECTOMY

History

It is to a Scottish surgeon, Patrick Heron Watson, that the honour of first performing total laryngectomy belongs. But on that occasion the operation was performed for syphilis (Foulis, 1866). It was Billroth of Vienna who first removed the larynx for cancer (Billroth, 1874).

At first, as might be expected, the results of operation were bad and not a single patient survived for one year in the first 25 cases recorded. Post-operative complications were frequent and severe, the most common causes of death being general septicaemia, spreading cellulitis or mediastinitis, septic pulmonary complications, haemorrhage and shock.

The first attempt to improve on these poor results was by performing the operation in two stages, the first consisting of the establishment of a tracheostomy, the larynx being removed later.

In 1905, le Bec used this technique, dividing the trachea and suturing it to the skin, while the cut lower end of the larynx was drained by a rubber tube brought through the skin above and to one side of the tracheostomy. The larynx was removed two or three weeks later when the tracheal opening had united with the skin. At this second operation the skin incision did not involve the tracheostomy opening and the larynx was removed from below upwards.

Single stage laryngectomy was suggested in 1921 by both Moure and Portmann and, since that time, most surgeons have practised a one-stage operation.

Pre-operative care

This does not differ in general from that involved in partial laryngectomy (p. 426). The patient should have a general medical examination which should include an electrocardiogram, chest x-ray, blood urea, complete blood count, serological tests, haemoglobin estimation and blood grouping.

If any general condition co-exists which might adversely affect the result, the operation would naturally be postponed until this problem had received adequate attention. The position with regard to his post-operative condition must be kindly and optimistically explained to the patient and to his relatives. The speech therapist introduces herself and the physiotherapist starts simple breathing exercises. At this time it often gives a patient further confidence if he can meet a patient who has achieved a good oesophageal voice after laryngectomy.

Anaesthesia

Some few surgeons may still prefer to perform the operation entirely under local anaesthesia and in fact attribute the reduction in their mortality very considerably to its use. On the other hand, the results obtained today by surgeons using modern general anaesthesia are in most respects superior to those obtained by surgeons using local anaesthesia only; and post-operative complications which can be attributed to the general anaesthetic as such are extremely rare if a skilled anaesthetist is employed. Where the standard of general anaesthesia available is unreliable, then no doubt careful sedation and local anaesthesia is preferable.

There is little objection to a suitable preliminary injection of Omnopon with scopolamine or atropine an hour before operation; any depressing effect it may have on the respiratory tract will have worn off before the end of the operation.

Local anaesthesia

This will be best obtained by the use of Xylocaine 1–2 per cent with the addition of a small amount of adrenaline—a strength of 1 :200,000 is sufficient.

The lines of the proposed skin incisions should first be infiltrated and then the region of the superior laryngeal nerves between the tip of the great cornu of the hyoid bone and the superior cornu of the thyroid cartilage. During the course of the operation further injections of this anaesthetic can be used around the trachea and in the neighbourhood of the recurrent laryngeal nerves, or in any other situation when anaesthesia seems to be incomplete.

A solution of 5 per cent cocaine on a pledget of cotton wool may be applied to mucous membranes both before and after opening of the pharynx.

Alternatively, regional anaesthesia of the cervical nerve trunks may be employed, together with the use of cocaine applied locally on a swab for the superior and inferior laryngeal nerves.

General anaesthesia

This will usually be induced by an intravenous barbiturate, such as thiopentone, with a suitable relaxant, followed by whatever inhalation anaesthetic is considered best for the particular patient (Coffin, 1955). Today it is frequently halothane with nitrous oxide and oxygen. Hypotensive techniques are often applicable.

If a preliminary tracheostomy has been performed, the anaesthetic will be given through this opening, using one of the short right-angled cuffed plastic tubes manufactured for positive pressure respiration. If the natural airway is adequate the anaesthetist may use an ordinary endotracheal tube (nasal or oral) which will be withdrawn when the larynx is mobilized by dissection and the right-angled plastic tube then inserted directly into the trachea via a tracheostomy before the operation proceeds further. It should be noted that there are some who hold the view that oral intubation of the cancerous larynx carries the danger of tracheal implantation of malignant cells, and for this reason it may be considered preferable to start all anaesthetic proceedings for laryngectomy with a preliminary tracheostomy using local infiltration. If the laryngeal airway is poor, then a preliminary tracheostomy under local anaesthesia is certainly essential for safety during induction of general anaesthesia. Whenever a tracheostomy becomes necessary it is considered wise to proceed at once to laryngectomy in view of the dangers of tracheal implantation due to the cannula.

Technique of operation

There are many variations in technique which may be employed and it is not possible in the scope of this work to go fully into the details of such variations. It must suffice to describe in detail the essential steps and to indicate briefly some of the most important alternative methods of procedure.

Position

The head is extended as for laryngofissure, with a sandbag beneath the shoulders.

Incisions

The classical approach of Gluck (1914) is still used with slight modifications (Fig. 184). It starts as a gently curved horizontal incision, convex downwards, at the level of the hyoid bone, extending laterally as far as the anterior border of the sternomastoid on each side. A vertical incision is now carried downwards about 2·5 cm. offset from the midline to the level of the first or second ring of the trachea. This incision should be made on the side where the maximum dissection is likely to take place; for example, if radical neck dissection is to be combined with resection of the larynx, so that the shorter flap will retain a good blood supply.

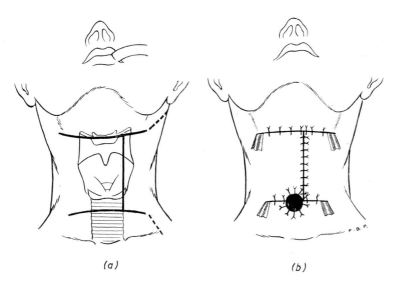

(a)   *(b)*

FIG. 184.—Total laryngectomy: (*a*) Gluck incision modified by offsetting the vertical component. Dotted lines show extensions required if neck dissection becomes necessary; (*b*) showing position of tracheostomy and lateral drainage.

A shorter convex upward-curving horizontal incision is then made across the lower end of the vertical incision, extending across the surface of the sternomastoid muscle for roughly half its width on either side. These incisions mark out two unequal lateral flaps which are dissected up to their bases and turned back. The flaps include all the superficial fascia, the platysma muscle and a few subcutaneous veins. These veins should be carefully secured and ligated as they are the most common source of a reactionary haemorrhage. In particular, the anterior jugular veins should be identified and tied. The flaps should then be covered in gauze moistened with normal saline solution.

This approach gives an excellent exposure for removal of the larynx and, with only slight modification, for pharyngolaryngectomy. The blood supply of the flaps is satisfactory, so that healing is good even after irradiation, and adequate drainage can be obtained at the extremities of the horizontal incisions as far from the tracheal orifice as possible. The main disadvantage of the incision is that the vertical component is close to the pharyngeal suture line and if this should break down a large pharyngeal fistula frequently results.

An alternative incision is illustrated in Fig. 185. This was first advocated by Francesco Durante (1905) and subsequently recommended by Gluck (1914) and by Sorenson (1930). The incision commences on the anterior border of the sternomastoid muscle about the level of the hyoid bone, passes down along the anterior border of the muscle for about 7·5 cm. and then curves across the middle line at the level of the second or third ring of the trachea.

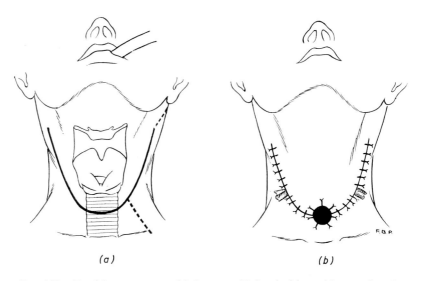

(a) *(b)*

FIG. 185.—Total laryngectomy: (*a*) Sorensen U flap incision with extensions for neck dissection; (*b*) showing position of tracheostomy and lateral drainage.

The advantages of this approach are that it gives adequate exposure, the suturing of the skin around the trachea is rather simpler than with two lateral flaps, adequate drainage can be provided on each side, well away from the trachea, the skin incisions are not so close to the pharyngeal suture line, and there is less scarring of neck tissues. This is a very satisfactory incision in all cases except in those following large doses of irradiation. In such cases the subcutaneous tissues are fibrosed and occasionally the tip of the flap may suffer loss of vitality and some necrosis.

If it should be found necessary to combine a radical neck dissection with either of these incisions, straight extensions can be produced from the nearest points to the mastoid process and to the centre of the clavicle.

A single vertical incision was at one time advocated (Jackson, 1940) and widely used. In theory ideal, and certainly practicable, it does not give sufficient exposure for the modern wide field operation nor allow easily for possible neck dissection.

Other incisions illustrated (Fig. 186) are used especially for combined total laryngectomy and radical neck dissection. The double Y incision of Hayes Martin (1957) is very effective and the exposure of neck and larynx adequate. Its one weakness is with surgery after a full course of irradiation to the neck. In such cases there is a tendency for skin breakdown at the upper and sometimes the lower incision junctions. This may result in the carotid arteries being at risk from exposure and delayed healing, the situation being further aggravated by any fistulous breakdown.

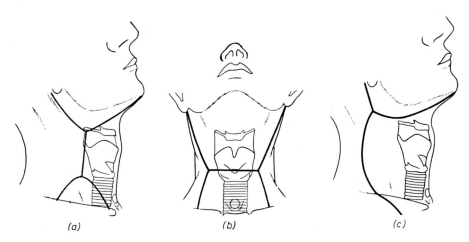

FIG. 186.—(a) Incision for combined total laryngectomy and unilateral radical neck dissection (Martin); (b) incision for combined total laryngectomy and bilateral simultaneous radical neck dissection (Martin); (c) Schobinger incision modified by Conley.

Recently the Schobinger flap as modified by Conley to overcome this weakness has proved very useful although the laryngeal exposure is sometimes more awkward (Fig. 186c).

Exposure of the larynx (Fig. 187).

The first step is to incise the deep fascia at the level of the upper border of the thyroid cartilage. A dissector is then passed, first beneath the sternohyoid muscle

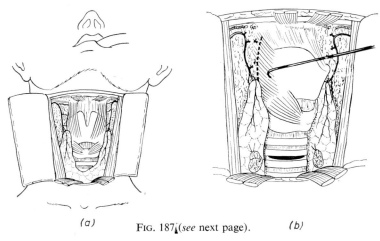

(a) FIG. 187 (*see* next page). (b)

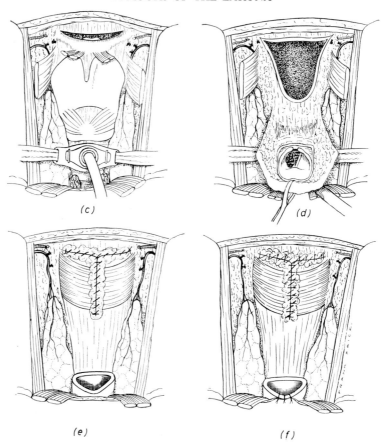

FIG. 187.—Steps in total laryngectomy: (*a*) incision, division of strap muscles and exposure of larynx, thyroid gland and upper trachea; (*b*) rotation of larynx to expose lateral muscular attachments—dotted line showing division of inferior constrictor muscle. Superior laryngeal vessels ligated and thyroid gland isthmus divided. Trachea opened; (*c*) anaesthetic tube inserted via tracheostomy. Pharynx opened through valleculae, above and behind hyoid bone; (*d*) whole larynx with hyoid bone drawn downward and forwards to expose tumour. Postcricoid mucosa divided transversely and pharyngeal mucosa peeled away from cricoid cartilage and out of pyriform fossae; (*e*) closure of pharynx after removal of larynx from stump of trachea. First layer of continuous chromic catgut to incorporate mucosal and muscle layers; (*f*) second layer of interrupted chromic catgut stitches binding all available connective tissues to re-inforce first layer. Commencing suture of skin margin to cut edge of trachea.

and the superior belly of the omohyoid muscle which are divided. The thyrohyoid muscle is now exposed and is similarly divided. It will be found to be as broad as the other two muscles together. Division of the thyrohyoid muscle will lay bare the thyrohyoid membrane. At this stage it will be convenient to expose and divide the internal laryngeal nerve and also the accompanying branch of the superior thyroid artery with its companion vein. These steps are then repeated on the opposite side.

The muscles should next be divided further down just below the lower border of the cricoid cartilage. Here lie the sternohyoid and sternothyroid muscles, the latter

442

being found to be much the bulkier of the two. Beneath the sternothyroid muscle the lateral lobe of the thyroid gland is exposed.

The sternomastoid muscles are now retracted laterally and the deep fascia covering the carotid sheath is incised longitudinally and with it the lower end of the superior belly of the omohyoid muscle. The deep fascia is removed together with any accompanying lymph nodes and stripped forwards towards the thyroid cartilage.

As the fascia is stripped forwards, the inferior constrictor muscle covering the posterior half of the thyroid ala must be identified. The fibres will be found to be running backwards and upwards. Care must be taken not to damage the muscle as it forms the most important structure in the repair of the pharyngeal wall. Its small nerve supply—the external laryngeal—can usually be seen and should if possible be preserved.

The lateral lobes of the thyroid gland are separated from the larynx on their inner aspect for some distance, but care should be taken not to strip them unnecessarily from the trachea. However, if there is the least chance of subglottic spread of disease, whether a neck dissection is performed or not, it is wise to remove the homolateral thyroid lobe and paratracheal lymphatics with the larynx.

It will now be necessary to divide the thyroid isthmus and expose the first five or six rings of the trachea. In addition some small vessels passing to the larynx will need to be ligated, particularly the cricothyroid arteries. This completes the exposure of the larynx which now needs to be freed from its posterior attachments.

Freeing the larynx

This is done while rotating the larynx first to one side then to the other. The first step is to divide the attachment of the inferior constrictor muscle to the thyroid cartilage. This is done with a knife, cutting vertically down to the cartilage, and the muscle is then dissected free from the lateral surface of the ala with a fairly sharp dissector. There is some advantage in removing the inferior constrictor muscle together with the perichondrium in one layer, as the stylopharyngeus muscle, which is intimately associated with the inferior constrictor, is attached to the posterior border of the cartilage and should be removed from its attachment to the thyroid cartilage in one layer with the inferior constrictor muscle. This can be done more easily if the dissection at this point is subperichondrial. When the posterior border of the cartilage has been freed it is a good plan to divide the superior cornu and remove it, taking care not to perforate the mucosa in so doing. The postero-superior border of the ala then forms a convenient angle for retraction. The mucous membrane of the pyriform fossa is exposed when the posterior border of the cartilage is reached and, by drawing the cartilage well across to the opposite side, the mucous membrane of the outer wall of the fossa can be easily separated from the deep surface of the cartilage.

Opening of the trachea

At this stage it is convenient to transfer the anaesthetic delivery tube from mouth to trachea, if a peroral tube was used, so that it is well free of the field during removal of the larynx.

The anaesthetist must be informed of this intention and should have prepared a sterile cuffed right-angled tracheostomy tube with a suitable connection to the main anaesthetic circuit. In addition, suction apparatus must be switched on and held ready.

Between its third and fourth rings the trachea is now opened through half its diameter, a black silk traction suture placed through the lower anterior cut edge, and the cuffed right-angle tube inserted as soon as the anaesthetist has withdrawn the original oral tube. During this manoeuvre opportunity is taken to remove all excess secretions from the trachea by adequate catheter suction. The cuff on the fresh tube is inflated and the tube itself rapidly connected to the anaesthetic circuit, being anchored in place by one or two skin stitches. Fresh sterile towels are placed in position and a small dry gauze pack inserted above the cuff in the cut end of the trachea.

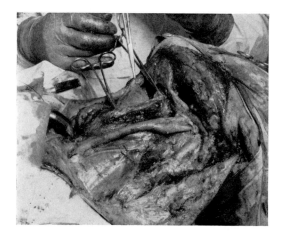

(a)

FIG. 188.—(a) Left radical neck dissection in continuity with total laryngectomy. The mucosal defect is identified by haemostat tips. The left vagus nerve has been sacrificed, but all other structures shown are normally preserved; (b) patient two weeks after the operation.

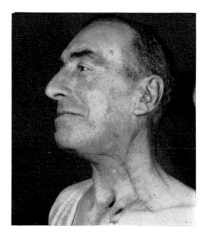

(b)

Removal of the larynx

The larynx can be removed either from above downwards or from below upwards (method of Perier). There is not much difference between the two methods regarding technical accomplishment, but most people prefer the former method as the growth can be seen more clearly from above and it is therefore easier to decide upon the amount of mucous membrane to be removed.

It is preferable to remove the whole hyoid bone with the larynx, since it ensures better clearance of the important pre-epiglottic space and also facilitates the final closure of the pharynx. Accordingly, sharp dissection is carried back through the muscle attachments along the upper surface of the bone until the submucosal layer in the valleculae is reached. The mucous membrane is then divided transversely with scissors passing across the middle line just in front of the tip of the epiglottis in such a manner that the epiglottis is removed but the mucous membrane of the vallecula is retained for purposes of suture. Naturally, if the growth is invading the epiglottis the incision in the mucous membrane may need to be modified.

As soon as the pharynx has been opened by this transverse incision, the epiglottis, which will be the most prominent object to be seen in the pharynx, is gripped securely with vulsellum forceps and drawn forwards. A careful direct inspection is now made of the larynx to assess the size and extent of the growth and to decide whether any modification is necessary in the amount of mucous membrane to be removed. The whole larynx is now drawn well forward by forceps on the hyoid bone or epiglottis. The mucous membrane is undermined and divided transversely on the upper part of the postcricoid area. The exact level of the incision will depend upon how much of the mucous membrane it is desired to remove. The lateral edges of the original transverse incision are then connected with this incision by dividing the intervening mucosa with curved scissors.

This division of the mucous membrane will pass across the top of the pyriform fossa, the mucous membrane of which was partially separated from the deeper surface of the thyroid ala at a previous stage. The mucous membrane from the pyriform fossa together with the mucous membrane from the back of the cricoid cartilage is now peeled away by careful gauze and occasional sharp dissection. This mucosal stripping is carried downwards as far as the lower border of the cricoid, or lower still if it is considered necessary to remove some of the trachea. No more mucous membrane should be separated than is necessary to allow division of the trachea at the desired level.

The larynx with its attached hyoid bone and muscle remnants is now removed by completing the tracheal division, if possible on a slightly forward bevel. The specimen should then be laid open posteriorly for inspection and photography before being immersed in fixative solution.

Closure of the pharynx

The opening into the pharynx is of roughly triangular shape and it is usually most convenient to suture it so that the resulting scar takes the approximate shape of the letters I or Y, depending upon the amount of mucosa available. There should be at least two layers of sutures; the first layer should aim at inverting the edge of the mucosa, and the second row of sutures should cover and re-inforce the first row, if possible completely. The best suture material is probably 2/0 chromic catgut on an atraumatic intestinal needle, although individual surgeons will have their own preferences. At this stage the extension of the head and neck should be reduced and a nasogastric feeding tube inserted by the anaesthetist.

If ample mucosa is available, the first or mucosal suture layer should consist of an inverting and continuous locking Connell type stitch inserted extramucosally as far as possible. Each bite should incorporate the divided constrictor muscles, adjacent connective tissue and fascia so that all dead space is eliminated and firm backing is given to the mucous membrane.

445

Where insufficient mucosa is available for the stitch pattern, a Y or T line must be the aim. Two similar Connell stitches are again used, the first starting inferiorly and crossing to the patient's right, while the second starts on the patient's left and crosses to the right, joining the ascending line at the middle of the Y.

A second reinforcing layer of interrupted chromic catgut or nylon stitches is then inserted, binding any remaining remnants of muscle and connective tissue firmly on to the reconstructed pharynx.

This part of the operation may be a little tedious but it is important that it should not be hurried, since careful suturing of the pharyngeal wall will make all the difference to the healing. When the pharynx has been sutured the surface should be lightly sprayed with a suitable antibiotic solution or powder.

Creation of tracheostome and skin closure

The anaesthetist should now ensure that the blood pressure is brought back to near normal limits. When all bleeding points have been satisfactorily controlled, the gauze pack is removed from around the trachea and a suction tube is inserted to remove any inhaled blood or mucus. If any doubt exists a bronchoscope can be passed and direct aspiration carried out.

The wound is again sprayed with antibiotic powder and the skin flap or flaps are returned to position. The remaining parts of the divided tracheal edge are now sutured to the skin, every endeavour being made to leave no raw edge exposed. Careful skin-to-mucosal suture of the tracheal edge will promote rapid healing and prevent subsequent cicatricial contraction of the tracheal orifice.

If the larynx is removed from below upwards, the trachea is divided as already described and is tethered to the skin by two fixation sutures. The larynx is then separated from the anterior wall of the gullet and hypopharynx by blunt dissection from below as far up as the arytenoids, and the pharynx opened at this point. The mucous membrane is then divided with scissors along the same lines as already described and the pharyngeal opening is sutured in the same way. There do not seem to be any particular advantages or disadvantages peculiar to either method. The removal from below is perhaps a little easier but it is not so easy to plan the mucosal incision as when the pharynx is opened through a superior pharyngotomy.

Before insertion of the subcutaneous and skin sutures an excellent practice is to tack down the skin flaps to the reconstructed pharynx and adjacent tissues with a few chromic catgut sutures.

The suture material for the skin and the tracheal orifice is a matter of personal choice but black silk is very satisfactory.

Adequate drainage of the wound is extremely important and is best dealt with by putting in lengths of soft latex tubing of the Paul or Penrose type at the lateral extremities of each of the horizontal incisions. These should be sutured to the skin and should project for some distance beyond it in order to conduct any exudate as far away from the tracheal orifice as possible. If a U-shaped incision has been made, drainage is most efficiently procured by inserting a strip of Paul's tubing about the middle of the incision on each side. If continuous suction drainage is to be used, special perforated plastic aspiration tubes are inserted in place of the drains.

Where a previous tracheostomy has been performed, the whole fistula including the surrounding skin should be excised with the laryngeal specimen. The siting of the main skin incisions at the start of the operation must be planned accordingly.

Post-operative care

This must be carried out under the personal supervision of the operating surgeon. In the first few days it is essential that a nurse be in constant attendance and preferably in an intensive care unit.

The immediate post-operative dressing should include a crepe bandage with a heavy pressure dressing of gauze and wool over the area of operation above the tracheal orifice. This will eliminate the dead space, ensure immobilization, tend to prevent exudates from collecting beneath the flaps and encourage their adherence to the pharynx. Alternatively, continuous suction drainage can be applied through perforated soft plastic suction tubes placed on each side beneath the flaps. If these are retained in place for 72 hours, only a light gauze dressing will be necessary.

A suitable size of laryngectomy cannula such as the Colledge pattern, modified to hold an extra long inner tube to carry it free of the heavy dressings anteriorly, should be used for the first few days (Fig. 189). This has been found to be an improvement on the older Moure–Lombard cannula. After the first three or four days, the inner tube can be omitted, although the cannula will need regular changing at least once daily.

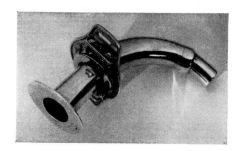

Fig. 189.—Colledge pattern laryngectomy cannula modified to hold temporary long inner tube for use with post-operative dressings.

Care of the tracheostome

The nurse should be provided with a bedside suction apparatus for keeping the tracheostome free of mucus without disturbing the patient by having to wipe it away. Handling of all suction tubing by the nurses must be as clean as possible. Catheters must be whistle-tipped and of soft rubber or plastic. Eight to twelve will be needed per patient if used again. The catheters are kept in a suitable antiseptic solution, used once only and then discarded into a separate receiver for sterilization or disposal.

The inner tube should be removed every hour or two for cleaning but the nurse must not interfere with the outer cannula; this should be removed by the surgeon at his discretion, for purposes of cleaning or change of dressing. Before operation, all nurses who are to be in attendance should be fully acquainted with the type of cannula to be used and have a duplicate demonstrated to them. A spare should be available at all times in the ward for changes of dressing.

After the stitches have been removed and the wound is healed, in about 6–9 days, a simple metal laryngectomy cannula of the Colledge type, omitting an inner tube, can be used, or a large size plastic Morant Baker cannula may be worn. The patient must be instructed how to clean and change these for himself. When it is evident that there is no tendency for the tracheal orifice to contract, usually after about 6–8 weeks, the cannula may be discarded completely in many cases and a buckle-shaped shield holding a disposable gauze swab can be worn round the neck to cover and protect the stoma. Alternatively, a wire mesh shield can be clipped on to the front of a laryngectomy cannula if this must continue to be worn (Fig. 191). A thin gauze veil may then be worn around the neck beneath the shirt.

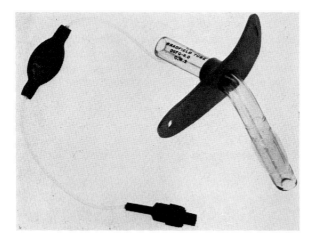

FIG. 190.—Plastic tracheo-stomy tube with inflatable cuff.

FIG. 191.—Tracheostome shields: (a) soft plastic buckle held by tapes around neck and covered with disposable gauze; (b) spring wire baffle clipped to flange of laryngectomy cannula.

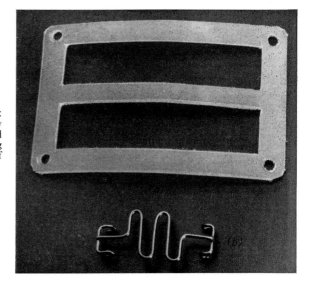

Care of the wound

If reasonable care has been taken both before and at operation, and if antibiotics are used, there is nowadays an excellent chance of healing by first intention. The drainage tubes must be removed after two or three days, if there is no longer any discharge of blood-stained serum from them. If there is any doubt, how-ever, as in post-radiotherapy cases, the drainage tubes are best left in position for an extra day or two. If the wound is going to break down, the most likely time is about the tenth day, when the sutures used for the pharyngeal wall will begin to slough out. The only sign of this may be a small leakage of saliva or mucus from one or other of the drainage areas, but within a day or two the other side will also leak and a large part of the incision may quietly gape open without any obvious signs of inflammation. The leaking saliva would appear in such cases to exert some sort of digestive action on the fibrinous exudate or young fibrous tissue of the wound. Fortunately by this time the tracheal stoma is often firmly healed and does not tend to break down, especially if it has been possible to make the opening in a part of the skin that has not been so extensively irradiated.

If leakage occurs, it is important that the nurse changes the dressings frequently, often three or four times daily, and the suction tube is now of great importance. Although plain dry dressings are most useful together with a suitable antibiotic spray to the wound itself, sloughing and infected wounds will require the additional use of antiseptic applications. Freshly prepared zinc peroxide cream has been found to be constantly effective in such cases. There is also less tendency to leak if the dressings are held firmly in place by a webbing band and buckle which can be quickly adjusted.

With modern antibiotics, sepsis is no longer the bugbear it was and the large fistulae associated with septic sloughing of the flaps, which were at one time not uncommon, now rarely occur. In the majority of cases and even after irradiation, fistulae will heal within a few weeks. Occasionally, however, a permanent fistula will remain, usually about the midline, requiring secondary closure by a suitable reconstructive procedure. No attempt at direct repair should be made until the tissues are well healed and the skin and mucous membrane in the fistula are united without intervening raw surfaces.

Antibiotic cover

Change occurs so rapidly in the use of these agents that it is not easy to lay down any permanent rules. At the present time, however, the safest routine would appear to be a Polymyxin-Bacitracin spray to the wound at the time of operation and at subsequent dressings, while a routine course of 250 mg. systemic tetracycline or ampicillin is also given six-hourly, commencing the day before operation and going on for at least two weeks afterwards, even if there is no pyrexia and the wound is healing well.

Naso-oesophageal feeding tube

This should be of soft rubber or plastic. The most practical size is a No. 12 or 14 F.G. whistle-tipped urethral catheter with a washer-type disc mounted at its outer end to prevent its disappearing into the nose. It is passed intranasally at the time of operation and should be left in until such time as the wound is healed, usually 6–7 days, but often longer in some irradiated cases. Saliva can be swallowed quite comfortably and the tube should be fixed to the nose with a strip of adhesive tape or a silk suture. The nurse in attendance must take care to see that the patient does not pull out the tube while he is coming round from the anaesthetic or subsequently.

A few surgeons dispense with feeding tubes altogether, starting small oral feeds at once or relying on intravenous nutrition for the first few days. The patient is certainly more comfortable, but it is felt that a feeding tube does diminish the likelihood of complications, especially after irradiation; it ensures adequate dietary intake, and should a fistula develop continued feeding will present no difficulty.

449

Chest complications

These depend almost entirely upon the presence of blood or inspissated secretions in the bronchi and are more often in the nature of a partial collapse with mild infection than an established bronchopneumonia. With careful technique they are now uncommon.

Treatment is, in the main, preventive. Omnopon may be given an hour before operation but on no account should any be given after this time because of its depressant effect on the respiratory system.

Cocaine should be employed conservatively on the tracheal mucosa and not so liberally that it runs down into the bronchi.

If there is any likelihood of blood in quantity having entered the trachea during operation a bronchoscope should be passed before the patient leaves the table and thorough aspiration carried out. If the operation is being done under general anaesthesia this must always be lightened before the end of the operation so that the cough reflex is present before dressings are applied.

The patient should be sat up as soon as possible after operation since coughing is much easier and more effective in this position than if the patient is recumbent. If there are any signs of post-operative pulmonary collapse or obstruction, then a bronchoscope should be passed for purposes of direct aspiration, while if broncho-pneumonia does develop it should be treated on general medical lines. A portable chest x-ray and an electrocardiograph the first day after operation are necessary routine measures.

Other complications

Reactionary haemorrhage may occur, particularly from veins in the skin flaps or in the region of the thyroid gland. If necessary, the wound must be re-opened and the bleeding vessel ligated.

Wound infection is today uncommon and if it arises it must be controlled on a routine bacteriological and suitable antibiotic basis.

Pulmonary and cerebral embolism have been recorded but though serious they are not of especial frequency following this operation. Probably the most serious complication which usually occurs without warning is cardiac infarction. A post-operative electrocardiograph the day after operation may be useful in this respect.

Pharyngeal fistula is the most common complication which one must endeavour to avoid. It occurs in at least 20 per cent of patients. The main factors in its prevention have already been considered.

In the majority of cases the fistula is small and heals within a few weeks without interference. If it persists, it may be closed by a simple plastic operation, in which the skin and mucosal surfaces are separated from each other, the mucosal layer carefully sutured so that the edges are turned into the pharynx and the skin sutured to cover it so that the edges are slightly everted. If possible the two suture lines should not lie over each other. If the opening is of larger size it may be necessary to incise the skin around the fistula and turn the skin inwards so that the anterior wall of the pharynx is now lined by skin. The raw surface remaining may be closed by turning down a rotation flap of skin from beneath the chin or from the side of the neck. If this is not possible the skin must be provided from else-where and it may be that a tubed pedicle or rotation flap from the anterior chest will be required. If this is likely to be necessary the pedicle must be planned and prepared beforehand so that it will be ready for use as soon as the edges of the fistula have healed, thus avoiding unnecessary delay.

Crusting of the upper part of the trachea is also a common post-operative complication. This is due to the unnatural drying of the secretions in the trachea because the inspired air is inadequately warmed or moistened. The crusts may be removed by cotton-wool swabs moistened with dilute bicarbonate of soda, and the tracheal surface should be sprayed every two or three hours with a similar 1 per cent solution, sometimes combined with Alevaire or Varidase if crusting is severe. Some degree of infective tracheitis is also present as a rule and may require the further use of systemic and local antibiotics. Care must be taken to see that inspired air is adequately humidified.

Swallowing after laryngectomy

As a rule this presents no difficulty. Even while a nasal feeding tube is in position a patient can swallow his saliva without difficulty and drink fluids quite satisfactorily, although the act of swallowing is painful for the first few days. If the operation has proceeded satisfactorily and a fistula is not anticipated, it is possible to remove the feeding tube after about six days, but if there has been previous irradiation it is much wiser to leave the tube in position for at least ten days, since it is often not until the tenth day or later that the pharyngeal wound breaks down. If the wound does break down, the tube should be left in position until the full extent and size of the fistula are revealed. If the fistula is small, it can probably be controlled during swallowing by pressure from a gauze pack, and if so the tube can be removed. If a large fistula persists, however, it is much wiser to continue using a tube until the fistula is repaired, although it may be more convenient to withdraw the tube and insert it for each feed. Occasionally a temporary gastrostomy may be less tiresome for the patient and facilitate healing.

Functional rehabilitation

All operations on the larynx and pharynx imply at least temporary interference with function, depending upon the amount of anatomical and neurological disturbance. When the act of swallowing is deranged it is usually due to immediate mechanical factors, such as oedema and distortion of the lumen with neuromuscular inco-ordination and all the discomfort of local movement. As healing proceeds these factors rapidly resolve and the patient quickly re-educates himself with minimum assistance, although the swallow may remain more of a voluntary effort than formerly. Occasionally, dysphagia will be more serious and persistent. In these cases further surgical measures may become necessary.

When the voice is impaired by operations on the larynx, the aid of a speech therapist is essential in restoring its quality and strength. After total laryngectomy a fair though gruff voice can be regained by learning oesophageal speech. This requires using the oesophagus as an air reservoir filled by voluntary effort from the pharynx or even by inflation through a prepared tracheo-oesophageal fistula, as was first suggested by Conley (1958). The air is then passed rapidly upward at will, causing the narrower parts of the lower pharynx to vibrate with the production of a low pitched sound.

Recently several further attempts have been made to aid voice production by means of a tracheo-oesophageal fistula carefully constructed in stages (Asai, 1965; Montgomery and Toothill, 1968). When successful this can certainly produce a stronger voice, but problems of management of the fistula with spillover from the

451

pharynx have been encountered, and there is the necessity to close the tracheostome when speaking.

Despite occasional reports there is at present no record of any effective and successful total laryngeal transplant having been carried out in the human. Work continues in animals but so far without much lasting success.

Alternatively, a patient may prefer or be obliged to use one of various types of mechanical speech aid now on the market. These comprise the portable transistorized electrolarynx acting through a vibrating disc placed against the skin of the neck (Barney, 1958) (Fig. 192). Modifications of the original Tapia artificial reed larynx operating from the tracheostome such as the van Hunen nylon membrane vibrator may be used, and also electrically operated mouth resonators activated by a small wire from pocket batteries, either carried externally, such as the Ticchioni pipe, or built into the upper denture (Tait, 1959).

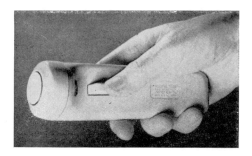

Fig. 192.—The Bell system transistorized electrolarynx to show the vibrating disc operated by a thumb switch.

To a large extent restoration of function depends upon the age, intelligence and determination of the patient, whatever aids may or may not be available. About 60 per cent of all "laryngectomees" achieve a useful oesophageal voice without artificial aids. However, any good speech rehabilitation programme must give instruction in artificial aids to those who require them in order to help prevent the lowering of morale and drift into depression that can easily occur in some of these patients (Martin, 1963).

Disability after laryngectomy

The main disability from which the patient will suffer after operation is naturally the loss of his normal voice. The sense of smell is also impaired only because there is no regular air current through the nose, but taste and the appreciation of flavours remain during eating and there is usually no complaint on this account. Some patients even resume smoking with evident satisfaction.

The patient must take care when having a bath or washing that water does not enter the tracheostome, and swimming must be prohibited.

Heavy lifting or strenuous digging is not possible as these actions entail fixation of the chest wall by closure of the larynx, but light digging is possible and occasionally the patient can partially close the tracheostomy opening by contracting any muscle remnants surrounding it. Several young women who have undergone this operation have subsequently married and borne children without difficulty (Shaw, 1965).

If radical neck dissection has been necessary, some reduction in the usefulness of the arm above the shoulder level may be expected, especially in the later age groups, together with a variable amount of persistent discomfort, more evident again in those whose range of movement is most impaired (Ewing and Martin, 1952).

Apart from these disadvantages, patients come to terms with their disability and live happy and useful lives, often carrying on with their previous work and usually independent of outside help.

RESULTS OF TREATMENT

Assessment of the relative values of the different forms of treatment for laryngeal cancer is not easy; authorities vary in their opinions as to the type of treatment that is suitable for any particular case; one surgeon may limit his selection of cases suitable for partial laryngectomy to those which are considered ideal for such an operation while another may be prepared to perform this operation on any case within the limits of practicability. Naturally the results of partial laryngectomy in the hands of the former are likely to be better than in those of the latter.

A surgeon may consider total laryngectomy to be the only method of treatment for all cases other than the early ones while his neighbour may decide to treat intermediate cases by some form of radiation and reserve radical operation for the very advanced cases. Variations in the practice of surgeons could be multiplied almost indefinitely and to this extent the value of the statistical results of treatment as between one group of cases and another must be to some extent discounted.

Even if all patients attending a particular clinic are included the results would not be comparable, since a clinic will tend to draw cases of a certain type from far afield because of some particular advantage or reputation which an individual or group in that clinic may possess. In addition, the nomenclature and classification of malignant disease in this region is not yet standardized although it is to be hoped that universal adoption of the T.N.M. system in reporting will greatly improve the comparative value of treatment results. There are also certain ethnic variations in sites of laryngeal cancer.

Despite these valid warnings in assessing results there is much that can today be stated with some confidence. It will already have been noted that great technical advances have been made in both surgery and irradiation for laryngeal cancer during the past 20 years. A quarter of a century ago radiotherapy was rightly condemned even for limited cordal cancer (Colledge, 1940); today, however, there are few who would disagree that it is now the treatment of choice in such lesions, and furthermore that modern radiation techniques still allow the surgeon to perform partial or total laryngectomy with success, should the tumour show a poor response or recur (Ormerod, 1958).

These conclusions can be illustrated more clearly by studying the results in some large series treated in recent years. McCabe and Magieski (1960), reviewing a series of 951 limited tumours of the larynx support irradiation for Stage 1 cordal tumours and surgery for the more extensive growths. They also averaged the results quoted by 13 surgeons and 14 radiotherapists writing on the treatment of limited cordal cancer between 1946 and 1959; five-year survival rates were 83 per cent and 75 per cent respectively. Lederman (1961) reviewed a personal series of 957 cases of laryngeal cancer going back to 1933 and all treated by irradiation. Stage 1 cases gave a five-year cure rate of 81 per cent although this dropped to 60 per cent in Stage 2 and significantly to 22 per cent in Stage 3 cases. Another approximately comparable large series of 683 patients with early cordal cancer treated by primary surgery showed 83 per cent of patients surviving five years free of disease but with impaired voice (Frazell and Gerold, 1960). Again, a recent series of 306 cases treated between 1948 and 1956 gave a five-year rate by irradiation for early glottic lesions of 85 per cent and an overall rate of 62 per cent for all cases treated by both main methods (Shaw, 1965).

For larger tumours, late Stage 2, Stage 3 and a few Stage 4 cases, there is also increasing evidence that prompt radical surgery, often with preliminary irradiation, will give the best results in terms of cure (Work and Boyle, 1961; Bryce, Ireland and Rider, 1963; Biller and colleagues, 1969). Coupled with this and with greater knowledge of the surgical pathology in relation to lymph drainage of all laryngeal regions (Ogura, 1951; Pressman and Simon, 1961), improved results are today being shown for extensive glottic and supraglottic tumours by combining resection of the primary lesion with elective neck dissection (Pietrantoni and Fior, 1958; McGavran, Bauer and Ogura, 1961). The former authors give a five-year rate of 48 per cent for supraglottic lesions treated by total laryngectomy alone, rising to 70 per cent if combined with homolateral elective neck dissection. It is also well shown by these authors that delay until nodes are palpable in these cases will halve the cure rate despite radical combined resection. In a series already mentioned, a crude five-year survival rate of 63 per cent was obtained for all tumours first treated surgically (mostly Stage 2 and 3) compared with 45 per cent for the same type of cases treated by primary irradiation (Shaw, 1965).

Recent results of using the more sophisticated modern techniques of partial laryngectomy, often combined with elective radical neck dissection in supraglottic lesions, have given at least 70 per cent five-year survivals with preservation of a laryngeal voice (Ogura and Mallen, 1965; Shumrick, 1969; Som, 1969).

All these results can certainly be criticized on many grounds, but they do illustrate certain trends developed through increasing experience of modern treatment potentials. First, that irradiation today gives excellent results in the early glottic tumours with absolute preservation of function. Secondly, that the balance of judgement between conservative and radical surgery of the larynx is becoming finer with the results of the former approximating the latter for supraglottic tumours.

Nevertheless the ultimate results of treatment still depend on the known clinical and pathological features of the tumour, the biological resistance of the host tissues, and upon the patient's sex, age and psychology.

PROGNOSIS

In general terms, the further from the vocal cords the worse the prognosis. This may be usefully illustrated by reference to figures derived from a recent study (Shaw, 1964). Approximate gross five-year survival rates were as follows:

85 per cent cases of early glottic cancer (Stage 1) treated by external irradiation.

65 per cent of more advanced cases of glottic cancer (mainly Stage 2 or 3) treated by total laryngectomy alone.

35 per cent of all cases of extraglottic or transglottic cancer of the larynx (mainly Stage 3) undergoing extended radical surgery.

This picture of prognosis matches closely the results according to stage reported by Smith and his colleagues (1961) in their detailed study of 600 cases of laryngeal cancer.

Glottic growths are the most common and have the most favourable prognosis, especially when strictly limited to one membranous vocal cord. Subglottic tumours are less favourable for reasons discussed already and because symptoms tend to be delayed. Patients with supraglottic tumours who used to have a poor prognosis now have a much improved outlook as a result of modern methods of partial laryngectomy and neck dissection.

Limited leucoplakia undergoing malignant change can best be treated by adequate surgical removal, as it is of uncertain radio-sensitivity.

Tumours showing numerous mitoses are often more radio-sensitive, but more commonly recur sooner, than well differentiated carcinoma.

Tumours occurring in the aged often tend to be very slow in their progress.

Left alone, an untreated glottic cancer may not cause death for three or more years after the first symptoms appear, whereas supraglottic and subglottic tumours will progress rapidly to fatal results in a few months.

REFERENCES

Abrikossoff, A. (1931). *Arch. Path. Anat.*, **280,** 723.
Alonso, J. M. (1957). *Ann. Otolaryng., Paris,* **74,** 75.
Asai, R. (1965). *Proceedings of the Eighth International Congress of Otolaryngology, Tokyo.*
Asherson, N. (1957). *J. Laryng.*, **71,** 730.
Auerbach, O. (1956). *New Engl. J. Med.*, **256,** 97.
— Hammond, E. C., and Garfinkel, L. (1970). *Cancer,* **25,** 92.
Barney, H. L. (1958). *Ann. Otol.*, **67,** 538.
Barsocchini, L. M., and McCoy, G. (1968). *Ann. Otol.*, **77,** 146.
Bayliss, R. I. S. (1957). *Proc. R. Soc. Med.*, **50,** 1.
Biller, H. F., Davis, W. H., Powers, W. E. and Ogura, J. H. (1969). *Laryngoscope,* **79,** 1387.
Billroth, T. (1874). *Arch. Klin. Chir.*, **17,** 343.
Birck, H. G., and Manhart, H. E. (1962). *Arch. Otolaryng.*, **77,** 603.
Bjork, H., and Weber, C. (1956). *Acta oto-rhino-laryng.*, **46,** 499.
Bocca, E., Pignatoro, O., and Mosciaro, O. (1968). *Ann. Otol.*, **77,** 1005.
Brindle, M. J., and Stell, P. M. (1968). *Clin. Radiol.*, **19,** 257.
Broders, A. C. (1920). *J. Amer. med. Ass.*, **74,** 656.
Broyles, E. N. (1941). *South. med. J.*, **3,** 239.
Bryce, D. P., Ireland, P. E., and Rider, W. D. (1963). *Ann. Otol.*, **72,** 416.
Cady, B., Rippey, J. H., and Frazell, E. L. (1968). *Ann. Surg.*, **167,** 116.
Capps, F. C. W. (1957). *J. Laryng.*, **71,** 709.
Coffin, S. (1955). *Anaesthesia,* **10,** 285.
Colledge, L. (1940). *J. Laryng.*, **55,** 443.
Conley, J. J. (1961). *Arch. Otolaryng.*, **74,** 21.
— de Amesti, F., and Pierce, M. K. (1958). *Ann. Otol.*, **67,** 655.
Coutard, H. (1939). *Surg. Gynec. Obstet.*, **68,** 467.
Creston, J. E. (1961). *Arch. Otolaryng.*, **74,** 556.
Crookes, J. (1953). *J. Laryng.*, **67,** 433.
Cummings, C. W., Montgomery, W. W., and Balogh, K. (1969). *Ann. Otol.*, **78,** 76.
Curwen, M. P., Kennaway, E. L., and Kennaway, N. M. (1954). *Brit. J. Cancer,* **8,** 181.
Durante, F. (1908). *Int. Clin.*, **1,** 122.
El-Mofty, A. (1959). *J. Laryng.*, **73,** 768.
Epstein, S. S., and Winston, P. (1957). *J. Laryng.*, **72,** 452.
— and Shaw, H. J. (1958). *Cancer N.Y.*, **11,** 326.
— Winston, P., Friedmann, I., and Ormerod, F. C. (1957). *J. Laryng.*, **71,** 673.
Ewing, M. R., and Martin, H. (1952). *Cancer, N.Y.*, **5,** 873.
Falbe-Hansen, J. (1955). *Acta oto-rhino-laryng.*, **45,** 388.
Finzi, N. S., and Harmer, D. (1928). *Brit. med. J.*, **2,** 886.
Foulis, D. (1866). *Trans. Int. Med. Congr., London,* **11,** 25.
Frazell, E. L., and Gerold, F. R. (1960). *Postgrad. med. J.*, **27,** 394.
Fust, J. A., and Custer, R. P. (1949). *Amer. J. clin. Path.*, **19,** 522.
Gluck, T. (1914). In *Handbuch der Speziellen Chirurgie* (Ed. by Katz, Preysing and Blumenfield). Wurzburg; Kabitzch.

Harrison, D. F. N. (1964). *Quart. J. Med.*, **33**, 25.
Hautant, A. (1937). *J. Laryng.*, **52**, 65.
Heath, D. (1961). *J. Laryng.*, **75**, 679.
Holborow, C. A. (1958). *Arch. dis. Child.*, **53**, 210.
Holinger, P. H. (1962). *Arch. Otolaryng.*, **75**, 105.
— Johnson, K. C., and Anison, C. C. (1950). *Ann. Otol.*, **59**, 547.
— — and Delgado, A. (1959). *Arch. Otolaryng.*, **70**, 555.
— — Conner, G. H., Conner, B. R., and Holper, J. (1962). *Ann. Otol.*, **71**, 443.
— Schild, J. A., and Maurizi, D. G. (1968). *Laryngoscope*, **78**, 1462.
Hollingsworth, J. B., Kohmoos, H. W., and McNaught, R. C. (1956). *Arch. Otolaryng.*, **52**, 82.
Howell, T. R., Gildersleeve, G. H., and King, E. A. (1968). *Amer. J. Roent.*, **102**, 938.
Howie, T. A. (1957). *J. Laryng.*, **71**, 249.
Isambert, A. (1876). *Ann. Mal. Oreille Larynx.*, **2**, 1.
Jackson, C. L. (1940a). *Arch. Otolaryng.*, **31**, 23.
— (1940b). *Surg. Gynec. Obstet.*, **70**, 537.
— and Jackson, C. (1942). *Diseases and Injuries of the Larynx*. New York; Macmillan.
Kirschner, J. A. (1969). *Ann. Otol.*, **78**, 689.
Kleinsasser, O. (1965). *Z. Laryng. Rhinol.*, **44**, 711.
Klopp, C. T. (1950). *Ann. Surg.*, **132**, 811.
Krishaber, L. (1879). *Gaz. Hebdom Mied Chir.*, **16**, 518.
Kuhn, A. J., Devine, K. D., and McDonald, J. R. (1957). *Laryngoscope*, **67**, 518.
Lavelle, R. J. (1969). *Brit. J. Cancer*, **23**, 709.
Le Bec, E. (1905). *Ann. Mal. Oreille Larynx*, **31**, 375.
Lederman, M. (1961). *Brit. med. J.*, **1**, 1639.
Lennox, B., Timperley, W. R., Murray, D., and Kellett, H. S. (1968). *J. Path. Bact.*, **96**, 321.
Leroux-Robert, J. (1956). *Ann. Otol.*, **65**, 137.
Lewis, R. S. (1961). *J. Laryng.*, **75**, 794.
Lindberg, R., and Jesse, R. H. (1968). *Amer. J. Roent.*, **102**, 132.
McAlpine, J. C., Radcliffe, A., and Friedmann, I. (1963). *J. Laryng.*, **77**, 1.
McCabe, B. F., and Magieski, J. E. (1960). *Ann. Otol.*, **69**, 1013.
McGavran, M. H., Bauer, W. E., and Ogura, J. H. (1961). *Cancer, N.Y.*, **14**, 55.
Mackenty, J. E. (1925). *Ann. Otol.*, **30**, 599.
MacNaughton, I. P. J., and Fraser, M. S. (1954). *J. Laryng.*, **68**, 680.
Majoros, M., Devine, K. D., and Parkhill, F. M. (1963). *Surg. Clin. N. Amer.*, **43**, 4, 1049.
Martin, H. (1947). In *Surgery of the Nose and Throat* (Ed. by J. D. Kerman) New York; Nelson.
— (1957). *Surgery of Head and Neck Tumours*. New York; Hoeber-Harper.
— (1963). *Cancer, N.Y.*, **16**, 823.
Mawson, S. (1961). *J. Laryng.*, **75**, 1076.
Moffitt, O. P. (1959). *Laryngoscope*, **69**, 1421.
Montgomery, W. W., and Toothill, R. J. (1968). *Arch. Otolaryng.*, **88**, 499.
Moore, I. (1920). *J. Laryng.*, **36**, 49.
Moure, E. J. (1921). *Presse Med.*, **57**, 561.
Negus, V. E. (1949). *Comparative Anatomy and Phsyiology of the Larynx*. London; Heinemann.
— and Thomson, St. C. (1955). *Diseases of the Nose and Throat* (6th ed.). London; Cassell.
New, G. B., and Erich, J. B. (1938). *Arch. Otolaryng.*, **28**, 841.
Norris, C. M. (1958). *Laryngoscope*, **68**, 1240.
— (1963). *Ann. Otol.*, **72**, 83.
Ogura, J. H. (1951). *Trans. Amer. Acad. Ophth. Otol.*, **55**, 786.
— (1955). *Laryngoscope*, **65**, 867.
— Mallen, R. W. (1965). *Trans. Amer. Acad. Ophthal. Otolaryng.*, **69**, 832.
— Biller, H. F., Calcaterra, T. C., and Davis, W. H. (1969). *Int. Surg.*, **52**, 29.
Ormerod, F. C. (1958). *Acta oto-rhino-laryng. belg.*, **6**, 527.
— and Shaw, H. J. (1956). *J. Laryng.*, **70**, 433.
Payling Wright, G. (1958). *Introduction to Pathology*. London; Longmans.
Pietrantoni, L., and Fior, R. (1958). *Acta Otolaryng.*, Suppl., 142.
Pinsker, O. T., and Proud, C. O. (1958). *Arch. Otolaryng.*, **67**, 268.
Portmann, G. (1921). *Presse Med.*, **57**, 561.
— (1939). *Treatise on Surgical Technique in Otolaryngology*. Baltimore; Williams and Wilkins.
Pracy, R. (1970). *J. Laryng.*, **84**, 37.
Pressman, J. J., and Simon, M. B. (1961). *Laryngoscope*, **71**, 1019.
Rabbett, W. F. (1962). *Laryngoscope*, **72**, 1760.
Salmon, L. F. (1957). *J. Laryng.*, **71**, 766.
Shaw, H. J. (1957). *Ann. R. Coll. Surg. Engl.*, **21**, 290.
— (1964). *Brit. J. clin. Pract.*, **18**, 249.
— (1965). *J. Laryng.*, **79**, 1.
— (1966). *J. Laryng.*, **80**, 839.
Shumrick, D. A. (1969). *Arch. Otolaryng.*, **89**, 629.
Siirala, U., and Siirala, O. (1966). *Acta otolaryng.*, *Stockh.* Suppl., **224**, 468.

REFERENCES

Smith, R. R. (1961). *Surg. Gynec. Obstet.*, **113**, 435.
Som, M. L. (1969). *Semon Lecture*, University of London.
Sorensen, J. (1930). *Quoted by* Thomson, St. C. and Colledge, L. (1930).
Stewart, E. F. (1960). *J. Laryng.*, **74**, 525.
Stewart, J. P. (1957). *J. Laryng.*, **71**, 718.
Strong, E. W., Hensche, U. K., Nickson, J. J., Frazell, E. L., Tollefsen, H. R., and Hilaris, B. S. (1966). *Cancer.* **19**, 1509.
Sullivan, R. D. (1960). *Cancer Chem. Rep.*, **10**, 39.
Tait, R. V. (1959). *Proc. R. Soc. Med.*, **52**, 747.
Taylor, J. N. S. (1965). *J. Laryng.*, **79**, 15.
Thomson, St. C., and Colledge, L. (1930). *Cancer of the Larynx.* London; Kegan Paul.
Trotter, W. (1926). *Brit. med. J.*, **1**, 269.
UICC (1962). *Report of Committee on Clinical Stage Classification* (p. 17).
— (1968). *Report of Committee on T.N.M. Classification*, Geneva.
Ungerecht, M. (1951). *Arch. Ohren-, Nasen- KehlkopfHeilk.*, **160**, 158.
U.S. Dept. Health, Educ. and Welfare (1964). *Smoking and Health.* A report of the Advisory Committee to the Surgeon General of the Public Health Service.
Welsh, L. W., and Welsh, J. J. (1961). *Laryngoscope*, **71**, 185.
Willis, R. A. (1953). *The Pathology of Tumours* (2nd ed.). London; Butterworths.
Wilson, C. P. (1955). *Ann. R. Coll. Surg. Engl.*, **17**, 1.
Winston, P., and Epstein, S. S. (1958). *J. Laryng.*, **72**, 452.
Work, W. P., and Boyle, W. F. (1961). *Laryngoscope*, **71**, 230.
Wynder, E. L., Bross, I. J., and Day, E. (1956). *Cancer, N.Y.*, **9**, 86.
Zalin, H. (1948). *J. Laryng.*, **62**, 621.
Zaprewski, A., and Sobocynski, A. (1957). *Larynogscope*, **60**, 290.

16

CERVICAL NODE DISSECTION

Maxwell Ellis

There are two conventional opinions on the management of cervical nodes in squamous cell carcinoma of the larynx and laryngopharynx.

In one school of thought, the very existence of cervical lymphatic tissue is almost a red rag to a bull and the nodes are ruthlessly hunted down and hopefully extirpated to the surgeon's best ability in all cases (except those of glottic cancer). The theory is that metastasis in the nodes is so frequent, clinically or microscopically, that it is unnecessary to be concerned by those cases where it would not occur. The operative injury to this group is disregarded and its infliction accepted as serving the interests of the presumed larger group—if the original assumptions are correct. This is the so-called "prophylactic", or "elective" or "functional" approach. It maintains a dignified silence about cases where cervical metastases occur after such excisions or contralaterally. Much worse, it assumes that a cancer cell must inevitably become a cancer mass, a theory for which the protagonists of the method have provided no evidence.

The second conventional approach is based on the assumption that metastatic cancer in the cervical nodes is not inevitable and that when it does occur it can be diagnosed early at a routine follow-up examination and excised, with a good prognosis. Undoubtedly, every surgeon treating cancer should have a good follow-up organization or he should not be dealing with cancer, much less writing about it. This method of operating only on clinical and not on hypothetical cancer has been the practice of many surgeons and clinics for years and has not proved less successful than the other.

Role of lymphocytes

There is much evidence for the existence of an immune reaction to cancer and evidence also that this reaction is mediated through the lymphoid cells (Alexander and Fairley, 1968). The successive groups of lymph nodes radiating from the site of the primary growth are not sumps into which cancer is deposited, but areas of anticancer activity each probably fortifying its proximal neighbour. In fact, the reactivity in these successive groups, in breast cancer, has been used as a prognostic index (Black and Speer, 1960). Thus lymph nodes may enlarge because of lymphoid hyperplasia, or sinus histiocytosis, an indication of activity, and a demonstration that the lymphocytes are fulfilling their proper function. Cancer cells found on histological examination of nodes are by no means certain to become cancer masses. The discovery of cancer cells in a node at any particular point of time is not necessarily a true indication of the dynamic process of cancer growth and immunological destruction which is occurring in the node. The cancer growth may well overcome the defences and become a clinical cancer mass. When it does, two further considerations arise. First, it is known that reducing the size of the cancer in the body improves the qualities of the defences against the residual growth. Secondly, the next group of lymph nodes and the still more distal ones wait to play their part in resisting the spread of cancer from the original and secondary sources. Thus, it is right to excise a group of cancerous lymph nodes, to reduce the overall mass in the body, but it may not be right to extend this incision to lymphatic areas still capable of cancer reactivity. In other words, there is a case for local excision rather than a block operation. Research in progress on lymphocyte function indicates a greater need to correlate clinical methods with what is already known and being discovered of cancer biology and immunology.

A voluminous literature on this fascinating and vitally important subject already exists, and this brief discussion is only intended to provoke thought and to stimulate a re-examination of what have become somewhat mechanical routine practices.

Scope of the operation

A block dissection consists of the removal in a single mass of all the lymph nodes in the anterior and posterior triangles of the neck, as well as their associated lymphatic vessels. To achieve this, all the cervical nodes and fascia of the neck must be removed in a single block from the clavicle below, to the base of the skull and the mandible above; and from the anterior border of the trapezius behind, to beyond the midline in front. Anteriorly the dissection must extend to the anterior belly of the digastric muscle on the opposite side.

The sternomastoid muscle, the internal jugular vein, the submaxillary salivary gland and the tail of the parotid gland are all included in the excision. The subdigastric lymph nodes, the most important group of all, cannot be satisfactorily removed unless the posterior belly of the digastric muscle and the stylohyoid muscle are divided close to their origins, and included in the excision.

The operation can be done on both sides, and it is not essential to preserve either internal jugular vein; however, the risk of troublesome venous congestion in the head can be reduced by separating the two operations by as many weeks as is safely possible.

The method of block dissection to be described is one which can be conveniently combined with excision, in continuity, of a primary tumour of the pharynx and larynx (*en bloc* dissection). The technique can readily be modified for local excisions.

The skin incision

A midline incision is advised (Fig. 193) for a laryngectomy or pharyngolaryngectomy and a decsription of the technique has been given elsewhere (Ellis, 1969). If an *en bloc* dissection of the lymph nodes is necessary it can readily be performed by means of a further transverse incision (Fig. 194). This extension is possible at any time during the operation, if previously unsuspected cancerous nodes are found.

From the midpoint of the midline incision another is made running horizontally and then upwards in a smooth curve to the mastoid process. Excellent access is obtained and the flaps are widely based and well nourished, an important factor if the area has been irradiated. One of the difficulties after a block dissection is to prevent serum collecting in the supraclavicular fossa, and the shape and weight of the large inferior flap tend to cause it to fall inwards and obliterate this space.

460

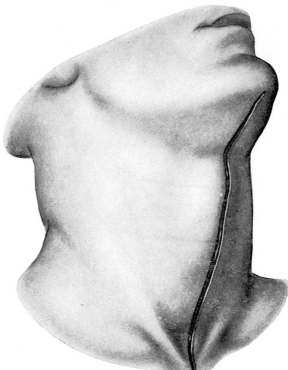

FIG. 193.—Midline incision for laryngectomy.

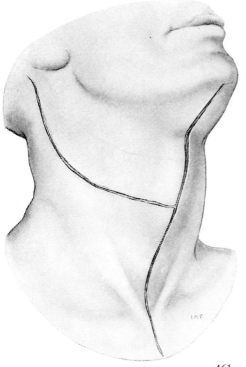

FIG. 194.—Incision for laryngectomy with block dissection.

461

The economy of these two incisions is valuable if repair operations later become necessary in a heavily irradiated case, as the skin of the neck is so little disturbed by incisional scars.

The platysma muscle is included in the skin flaps, for if widespread involvement of the platysma is found, the operation should be abandoned. A local area of the platysma may be invaded by growth, and the overlying skin can then be excised completely and replaced later with a flap rotated into the defect, or by a Thiersch graft.

Reflection of the skin flaps

The flaps are dissected back to expose the whole field from the clavicle and manubrium to the mastoid process and the mandible, and from the anterior border of the trapezius to the lateral border of the opposite infrahyoid muscles (Fig. 195). In reflecting the superior flap the mandibular branch of the facial nerve should be identified and spared. It runs deep to the platysma crossing the facial artery and vein just above the level of the lower border of the mandible. The cervical branch is almost invariably divided.

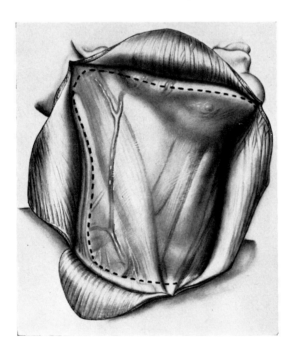

FIG. 195.—Reflection of the skin flaps.

The inferior and lateral dissection

The cervical fascia is incised over the clavicular origin of the sternomastoid muscle, along the clavicle to the anterior border of the trapezius muscle and then medially to the medial border of the opposite sternomastoid muscle (Fig. 196). The sternal and clavicular heads of the sternomastoid muscle on the side of the dissection, and the sternal head of the opposite sternomastoid muscle, are divided close to their origins. The omohyoid muscle is divided where it passes deep to the trapezius. The external jugular vein, the transverse scapular vein and the transverse cervical vein are encountered at the posterior border of the clavicular head of the sternomastoid, and must be picked up and ligated.

The lower end of the internal jugular vein is carefully dissected out of the carotid sheath, and completely freed for about 2 cm., as near as possible to the subclavian vein. The vagus nerve is identified in the carotid sheath and is left undisturbed. Throughout the dissection it should be handled as little as possible and always very gently. The freed portion of the internal jugular vein is doubly ligated and then divided.

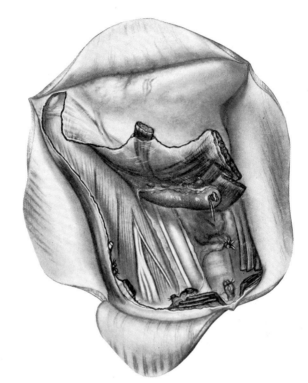

FIG. 196.—The inferior and lateral dissection.

The tissue thus separated inferiorly can now be swung upwards and medially, progressively easing the internal jugular vein out of the carotid sheath, as the dissection proceeds superiorly along the border of the trapezius muscle.

The fascia along the anterior border of the trapezius is incised and the dissection carried across the floor of the posterior triangle. The accessory nerve is divided as it enters the trapezius at the junction of the upper two-thirds and lower one-third, and just below it the transverse cervical vessels are picked up and ligated. Successively, working medially, the scalenus medius muscle, the trunks of the brachial plexus and the scalenus anterior muscle are exposed and cleaned, preserving the phrenic nerve which runs downwards and medially on the surface of the scalenus anterior.

The superior dissection

The attachment of the cervical fascia is divided in the whole length of the exposure, from the mastoid process and along the mandible to just beyond the midline (Fig. 197). The facial artery and vein are closely attached to it at the anterior border of the insertion of the masseter muscle and must be ligated and divided. Near the midline several smaller vessels are encountered. Beginning laterally, the levator scapulae and the splenius muscles are exposed in the apex of the posterior triangle, and the sternomastoid muscle is divided at its insertion and retracted medially. The accessory nerve is thus again exposed, passing into the under surface of the muscle, and superficial to the internal jugular vein, and it is again divided.

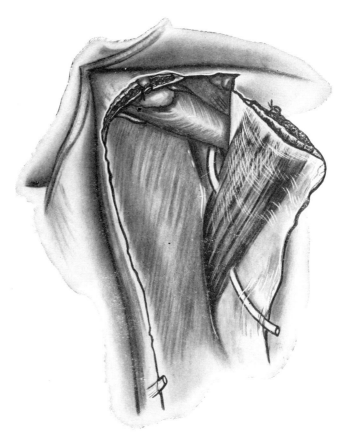

FIG. 197.—Division of the facial vessels and sternomastoid muscle.

The dissection is next carried medially across the tail of the parotid gland and deepened until the posterior belly of the digastric muscle is clearly defined (Fig. 198). A number of large veins are encountered and must be carefully isolated and ligated. The main trunks are the posterior auricular vein, the posterior facial vein and its posterior and anterior divisions inferiorly, the common facial vein and the external jugular vein. The posterior border of the submaxillary salivary gland is then revealed.

The digastric muscle is divided close to its origin in the digastric fossa. The occipital artery running near its lower border and the posterior auricular artery near its upper border must also be picked up and ligated. The stylohyoid muscle is divided near its origin from the styloid process. The internal jugular vein and the glossopharyngeal and hypoglossal nerves are now exposed (Fig. 199). The former nerve comes from between the vein and the internal carotid artery deep to the styloid process, whilst the latter is larger and lower in the neck, running downwards and then forwards superficial to the external carotid artery, and just above the greater cornu of the hyoid bone.

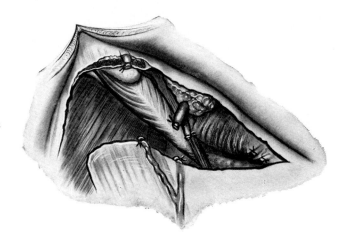

Fig. 198.—Dissection across the parotid tail.

The internal jugular vein, often greatly distended, especially if hypotensive drugs have not been used, is carefully isolated and doubly ligated as near to the base of the skull as possible.

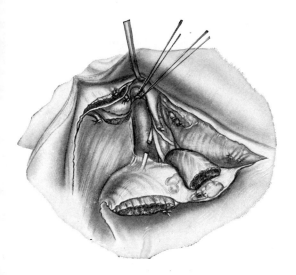

Fig. 199.—Ligation and division of the internal jugular vein.

The whole mass of tissue, comprising the fascia and cellular tissue of the posterior triangle, the posterior belly of the digastric, the stylohyoid, the omohyoid and the sternomastoid muscles, and the excised segment of the internal jugular vein,

465

can now be reflected medially to the line of the external and common carotid arteries.

The submaxillary salivary gland, which is now fully exposed (Fig. 200), is stripped forwards and downwards, ligating and dividing the facial artery again, near its origin from the external carotid artery. The lingual artery sometimes loops up into

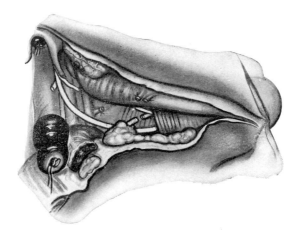

FIG. 200.—Dissection of the submaxillary salivary gland.

the field of the dissection at the posterior border of the hyoglossus muscle, but it can usually be spared. The duct of the salivary gland is separated from the lingual nerve and divided where it dips deeply between the hyoglossus and mylohyoid muscles.

FIG. 201.—Division of the anterior belly of the digastric muscle.

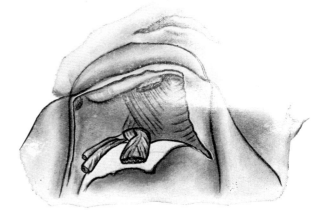

Anterior dissection

The anterior belly of the digastric muscle is divided at its origin from the lower border of the mandible near the midline.

The fascia is now incised along the medial border of the opposite anterior digastric belly down to the greater cornu of the hyoid bone (Fig. 201).

The fascia and nodes are cleared from the mylohyoid, and the anterior dissection is then continued downwards from this point to the inferomedial angle of the wound, including the anterior belly of the omohyoid muscle. The mass is removed in one block.

Lateral lobe of thyroid gland.

The dissection should include the lateral lobe and isthmus of the thyroid gland. Therefore, the superior thyroid artery is identified where it originates from the external carotid artery, just below the greater cornu of the hyoid bone, and it is ligated and divided. Inferiorly, behind the common carotid artery, at the level of the cricoid cartilage, the inferior thyroid artery must be found and ligated (Fig. 202).

The isthmus of the thyroid gland is divided near its junction with the opposite lateral lobe, and the cut surfaces are transfixed with a thread suture, encircled and tied. The fascial plane behind the thyroid gland is now entered, exposing the lateral aspects of the pharynx, larynx and trachea.

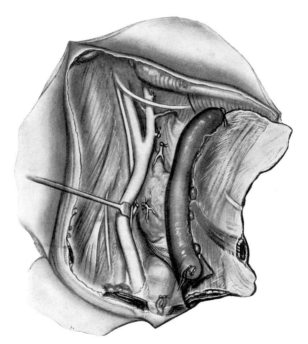

FIG. 202.—Ligation and division of the superior and inferior thyroid vessels; dissection of the lateral lobe of the thyroid gland.

Excision completed

The larynx on this side is freed by incising the inferior constrictor muscle, dividing the superior and recurrent laryngeal nerves, and detaching the muscles from the hyoid bone. The larynx is isolated on the opposite side and removed from above downwards (Ellis, 1969).

The complete excision will now include the lymph nodes and cellular tissue in continuity with the larynx (and laryngopharynx) (Fig. 203).

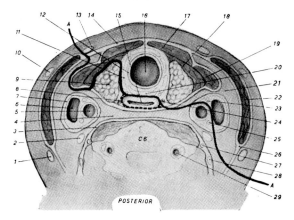

ANTERIOR

POSTERIOR

FIG. 203.—*En bloc* dissection of larynx with cervical lymph nodes.

1. Posterior jugular vein
2. Sympathetic trunk
3. Prevertebral fascia
4. Retro-oesophageal space
5. Common carotid artery
6. Internal jugular vein
7. Carotid sheath
8. Recurrent nerve
9. Thyroid gland
10. External jugular vein
11. Crico-arytenoideus posticus
12. First tracheal ring
13. Anterior jugular vein
14. Pretracheal fascia
15. Oesophagus
16. Trachea
17. Sternohyoid
18. Sternothyroid
19. Omohyoid
20. Cricoid cartilage
21. Lymph node area
22. Sternomastoid
23. Descendens hypoglossi
24. Inferior thyroid artery
25. Vagus
26. Investing fascia
27. Phrenic nerve
28. Brachial plexus
29. Vertebral dorsal vessels

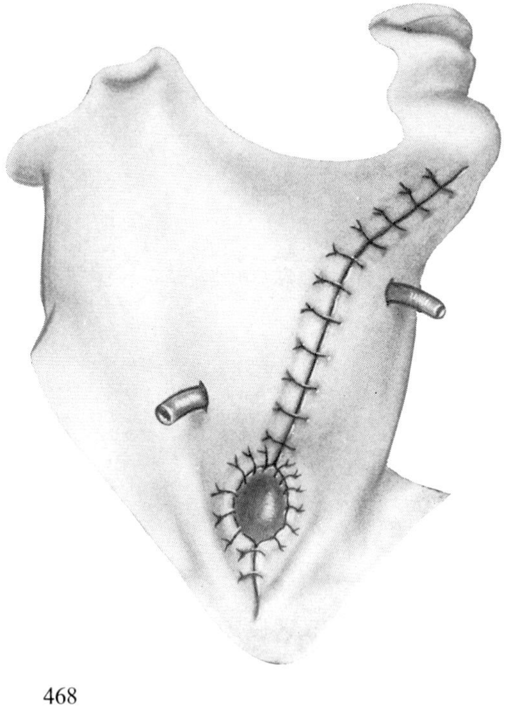

FIG. 204.—Closure and drainage of the laryngectomy.

In a laryngectomy, the tracheostome is fashioned in the lower part of the midline incision (Fig. 204).

If a complete pharyngeal segment is excised with the larynx, as a planned procedure, the original incisions are slightly different (Fig. 205) and the final closure will vary with the method of repair adopted. A primary Thiersch graft replacement will appear as in Fig. 206, whilst with a delayed repair an oesophagostome is created

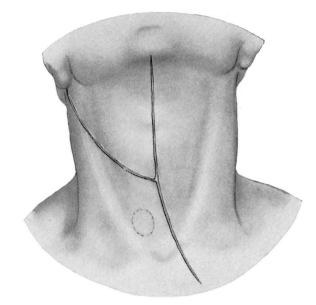

FIG. 205.—Alternative incision for *en bloc* neck dissection.

if possible in the lower curved part of the midline incision, obtaining as much skin bridge as possible between the two stomata. If this cannot be done the oesophagostome must be fashioned in a buttonhole incision. It is an advantage to bury the oral pharyngostome until ready for the final stage of reconstruction (Ellis, 1963).

Closure

Before closing the wound, it is of the utmost importance to secure haemostasis.

A Penrose drain can be left in the wound from near the angle of the jaw emerging through a stab incision in the lower flap (Fig. 207). Suction drainage can be used if continuous nursing supervision is available. A firm bandage must be applied over a well-padded dressing of gauze and wool.

The skin incisions are closed with interrupted sutures of silk or thread, and a controlling plaster cast is applied as soon as the patient has recovered consciousness if suction drainage is not employed.

Block dissection only

Block dissection of the lymph nodes and lymphatic tissues may be needed if cancerous nodes appear after successful irradiation of the primary growth or after its successful excision. The incisions advised are shown (Figs. 208 and 209). If no previous operation has been performed, these incisions leave the skin of the centre

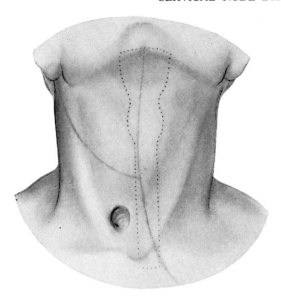

FIG. 206.—Primary Thiersch graft replacement in closure.

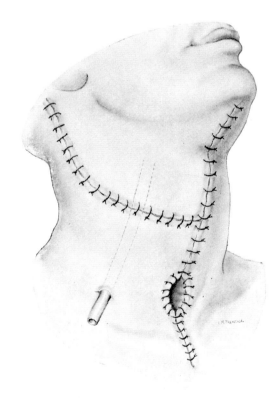

FIG. 207.—Closure of laryngectomy with block dissection. Penrose drain.

470

of the neck untouched in case a subsequent recurrence demands operation. When the primary has already been excised, the incisions provide a clear means of access.

The steps of the dissection are as already described. The lateral lobe of the thyroid

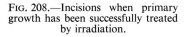

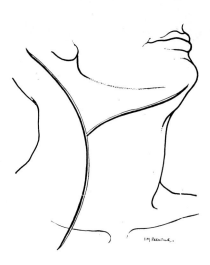

FIG. 208.—Incisions when primary growth has been successfully treated by irradiation.

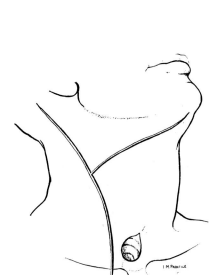

FIG. 209.—Incisions when primary growth has already been successfully excised.

gland may be left behind if desired, but in a post-irradiated case the gland is likely to be fibrotic and relatively useless and can profitably be removed, whilst it may already have been removed in a post-laryngectomy case.

The methods of wound drainage and suture are as before.

REFERENCES

Alexander, P., and Fairley, G. H. (1968). In *Clinical Aspects of Immunology* (Ed. by P. G. H. Gel and R. R. A. Coombs). Oxford; Blackwell.
Black, M. M., and Speer, F. D. (1960). *Surgery Gynec. Obstet.*, **110**, 477.
Ellis, M. (1963). *J. Laryng.*, **77**, 872.
— (1969). In *Operative Surgery* (Vol. 10, Ed. by C. Rob, R. Smith, S. Duke-Elder and M. Ellis), London; Butterworths.

17

SKIN GRAFTING

R. L. G. Dawson

When discussing skin grafting it is also necessary to include the subcutaneous tissue as well. The skin is made up of the epidermis, with the malpighian layer, and the dermis containing elastic and fibrous tissue in which also lie the hair follicles, sebaceous glands and the sweat glands. Immediately beneath the dermis lies the subdermal plexus of blood vessels, then the adipose tissue, separated from the muscular and skeletal parts of the body, in most places, by the superficial and deep fascia.

TYPES OF SKIN GRAFT
Various forms of skin graft are available for use in surgery of the head and neck:

The thin split-skin graft

This is taken with the unguarded Blair knife, the guarded Humby Braithwaite, or Watson knife, or with an electric dermatome. Essentially it is a thin graft and one can usually read the hands of a watch through it. When the graft is taken it is cut just below the malpighian layer of the epidermis, and through the hair follicles, sweat glands and sebaceous glands, and it is these structures which revert back to their original origin during the healing process, and produce a new epidermis. The graft, described by Thiersch, of skin sliced across the tops of the rete pegs of the malpighian layer, is difficult to obtain. The split-skin graft is thicker than that described by Thiersch. The inner side of the upper arm is a suitable donor site for small hairless grafts, and if skin is taken from this area it does not interfere with the early discharge of the patient from hospital. For large areas of skin graft the inner and posterior aspect of the thighs are the most useful sites, but the patient has to remain in hospital for a greater length of time, with subsequent difficulty in walking, till the area is healed in about ten days. The skin is put on the stretch when it is sliced at a constant level with one or other of the various cutting instruments available. The donor area is subsequently dressed with tulle gras, gauze, and much wool covered by a crêpe bandage. The donor area is not disturbed for ten days, and at the end of this time it will be found that, except when a thick graft has been taken, complete healing has occurred. The patients will not lose their superficial scarring for about nine months to a year afterwards.

Where a thicker skin graft has been taken, more of the sebaceous glands, hair follicles and sweat glands have also been removed and therefore the healing is slower, taking two to three weeks. The three-quarter thickness graft is often taken with a guarded knife with a fixed grafting space which prevents the knife going too deep. The Padget dermatome is a metal drum adhering to the skin of the abdomen or buttock with Bostik. When adhesion has taken place the drum is rotated and a knife set at a fixed distance from the drum is passed backwards and forwards, so slicing the skin as it is lifted by the drum off the donor site. These donor sites take longer to heal than those that have given a thin split-skin graft, and such skin is usually only used as a definitive repair.

The Wolfe graft

This is a whole thickness skin graft including all the dermis but the subdermal fat and subdermal plexus have been removed. The donor sites for this graft are preferably the post-auricular region, which produces a graft of identical colour match to the rest of the face, but can only produce a relatively small graft; the supraclavicular region where the colour match is very good, but not so perfect as the post-auricular region; and the abdomen where the skin is thick and a large amount can be taken, but the colour match is poor for the face or neck. The

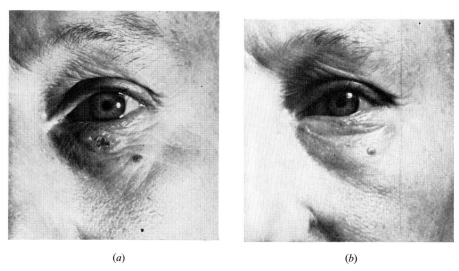

(a)   (b)

Fig. 210.—(a) A patient with a basal-celled carcinoma of the lower eyelid; (b) same patient after a post-auricular Wolfe graft.

donor areas of these grafts can be closed by direct approximation in the post-auricular region and in the supraclavicular region, but unless the grafts are small a thin split-skin graft is needed to close the donor area on the abdomen. In the post-auricular region the sulcus is distended with normal saline and then a pattern of the defect is marked out, remembering that the skin on the back of the ear is thinner than the skin over the mastoid process. This is particularly important where a definitive post-auricular Wolfe graft is being used to correct an ectropion on the lower eyelid. The thick skin is always placed along the malar line whereas the thinner skin is placed along the lid margin. The donor area from the post-auricular region is closed by a running subcuticular catgut suture. This has the effect of pinning the ear back and obliterating the post-auricular sulcus. It is necessary to trim every scrap of fat off the undersurface before using the graft, otherwise small areas of necrosis will occur.

Free eyebrow grafts

Free eyebrow grafts can be taken from the occiput and inset into a prepared bed along the supra-orbital margin. There is about 50 per cent survival of the hair follicles and because of this a graft is taken that is wider than necessary. The donor areas are closed by direct approximation. Care has to be taken to put the grafts on the right way round, otherwise the hair will grow in towards the centre of the face instead of towards the lateral side, and as the hair is not "terminal hair" constant trimming is necessary.

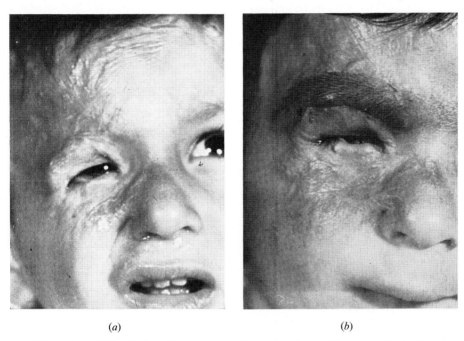

(a)   (b)

FIG. 211.—(a) A child with facial burn scars and loss of eyebrow; (b) same patient with a free eyebrow graft in place.

Local flaps

Here we are dealing with a graft which by definition always remains attached to a blood supply while it is being moved. This is in contradistinction to a free skin graft where the graft is lifted completely away from its blood supply and put down on a new bed and must take up its humoral nourishment initially by "plasmatic" circulation, but by the end of 48 hours new capillaries have grown in from the donor site to maintain the nourishment of the graft. With local flaps which are composed of skin, subdermal plexus and subcutaneous tissue, a variety of types are used.

The Z-plasty

This is probably one of the most useful operations in plastic and reconstructive surgery, and in principle the surgeon sutures into a defect two sides of a triangle, where one previously existed. The angle at which the flaps are cut and the amount of mobilization necessary beyond the base line of each flap depends upon the site and extent of the contracture. By increasing the length of a certain incision, by Z transposition, the surgeon uses the excessive tissue on either side of a linear contracture to make good a lack of tissue in the centre of the area. On the head and neck, where there is a good vascular supply, the surgeon is able to take greater risks with the blood supply, using much narrower and longer flaps than he could on the trunk. Sutures are usually removed in seven days and the early removal of sutures, compared with other parts of the body, is general for most areas of the head and neck.

The transposition flap

This is a local flap with a good base through which the blood supply can come and go, but which is moved from one part of the anatomy to close a defect in a neighbouring part. The defect is not suitable for a split-skin graft because of bare bone, or because the receiving area has been irradiated and therefore is not a good bed upon which a free skin graft can survive. The flap can be used to cover a cavity, or to produce the necessary bulk in a defect. The defect left by the movement of the flap can be grafted with split skin in a less conspicuous area. The transposed flap transposes a defect from one neighbouring area to another, by a

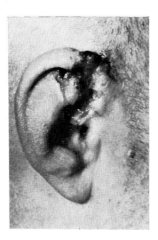

Fig. 212.—(*a*) A carcinoma of the ear.

simple movement of the flap. Occasionally the defect left by the transposition can be filled up by neighbouring skin without the necessity for a split-skin graft. This flap can be used on the neck, cheeks, and scalp, and a common scalp flap is one that is used to cover the defect over the mastoid process and the neighbouring area after the wide removal for a tumour. The scalp is rotated down to fill the defect, and split skin is used to cover the pericranium of the donor area (Fig. 212).

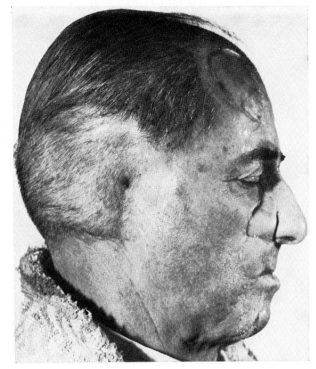

Fig. 212.—(*b*) Same patient after excision and a transposition scalp flap to cover the bare bone.

Rotation flaps

These are used extensively on the cheeks and the neck to fill a defect left by excision of a new growth, haemangioma, or deep scarring. For every centimetre of defect to be closed there must be an 8 cm. circumference of the flap. After the flap has been marked out the operator must test, with a piece of gauze, the extent of rotation from the centre of the base line of the flap. Additional length to the flap can be obtained by the "back cut" at the furthest end of the incision, and also by removing a wedge from the peripheral side of the incision. The "back cut" will open up and produce additional length to twice the length of the cut, whereas closure of the wedge incision will narrow the peripheral margin of the flap incision according to the size of the base of the wedge. In all local flaps a good and extensive subcutaneous mobilization of tissues must be performed beyond the base of the flap (Fig. 213).

The Abbé and Estlander flaps

These are used in reconstructing the lip. The Abbe flap (Fig. 214) is most often used where there is a tight upper lip and a relatively redundant lower lip, in certain cases of cleft lip, particularly where there has been the old straight suture repair performed. A triangular flap of the lower lip based on one side of the labial artery, is rotated through 180 degrees from the lower lip and inset into the defect created in the upper lip. The donor area in the lower lip is repaired by direct approximation

477

of the tissues in three layers and the flap is inset into the defect in the upper lip; the bridge between the upper and lower lip containing the labial artery and vein remains for the necessary three weeks until such time as the receiving tissues of the upper lip have produced a satisfactory blood supply for the flap. A subsequent

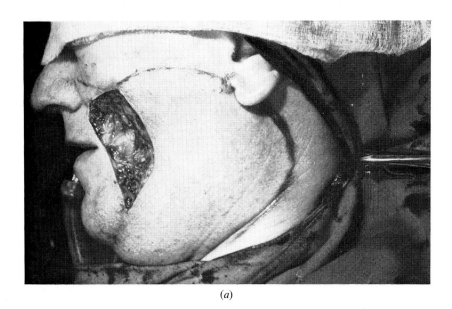

(a)

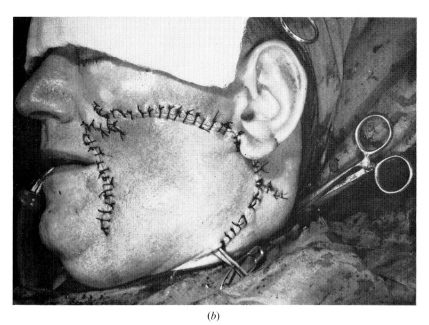

(b)

FIG. 213.—(a) Excision of a basal-celled carcinoma of the cheek and the rotation flap designed; (b) the rotation flap in place.

"Cupid's bow" operation and general tidying up of the scar is usually needed. The worst feature about this operation is the almost invariably ugly scar of the lower lip.

The Estlander flap is similar to the Abbé flap, used either from the lower lip to the upper lip or vice versa, and using the labial artery to keep the flap viable during the three weeks of being inset into the opposite lip. It is a laterally situated flap.

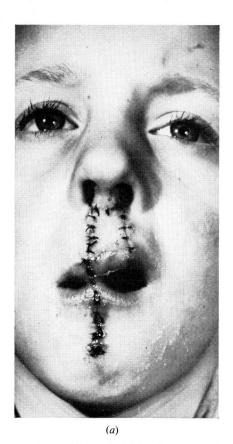

(a)

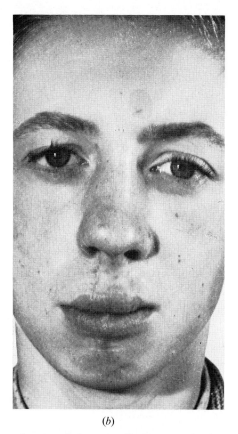

(b)

FIG. 214.—(a) The Abbé flap in place to increase the size of the upper lip from a redundant lower lip; (b) same patient showing the fullness achieved by the Abbé flap operation.

The "fan-flap" of Gillies (Fig. 215), a more extensive procedure, is used where there has been a defect created of more than one third of the lip. If the defect is a third or less a good cosmetic and functional result can be achieved by direct approximation. If it is more than one third, one side has to be mobilized along the buccal sulcus and around the commissure into the other lip, and the whole area divided through skin, muscle and mucous membrane and rotated into place. The mucosa, muscle and skin of the defect is repaired by direct approximation. A commissurotomy is often needed afterwards. Other local flap reconstructions are sometimes necessary, but it is better to avoid the Dieffenbach flap because this is rotated

479

from the cheek to the midline, and the patients almost invariably end up with a small gutter in the centre of the lower lip which tends to dribble.

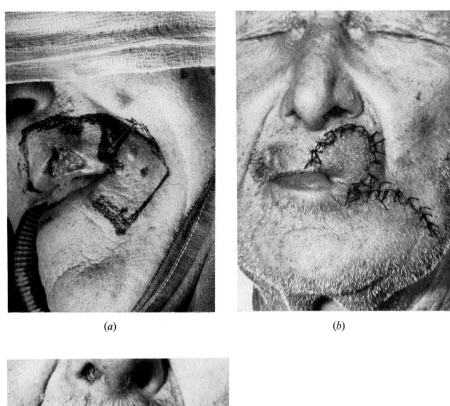

(a)

(b)

(c)

FIG. 215.—(a) A recurrent carcinoma of the upper lip with the excision and the proposed "fan-flap" marked out from the lower lip; (b) the excision has been performed and the "fan-flap" is in place; (c) same patient showing the degree of mouth opening that is possible.

Abdominal flaps

Where there is no available local tissue, skin and fat have to be brought in from a distance. By this method a total cheek reconstruction can be performed using an abdominal flap (Fig. 216), initially attached to the wrist, outlined and trained so that it is receiving all its blood supply from the wrist attachment. When this has been achieved, after about five weeks of wrist attachment, the flap is taken off the trunk, the donor area grafted and the flap, still attached to the wrist, is sutured into the planned defect on the cheek. This is a good repair, but can be difficult for the patient because of the positioning of the limbs when the flap is being migrated. The colour match is not good.

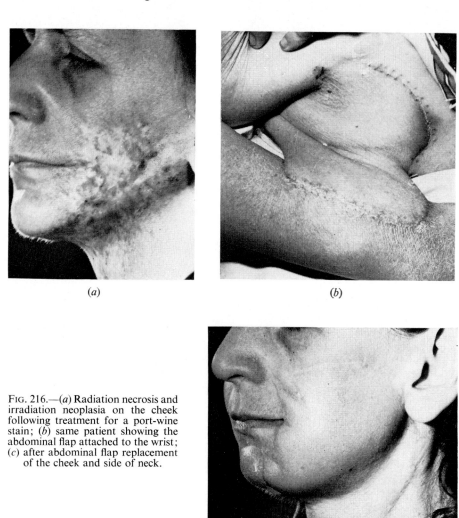

(a)

(b)

FIG. 216.—(a) Radiation necrosis and irradiation neoplasia on the cheek following treatment for a port-wine stain; (b) same patient showing the abdominal flap attached to the wrist; (c) after abdominal flap replacement of the cheek and side of neck.

(c)

Tubed pedicles

Finally, tubed pedicles (Fig. 217) can be used. They can be raised from the neck, and are a good colour match, but the extent and size of the tissue available is not great. For any relatively large repair it is best to use the anterior-thoracic tubed

481

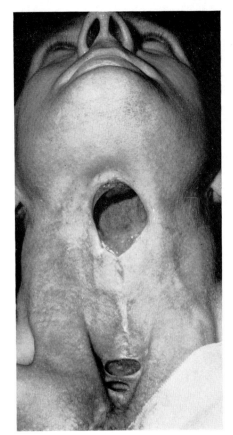

Fig. 217.—(*a*) Post-pharyngolaryngectomy. The bridge between the tracheostome and oesophagostome should be larger.

(*a*)

Fig. 217.—(*b*) An anterior thoracic bipedicled tubed flap is raised 7·5 cm. wide, 20 cm. long. The donor area is grafted with split skin from the thigh.

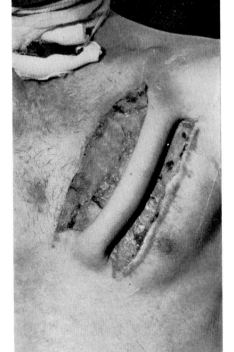

(*b*)

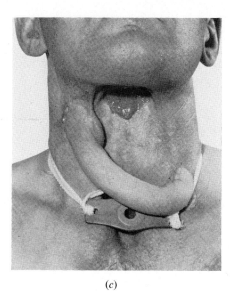 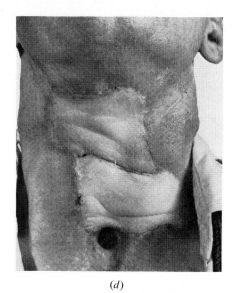

(c) (d)

FIG. 217.—(c) The tubed pedicle has been transferred to low down and high up on either side of the neck; (d) the tubed pedicle has been divided and spread over the new oesophagus that has been made by inturning the neck skin to make a tube. Continuity of the oesophagus has now been re-established.

pedicle, which can be raised in men. For women it is best to use a lateral thoracic one which is not so disfiguring but more difficult to manage because the tube cuts across the general direction of the blood supply to the skin. The anterior-thoracic and lateral-thoracic tubes are extremely useful for repair after total pharyngo-laryngectomies or following mandibulectomy and removal of covering in the chin area.

PRINCIPLES OF SKIN GRAFTING

The principles of skin grafting can, therefore, be listed as follows:

(1) Where skin has been lost, restore it with free skin grafts.

(2) Where skin and subcutaneous tissue have been lost, make good the loss with local or distant flaps or with tubed pedicle repairs.

(3) Free skin grafts do not survive on heavily irradiated tissues, therefore flap repairs must be performed in these areas.

(4) Temporary skin grafting should be used:

(a) on infected surfaces;

(b) where definitive flap surgery will be needed later, to restore appearance and function and contour;

(c) application of a temporary graft to achieve healing minimizes subsequent contracture.

(5) Definitive free skin grafting can be used on clean non-infected surfaces.

(6) Thin free skin grafts contract up to 60 per cent of their original size. Therefore an excessive amount of skin must always be let in to an area, and the deformity markedly overcorrected.

(7) Thick, three-quarter skin grafts contract only a little.

(8) Wolfe grafts do not contract at all.

(9) The colour match.

(*a*) A post-auricular Wolfe graft shows the best colour match, but one must beware of putting these grafts on prominent parts such as the nasal bridge and the prominence of the malars. These grafts become excessively red in these areas and never settle down to a normal colour match with the rest of the skin. The ideal places for the post-auricular Wolfe graft are on the side of the nose, the inner canthal region and the lower eyelids.

(*b*) Supraclavicular skin produces a good colour match.

(*c*) Thin split-skin grafts are necessary for reconstruction of the upper eyelids but they will always remain paler than the normal lids. The post-auricular Wolfe graft shows a very good colour match for the lower eyelids, and has a stability in it which allows the lid to remain in contact with the globe of the eye.

(*d*) The worst colour match is abdominal skin, which is much too pale and may remain so always, but just occasionally an over-reaction to colour is met, and the grafted tissues eventually become much too bright a pink.

(10) When performing any type of free skin graft or flap surgery, it is essential to obtain absolute haemostasis; particularly is this so when using free skin grafts, because any small amount of haematoma will cause a necrosis of the skin over-lying it. It is recommended that the graft bed be washed out with thrombin before pressure fixation is applied.

(11) Meticulous suturing is required for definitive grafts and flaps. Temporary skin grafts can usually be laid on granulating areas and maintained in place with a pressure bandage. The fixation of definitive grafts is performed by using long tie-over stay sutures over a wad of flavine wool, followed by either bandaging or Elastoplast fixation, the Elastoplast being applied in layers in all directions. For definitive grafting the first dressing should be performed in ten days. For temporary grafting on infected areas, three days is enough. If the dressing is not changed reasonably early, death of the grafts may occur through infection. In definitive free skin grafting, besides the long tie-over stay sutures, a continuous everting mattress suture of fine silk is used. This not only maintains perfect apposition of the skin edges, but also acts as a haemostatic suture.

(12) For cavity grafting with epithelial inlays, or inlays to deepen the buccal sulcus, for example in retrognathism where a prosthesis is to be worn, the cavity must be made much larger than will ultimately be needed. The cavity is distended with a gutta percha mould supported by a tray fixed to cast silver cap splints, attached to the mandible. The skin is then placed over the mould, its raw side outwards, the mould fitted into the cavity, and Elastoplast used to strap the covering skin down against the mould. Under general anaesthesia the first dressing is performed, with a change of the mould, at the end of three weeks, after which time the patient is instructed to take the mould out daily, to clean the cavity and to re-insert the mould quickly. If during the early weeks the mould is out for more than five minutes, contracture is liable to occur with the impossibility of putting the mould back in place again. As the months go on, however, the cavity becomes

much softer and the potentiality of the skin graft to contract, much less. At the end of six months, when the young fibroblasts have matured to fibrocytes, no further contracture will occur, and at this time a definitive prosthesis can be fitted to maintain the cavity to the right size. It is desirable where possible to take the skin from a non-hairbearing area.

(13) Infection of the receiving area must be avoided wherever possible and for cavity grafting it is advisable to give the patient parenteral antibiotics. Where skin grafts are used for temporary covering in order to achieve healing, the appropriate antibiotic is given. An absolute contra-indication to free skin grafting is the presence of a haemolytic streptococcus which will cause complete failure of the survival of skin grafts in nearly all cases. Therefore infections have to be treated initially, until three clear swabs have been obtained. After successful grafting, when the surface is dry, daily massage with lanoline not only promotes more rapid softening in the area and therefore flattening of otherwise slightly ridged grafts, but also keeps the skin grafts from appearing too dry and scaly.

(14) When a cheek is to receive a definitive three-quarter thickness or Wolfe graft, the upper and lower teeth must be fixed together. This is usually done with cast metal silver cap splints. The inside of the cheek is filled out with a bung of gutta percha. The graft is then sutured on to the cheek and can be dressed firmly down against the gutta percha mould lying in the oral cavity. In this way a firm base is obtained with the minimal risk of haematoma formation. The gutta percha bung and the interdental fixation can be removed at the end of three weeks. The patient takes a liquid diet in the meantime.

(15) Z flaps are used either for the correction of a linear scar, or where the incision has to go across a depression, or where, if a linear incision is made subsequent scar contraction will cause a linear contracture. Upon the amount of lengthening of the scar that is needed in order to avoid bowstringing depends the angle at which the Z flaps are constructed. Initially an incision is made along the scar and from either end in different directions, at certain angles, incisions are made so that two triangular flaps are fashioned. These are undermined fairly extensively into the base of the flap as well. After all scar on the base has been removed, these two flaps are transposed one to the other so that the whole direction of the scar is changed and the main scar takes on a more transverse instead of vertical direction. The maximum amount of correction can be obtained by making the secondary incisions at either end of the original incision at 90 degrees to the original incision. When these flaps are transposed maximum lengthening occurs. It is, however, unusual to use such a wide angle and the usual angle is at 45 degrees to the initial incision.

(16) The transposition flap is used to fill defects where full thickness of skin and fat is needed, where the use of free graft is not possible, either because of the final cosmetic result, or because a free graft would not survive on the receiving tissue. The flap is constructed so that it can move across to fill the defect. The dimensions of the flap must be such that a good blood supply is possible through the base of the flap. This is usually easy on the face and neck, but on the rest of the body a 1×1 dimension can be regarded as safe. The defects resulting from the movement of the flap to fill the proposed area can either be covered with a skin graft, or a further flap can be lifted to fill the defect.

(17) The rotation flap: the most frequent sites for the use of such flaps in head and neck surgery are on the neck or on the cheeks, and occasionally when the defect

is not very large a pure rotation flap can be used for the frontal region and temporal region. The flap is stretched into place, having been lifted, and the base undermined. The incision is usually closed with the assistance of a "back cut" into the base of the flap to lengthen the cut edge on the flap side, or the removal of a wedge from the cut edge on the outer side to shorten that edge.

All these flaps must be drained for 48 hours post-operatively. Cheek flaps may be constructed either along the malar line and then down the pre-auricular sulcus to below the angle of the mandible, for a distally based flap, or down the naso-labial fold and across the mandible midway between the chin and the angle, with the insertion of a Z-plasty to avoid contracture across the submandibular depression. This is an ascending flap based on the pre-auricular region. The neck flap is safest when it is based laterally but the vascular supply is so good that it can very often be based medially, almost on the midline of the neck. It is not, however, advisable to go across the midline of the neck in constructing a rotation flap and base it on the opposite side, for vascular trouble may occur at the very end of the flap, which is usually the most important and most necessary point.

(18) The Imre flap is used in reconstructive procedures on the lower eyelid and can be based either laterally or medially, the incision passing along the eyelid edge and then along the malar line. This flap of eyelid skin can be raised and advanced so that it can fill up a defect either on the inner side or the outer side of the lower eyelid.

(19) The Tripier flap is a bipedicled bucket-handle flap of upper-lid skin which is sometimes used to reconstruct defects in the lower eyelid, particularly in the centre. It is raised, swung down across the palpebral fissure and sutured into place. The donor area is closed by direct approximation. Subsequently a minor procedure is often needed to divide the base on each side, on the upper lid, and to make the inner canthal regions more pleasing in appearance. This flap provides a full thickness graft of eyelid skin with a small amount of underlying fat, and is really a better procedure than using a forehead flap, providing the defect is only a small one. It cannot be used for large defects.

(20) The flap from a distance: if, for example, a cheek has to be completely recovered for a deformity with scar contracture, or for new growth or for damage following therapeutic irradiation, a pattern of the normal cheek is usually made, and this is then reversed to produce the size of the flap needed to reconstruct the damaged cheek. It is then marked out on the abdomen and the distal part of the flap is raised and attached to the wrist. The wrist skin is turned back to line the abdominal skin. The remainder of the flap that will ultimately be lifted is marked out by fine incisions around the periphery, which will form permanent marks to be used in three weeks' time. At the end of three weeks, the flap is "delayed". This means that an incision is made around the previous marks, and the flap raised as far as its attachment to the wrist. It is then sutured back into the same position, and a drain is inserted for two days. This procedure is performed in order to train the blood supply, and venous drainage, that is to be conveyed only through the wrist attachment. In a further week the flap is ready to be cut entirely off the abdomen and is inset into the damaged cheek after excision has been made according to the pattern of the flap. The donor area on the abdomen is covered with a split-skin graft removed from the thigh. The arm and wrist, with the abdominal

flap attached, are then fixed to the head with 7·5 cm. Elastoplast, and the arm remains attached to the head for the three weeks that the flap is lying in place before division. Care must be taken that there is no angulation of the flap and that no shearing occurs on the attachment to the wrist by an alteration in the head and arm position. This must be watched carefully and inspected very frequently for the first three days. The drainage tube is inserted for two days. Three weeks later the wrist attachment is divided, the wrist wound closed and the cheek wound closed with the new flap in position. About six months later further scar excision and adjustment of the flap may be needed.

(21) The tubed pedicle can be used for reconstruction on most parts of the face but it has certain definite uses—for example to close a large hole in the cheek, where one end of the tubed pedicle is attached to the inner side of the cheek to form a lining, and the other end of the tubed pedicle is attached to the outer side of the cheek to form a cover.

It can be used safely for reconstruction after total pharyngolaryngectomy. In men the tube is usually raised in the anterior-thoracic region and gets its blood supply from the acromio-thoracic axis and from the perforating branches of the internal mammary. In a woman a lateral-thoracic tube is preferable, as in this way the front of the upper thorax is not marked. The dimensions of the tube are usually 20 cm. by 7·5 cm. These are the initial dimensions, but in some cases the tube may need to be subsequently lengthened. The thoracic skin is marked out and then raised at the junction between the superficial and deep fascia and left attached at either end. The central part is then sutured upon itself to form a tube with continuous medium silk. The donor area, in the anterior-thoracic region, is grafted with a split-skin graft to the thigh; in the lateral-thoracic region the donor area can usually be closed by raising the breast. At the end of three weeks the lower pole of the tube is detached and re-attached to the side of the neck just lateral to the tracheostomy and the oesophagostome. After another three weeks the upper pole of the tube is "delayed" for one week and then detached and inserted into the upper part of the neck on the opposite side but below the level of the pharyngostome. Three weeks later the tube is divided, and opened out, to be turned into the shape of strap flaps, there being two portions now, one to cover the upper part, and one to cover the lower part of the inturned skin of the neck. The skin of the neck is lifted by incision down each side after a medium bore stomach tube has been passed through the nose. The edges of the neck skin are then undercut and turned over on themselves and sutured together in the midline with catgut, so they form a tube joining the oesophagostome and the pharyngostome. The spread tubed pedicle is now laid across the defect in its two parts, the upper and lower part, so that the only situation where the suture line for the lining reconstruction and the suture line for the cover are in direct approximation is in the centre, at one point. This reconstructive procedure is carried out and finished within six months of the total pharyngolaryngectomy. The patients are fed by tube for ten days. Following this they should be eating a soft diet in the normal way. With this method contractures are not met with nor is there any operative mortality. This series of relatively minor procedures is performed over the space of about three months.

18

PRINCIPLES OF RADIOTHERAPY AND CHEMOTHERAPY IN MALIGNANT DISEASE OF THE HEAD AND NECK

D. F. N. HARRISON

INTRODUCTION

X-rays were discovered by Roentgen in 1895. The following year Becquerel described the radio-activity of uranium and a year later Thompson discovered the electron. However, it was the latter who pioneered the fundamental investigations which led to the eventual understanding of the principles of ionization and the physical properties of x-rays. Roentgen lost interest in his discovery and returned to research in general physics. In 1934 Joliot and Curie discovered a means of making an element radio-active. They exposed boron to a stream of alpha particles (helium nuclei); nitrogen was produced which was radio-active and changed into carbon (Raven, 1959). Most radio-active isotopes emit beta-rays but two at least emit the more important gamma-rays. These are cobalt and caesium and, as they are readily available, now form an important source of gamma-rays for medical radiotherapy. The development of nuclear fission has resulted in the availability of artificial radio-isotopes in large quantities and offers a means whereby neoplastic cells might be induced to take up selectively enough radio-active material to result in cell death. ^{131}I and ^{32}P are both used in this manner and have produced encouraging results in carcinoma of the thyroid and leukaemia, respectively.

Over 1,000 radio-isotopes are now in use but most are employed in industry or as tracers in medical research. The radiations at present used in the treatment of human cancer are only a part of the electromagnetic spectrum (Fig. 218). All the radiations at the higher end of the spectrum are referred to as "ionizing radiations" because of the effects they produce after interaction with matter (atoms or molecules). Energy is transferred from the radiation to the body and a chain of events is instituted which may eventually lead to cell death.

PRODUCTION OF IONIZING RADIATIONS

Radiations suitable for use in the treatment of cancer can be produced in two ways:

(1) X-rays resulting from the interaction of high-speed electrons with a target.

(2) By the breakdown of unstable radio-active isotopes, emitting gamma-rays.

Both x-rays and gamma-rays have identical physical properties and in 1928 the first unit of dosage was formulated—the roentgen (r). An additional unit—the

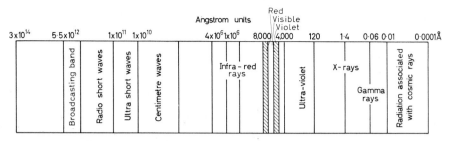

FIG. 218.—Electromagnetic frequency spectrum.

rad.—is also employed as a measure of the absorbed dosage per unit mass imparted by the ionizing particles to the irradiated tissue. Both units are of course complementary.

The wavelength of the radiation delivered to the tumour area is probably unimportant and in general either x-rays or gamma-rays could be used against any human cancer, the choice depending upon which is most convenient for each specific case. The choice then depends primarily on the physical and mechanical factors which affect the actual application of the radiation.

If an electron is passed between two points maintained at a high potential difference then it will be accelerated. For example an electron accelerated through 30,000 volts reaches a speed of approximately 96,000 km./sec. (Raven, 1959). When a beam of these high speed electrons is allowed to strike a metallic target such as tungsten, high frequency ionizing radiations are produced together with much dissipation of energy in the form of heat. As the accelerating voltage is increased more and more of the electron energy is transformed into x-rays and less into heat. The accelerating voltage may be produced by a simple transformer–rectifier system giving a maximum of 250 kV. High voltages result in difficulties of insulation. The van de Graaf generator is based on the principle of the Wimshurst-machine, and allows an accumulation of electrostatic charge eventually resulting in voltages of over 2,000,000 (2 MeV). If the electrons are accelerated in a circular orbit utilizing a changing magnetic field and then allowed to bombard a suitable target, x-rays are produced with energies of up to 50,000,000 V (50 MeV). This principle is employed in the betatron and, in a modified form, in the synchrotron. An alternative principle is used in the linear accelerator where the electrons are accelerated along a wave guided by high frequency radio-waves and values of 4–5,000,000 V are possible. There is obviously a tendency to use higher and higher voltages to produce x-rays, thus giving greater energy, better penetrating power and therefore better dose distribution to the deeper tissues of the head and neck.

Radio-active sources

The spontaneous disintegration of certain radio-active elements such as radium leads to the emission of alpha particles and the more important high speed electron —the beta particle. As a result of the latter emission a new element is formed and this frequently loses energy by the emission of electromagnetic gamma-rays—these are identical with x-rays. The rate of decay for any radio-active element is constant and is usually expressed as its "half-life". This is the time required for half the atoms in any given mass to break down (Table I).

TABLE I

Radio-active element	Half-life
Radium	1590 years
Caesium-137	33 years
Cobalt-60	5·2 years
Phosphorus-32	14·3 days
Iodine-131	8 days
Radon	3·83 days
Yttrium-90	64 hours

Originally use was made of the beta-ray emission of radium but in modern radiotherapeutic practice the radium is usually screened to allow only the gamma-rays to pass through. One of the decay products of radium is radon, a gas with a half-life of under four days. It also emits gamma-rays and has considerable clinical use for interstitial irradiation. Transportation requires only minimal precautions and the exhausted radon seeds may be left *in situ* if removal is contra-indicated. With the development of nuclear fission it became possible to manufacture artificial radio-active isotopes of most natural elements. Many of these are unstable and some emit gamma radiation in such quantities as to be useful for radiotherapy. Cobalt-60 is highly active and is used in telecurie units to give radiation equivalent to a 5 MeV x-ray tube.

Caesium-137 is a by-product of the fission of uranium and plutonium, and it is therefore obtainable by extraction from the waste material from nuclear reactors. It requires a large source in order to give adequate radiation but of course is more easily available than cobalt-60.

BIOLOGICAL EFFECT OF RADIATION

The value of radiation in the treatment of cancer depends upon its capacity to destroy the malignant growth *in situ* without, at the same time, producing irreversible destructive changes in the surrounding tissues. The permanent effect of radiation on tumour cells has been shown to be damage to the nucleus and cell death. Reversible effects are suppression of mitosis and cessation of tissue growth and this is related primarily to the dosage of radiation which has been given. It is well known that tumours show varying sensitivity to the same radiation dose. Factors such as: (*a*) differences in growth rates, (*b*) cell sensitivity, and (*c*) time to recover from suppression of mitosis, all influence the general sensitivity of the growth, but in addition, changes in the surrounding tissues (the indirect effect of radiation) may also be of importance by reducing the tumour blood supply. The fractionation of the radiation dose is intended to control both these direct and indirect effects, the ultimate aim being to deliver the highest possible dose to the tumour without damaging the surrounding "apparently" normal structures.

Radium emits both gamma- and beta-rays at an intensity of radiation which is low compared with x-rays. Consequently during radiation treatment the cells recover more quickly from the mitosis suppressing effect, and with fractionated dose therapy cell degeneration proceeds continuously. The biological effect produced in the tissue bed by this therapy favours the treatment of large skin lesions or deep seated neoplasms where the tumour bed is composed of different tissues, such as in carcinoma of the larynx. With supervoltage therapy the dosage increases with depth; consequently tissue damage is minimized at the surface, thus avoiding the more severe skin reactions so frequently seen with high voltage therapy. Energies in excess of 1 MeV will also produce decreased bone damage since there is less discrepancy between bone and soft tissue absorption.

METHODS OF RADIATION THERAPY

The decision as to whether any particular neoplasm should be treated primarily with radiotherapy or radical surgery is one which should be taken at a combined consultative clinic. Patients with obviously incurable neoplasms who are subjected to ill-advised or over-enthusiastic therapy under the guise of palliation, can have their lives made intolerable by severe skin infections, radiation sickness or suppurating cavities. "It is a wise doctor who knows when not to treat his patient".

Radical excision of all visible tumour and its lymphatic drainage field is frequently possible in neoplasms of the head and neck. In many regions this is accompanied by considerable deformity of large pharyngolaryngeal defects, the closure of which necessitates many reparative operations. In sites such as the nasopharynx, ethmoid or middle ear, radical excision may be impossible and radiotherapy is invariably the treatment of choice. It is not proposed to discuss the various indications that must be considered before deciding whether radiotherapy or surgery is indicated in the many varied neoplasms encountered in the head and neck. However, if radiotherapy is to be given then the radiotherapist must decide whether the treatment is to be by external irradiation, x-rays or gamma-rays, by surface or intracavitary radium or by interstitial radium or radio-isotope therapy. The decision is naturally determined by the histology of the tumour, its site and extent.

X-rays

It has already been said that gamma-rays and x-rays are identical, although produced in different ways. The penetrating powers of x-rays depend upon the voltage at which they are produced. Low voltage therapy units generate rays up to 100 kV and are used almost exclusively for skin tumours. The most common machines in radiotherapy departments, however, are the high voltage 250 kV generators. Unfortunately, they tend to produce severe skin and mucosal reactions, and there is considerable absorption of radiation energy by bone. Supervoltage therapy was developed in the hope of avoiding these side effects and machines such as the linear accelerator (Fig. 219) and betatron produce electron speeds which correspond to voltages of the order of 8,000,000 V.

Radium

The alpha-radiation emitted by radium is of no value in cancer therapy and the beta rays are of use only when emitted by certain specific isotopes such as ^{32}P and ^{131}I. Although the gamma-rays given off by radium are identical with x-rays but at lower voltage, the source is of course much less cumbersome and may consist of only a few milligrammes of radium or, at the most, several grammes. Radium then is an excellent means of introducing a source of gamma-rays into cavities or directly into tissues, such as the tongue. Filters eliminate all radiation except the gamma-rays. Both radium needles and radon seeds are of value in treating head and neck cancer, although the needle pallisade (Finzi–Harmer technique) is no longer used in the management of glottic carcinoma.

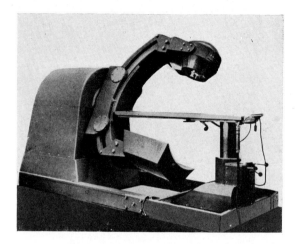

FIG. 219.—Linear accelerator. *(Reproduced by courtesy of Mount Vernon Hospital.)*

By enclosing large quantities of radium in a shielded container, possessing only one small aperture, it has been possible to produce a beam of gamma-rays approximately equivalent to a 1,000,000 V x-ray machine. This radium bomb is still in use for treating carcinoma of the larynx but cannot compete with the energies produced by modern supervoltage machines.

Megavoltage therapy

This term was developed to meet the requirements of gamma-radiation produced by teletherapy units and x-rays from the bigger supervoltage machines. The production of cobalt-60 from the uranium pile provided a source of gamma-rays, comparable with that produced by the more expensive and bulky x-ray machines working at over 1,000,000 V (Fig. 220). The maximum dosage from a cobalt unit is developed at about 4 mm. below the skin surface. This ensures that the skin dose is less for a given maximum dose in the deep tissues. Deep seated tumours, such as occur in the head and neck, are treated more easily and with less unpleasant side effects for the patient. Energy absorbed by bone is the same as for the tissues but it is essential to realize that there is no fundamental difference in effect upon the tumour cells. Both caesium-137 and iridium-192 have been used for beam radiation but as yet are not serious competitors to cobalt-60.

It was hoped that the systemic administration of radio-isotopes might result in the selective destruction of malignant cells. For successful use of these preparations there must be: (1) a high uptake of the radio-active element by the cancer cell; (2) small or no uptake by normal cells; and (3) sensitivity of the malignant cell to the dose of radiation delivered. Unfortunately, only ^{131}I has been of real value but further developments using sophisticated immunological techniques may prove more successful.

Despite these tremendous technical developments in radiotherapy over the last 20 years, the cure rates for patients with cancer have not improved to any real extent. Attempts have been made to increase the sensitivity of the malignant cell to ionizing radiations by the use of drugs such as synkavit, insulin and steroids but

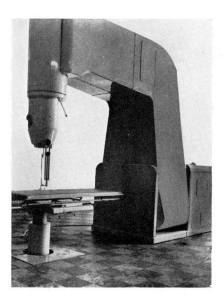

FIG. 220.—Cobalt bomb. (*Reproduced by courtesy of Mount Vernon Hospital.*)

with little success. It has been shown that anoxic cells are less easily damaged by radiation and the introduction of hyperbaric oxygenation radiotherapy by Churchill-Davidson, Sanger and Thomlinson (1955) may yet prove to be of value in the treatment of human cancer.

CHEMOTHERAPY

Despite advances in surgical technique and radiotherapy, the prospect of a permanent cure for the majority of patients with cancer of the head and neck remains extremely small. Modern anaesthetic techniques have allowed the most radical of surgical procedures to be carried out safely, and although radiotherapy still plays a dominant rôle in the treatment of cancer in certain sites, such as the nasopharynx, the general outlook is depressing. In recent years an intense search has been carried out for means whereby the prognosis for patients with head and neck cancer might be improved, the emphasis being directed towards the development and usage of a variety of chemotherapeutic agents. The success of chemotherapy against bacteria and protozoal infections stimulated research into the possibility of attacking the cancer cell by means of cytotoxic agents. Unfortunately, although vast numbers of these drugs have been synthesized and tested, none have had the dramatic success experienced by their predecessors against bacteria. Yet some do alleviate the sufferings of patients with advanced cancer and may prolong life for many years. The final attack against human cancer may lie in techniques and methods as yet unthought of; meanwhile the clinician, radiotherapist, surgeon and bio-chemist must utilize every available weapon in their efforts to cure the patient of his neoplasm.

Historical review

Since earliest times attempts have been made to destroy superficial cancers by the topical application of a wide variety of preparations, the use of ointment for ulcerating skin tumours being described in detail in Egyptian papyri. Present-day cancer chemotherapy probably dates from the observations of Gilman and Philips in 1946, that nitrogen mustards caused regression of not only certain experimental tumours but also human lymphosarcoma and Hodgkin's disease. These findings were stimulated by a report four years previously by a U.S. Medical Officer, Alexander, who had noticed that the survivors from a Liberty ship sunk whilst carrying 250,000 Kg. of mustard gas, were dying of agranulocytosis. Clinical trials were started immediately, the compounds being given systemically. Although regression of the tumour mass often occurred, the mustards were not tumour specific and appeared to exert their greatest effect upon all rapidly growing tissues, even in doses exhibiting no tumour-inhibiting effect; serious and often irreversible damage was caused to the bone marrow and the gastro-intestinal tract.

In an attempt to minimize toxicity and yet increase the tumoricidal action, intra-arterial administration of nitrogen mustard was investigated (Klopp and his colleagues, 1950; Sullivan and his colleagues, 1953). Unfortunately, leakage into the systemic circulation continued to produce serious marrow depression. Creech (1958) attempted to overcome these problems by isolating the tumour-bearing area from the systemic circulation and then perfusing the blood supply to the tumour with a pump oxygenator system (Fig. 221). This technique has proved successful in the limbs but is virtually impossible to apply to the head and neck.

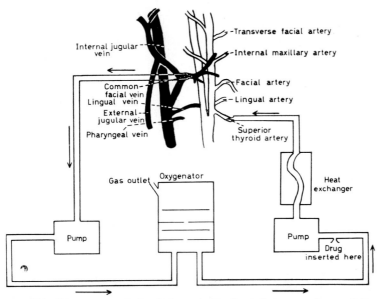

FIG. 221.—Extracorporeal circulation suitable for infusing neoplasms of the head and neck.

495

Even if both carotid arteries and internal jugular veins are cannulated, the extensive vertebral venous system is ignored and there is inevitably serious leakage into the systemic circulation. In recent years most workers with cancers of the head and neck have given cytotoxic agents either by continuous intra-arterial infusion (with or without a systemic antidote) or by intermittent intra-arterial injection. Use is thus made of the readily accessible blood supply of the majority of head and neck tumours, although neoplasms which are localized to areas outside the distribution of the external carotid artery are not really suitable for regional chemotherapy (Nahum, 1963).

Selection of patients

The decision to treat any patient with a new, and potentially lethal, form of therapy can only be taken after serious consideration of each individual case. Only then, when knowledge of the natural history of the disease is weighed against expected relief and possible toxic side effects, can a conscientious decision be taken. There is considerable confusion as to the rightful rôle that chemotherapy should play in the management of cancer of the head and neck. Chemotherapeutic success depends largely upon concentrating enough of the active agent within the tumour area—but without producing fatal systemic effects. Although avascular necrotic tumour tissue can be excised, previous radical surgery or radiotherapy invariably destroys much of the regional blood supply, making it virtually impossible to bring sufficient cytotoxic agent in contact with the neoplastic cells. However, the published reports hardly justify at present the thesis that all neoplasms of the head and neck should be treated primarily with chemotherapy. The majority of patients receiving cytotoxic drugs today have already failed to respond to more orthodox therapy and face a prolonged period of pain, suppuration and deformity until inhalation, bronchopneumonia or secondary haemorrhage terminates their existence. Enthusiastic attempts to improve the prognosis and well-being of these unfortunate people is praiseworthy but unjustifiable if resulting in severe toxic side effects or increase in pain and discomfort. If these principles are considered in each patient there is rarely difficulty in selecting patients for treatment or evaluating the success of therapy.

The prospect of a permanent cure for a patient with a neoplasm of the head and neck is little more than it was 20 years ago. It would appear that only a completely new approach to the problem can offer any real hope of an improvement in the management of a condition in which less than 30 per cent of patients can expect to be alive five years after confirmation of their disease. Chemotherapy is only of limited value in the "failed" case and future improvement probably lies in a combination of this form of therapy with surgery or radiotherapy, used as an initial form of treatment.

Choice of drug

No cytotoxic agent at present in use against human cancer is curative and most do not even control the disease for more than a few months. Two main groups of drugs are available for the treatment of head and neck malignancies: (*a*) biological alkylating agents; (*b*) anti-metabolites.

Biological alkylating agents

This large group, which includes nitrogen mustard and its derivatives, are chemically highly reactive compounds and general cell poisons. Consequently they

PLATE IX

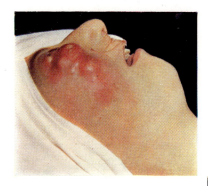

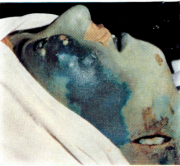

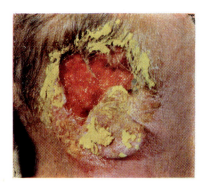

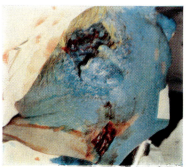

The use of Disulphine Blue as a tracer dye.

attack both normal and neoplastic cells. The main action is to alter essential cellular constituents, such as nucleic acid and enzymes by alkylation processes which lead inevitably to cell death. The damage they produce is somewhat similar to that following irradiation and consequently they are sometimes referred to as radiomimetic substances.

Amongst these agents are the nitrogen mustards (Fig. 222) with their active warhead $N(CH_2CH_2 CL)$—for example, nitrogen mustard, the methane sulphonates such as myleran, the ethylenimines, thiotepa, and finally the epoxides such as ethoglucid (Bergel, 1961).

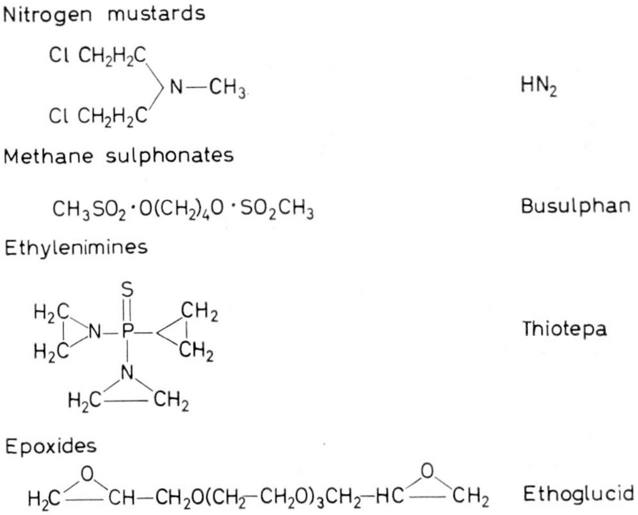

FIG. 222.—Biological alkylating agents.

Unfortunately, normal cells depend as much upon the integrity of their nucleoproteins as do malignant cells and the use of active non-specific alkylating agents is always accompanied by some damage to normal tissues. Systemic chemotherapy with any of these agents is invariably accompanied by bone marrow depression and ulceration of the intestinal mucosa. By administering the drug directly into the blood supply to the tumour area, as is practised in head and neck malignancies, a high concentration of drug may be safely given to a small volume of tissue. This results in tissue damage being restricted to the infused area and minimal systemic side effects. However, leakage into skin and destruction of tumour with surrounding normal tissue is invariably accompanied by blistering and oedema (Fig. 223).

When the neoplasm is situated in the tongue or laryngopharynx it may necessitate tracheostomy. Unfortunately, rapid destruction of tumours in this region may also result in inhalation bronchopneumonia, uncontrollable haemorrhage or the production of large tracheo-oesophageal fistulae. In an attempt to avoid these lethal side effects, biochemists have synthesized a variety of alkylating agents composed of "warheads" and "carriers" (Fig. 224). The mustard warhead is attached to a selection of molecular structures related to naturally occurring substances, which transport the active cytotoxic agent to the site of action where it is liberated by cellular enzymes. The N-phosphorylated nitrogen mustards—for example,

497

cyclophosphamide—are thought to be activated by phosphatases and phosphamidases. These enzymes are abundant in some malignant tumours and in the liver. Phenylalanine mustard (Melphalan) is believed to be taken up preferentially by those cells actively engaged in the production of the pigment melanin and where

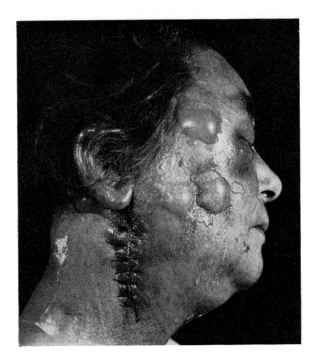

Fig. 223.—Vesiculation and oedema of facial skin after intra-arterial injection of an alkylating agent—ethoglucid.

they are malignant some degree of specificity of action may result. Both these drugs have been widely employed in malignancies of the head and neck, since they are completely stable in aqueous solution and non-vesiculating. Cyclophosphamide can be given by any route—intravenously, intra-arterially, intramuscularly, per-orally and by direct injection into the tumours. Dosage may vary from 4mg./kg./day for maintenance therapy to single intravascular injections of 60 mg./kg.

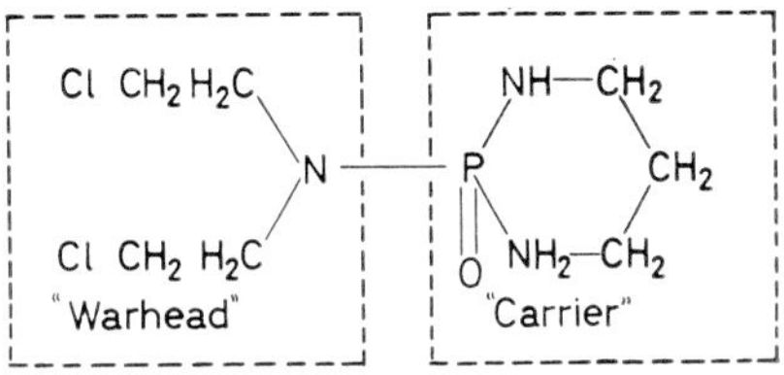

Fig. 224.—Formula of cyclophosphamide.

$$Cl\ CH_2H_2C \diagdown$$
$$N$$
$$Cl\ CH_2\ H_2C \diagup$$
"Warhead"

$$NH—CH_2$$
$$P \diagdown CH_2$$
$$\underset{O}{\|} NH_2—CH_2$$
"Carrier"

Anti-metabolites or metabolic antagonists

Substances which structurally resemble vitamins, co-enzymes or normal intermediary metabolic products but differ sufficiently to act as competitive inhibitors of essential metabolic processes, are called anti-metabolites. The most important in cancer chemotherapy are the anti-folic acid compounds such as methotrexate and the pyrimidine analogues—5-fluoro-uracil (Fig 225). Since these drugs act by competing with normal metabolites for cell enzymes, they must of necessity remain in contact with the tissues for days or weeks if sufficient numbers of cells are to be exposed to their metabolic blocking action.

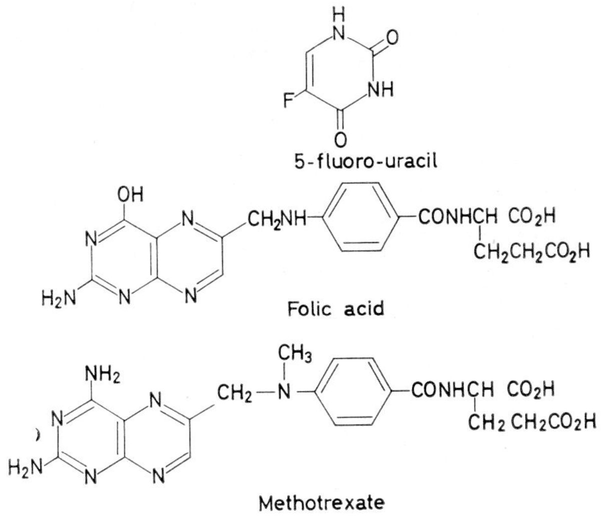

FIG. 225.—Formula of some anti-metabolites.

5-fluoro-uracil

Folic acid

Methotrexate

Sullivan and his colleagues (1959) described the first group of patients treated by continuous infusion of the anti-metabolite methotrexate, together with intra-muscular injections of systemic protective doses of the specific metabolite folinic acid (citrovorum factor). The rationale behind the giving of the antidote to the cytotoxic agent lay in the necessity for prolonging the duration of the arterial injection without increasing systemic toxicity. By giving intermittent intramuscular injections of the specific metabolite it proved possible to protect the patient without reversing the local anti-tumour effect. Methotrexate has been more widely used in malignancies of the head and neck than any other cytotoxic agent but although initial improvement is obtained in a large proportion of cases, recurrence takes place within a few months and the technique of administration carries with it a high morbidity and mortality rate.

Methods of administration

Although the prognosis for patients with malignancies of the head and neck is poor there are certain advantages to be gained by treating them with chemotherapy.

First, the survival time even of advanced cases can be measured in months, giving the chemotherapeutic agent a reasonable opportunity of producing an effect. Secondly, in most cases the tumour mass can be easily seen and any change in size and appearance will be obvious. Thirdly, use can be made of the fact that most neoplasms in this region are supplied by branches of the external carotid artery. This vessel is readily available to the surgeon, although previous radio-therapy or radical surgery may have destroyed much of the normal regional blood supply.

Goldacre and Sylven (1962), working with experimental tumours, showed that although small tumours are well vascularized and stain readily when vital dyes are given systemically, larger tumours frequently have a necrotic avascular area which does not stain. Biopsy shows that within this area there remain cells which, histologically, appear both malignant and viable. This may explain the re-growth of tumours which frequently occurs even after an initially satisfactory response to chemotherapy—a growth initiated by active malignant cells lying in an avascular and untreated area. All necrotic tumour material should be removed prior to therapy; this reduces the bulk of tissue requiring treatment, ensures that most of the visible neoplasm is well vascularized and minimizes the risk of toxic absorption or inhalation bronchopneumonia from sloughing of necrotic tissue.

Extracorporeal perfusion

This implies the continuous artificial circulation of cytotoxic drugs through a region. In some parts of the body it is possible to isolate completely the regional from the systemic circulation and the dosage of drug used is limited only by local tissue tolerance (Westbury, 1963). Imperfect isolation results in leakage into the general circulation. In the head and neck the afferent vessel cannulated is the external carotid artery and the efferent vessel usually the common facial vein (*see* Fig. 221). The collateral circuit consists of the external, anterior jugular and vertebral veins. All these veins must be occluded but the abundant cross collateral circulation in this region ensures that tumours near the midline receive blood from the opposite side and leakage is inevitable. Bilateral cannulation is possible but this technique is unsatisfactory and almost impossible after prior radiotherapy or radical surgery.

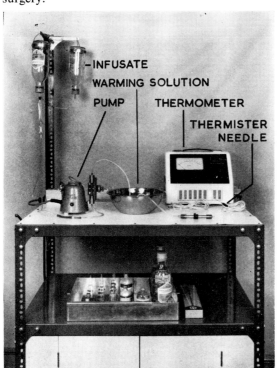

FIG. 226.—Equipment used for cotninuous intra-arterial chemotherapy. (*Reproduced by permission of the Royal National Throat, Nose and Ear Hospital.*)

Continuous intra-arterial infusion

The technique of long-term infusion can be used for any region where the tumour is supplied by one or two primary arteries. It is more suitable to the anti-metabolite group of drugs than the short-acting alkylating agents. The external carotid artery is exposed by a small skin incision and usually cannulated via its superior thyroid branch. A narrow portex tube is used and the catheter tip manipulated until it lies close to the opening of the vessel to be infused. Gentle instillation of 5 per cent fluorescin enables the area to be treated to be sharply demarcated when the patient is viewed under ultra-violet light. Retrograde catheterization of the external carotid artery via its superficial temporal branch avoids a neck incision but difficulty may be experienced in passing the catheter beyond the zygomatic arch. However, this may be the only possible approach if the cervical lymph glands are involved. The anti-metabolite is then placed in a bottle and suspended sufficiently high above the patient to exceed the blood pressure or a specially designed pump may be placed by the bedside (Fig. 226). On completion of the infusion the catheter is removed by firm traction and the site of exit compressed. This method, although popular, is associated with considerable morbidity, especially in the aged and the arteriosclerotic. Septicaemia, haemorrhage, leakage around the catheter and hemiplegia occur frequently and may result in death.

Intermittent intra-arterial injection

Many alkylating agents have half-lives of only a few minutes and are thus particularly suitable for this method where the drug is in contact with the neoplasm for only a short time. In order to minimize leakage of these highly reactive drugs it is desirable to administer the smallest effective dosage possible. This can only be

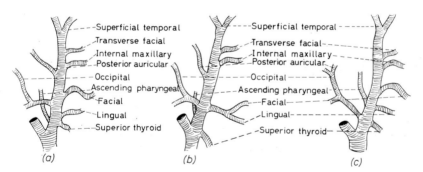

FIG. 227.—Variations in branching of the external carotid artery: (*a*) is the more common normal arrangement; (*b*) shows the superior thyroid arising from the common carotid (16 per cent of cases) and the lingual and facial arteries having a common stem (20 per cent of cases); and (*c*) the posterior auricular artery is a branch of the occipital.

done by isolating the arterial supply to the tumour area after open exposure of the carotid tree. Any branches leaving the external carotid artery and the upper 2·5 cm. of the common carotid artery are identified and those not required for infusion, temporarily occluded. It is only by this direct exposure that the many variations in the branching of the external carotid artery can be appreciated (Fig. 227). Injection of a tracer dye—methylene blue (or Disulphine blue for more permanent viewing,

Plate IX)—enables inaccessible areas such as the nasopharynx or pyriform fossa to be visualized and also ensures that unwanted tissues are not infused. The alkylating agent is now injected and the needle then removed. Pressure over the puncture site produces haemostasis and the neck incision is closed. The injection may be repeated as often as required (Harrison and Tucker, 1964).

The main systemic complication of all active cytotoxic agents is haematopoietic depression but gastro-intestinal and cerebral toxicity frequently occur with high doses of most alkylating agents. These are the limiting factors in determining dosage and since leakage is inevitable when treating neoplasms occurring in the head and neck, protection of bone marrow is important. Bone marrow may be aspirated and stored prior to chemotherapy, being replaced 12 hours later. However, such measures which also include the use of abdominal tourniquets and leucophoresis have proved to be of only minimal benefit. Harrison (1966) described the protective value of whole-body hypothermia, in which intra-arterial injections of alkylating agent were given in high dosage without producing severe leucopenia or cerebral toxicity. By depressing the mid-oesophageal temperature to 38°C, cerebral and marrow metabolism is decreased and the blood flow to the marrow spaces reduced. By the use of this procedure neurotoxic drugs, such as Epodyl, can be given with safety to patients with advanced tumours of the maxilla, nasopharynx and middle ear. No cures are claimed but lengthy relief from the pain, common to tumours involving bone, occurs in most patients.

Combined therapy

Attempts at improving the cure rate of head and neck cancer by combining chemotherapy, radiotherapy and surgery are theoretically attractive. In various parts of the world randomized trials using two or all three modalities are in progress, and preliminary reports suggest that in sites such as the larynx, pre-operative radiotherapy increases the long term cure rate.

A synergistic effect between radiotherapy and cytotoxic drugs in some tumours has been suggested. Chemotherapy, given orally or intra-arterially, may precede radiotherapy or be combined with a programme of fractionated dosage. Clinical trials using various combinations are in progress particularly in neoplasms of the maxillary antrum and ethmoidal labyrinth, where the prognosis is extremely poor. Such techniques are complicated and dangerous; only long term follow-up and evaluation will reveal their true worth.

Despite the multiplicity of drugs now available and the many ingenious techniques employed for their utilization, chemotherapy has proved to be disappointing in the management of most head and neck cancers. Long term palliation is possible in many cases if treatment is undertaken by experienced physicians. However, toxic side effects may be severe and the patient's condition can easily be worsened. The future would appear to lie in combination therapy perhaps using more selective agents, but it appears certain that major advances will be dependent upon the development of a more rational basis for both the design and application of these drugs.

REFERENCES

Bergel, F. (1961). *Brit. med. J.*, **2**, 399.
Churchill-Davison, I., Sanger, C., and Thomlinson, R. H. (1955). *Lancet*, **2**, 1091.
Creech, O. (1958). *Ann. Surg.*, **148**, 616.
Gilman, A., and Philips, F. S. (1946). *Science*, **103**, 409.

REFERENCES

Goldacre, R. J., and Sylven, B. (1962). *Brit. J. Cancer*, **16**, 306.
Harrison, D. F. N. (1966). *J. Laryng.*, **81**, 173.
— and Tucker W. N. (1964). *Brit. J. Cancer*, **18**, 74.
Klopp, C. T., Alford, T. C., Bateman, J., Berry, G. N., and Winship, T. (1950). *Ann. Surg.*, **132**, 811
Nahum, A. M., and Rochlin, D. B. (1963). *Amer. J. Surg.*, **105**, 759.
Raven, R. W. (1959). *Cancer* (Vol. 5). London; Butterworths.
Sullivan, R. D., Miller, E., and Sikes, M. P. (1959). *Cancer*, **12**, 1248.
— Jones, R., Schnabel, T. G., and Shorey, J. M. (1953). *Cancer*, **6**, 121.
Westbury, G. (1963). *Ann. R. Coll. Surg. Engl.*, **32**, 358.

19

INTUBATION OF THE LARYNX, LARYNGOTOMY AND TRACHEOSTOMY

Douglas Ranger

INTRODUCTION

The physiological role of the nasal mucosa in respiration has been well documented. Nevertheless, circumstances sometimes make it necessary to bypass the nose and mouth to establish respiration between the outside air and the trachea. These circumstances may arise with dramatic suddenness or develop gradually. In progressive disease they can often be anticipated before they occur. They may be temporary or permanent, and when temporary the duration varies from a few minutes to several months.

These situations can be dealt with by the introduction of a tube via the natural passages through the larynx into the trachea (intubation), by opening the larynx through the cricothyroid membrane (laryngotomy), or by establishing an airway from the outside air through the neck directly into the trachea itself (tracheostomy). Each of these methods has its own particular advantages and disadvantages which will be considered in more detail later. However, to generalize, there are many situations in which intubation of the larynx or tracheostomy may be regarded as alternative methods of treatment initially and for a period of time afterwards. On the other hand laryngotomy differs from both of those procedures in that it is used only as a very temporary expedient to establish an airway quickly, in the few emergencies in which intubation is impossible and conditions are such that tracheostomy would be a more hazardous immediate procedure. Once the emergency situation has been resolved an elective tracheostomy is performed and the laryngotomy closed.

Accordingly intubation and tracheostomy will be discussed first and then laryngotomy will be considered later.

INDICATIONS FOR INTUBATION AND TRACHEOSTOMY

By far the commonest indication for intubation of the larynx is the administration of an endotracheal general anaesthetic. This is considered in detail in all standard textbooks of anaesthesia and requires no further comment here. Tracheostomy may be performed as a preliminary to operations on the larynx or pharynx and its use for this purpose will not be discussed further in this chapter.

In a wide variety of other diseases intubation and tracheostomy can increase respiratory efficiency in different ways and consideration will be given later to their place in various diseases. However, the general indications for intubation or tracheostomy may be summarized as:

(1) Respiratory obstruction.
(2) Secretions retained in the lower respiratory tract.
(3) Inhalation of fluids into the trachea.
(4) Respiratory insufficiency.

These are now considered in more detail.

Acute laryngeal or tracheal obstruction

Obstruction of the laryngeal airway may be unexpected and may occur with dramatic urgency when the larynx is injured, when a foreign body impacts in the larynx or when the laryngeal sphincter becomes firmly closed by spasm. Obstruction develops very rapidly as a result of oedema from burns or in angioneurotic and allergic conditions, and occurs quickly in inflammatory states such as acute epiglottitis and laryngotracheobronchitis. Paralysis of both vocal cords abolishes the movement of abduction which normally accompanies inspiration, and the respiratory obstruction resulting from sucking-in of the laryngeal structures may develop rapidly. Cysts and tumours of the thyroid gland may compress the trachea, and haemorrhage into such a cyst can cause acute severe obstruction. In addition the upper airway may be obstructed by inflammatory or neoplastic swellings of the mouth or pharynx, or by fractures of the mandible allowing the tongue and soft tissues to fall backwards. The same situation has been known to occur in bilateral hypoglossal nerve paralysis but such an event is rare in a conscious patient.

Secretions retained in the lower respiratory tract

In a wide variety of conditions there may be inadequate clearance of secretions from the lungs and these then produce an obstruction of the lower airway with consequent hypoxia and carbon dioxide retention. This leads to mental confusion and possibly coma, with reduction of the cough reflex and further accumulation of secretions, and so a vicious circle is created. If infection supervenes the secretions are greatly increased and the deterioration is more rapid.

It is essential that secretions retained in the bronchial tree should be removed. In some patients this can be achieved simply by posturing and by physiotherapy. In others, clearance by bronchoscopy may be adequate to break the vicious circle and allow the patient to recover sufficiently to clear his own secretions subsequently with the assistance of posture and physiotherapy. However, whenever these measures are inadequate or it is obvious that the primary cause of the condition will persist, repeated aspirations will be required and these can most easily be carried out after intubation or tracheostomy. In many patients either route will prove to be adequate but aspiration via a tracheostome is more efficient in that the catheter can be directed into each main bronchus separately whereas this is more difficult when the catheter is passed down an endotracheal tube.

Inhalation of fluids into the trachea

The importance of removing secretions from the lower respiratory tract has just been stressed. It is equally important to prevent fluid from entering the trachea and bronchi and this can be effected by inserting a tube with a cuff which can be inflated to provide an airtight seal.

This procedure may be required when there is bleeding into the lumen of the larynx or trachea from an injury or tumour. Severe haemorrhage from similar lesions in the mouth or pharynx may also necessitate treatment in this way. Paralysis of the protective sphincter mechanism of the larynx leads to aspiration of pharyngeal secretions and of food but the airway will still be kept clear if there is an adequate cough reflex. However, if this fails a cuffed tube will be needed. Pharyngeal paralysis and oesophageal obstruction produce pooling of secretions and food in the hypopharynx and a tendency to spill over into the larynx. Again the cough reflex may be sufficient to expel the secretions from the respiratory tract satisfactorily but, if not, a cuffed tube will be required.

Normally, the entrance of anything except air into the larynx provokes a brisk cough reflex. In patients with a laryngeal paralysis there may well be an accompanying sensory loss and the reflex may not be brought into action. Even when there is no damage to the sensory nerve pathways the repeated inhalation of secretions through the larynx induces a state of tolerance and the cough reflex may gradually fail.

Respiratory insufficiency

Any of the conditions mentioned above may give rise to a state of respiratory insufficiency. However, even when there is no obstruction of the airway and no secretions are retained in the bronchial tree respiration may still not be adequate to meet the requirements of the patient. Such a state may be caused by pulmonary, circulatory or muscular disease and may also occur in patients critically ill from other causes, such as gross disturbances of biochemical balance, when the continuous effort of breathing cannot be sustained. Under such circumstances intubation or tracheostomy will be required in order to allow the institution of intermittent positive pressure respiration. Mechanical ventilation of the lungs in this way is also indicated in patients with respiratory paralysis. In some conditions it is desirable to induce a respiratory paralysis by means of drugs and then provide controlled respiration for the patient.

In normal adults the dead space in the respiratory tract measures about 150 cm³. A tracheostomy will reduce this by about half but this will have only a marginal effect on the ratio of the physiological dead space to the tidal volume, especially in patients with emphysema where the dead space may amount to 500 cm.³ or more.

Intubation or tracheostomy

In some situations it may be possible to treat a patient either by intubation or by tracheostomy and a decision has to be made between them. The chief advantage of intubation lies in the fact that this technique provides a rapid method of treatment without the need for any incision and pulmonary infection is less likely to develop. The disadvantages of intubation are due to the fact that, even with skilled nursing, the tubes may become obstructed or displaced and that these complications are more difficult to deal with than similar situations arising in connection with a tracheostomy tube. Also, although opinions vary considerably about the length of time during which an endotracheal tube may be retained without trouble, some of the complications are directly related to the duration of intubation.

In contrast those complications of tracheostomy which are not common to both procedures are associated with the operation itself and the tube may be retained

permanently if necessary. With a suitable careful technique the operative complications can be avoided. In addition, as has been mentioned already, tracheostomy
allows more efficient aspiration of the bronchial tree than can be achieved with
intubation.

In any particular patient the decision will be made on an assessment of the
patient's condition and an estimate of the time for which it is expected that a tube
of one type or another will be required. Even if a tracheostomy seems to be clearly
indicated there may well be advantages in preliminary intubation. Not only will
this be desirable for the purpose of administering an anaesthetic during the performance of the tracheostomy but it will enable the patient's general condition
to be improved if this is necessary and allow more time for adequate assessment of the patient. In addition intubation will enable the patient to be transported
safely to surroundings suitable for carrying out the tracheostomy.

In a number of conditions it may well be reasonable to treat the patient initially
by intubation via the nose or mouth and reserve a decision about tracheostomy
until the need for it becomes clearer. However, as soon as a decision has been made
that a tracheostomy is necessary then it should be performed without any further
delay in order to avoid as far as is possible those complications which occur as a
direct result of prolonged intubation through the larynx.

Clinical applications

Consideration will now be given to the roles of tracheostomy and intubation
in various clinical states. It is impossible to cover in detail all conditions in
which they may be required and conditions of similar type will be considered
together.

Upper respiratory obstruction

The best method of dealing with an acute laryngeal or tracheal obstruction will
depend on the circumstances under which the obstruction occurs. When the trouble
arises outside hospital and away from any surgical instruments anyone who is
present must improvise to the best of his ability and it is impossible to discuss here
the management of the patient under such varied conditions. When the obstruction
occurs in a situation where full facilities for treatment are available it is considered
that in most conditions the best initial treatment is per-oral intubation using a
laryngoscope to visualize the larynx. In most patients in this category it will be
possible to pass a laryngoscope into the mouth and depress the tongue sufficiently
to see the laryngeal inlet and pass an endotracheal tube. One exception to this has
already been mentioned in Chapter 12; obstruction resulting from injury may be
accompanied by so much distortion of the larynx that it might be very difficult to
recognize the structures and intubate the larynx successfully. Under these circumstances it is recommended that an immediate tracheostomy should be carried out.
Another condition preventing intubation is severe trismus.

In those obstructive conditions which develop slowly and in which respiratory
difficulty can be anticipated, a tracheostomy should be performed early, before
dyspnoea or cyanosis develops. Either of these signs occurring at rest must be
regarded in most patients as a clear indication for tracheostomy unless the obstruction can be relieved quickly with no chance of recurrence. No sedative must ever
be given unless the patient can be kept under careful observation, in case such a
course of action leads to an impairment of respiration.

Coma

In comatose states secretions tend to accumulate in the bronchial tree. In many patients this can be prevented and the chest kept clear by posturing and by physiotherapy. However, in some patients these measures may prove inadequate or posturing may be prevented by the presence of other lesions. In such patients intubation or tracheostomy is indicated.

If, when the patient is first seen, it seems likely that the coma will persist and if it is evident that posturing will prove inadequate then a tracheostomy should be performed early before any degree of hypoxia can occur from secretional obstruction and before any infection develops. This is of importance because hypoxia alone may produce a state of confusion and later coma which may be attributed to the original lesion, and the correct diagnosis and vital treatment overlooked.

Coma from head injuries may be complicated by damage to other structures, such as a fractured femur, which may prevent turning of the patient. These patients are best treated by tracheostomy at the outset.

When coma occurs in patients suffering from chronic respiratory disease the problem of keeping the bronchial tree clear will be greatly increased and a tracheostomy is likely to be required.

Chest injuries

In crush injuries of the chest the prognosis has been improved immeasurably by positive pressure respiration. Sucking pneumothorax and flail chest are absolute indications for mechanical ventilation after intubation or tracheostomy.

Tetanus and status epilepticus

In mild and moderate degrees of tetanus or status epilepticus sedation may provide an adequate method of treatment. When the spasms are severe there is so much interference with respiration that respiratory insufficiency is likely to develop. In these patients treatment with muscle relaxants and positive pressure respiration applied through a cuffed tube provides the best method of maintaining adequate respiration and keeping the lungs clear.

Poliomyelitis and polyneuritis

Although it is possible to manage some patients with respiratory paralysis in a tank respirator or cuirass, the nursing problems are so much greater under those circumstances that positive pressure respiration via a cuffed tube is preferable. When there is a combination of respiratory paralysis and bulbar involvement, pharyngeal secretions tend to be aspirated with respiration and a cuffed tube with positive pressure respiration is clearly indicated.

Respiratory disease

Respiratory insufficiency may develop in any patient who develops an acute severe respiratory infection and becomes unable to eliminate the secretions from the bronchial tree by coughing. Such a state is especially liable to develop in patients who have a pre-existing chronic bronchitis and emphysema and develop an acute bronchitis or pneumonia. It is also prone to occur in patients who have had a previous severe debilitating illness so that they rapidly become fatigued and are unable to continue coughing. Elderly patients form a high proportion of this group. Pain in the abdomen from injury or operation may inhibit the cough, and pleural involvement from pneumonia may act in the same way. Sedation may be a precipitating factor in some patients.

In any of these conditions intubation or a tracheostomy may be needed to ensure elimination of secretions and adequate ventilation.

TRACHEOSTOMY

From the time of the first tracheostomy (in or before the first century B.C.) until about 1930 this operation was performed almost exclusively for laryngeal obstruction. Nowadays, this is only one of several indications for the procedure and most patients who have the operation have no obstruction in the larynx or trachea.

Whatever the indication the operation is best performed as an elective procedure under endotracheal general anaesthesia in a properly equipped operating theatre. Even then certain hazards can be encountered but the difficulties are greatly increased if the operation has to be carried out as a matter of urgency or if the facilities are inadequate. For these reasons, as has already been pointed out, intubation for a period before operation may be an advantage.

Operative technique

The degree of urgency with which the operation has to be performed will determine many of the details of the operation. Therefore operative technique will be considered under three separate headings. Whenever possible the operation is best performed as an elective procedure in a non-obstructed patient.

Emergency operation

If a patient must have an airway established urgently because of complete or almost complete respiratory obstruction, and if it is impossible for some reason to relieve the obstruction in any other way such as by intubation or laryngotomy, then an emergency tracheostomy will be required. Under these circumstances all that can be done is to make whatever arrangements are feasible for the head to be kept as steady as possible in the midline, to palpate the thyroid and cricoid cartilages with the fingers of one hand and—with a knife in the other—to make a vertical incision downwards from the thyroid cartilage in the midline of the neck. At this stage the wound will fill with dark blood but time will not permit any steps to be taken to control the haemorrhage. However, if an assistant and a suction apparatus happen to be available these are an invaluable asset. At this stage it should be possible to feel the cricoid cartilage and the cartilaginous rings of the trachea with the fingers of one hand in the wound and the best that can be done then is to make a vertical incision through two or three rings of the trachea. A slight twist of the knife blade will open the trachea and the patient will usually then splutter and cough through the blood. A tube of some sort should be inserted into the trachea as soon as possible and blood sucked out, if necessary by the operator applying oral suction to the end of the tube or to a catheter introduced through it. Inflation of the lungs may be needed and in an emergency this can be carried out by mouth-to-trachea respiration. Once an airway has been established and the immediate emergency overcome the tracheostomy should be re-fashioned as in the elective operation described on p. 511.

Intermediate operation

In some patients there may not be quite the same need for haste in performing the tracheostomy and there might be time to transfer the patient to the operating theatre but it may be considered unwise to administer a general anaesthetic or attempt intubation in case such procedures precipitate a complete obstruction. Under these circumstances it will be necessary to carry out the operation under a local anaesthetic. Under such conditions tracheostomy can, of course, be performed adequately in the way described below, but the difficulties for the patient and for the operator are much greater than if the procedure can be undertaken on a fully oxygenated and relaxed patient having a general anaesthetic administered through an endotracheal tube. This is the ideal which should be aimed at and practised unless conditions make it impossible.

Elective operation

When a tracheostomy is performed on an anaesthetized intubated patient the first step is to position the head correctly without any rotation and without too much extension. A little extension helps to keep the chin up and out of the way but if the movement is excessive an undue length of trachea may be drawn upwards into the neck. This will not interfere with the operation, and may even aid it a little, but it may increase the obstruction and the subsequent management of the patient will be rendered difficult unless the opening into the trachea is made to suit the position in which the patient will lie or sit post-operatively. In young patients it is sometimes possible to extend the neck to such a degree that an opening can be made so low in the trachea that it comes to lie behind the manubrium when the head is flexed. This must, of course, be avoided. Ideally the tracheal opening should be at the level of the third cartilaginous ring. An opening higher than this may give rise to subglottic stenosis while one which is lower may not only prevent proper fitting of the tube but also allow an insufficient distance between the tracheal stoma and its bifurcation. This latter point is of special importance when a cuffed tube is to be used. In some patients the tracheal rings are close together and portions of two of them will need to be excised. In that case the third and fourth rings will usually be the most suitable but in patients with a short neck it may be necessary to make the opening through the second and third rings. *The first ring should always be left intact to avoid the risk of subglottic stenosis.*

A vertical skin incision is still sometimes advocated because it is regarded as being easier and is said to allow better drainage of the wound. However, a transverse incision has the compelling advantage that it allows much more satisfactory closure of the skin edges to the tracheal opening and this makes the management of the patient after operation safer and easier. For this reason a transverse incision should be used. Adequate drainage of the wound is not a problem and even if the operation is made fractionally more difficult this cannot outweigh the advantage of increased safety for the patient. The cosmetic advantage of a transverse incision is also of some importance, especially in women. Although the scarring after tracheostomy is caused mainly by the presence of the tracheostomy tube—and this is independent of the incision used—the scar can be excised more inconspicuously when the original incision has been transverse (Fig. 228).

After a short collar incision has been made approximately 2 cm. below the cricoid cartilage through skin, subcutaneous fat and deep cervical fascia, the flaps are raised a short distance and the infrahyoid muscles exposed. The interval between the right and left sternohyoid muscles is defined and the two muscles separated and retracted. The sternothyroid muscles on a deeper plane are dealt with in the same way. After these muscles have also been retracted the thyroid gland and trachea will be visible. The anatomical variations at this stage are considerable. In some patients the lateral lobes of the thyroid gland are small and situated well to the sides of the trachea with only a very narrow isthmus crossing the

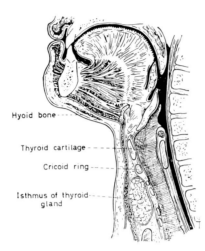

Hyoid bone

Thyroid cartilage

Cricoid ring

Isthmus of thyroid
gland

FIG. 228.—Diagram to show the surgical anatomy of the trachea and larynx.

trachea away from the position where the opening will be made. In the majority of patients, however, the thyroid isthmus is of such a size or in such an area that it will interfere with the tracheostomy, and in that case it needs to be divided and retracted. Division of the thyroid isthmus is usually best carried out by means of the diathermy knife in order to prevent haemorrhage. The cut edges may also be oversown, or simply ligated if the isthmus is narrow.

FIG. 229.—The incision in the trachea for tracheostomy.

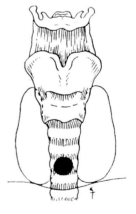

The trachea is now exposed and the third tracheal ring identified (Fig. 229). It is necessary to make a circular opening into the trachea of the same size as the tracheostomy tube to be introduced. A simple vertical incision in the tracheal wall is unsuitable because it makes it much more difficult to replace a tube that becomes dislodged in the early post-operative period and pressure of the tube may well lead to necrosis of the cartilage. A circular opening which is too small will often result in the upper edge of the stoma being forced inwards by the tube and this will give rise to stenosis. An opening which is too large will allow blood from the wound to run easily into the trachea and also encourage surgical emphysema. However, if a cuffed tube is to be used these dangers will be obviated and in such a case it is necessary to make the opening large enough to permit the easy passage of the cuff into the trachea. Attempts to force it through a narrow opening may lead to the fracture or displacement of a cartilage or to a puncture of the thin-walled cuff.

At this stage, before the trachea is opened, all bleeding points must be dealt with and a tracheostomy tube of the appropriate size selected for insertion. A sucker should also be to hand to prevent any blood from the cut edges of the trachea entering the lumen and also to aspirate any retained secretions from the bronchial tree. A circular area, the size of the tube, is then excised from the anterior wall of the trachea, care being taken to retain the excised portion firmly with a pair of forceps before its final separation, in order to prevent any possibility of its being inhaled. The skin edges are then sutured to the edges of the tracheal opening with fine catgut on an eyeless needle, the tracheostomy tube inserted and, if necessary, the rest of the incision loosely closed with further sutures. The incision should not be tightly sutured because of the risk of air from the trachea being trapped in the wound and giving rise to surgical emphysema.

It is sometimes advocated that a window should be cut in the tracheal wall in such a way that a flap of tracheal wall is left hinged inferiorly (Bjork, 1960). This flap is then sutured to the lower skin edge. However, if this flap of tracheal wall were to become detached from the skin and forced inwards into the tracheal lumen, a fatal obstruction could occur and has been known to do so. It is simpler and safer to excise completely a circular area of tracheal wall and then suture the skin edges around the opening (Hewlett and Ranger, 1961). This ensures faster healing; it prevents the risk of the tube being extruded from the trachea post-operatively and coming to lie in the pre-tracheal space; it reduces the risk of haemorrhage from the wound into the trachea; and it reduces the risk of surgical emphysema in the tissues of the neck.

The tube is retained in position by tapes around the neck. Any dressing around the tube must be large so that there is no possibility of the dressing becoming hidden under the flange of the tube and forced into the tracheal lumen if the tube becomes slightly extruded and then pushed back into position. Fatalities have occurred in this way. The safest method of all is to secure any dressings with tape passed around the neck. If secretions coughed out of the tube are copious it is often an advantage to fasten a bib of waterproof plastic material below the tracheostome but precautions must be taken to ensure that this plastic cannot flap over the opening on inspiration.

Post-operative management

The purpose of a tracheostomy is to provide a route for respiration and for aspiration directly into the trachea. This can be achieved only if the tube is retained in its correct position and if the patency of the tube and of the trachea is maintained. The tracheostomy may also be used as a means of providing other treatment for the patient and positive pressure respiration provides a good example.

513

However important this may be the details of these additional forms of therapy are beyond the scope of this chapter and will not be discussed here. It is proposed to give details of the care of the tube itself and of the trachea.

Tube position

Retention of the tracheostomy tube in its correct position is best achieved by careful attention to the operative details already described. If the opening in the trachea is made at the correct site, if the skin edges are sutured to the tracheal stoma, if a tracheostomy tube of appropriate size and shape is chosen for the patient, and if the flange is secured with tapes passing around the neck, then the tube will remain in position without any difficulty. If, despite performing the operation as described, the tube tends to become displaced then this almost certainly indicates that the tube chosen is not suitable for that particular patient. Tubes are available not only with different sizes of lumen but also with different curves and it should be possible to find one to fit every patient. If there is any doubt as to whether the tube is fitting correctly a lateral soft-tissue x-ray of the neck should be taken. This will show the position of the tube in the trachea and will reveal any fault of alignment. Another tube of a different design which overcomes this difficulty can then be inserted.

Tube patency

The tracheostomy tube can become obstructed by an inflated cuff over-riding the end of the tube or by secretions drying within the lumen. Obstruction by an inflated cuff is due to a detachable cuff slipping off the end of the tube or by the cuff having to be grossly over-inflated because too small a tube has been used. This accident can be prevented by using tubes in which the cuff is attached and by choosing one of a suitable size.

Obstruction of the lumen of the tube by dry secretions can be largely prevented by adequate humidification of the inspired air and by aspiration of the secretions from the trachea. When room air is being inhaled the need for humidification will vary a lot depending on atmospheric conditions but some additional moisture should always be provided for a time after tracheostomy until the trachea has adapted itself to the loss of the moistening effect of the upper respiratory tract. The most efficient humidification is provided by a heated, thermostatically controlled bubble humidifier or by a nebulizer, and one of these methods should be used wherever possible in patients breathing room air and in every patient having positive pressure respiration. If the secretions are particularly tenacious and difficult to eliminate an aerosol of Ascoxal is often helpful.

Aspiration of secretions from the trachea should be undertaken as often as required. It must be carried out by using a sterile catheter which must not be allowed to become soiled before it enters the trachea. If a catheter becomes contaminated from outside sources it must be discarded. Suction should be continued for only short intervals at a time and steps taken to aspirate from both bronchi. This is best achieved by using a catheter with a slightly angled tip which can be directed to each bronchus.

The above measures will often keep the lumen of the tube free from dried secretions but if these develop it will be necessary to remove the tube and clean it. Metal tubes are made double, one inside the other, and the inner tube should project about 3 mm. below the lower opening of the outer tube. This allows the inner tube with its dried secretions to be removed while the outer tube remains *in situ* ready to receive the inner tube after cleaning. In this way there is no difficulty in replacing the tube.

Plastic and rubber tubes are single and when they are removed they have to be replaced through the tracheal stoma. In the early stages after operation there will be a tendency for the divided thyroid isthmus and infrahyoid muscles to close over the opening when the tube is removed, but this does not occur when the skin edges have been sutured to the trachea as previously described or when these structures have been sutured to the sternomastoid muscles, away from the opening. When this technique has been used there is little difficulty in changing the tube at any time. Before removing the tube it is best to have a second tube available identical with the one to be removed. Adequate illumination is needed. Tracheal dilators are inserted alongside the tube which is then removed and the second tube is inserted immediately. After cleaning the original tube it is retained by the patient's bed ready to be re-inserted if it is necessary to change the tube once more.

After an interval of some days fibrosis around the tracheostomy prevents the tracheostome from becoming covered by the thyroid gland or muscles but the opening tends to contract once the tube has been removed and sometimes this can happen with alarming speed. Accordingly it is recommended that there should always be a second tube ready for insertion immediately the first one is removed.

If the operation has been performed because of a laryngeal obstruction it is possible that there might be sufficient lumen to allow expiration through the larynx even though inspiration is impeded. However, in the first few days after operation any resistance to the act of expiration or coughing might force air to escape through the tracheal stoma into the tissues of the neck producing a surgical emphysema. Accordingly, during that period the tube must not be blocked off at any stage of the respiratory cycle. However, when the tissue planes have become sealed off after some days it may well be possible to fit the tracheostomy tube with a valve (Fig. 230) which opens on inspiration but closes on expiration. In this

Fig. 230.—Inspiratory valve showing front and sectional views.

way during expiration the air passes upwards alongside the tube and through the glottis so that the patient can speak in the same way as previously, even though air is drawn into the lungs through the tracheostomy tube. Valves of this type can be used in metal, plastic or rubber tubes but, of course, cannot be employed in association with a cuffed tube.

Tracheal patency

Just as secretions may dry on the inside of the tracheostomy tube, so crusting may occur in the trachea unless the air is humidified adequately. If crusts have been allowed to form there is the danger that they may be dislodged and inhaled into the bronchi and deaths have occurred from this cause. Accordingly every precaution must be taken to avoid crusting but if it does occur the crusts should be removed via a bronchoscope, which can usually be passed quite easily through the tracheostomy if the chin is turned slightly to one side.

Pressure from the cuff can produce necrosis of the tracheal mucosa which may then be shed as a cast and inhaled into the bronchial tree or which may predispose to the formation of crusting on its surface. This pressure necrosis can be avoided by using a cuff of adequate length and ensuring that it is never inflated more than is required to produce a reasonably airtight seal under normal inflation pressures. Periodic deflation of the cuff for short periods of time is probably unnecessary if the above precautions are observed. A cuff which is very short requires a much higher pressure to produce an adequate seal and should be avoided.

Very occasionally a standard type of tracheostomy tube may not be long enough to relieve an obstruction as, for example, where the upper trachea is compressed from without by tumours of the thyroid gland or upper oesophagus. In such instances, a Koenig's tube may be required. This has a spiral wire extension with an olive-shaped distal extremity.

Decannulation

Once the need for a tracheostomy has passed, the tube should be removed. If it has been present for only a short time this will present no problems. The patient will welcome the return of natural breathing and the stoma will contract and heal over quickly—even though the skin edges were sutured to the trachea. The resulting scar is not usually unsightly but if necessary the appearance can be improved by simple scar excision.

In contrast, when the tracheostomy has been present for a long time decannulation may be very difficult, especially in children. The patient will have become used to breathing through the tube with its diminished resistance and will find some difficulty in accustoming himself suddenly to the increased resistance associated with breathing through the natural passages. He may also need a little time to become adjusted to the sensation of air passing once more through the larynx, mouth and nose. This re-adaptation can be achieved best by gradually reducing the size of the tube so that decreasing amounts of air pass through the tube and increasing quantities traverse the larynx.

COMPLICATIONS OF INTUBATION AND TRACHEOSTOMY

A number of complications which may occur during and after the operation of tracheostomy have been mentioned already during the discussion of operative technique and post-operative management. It is now necessary to discuss them in some detail and also to deal with those complications which may follow intubation. It is not possible to give a complete list of every complication which could possibly occur but Table I includes the most common and important ones. Those complications which may occur with either intubation or tracheostomy are given first.

As will be seen, many of the complications may occur with either procedure but not necessarily with the same frequency and the effects may not be equally severe. They will now be considered in more detail.

Apnoea

In patients who have had a laryngeal obstruction for a long time the sudden reduction of carbon dioxide tension consequent on intubation or tracheostomy may produce apnoea. The administration of 5 per cent carbon dioxide in oxygen for a few hours may be necessary.

TABLE I

COMPLICATIONS OF INTUBATION AND TRACHEOSTOMY

Intubation		Tracheostomy
	Apnoea	
	Displacement of the tube	
	Blockage of the tube	
	Tracheitis	
	Pulmonary infection	
	Ulceration of the Trachea	
	Stenosis of the trachea	
	Erosion of an artery	
Laryngeal oedema		Haemorrhage
Laryngeal ulceration		Surgical emphysema
Subglottic stenosis		Pneumothorax
Nasal or oral ulceration		Subglottic stenosis
Dysphagia		Difficult decannulation

Displacement of the tube

An endotracheal tube passing through the mouth or nose, or a tracheostomy tube, may be displaced by the patient coughing, by the traction of tubing connecting the tube to a respirator or by the patient's hand. Intermittent positive pressure respiration may be a factor in some displacements. An endotracheal tube passed through the nose is less likely to be displaced than an oral tube but either should be anchored firmly to the patient by tapes passing round the head. Swallowing movements and movements of the jaws and lips may play some part in the displacement of oral tubes.

Displacement of tracheostomy tubes should be prevented by the measures already discussed in the section on operative technique, particularly by correct siting of the tracheostomy, by suture of the skin edges to the tracheal opening and by using a correctly fitting tracheostomy tube.

If the skin has been sutured to the tracheal opening at tracheostomy then displacement of the tube is immediately obvious and readily correctable. If the skin has not been sutured to the tracheal stoma then the tube may come to lie in the pretracheal space and this is not always clear at an early stage.

Displacement of an oral or nasal endotracheal tube may not be readily detected and when it does occur it is more difficult to replace rapidly than a tracheostomy tube. As a result tube displacement is a more serious complication of intubation than of tracheostomy and leads to more serious complications.

Blockage of the tube

Either type of tube may become blocked by inspissated secretions but this is more likely to occur with endotracheal tubes because of their length and because of the greater difficulty of changing them. This is the most frequent of the severe complications of intubation and accounts for the majority of the deaths associated with this procedure.

Adequate humidification and regular frequent suction minimize the risk of blockage of the tube but cannot eliminate it because the action of suction itself tends to produce some drying of secretions and if these are viscous they tend to adhere firmly to the walls of the tube.

Any tendency to blockage of the tube should be dealt with by replacing the tube with a new one before the obstruction becomes severe.

Tracheitis and pulmonary infection

Infection may be present in the bronchial tree before a tube is introduced and may have been the precipitating factor which made the procedure necessary. Infection may also be introduced during aspiration and the need for adequate care and sterility during the procedure has already been stressed. Any pressure necrosis of the tracheal wall will predispose to the occurrence of infection while infection itself makes it more likely that ulceration may occur from pressure of the tube. Antibiotics will be required if infection is present before intubation or tracheostomy or develops subsequently.

Ulceration of the trachea

The trachea may become ulcerated as a result of necrosis from the pressure of the tip of the tube impinging on the tracheal wall or from the pressure of the inflated cuff.

Pressure from the tip will occur if a tube with too great a curve is used so that the beak of the tube impinges on the anterior wall. This will be more likely to happen with hard tubes than with soft ones especially if the tip is not smooth and bevelled. The best way of avoiding such a complication is to have lateral soft tissue radiographs taken with the patient in the normal resting position. If x-rays show that the tube is impinging on the tracheal wall then a tube of different shape or different dimensions should be used. If it is ever necessary to shorten a tube to ensure a suitable fit then the cut surface must be carefully smoothed off.

Pressure from the inflated cuff rapidly leads to cytological evidence of damage to the epithelial cells of the tracheal mucosa and is equally liable to occur with intubation or tracheostomy. However, although such damage is evident within a matter of hours ulceration of the tracheal mucosa can be avoided in almost all patients with careful attention to detail. A cuffed tube should not be used unless it is necessary and if such a tube is inserted the cuff should not be inflated unless it is clear that inhalation of fluids is occurring or that it is needed for applying intermittent positive pressure respiration. The largest tube which fits the trachea comfortably should be used and when the cuff is inflated this should be done very gradually until an air-tight fit is obtained with minimal pressure. The volume of air required should be noted and if it should be necessary to deflate the cuff the same volume is used for re-inflation.

Opinion varies about the value of periodic regular deflation of the cuff and also the placing of pads under the flanges of the tube at intervals in order to alter the position of the cuff in the trachea. Deflation for periods of a few minutes every hour is a procedure which is practised in some centres but theoretical considerations suggest that this is unlikely to be of any real value and practical experience in a large number of clinics shows that tracheal complications from the cuff can be avoided successfully even when the cuff is maintained in an inflated state, provided the precautions about size of tube and cuff pressure which have been mentioned already are carefully observed. Although the position of the cuff in the trachea can be altered to some extent by placing pads under the flanges of the tube it is impossible to avoid some overlap of the areas of tracheal wall in contact with the cuff and this will prevent the measure being fully effective.

Infection is one other important factor in the aetiology of tracheal ulceration and should be avoided by the measures mentioned already.

Stenosis of the trachea

Stenosis may follow any ulceration of the trachea and should be avoided by the measures mentioned above. In addition, fibrous strictures may develop in the sub-glottic region as a result of making the tracheostomy opening too high (Fig. 231) and it has already been stressed that the first tracheal ring must always be preserved intact if this risk is to be avoided.

A stricture may also develop just above the tracheostome as a result of the cartilaginous ring above the opening being forced inwards by an ill-fitting tube. This is prevented by selecting the appropriate tube for the patient and making the opening in the trachea the right size for the tube.

Erosion of an artery

Fatal erosion of large arteries has occurred from the pressure of tubes. The tip of the tube may ulcerate the anterior wall of the trachea at the point where it is crossed by the innominate artery and such a risk should be avoided by the selection of a suitable tube and x-ray assessment of its position.

In a few patients the right common carotid artery crosses the trachea in the neck and could be opened inadvertently at operation or become ulcerated from pressure of the tube. Jarvis has described one fatality resulting from this cause in a child and the author has found the right common carotid artery crossing the trachea obliquely at the level of the second tracheal ring in a woman aged 44.

Special complications of intubation

Having considered those complications which may occur from the insertion of a tube into the trachea either via the natural passages or after a tracheostomy it is necessary to mention the problems particular to intubation via the nose or mouth.

Laryngeal oedema

Any tube which traverses the larynx is liable to produce laryngeal oedema and the longer the tube is retained in position the more likely is this to happen. The following facts are relevant:

(1) The material of which the tube is made.
(2) The size of the tube relative to the larynx.
(3) The presence of any laryngeal disease.
(4) The amount of movement occurring between the larynx and the tube.

Tubes which are made of extremely smooth non-irritant plastic materials are tolerated much better than others as has been shown by Jackson Rees and Owen-Thomas. The tube must be of sufficient size to allow adequate respiratory exchange and facilitate suction but unduly large tubes should be avoided and if, in any emergency, such a tube has had to be forced through the larynx it should be exchanged for a more appropriate one as soon as circumstances permit. Inflammatory conditions in the larynx make it more likely that reaction from the tube will occur earlier than would be the case otherwise and should be controlled by suitable antibiotics.

However, even when an extremely smooth tube of suitable size is retained in the larynx without any infection, there may be considerable variation in the period during which tubes can be left in the larynx without reaction occurring. In many instances the differences are dependent on the amount of movement which takes place between the larynx and the tube. When the larynx is completely paralysed, as may occur in paralysing diseases and profound coma, the only movement occurring may result from the slight movement consequent on the intermittent positive pressure respiration. On the other hand in some patients there may be frequent active laryngeal movements and the oedema is likely to develop much sooner. Campbell has reported that in a series of over 200 intubations oedema of the glottis was present in 100 per cent of those patients in whom the intubation time exceeded 48 hours. More extensive oedema will occur in the subglottic and supraglottic regions when the reaction is greater.

Laryngeal ulceration

Ulceration of the larynx from the pressure of an indwelling tube may occur and the most likely areas to be affected are the posterior parts of the vocal cords. This may lead to the formation of granulomata which will usually require removal although some will resolve spontaneously or with steroids.

Subglottic stenosis

Oedema of the glottis and subglottic regions will usually subside rapidly after the tube is removed but in a proportion of patients a subglottic stenosis develops for which a subsequent tracheostomy will be required.

Nasal and oral ulceration

Prolonged pressure from a tube may ulcerate the nasal mucosa but this seldom causes any disability and healing usually occurs rapidly when the tube is withdrawn. Ulceration of the corner of the mouth with oral tubes can be avoided by alteration of the position of the tube from time to time.

Dysphagia

A proportion of patients requiring intubation are unable to swallow because of the basic underlying pathology. In the others the presence of an indwelling endotracheal tube does produce some difficulties with swallowing and in some patients a nasogastric tube will be required.

Special complications of tracheostomy

Apart from the complications which are common to intubation and tracheostomy there are some which occur only in association with tracheostomy. These will now be considered.

Haemorrhage

If bleeding points are dealt with adequately during the operation especially in the thyroid isthmus and haemostasis secured before the trachea is opened there should be no trouble from bleeding. If reactionary or secondary haemorrhage does occur, blood may enter the trachea alongside the tube and steps must be taken to prevent further bleeding into the bronchial tree. As an immediate measure a cuffed tube can be inserted. Then the wound should be opened and the source of bleeding dealt with.

Haemorrhage from erosion of a major artery in the neck has been considered previously.

Surgical emphysema and pneumothorax

These complications account for some post-operative deaths after tracheostomy and are especially liable to occur in children. In some patients they may develop during expiration in the presence of some degree of obstruction, but usually air is sucked through the wound and neck into the mediastinum on inspiration. Subsequent rupture into the pleural cavity may occur. This risk of inspiratory emphysema and pneumothorax is greatly increased if there is any obstruction of the trachea or tube and this point is well stressed by Reading (1958). This dangerous complication can be prevented by avoidance of any unnecessary dissection of tissue planes during operation, by maintaining a clear airway during and after operation, and by suturing the skin edges to the tracheal opening. In infants this latter procedure must be done with extreme care to avoid subsequent narrowing of the trachea.

Subglottic stenosis

Fibrous strictures may develop in the subglottic region as a result of making the tracheostomy opening too high (Fig. 231) and it has already been stressed that the first tracheal ring must always be preserved intact if this risk is to be avoided.

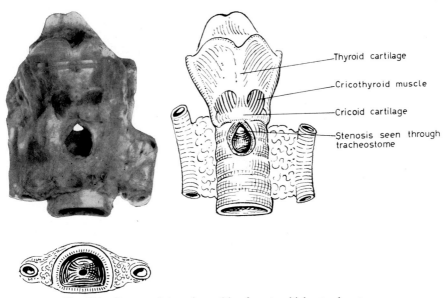

Thyroid cartilage

Cricothyroid muscle

Cricoid cartilage

Stenosis seen through tracheostome

FIG. 521.—Laryngeal stenosis resulting from too high a tracheostomy.

A stricture may also develop just above the tracheostome as a result of the cartilaginous ring above the opening being forced inwards by an ill-fitting tube. This is prevented by selecting the appropriate tube for the patient and making the opening in the trachea the right size for the tube.

Ulceration of the trachea by pressure from the tip of the tube or by excessive pressure from a cuff may give rise to stricture formation. Prevention is ensured by selecting a tube which fits well in the trachea and by not over-inflating the cuff.

Difficult decannulation

After a patient has been breathing through a tracheostomy tube for a long time decannulation may present difficulties because of the need of readjustment to the passage of air through the larynx. This is especially liable to happen in children. The first essential in any such difficulty is to assess the laryngeal airway and establish that there is no stenosis preventing decannulation. Providing the laryngeal airway is adequate the patient must become accustomed to increasing amounts of air passing through the larynx and become decreasingly dependent on the tracheostomy by gradually reducing the size of the tracheostomy tube. In some patients it may be helpful to administer drugs to allay anxiety.

If the tube has been in place for a long time a fistula will probably remain when it is finally removed because the edges will have become soundly epithelialized. The fistula should be allowed to contract as much as possible by leaving it covered by a dressing for a few weeks and then the track should be excised and the fascia and skin sutured over the opening.

LARYNGOTOMY

The interval anteriorly between the thyroid cartilage above and the cricoid cartilage below is narrow and only relatively small tubes can be introduced in this situation. An oval tube will help but there is also the disadvantage that no tube can be retained for long in this situation without producing stenosis. Nevertheless the laryngeal cartilages are usually readily palpated and the cricothyroid membrane is more superficial than the trachea and unlikely to be covered by any part of the thyroid gland or crossed by any large blood vessels. Accordingly, in an emergency when an airway has to be established without delay it may be quicker and safer to perform a laryngotomy through the cricothyroid membrane than to attempt a tracheostomy. This is especially so when the operation has to be performed without proper facilities. Laryngotomy is never an elective procedure.

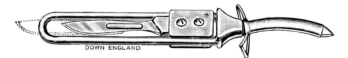

Fig. 232.—Cawthorne's instrument for emergency laryngotomy.
(*Reproduced by courtesy of Down Bros. and Meyer & Phelps Ltd.*)

The indication for laryngotomy is a sudden laryngeal obstruction when relief by intubation is not possible. The need is most likely to arise in situations where full surgical facilities are not available and the surgeon often has to improvise with any knife which happens to be available. Even sharp scissors can be used but the most nearly ideal instrument for such an occasion is provided by the combined knife and laryngotomy tube described by Cawthorne (1964) (Fig. 232). This is small and easily carried in a pocket or handbag.

Operation

The patient's head should be extended in the midline without any rotation and, if possible, retained there by an assistant. The laryngeal cartilages are palpated and the interval between the thyroid and cricoid cartilages identified. A transverse incision is then made in this situation and the cricothyroid membrane opened either at the original stroke of the knife or at a second attempt after separating the skin incision with the fingers of the other hand. If a laryngotomy tube is to hand (Fig. 233) it should then be inserted but if not the incision must be kept open in any way possible. Initially, a slight rotation of the knife blade will serve to separate the cartilages and provide an airway.

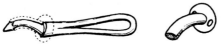

FIG. 233.—Laryngotomy tube with introducer. Note the oval section.

When the sudden emergency has been overcome and an airway established it will be necessary to replace the laryngotomy with an elective tracheostomy unless the obstruction was only brief and no further obstruction is likely to occur. However, a much more satisfactory tracheostomy stoma can be fashioned when the operation is undertaken as a planned procedure than when it is carried out hurriedly in the severely obstructed patient.

REFERENCES

Bjork, V. O. (1960). *J. thorac. cardiovasc. Surg.*, **39**, 179.
Cawthorne, T. (1964). *Lancet*, **1**, 1081.
Hewlett, A. B., and Ranger, D. (1961). *Postgrad. med. J.*, **37**, 18.
Jackson Rees, G., and Owen-Thomas, J. B. (1965). *Brit. J. Anaesth.* **38**, 901.
Jarvis, J. F. (1964). *J. Laryng.*, **78**, 781.
Reading, P. (1958). *J. Laryng.*, **72**, 785.

20

NEUROLOGICAL AFFECTIONS OF THE LARYNX

JOHN BALLANTYNE

The larynx may be affected by a wide variety of neurological lesions, either organic or non-organic; and these may produce either sensory or motor disorders, or a combination of both.

SENSORY DISORDERS OF THE LARYNX

These include anaesthesia, hyperaesthesia and paraesthesia.

Anaesthesia of the larynx

This may be defined as a loss of sensation in the laryngeal mucosa due to lack of sensory innervation. The laryngeal reflexes are also affected. Unilateral anaesthesia is usually symptomless and will therefore escape detection unless special tests are carried out; the consequences of bilateral anaesthesia are always serious but in most instances it forms but a part of a much more extensive neurological lesion, both sensory and motor, of the pharynx and larynx. Hence, for practical purposes, anaesthesia of the larynx never forms a complete clinical entity.

Aetiology.—Common sensation in the larynx is supplied by the internal branch of the superior laryngeal nerve, and the main trunk of this nerve may be involved in a variety of traumatic, inflammatory and neoplastic lesions in the neck; the vagus nerve itself may be attacked by similar lesions higher in the neck, and other cranial nerves are simultaneously involved, with increasing frequency, as the jugular foramen is approached. The resulting lesions may give rise to anaesthesia of the mouth, palate and pharynx, as well as the larynx, together with motor paralysis due to involvement of adjacent motor nerves. In most of these cases the anaesthesia is unilateral.

Bilateral lesions, however, are usual in most other cases. A transient anaesthesia follows the local application of analgesic solutions, and one of the most common forms of recoverable anaesthesia used to be that due to the peripheral neuritis of diphtheria, now fortunately a relatively rare disease; a toxic neuritis may also result from lead poisoning but this has always been rare.

The most serious causes of bilateral anaesthesia are such bulbar lesions as tabes and gummata (now rare); syringobulbia; disseminated sclerosis; occlusion of the posterior inferior cerebellar artery; and haemorrhage and tumours of the brain stem.

Clinical features.—As already stated, unilateral anaesthesia of the larynx may cause little or no trouble, but the ever-present danger in a bilateral lesion is that of inhalation of foreign matter, particularly food and drink, with ultimate death from pulmonary infection. This is due to loss of the protective reflexes of the larynx.

Prognosis.—The outlook in these cases depends, naturally, on the amenability to treatment of the causative lesion. When diphtheria was a common disease, recovery from the peripheral neuritis was expected within five or six weeks. In bulbar lesions the chances of recovery are always very poor.

Treatment.—The treatment is that of the causative lesion, whenever this is possible, but in many instances (especially in affections of the central nervous system) one can expect to do no more than to prolong life by the use of a feeding tube or gastrostomy.

Hyperaesthesia and paraesthesia of the larynx

Excessive and abnormal sensations in the larynx are referred to, respectively, as hyperaesthesia and paraesthesia.

Aetiology.—Hyperaesthesia and paraesthesia of the larynx occur most commonly in women, especially at the time of the menopause. They may also be due to excessive smoking and drinking; to vocal or mental fatigue; to atrophic rhino-laryngitis; or to infection in the nose and throat, teeth, or sinuses; they may, indeed, be entirely psychosomatic (p. 539). It must not be forgotten, however, that excessive sensitivity in the larynx may precede a tuberculous lesion in the larynx, and that malignant lesions of the larynx and laryngopharynx may be heralded by a relatively long period of vague symptoms. It is therefore incumbent upon the laryngologist always to exclude an infective or neoplastic lesion of the upper or lower respiratory tract before he labels the patient as a "neurotic".

Clinical features.—The patient will commonly experience sensations of tickling or pain, burning or tightness, soreness or rawness; but the most common complaint is of an uncontrollable desire to cough and hawk, and to dispel a "frog in the throat".

Treatment.—After treating any infection in the nose, throat or teeth, and after excluding any of the more serious conditions referred to above, the patient must be firmly re-assured.

Excesses of alcohol and tobacco should be avoided, and hawking and hemming discouraged.

Simple antiseptic lozenges may help to allay irritation, but otherwise local treatment to the larynx is to be discouraged, as it serves only to focus the patient's attention even more on the hypersensitive larynx.

MOTOR DISORDERS OF THE LARYNX

These may be either spasmodic or paralytic.

Spasmodic disorders of the larynx

These may occur in children or in adults.

526

Laryngeal spasm in infants and children—laryngismus stridulus

This is a spasmodic condition occurring in infants and young children, more commonly in boys than in girls, and characterized by the sudden onset of an afebrile attack of severe inspiratory stridor.

Aetiology.—Laryngismus stridulus was a relatively common condition in the days of undernourished, "rickety" children but today it is fortunately rare.

It used to be thought that it was due to a collapse of the soft tissues of the larynx out of sheer feebleness, but essentially it is due to a narrowing, transient or constant, of passages with muscular walls. The relatively small passages in infants and children are more easily blocked than they are in the adult. The causes are:

(1) Swellings, which may be (*i*) inflammatory (viral or bacterial), (*ii*) allergic (as in angioneurotic oedema) or (*iii*) traumatic (as after intubation). (2) Collapse or sagging of the walls of the passages as the result of unilateral or bilateral paralysis. (3) Contractions, or scarring. (4) Active contractions due to (*i*) tetany or tetanus, (*ii*) laryngeal crises of tabes, very rarely, or (*iii*) hysteria, either as an overlay to any of the above causes or in a pure form by itself.

A similar stridor may occur during measles, whooping cough or simple laryngitis. It should be easily distinguished from the febrile illness of diphtheria, but a foreign body must be excluded in a first attack.

Clinical features.—Characteristically the attacks of stridor begin some time between the fourth month and the second year of life.

The attack comes on suddenly, not uncommonly during sleep, with a crowing inspiratory stridor which wakens the child in a panic-stricken fight for breath. The terror of suffocation is accompanied by dilatation of the pupils, and the nostrils are flared. The chest heaves and these violent efforts at inspiration are followed by cyanosis and sometimes by carpopedal spasms.

Respiration may cease entirely for a few seconds and, after a variable time, usually lasting between a quarter of a minute and two minutes, a long deep breath ushers in the end of the attack and the exhausted child falls asleep.

Treatment.—During the attack, every effort should be made to allay the fears of the child and his parents. The tongue should be pulled forwards, cold water splashed on his face and chest, and oxygen administered if available.

If breathing does not resume spontaneously after the attack has passed, artificial respiration should be applied and, very rarely, tracheostomy may be required.

Between attacks, the essential treatment is directed to the cause. This will include treatment with the appropriate vitamins, preferably under the direction of a paediatrician.

Laryngeal spasm in adults

This may present in a number of ways: as a laryngeal cough, glottic spasm or laryngeal vertigo.

Laryngeal cough.—Expiratory spasmodic contractions of the adductor muscles of the larynx may be caused by irritation from infections in the nose and sinuses, nasopharynx and oropharynx; and a laryngeal cough may also be caused by compression of the vagus trunk or the recurrent laryngeal nerves by an intrathoracic aneurysm, or by tumours in the thyroid gland, oesophagus or mediastinum.

Laryngeal spasm due to progressive compression of the vagus may lead to paroxysmal attacks of coughing with inspiratory stridor and dyspnoea, and the cough is typically "brassy" in character during the stage of irritative pressure.

When one or both recurrent laryngeal nerves are completely paralysed, the cough becomes hollow and blowing—the so-called "bovine" cough.

Glottic spasm.—This may be due to reflex spasm from the inhalation of a foreign body, or simply from "getting something down the wrong way". The spasm in these cases will pass off as soon as the foreign body has been expelled or passed through the glottis.

The laryngeal crises of tabes were well recognized when syphilis was a common disease, and indeed glottic spasm was sometimes its first manifestation, spasm may also occur in other lesions of the central nervous system, such as disseminated sclerosis, bulbar palsy, tetanus and tabes. In all such cases, the lesion tends to produce a combined spasm of the larynx and pharynx which is usually a precursor of paralyses and other more widespread lesions.

Clinical features. Glottic spasm causes first an irritating cough, followed by inspiratory stridor. In severe cases, this may proceed to a feeling of asphyxia, with marked distress and great air-hunger, and in rare instances there may even be loss of consciousness. In such extreme cases, consciousness is regained as the spasm relaxes.

Treatment. Simple spasm is relieved by spraying the larynx with a few drops of 10 per cent cocaine; and the laryngeal crisis of tabes can be helped by sedation, or the inhalation of amyl nitrite.

If a foreign body is suspected a direct endoscopy may be required urgently, and tracheostomy is occasionally necessary.

Laryngeal vertigo.—The so-called "laryngeal vertigo" is a rare condition in which a bout of coughing is followed by a temporary loss of consciousness. Alternative names include laryngeal epilepsy; laryngeal or post-tussive syncope; and ictus laryngis.

Aetiology. The cause of this condition is not known with certainty. Charcot, who first described and named it in 1876, regarded it as a true vertigo, analogous to Menière's disease; others have considered it to be a form of petit mal. But the most likely explanation would appear to be that advanced by Sharpey-Schafer in 1953: "Persistent paroxysms of coughing would cause a rise in intrathoracic pressure which, in its turn, would obstruct the return of blood to the right side of the heart, thus indirectly reducing the supply to the left side". This sudden lowering of arterial pressure leads to a sudden decrease in the vascular supply of the brain, with subsequent anoxia and syncope.

Clinical features. Laryngeal vertigo occurs almost exclusively in men, usually of the plethoric type and usually between the ages of 35 and 70.

The patient is seized with a sudden violent bout of compulsive coughing, which may be initiated by smoking or drinking, by infection in the nose or throat, or indeed by anything which produces irritation of the larynx. The coughing ends suddenly with a glottic spasm; subjective dizziness follows and there may be transient loss of consciousness, with falling to the ground, and disturbed vision and epileptic convulsions. The face may be pale or cyanosed but consciousness usually returns quickly. The feeling of panic which often accompanies these seizures may itself provoke autonomic failure proceeding to fainting.

The occurrence of these attacks, which may resemble the laryngeal crises of tabes, shows no regular pattern, with wide variation between one attack per day and one in a lifetime.

Treatment. Recovery is the rule and treatment is therefore rarely necessary. Every effort must be made to remove any possible source of irritation to the larynx, and the consumption of tobacco and alcohol should be strictly curtailed.

During an attack the patient should be recumbent and the collar loosened; an inhalation of amyl nitrite may be helpful.

Paralytic disorders of the larynx

Paralysis of the larynx may exist alone, or as part of a wider symptom-complex.

The term "laryngeal paralysis" can be applied correctly only to those cases in which some or all of the intrinsic muscles of the larynx are paralysed by physical or functional interruption in their motor nerve supply. The intrinsic muscles of the larynx, and their actions, are described in Volume 1; so also are their nerve supply. It might not seem amiss, however, to revise certain aspects of applied anatomy at this point.

The vocal cords may be brought together (adduction); they may be separated (abduction); and they may be tightened or tensed (tension).

The *adductors* are the lateral crico-arytenoid, the interarytenoid and (to a slight extent) the thyro-arytenoid muscles.

The sole *abductor* is the posterior crico-arytenoid muscle.

The *tensors* are the thyro-arytenoid (internal tensor) muscle, including its "vocalis" fibres; and the cricothyroid (external tensor) muscle.

All the intrinsic muscles of the larynx are supplied by the recurrent laryngeal nerve, with the single exception of the cricothyroid muscle, which is supplied by the motor fibres of the superior laryngeal nerve.

Since all true paralyses of the larynx are due to lesions of one or both of these nerves, they are described according to the nerve involved, and not according to the muscle(s) paralysed thereby.

Lesions of the peripheral motor nerves to the larynx

Unilateral recurrent laryngeal nerve paralysis.—In the present context, this term is used to describe a paralysis of the recurrent laryngeal nerve, distal to its point of separation from the vagus trunk.

This is the most common form of laryngeal paralysis, and it is twice as common in men as in women.

Aetiology. Operations upon the thyroid gland still constitute the greatest hazard to the recurrent laryngeal nerve, and it is important that the larynx should always be inspected before and after thyroidectomy by indirect (mirror) laryngoscopy. There is, furthermore, a growing feeling among thyroid surgeons that the incidence of these injuries could be reduced if a diligent search were made routinely for the nerves at the time of operation.

Williams (1958) reported his findings in 100 operations for benign, non-recurrent goitres. No paralysis was found in any single case on pre-operative indirect laryngoscopy; nor was any lesion found in the immediate post-operative period. However, four or five days later, paralysis of one vocal cord occurred in no fewer than seven cases, five of which made a complete recovery. In the remaining two cases the paralysis was permanent. It was known that the nerve was *not* divided or crushed or traumatized in any way at the time of operation, and Williams felt that oedema was the most likely cause of early post-operative paralysis. Later, of course, fibrosis may occur.

Two years later, Hawe and Lothian (1960) had exposed the recurrent nerve in as many as 1,011 operations, with paralysis in 28, of which only three proved permanent. Indirect laryngoscopy had been performed pre-operatively, and direct endoscopy was performed routinely on the table at the end of the operation. If a cord was paralysed the corresponding nerve was examined immediately. In two instances, the nerve was included in a ligature but recovery occurred in both, between four and twelve months after the operation.

Blackburn and Salmon (1961) analysed their findings in 250 thyroidectomies, pre- and post-operative inspection of the larynx having been made in every case. There were five cases of permanent, and four cases of temporary, unilateral paralysis of the recurrent laryngeal nerves. Blackburn and Salmon considered exposure of the nerve to be the best safeguard against injury.

Carcinoma of the thyroid, and of the lower pharynx or upper oesophagus, may invade the nerve in the neck or mediastinum.

In the thorax, the left recurrent laryngeal nerve is, of course, much more susceptible to damage, and it is estimated that in all cases of unilateral paralysis it is involved twice as often as the right. In this part of its course it is particularly likely to be affected by carcinoma of the bronchus, with secondary involvement of the mediastinal glands, and by carcinoma of the oesophagus; and in both of these conditions the paralysis indicates inoperability of the causative lesion.

Less common thoracic lesions which lead occasionally to laryngeal paralysis are enlargement of the left auricle due to mitral stenosis; congenital heart disease; aneurysms, usually syphilitic and now very rare; bronchiectasis; and various adenopathies.

In about one-quarter to one-third of all cases of recurrent laryngeal paralysis, no definite causative lesion can be found, and in such instances it is thought to be often due to peripheral neuritis which may be caused by a virus infection of the influenzal or herpetic type, by an infective lesion, due to streptococcal or diphtheritic infections, by chemical toxins, such as lead, or by avitaminosis, as in the polyneuritis of beri-beri.

Spontaneous recovery may take place in this "idiopathic" type after many months.

Clinical features. Respiration is unaffected, and a unliateral paralysis may be quite asymptomatic, perhaps after a transient hoarseness. However, the hoarseness tends to persist in about one-third to one-half of all cases.

In cases of bronchial carcinoma a very long interval may elapse between the onset of a left recurrent laryngeal palsy and the radiological or bronchoscopic evidence of the neoplasm.

The presence or absence of hoarseness depends upon the position of the paralysed cord and the ability of the unparalysed cord to compensate when the paralysed cord is not quite median.

A small number of patients complain of weakness and tiredness of the voice.

The paralysed cord usually lies in the median or paramedian position (Fig. 234) when the recurrent laryngeal nerve alone is paralysed, the superior laryngeal nerve remaining intact, for this latter nerve innervates the cricothyroid muscle which is not only a gross tensor of the cord but has also an adductor function.

It has been recognized for many years that, in the earlier stage of a progressive organic lesion of the recurrent laryngeal nerve, movements of abduction are abolished before movements of adduction; and that when spontaneous recovery occurs, movements of adduction return before those of abduction. Unless, therefore, the lesion is so gross that complete paralysis occurs at once the abductors are the only muscles affected for some time.

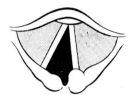

FIG. 234.—Left recurrent laryngeal nerve paralysis (indirect laryngoscopy).

This, very briefly, is "Semon's law" and Negus believes that this train of events can be explained by the later evolution, the lesser importance and the consequent greater vulnerability of the abductors.

However, the tenets of Semon's law have been seriously challenged, and Maxwell Ellis (1954) has been one of the most lucid exponents of this challenge. In the first instance, he argues, there is no direct evidence that the fibres which go to the abductor muscles and those which pass to the adductor muscles have any special grouping within the trunk of the recurrent laryngeal nerve; and in any event, he says, a partial lesion of such a small nerve is an extremely unlikely event. It appears to him much more likely that any lesion of the nerve will involve all its fibres.

According to Ellis, the shape of the larynx and the size and power of its intrinsic muscles are as much personal qualities as the configuration of the facial bones, and he believes that these normal physcial factors will determine to some extent the position of a paralysed vocal cord resulting from the weight of the toneless, paralysed muscles which drag on the arytenoid cartilage. Furthermore, he says, this position is modified also by the external pull of the active cricothyroid muscle, and all these tensions determine whether the cord sags into a median or a paramedian position; but it invariably lies at a lower level than normal.

After a time, certain associated changes take place which further modify the position of the paralysed cord. Contractures develop in the paralysed muscles, and fibrosis and permanent shortening follow; fibrous tissue is also laid down in the capsule of the crico-arytenoid joint, and sometimes in the joint cavity itself, leading to restricted movements and occasionally to fibrous ankylosis.

In any event, the paralysed cord nearly always comes to be ultimately in or near the midline, and at a lower level than the unaffected cord.

Treatment. The prognosis and treatment of unilateral recurrent laryngeal nerve paralysis both depend upon its cause.

Spontaneous recovery may occur in the so-called idiopathic type, due to peripheral neuritis, as long as two years after the onset of the paralysis; but in most other cases recovery is not to be expected and treatment of the cause is impossible.

In any event the disability caused by unilateral paralysis is usually very slight, and this may often be helped by a speech therapist.

Bilateral recurrent laryngeal nerve paralysis.—This has far more serious consequences than unilateral paralysis but is fortunately less common.

Aetiology. The causative lesions of bilateral paralysis are, in the main, the same as those which may cause the unilateral lesion (p. 529), and here again it most commonly follows surgical removal of the thyroid gland. Both recurrent laryngeal nerves may be injured at the same time, or paralysis of one nerve during a partial thyroidectomy may be followed by injury to the nerve of the opposite side at a second or subsequent operation upon the gland; in some of these latter instances the unilateral paralysis may have escaped notice at the earlier operation, only to be detected when further thyroid surgery converts it to an obvious bilateral involvement.

Williams (1959) reported a series of 115 cases of recurrent laryngeal nerve paralysis of known aetiology, seen at the Royal National Throat, Nose and Ear Hospital. In 22 (19 per cent) of these cases, the paralysis was bilateral; and, of these, 18 followed thyroidectomy, 2 were due to peripheral neuritis, and 2 were due to carcinoma, of the oesophagus and thyroid gland respectively.

Clinical features. The effects produced by a bilateral recurrent laryngeal nerve paralysis depend, of course, on the position of the vocal cords, but they tend to be more serious when the onset is sudden than when it is gradual. For example, a bilateral paralysis following immediately upon operation for thyroidectomy may demand urgent relief by tracheostomy, whereas that due to compression by a tumour or an aneurysm will often produce *dyspnoea* and *stridor* only on exertion, or when the narrow glottic chink is further narrowed by an acute inflammatory laryngitis.

The nearer the cords approximate to the midline, the greater is the respiratory distress and the better is the voice; the more the cords separate away from the median position, the better is the laryngeal airway, but the weaker the voice becomes.

On examination with the laryngeal mirror, the vocal cords are seen to lie in or near the midline, most commonly in the paramedian position (Fig. 235).

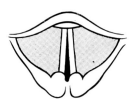

FIG. 235.—Bilateral recurrent laryngeal nerve paralysis.

This condition must be distinguished (by palpation) from fixation of the crico-arytenoid joints, such as that seen in certain "rheumatic" conditions.

Treatment. In some cases of bilateral paralysis especially in those of gradual onset, no surgical relief may be sought or required for many months or even years. Sooner or later, however, some form of surgical treatment will usually become necessary.

Tracheostomy may have to be performed as an emergency procedure in cases of sudden onset, as after surgical or accidental trauma to both recurrent laryngeal nerves, or in cases of long-standing bilateral paralysis where an acute inflammatory lesion in the larynx has supervened with the urgent onset of dyspnoea. It should also be performed, in the first instance, in all cases of bilateral paralysis of relatively short duration, even those following thyroidectomy in younger patients, as spontaneous recovery, either partial or complete, may take as long as six months to occur in cases where the nerves have become paralysed by fibrous scarring rather than active section. Indeed recovery has been reported after two years.

When the causative lesion is incurable the tracheostomy will, of course, be permanent, but when it is non-lethal—and especially in younger patients—other forms of surgical relief must be considered, particularly in traumatic cases.

Excision of one vocal cord.—Simple excision of one paralysed cord, following the lines of stripping of the ventricle in "roaring horses", has not proved satisfactory, mainly because the extra space afforded by the excision tends to fill up again in time with fibrous tissue.

There are, moreover, several modifications of this principle which still have their advocates.

As long ago as 1932, Hoover described an operation in which, after a preliminary tracheostomy, he carried out a submucous excision of one vocal cord through a laryngofissure. The whole of the cord was removed, including the thyro-arytenoid and lateral crico-arytenoid muscles.

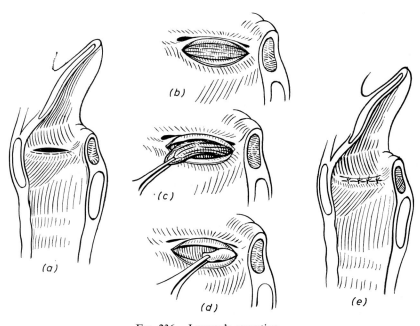

FIG. 236.—Lawson's operation.

Lawson (1965), of Manchester, has modified Hoover's operation and he described his technique at a meeting of the Section of Laryngology of the Royal Society of Medicine. He makes an incision along the whole length of the vocal cord, 1 mm. above and 1 mm. below the edge of the cord (Fig. 236). The mucous membrane is then dissected upwards and downwards, with fine ophthalmic scissors, to form an upper and a lower mucosal flap, 1 cm. above and below the cord. The arytenoid cartilage is removed together with the thyro-arytenoid and lateral crico-arytenoid muscles, and finally the flaps are sutured together accurately. No pack is used.

Unfortunately the voice is often very poor after submucous resection of the cord.

Cordopexy.—Transposition of one vocal cord is the operation of choice in these cases, if and when operation is to be undertaken.

King (1939) described an operation which was designed to rotate one of the paralysed cords outwards and hence to improve the airway (Fig. 237).

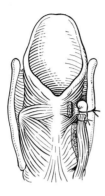

FIG. 237.—King's operation.

Using a collar incision, the larynx is approached from behind, after the inferior constrictor muscle has been detached from the posterior border of the thyroid ala. After exposing the pharyngeal mucosa it is gradually retracted until the arytenoid cartilage comes into view. This is mobilized by opening the capsule of the crico-arytenoid joint, and a suture is passed through the cartilage and outwards through the posterior part of the ala. This rotates the cartilage outwards, together with the posterior end of the cord. A second suture is so placed as to attach the arytenoid to the shortened anterior belly of the omohyoid muscle, in the hope that its contractions will cause further rotation of the arytenoid. This does not really work.

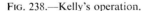
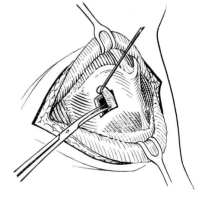

FIG. 238.—Kelly's operation.

Two years later Kelly (1941) reported a modification of King's operation in which the arytenoid cartilage was approached through a square window in the posterior part of the thyroid ala, about 1 cm. across (Fig. 238). After exposure of the arytenoid cartilage, it is dissected out and removed and a suture is passed through the posterior end of the cord. This draws it outwards and fixes it to the internal or external perichondrium of the ala.

Removal of the arytenoid cartilage gives added space for respiration, but the voice tends to be weaker.

De Graaf Woodman (1946) described his operation in 1946 (Fig. 239). This is the method of choice when radical surgery is indicated.

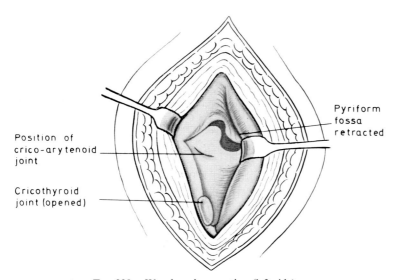

Position of crico-arytenoid joint

Cricothyroid joint (opened)

Pyriform fossa retracted

FIG. 239.—Woodman's operation (left side).

After a preliminary tracheostomy, an incision is made along the anterior border of the sternomastoid, from the top of the thyroid cartilage to the lower border of the cricoid.

The inferior constrictor muscle is separated from the posterior border of the thyroid ala and the inferior cornu, by making a vertical incision down to and through the perichondrium.

Hugging the cartilage closely, the surgeon elevates the periochondrium around its posterior edge and on to its medial aspect.

The cricothyroid joint is separated and the incision is carried on through the perichondrium on the lateral wall of the cricoid cartilage, continuing vertically upwards until the crico-arytenoid joint is encountered. The joint is not separated until the subperichondrial dissection of the arytenoid cartilage has been accomplished. The joint is then disarticulated and all the arytenoid removed except its free anterior part which is stitched to the inferior cornu of the thyroid.

Tracheostomy versus cordopexy.—The choice of treatment in cases of bilateral recurrent laryngeal nerve paralysis usually lies between tracheostomy and cordopexy.

Naturally the choice is determined to some extent by the cause of the paralysis, and it goes without saying that cordopexy is never indicated in inoperable neoplastic cases. Nor should it be performed, even in traumatic cases, less than nine months (and possibly even longer) after the onset of the paralysis, as spontaneous recovery

535

may take place even after so long an interval as this. The difficult choice comes after this. Should the patient be left with a permanent tracheostomy, or should a cordopexy be performed?

It has been argued that the younger patient does not look forward to a life with a tracheostomy tube. This may be so, and there is no doubt that activity must inevitably be restricted in certain ways: for example, the patient cannot swim. But with a valved inner tube, respiration is unimpeded and, above all, speech is normal or near normal. And this, surely, is just as important to an active young person as an unrestricted airway with an imperfect voice.

Cordopexy will, of course, allow the patient to dispense with the tube, and this in itself is the only advantage of the operation. But it is never possible to predict with certainty the results of a transposition operation, in terms of voice, and very often it is very poor. Increased airway must inevitably be gained at the expense of voice, and however satisfactory the position of a cord may appear to be on completion of the operation, further changes inevitably occur as the tissues settle down from the operative interference, and it can be generally stated that if the voice is entirely satisfactory, the airway is likely to be not much more than just adequate.

In those who depend on their voices for their living, therefore, a permanent tracheostomy is to be preferred to a cordopexy. An exception may be made where adduction of one of the paralysed cords is unusually good.

The patient must always be advised, but the final choice should always depend, to some extent at least, on his own feelings after he has been told of all the factors involved.

Paralysis of the superior laryngeal nerve.—Because of its relatively short course, an isolated paralysis of the superior laryngeal nerve is very rare; it is less uncommon, however, as part of a complete paralysis.

The motor division of the nerve supplies only one muscle, the cricothyroid, which is the "external tensor" and also helps to adduct the vocal cord. When this division alone is affected, if indeed this ever occurs, there will be only a paralysis of the cricothyroid; but if the whole trunk of the superior laryngeal nerve is involved, there will be anaesthesia in addition to the paralysis.

Aetiology. Among the more common causes of this rare condition are direct injury, due to surgical or accidental trauma; toxic neuritis (sometimes from diptheria when that was a much more common disease than it is today); enlargement of the cervical glands; and neoplastic conditions. Serological tests for syphilis should always be carried out.

Clinical features. The condition may affect one or both sides. Respiration is unaffected but the voice is rough and feeble and it tires easily; it is also said to be at a lower pitch than usual.

When anaesthesia is present as well as paralysis, the inhalation of food, fluids or pharyngeal secretions will give rise to cough, especially in bilateral cases. This association used to be seen most commonly in diphtheritic cases.

Paralysis of the superior laryngeal nerve prevents the cricothyroid muscle from fixing the thyroid upon the cricoid cartilage, and there is therefore no resistance to the pull of the thyro-arytenoid muscle. The unopposed thyro-arytenoid muscle is unable to harden the edge of the cord and this is said to produce wrinkling of the cord. However, the condition rarely occurs without concomitant paralysis of the recurrent laryngeal nerve and it has been disputed whether the appearance of a wavy cord is, in fact, ever really seen.

It is said that the glottic aperture is askew in unilateral cases (Fig. 240).

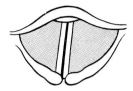

FIG. 240.—Left superior laryngeal nerve paralysis (indirect laryngoscopy).

Treatment. Treatment depends upon the cause. Some degree of spontaneous compensation may occur and, as a rule, the now rare diphtheritic cases recover. When anaesthesia accompanies the paralysis, an oesophageal feeding tube or gastrostomy may be necessary.

Combined paralysis of the superior and recurrent laryngeal nerves.—A combined paralysis may be caused by separate lesions in the respective nerves or, much more commonly, by lesions of the vagus nerve above the level at which the superior laryngeal nerve is given off. It may be unilateral or bilateral.

Aetiology. A combined paralysis may result from lesions in the upper part of the neck or in the region of the jugular foramen; in bilateral cases the lesion is usually at the bulbar level. Hence involvement of other cranial nerves will often co-exist.

Clinical features. In *unilateral* cases, the voice is husky but is very weak and easily fatigued. Respiration is not affected, and the glottic reflex is preserved by the bilateral sensory innervation of the larynx.

The vocal cord lies in a position intermediate between that of phonation (midline) and that of quiet inspiration (moderate abduction). This *intermediate* position is sometimes referred to as the "cadaveric" position, as every muscle is inactive as in death.

In *bilateral* cases, the voice is almost non-existent and is accompanied by great air-waste. There is a monotonous lack of change in vocal pitch. Expectoration is difficult and tracheobronchial secretions accumulate, with the production of wheezing. The glottic airway is not impeded.

Treatment. In unilateral cases, implantation of bone or cartilage into the paralysed cord has been reported to produce a good speaking voice.

In bilateral cases of combined paralysis, complete loss of sensation may necessitate tube-feeding or gastrostomy, and repeated aspiration of tracheobronchial secretions, preferably through a tracheostomy, may prolong life.

Lesions in the central nervous system

Motor paralyses of the larynx may be caused by lesions in the central nervous system. These are of two types: supranuclear and nuclear.

Supranuclear lesions.—Since the larynx is represented on both sides of the motor area of the cortex, a supranuclear paralysis due to a cortical lesion can occur only when that lesion is large enough to involve the laryngeal centres on both sides.

However, when the corticospinal fibres converge from each cortex into the brain stem, a relatively small lesion may be bilateral and effective.

Nuclear lesions.—Involvement if the nucleus ambiguus in diseases affecting the brain stem or bulb may produce a bilateral or, less often, a unilateral paralysis. This is usually accompanied by other signs of the causal disease, as described below.

Associated paralyses of the last four cranial nerves

The last four cranial nerves are not uncommonly involved together in a variety of pathological lesions. The ninth, tenth, and eleventh nerves share their origins in the nucleus ambiguus; they are closely related within the skull, and they have a common exit from the skull.

Although the twelfth cranial nerve has a separate exit from the skull, it is in close relationship to the other three nerves centrally, intracranially and below the base of the skull.

Paralysis of the glossopharyngeal nerve.—This causes loss of sensation over a variable portion of the tonsils and fauces, and there is loss of taste over the posterior one-third of the tongue.

Paralysis of the vagus nerve.—This causes paralysis of the palatal and pharyngeal muscles, as well as the laryngeal manifestations already described. Unilateral paralysis of the soft palate is usually symptomless but the palate is drawn to the opposite side; bilateral paralysis causes a nasal intonation (rhinolalia aperta) and regurgitation of fluids through the nose.

Unilateral paralysis of the pharyngeal muscles causes a varying degree of dysphagia and the posterior pharyngeal wall moves to the opposite side—the so-called "curtain movement"; bilateral paralysis produces severe dysphagia.

Paralysis of the accessory nerve.—That part of the nerve which is functionally differentiated from the vagus arises from the cervical spinal cord and it supplies the sternomastoid muscle and the upper part of the trapezius muscle. The sterno-mastoid rotates the head to the opposite side; paralysis of the trapezius causes a flattening and weakness of elevation of the shoulder, and often some slight winging of the scapula at rest.

Paralysis of the hypoglossal nerve.—Unilateral paralysis of this nerve causes slight dysarthria, and the tongue protrudes to the weakened side. Bilateral paralysis causes severe dysarthria and difficulty with the performance of the first part of the act of swallowing. Atrophy of the tongue musculature occurs, with the formation of broad wrinkles in the mucosa. There is partial or complete inability to protrude the tongue.

The associated lesions of the last four cranial nerves may be either unilateral or bilateral, and a number of syndromes have been named after those who first described them. These include: (1) Tapia's syndrome, with paralysis of the tongue and larynx on the same side, due to involvement of the tenth and twelfth cranial nerves; (2) Avellis' syndrome, a palatolaryngeal hemiplegia due to simultaneous affection of the tenth cranial nerve, and the palatal branch of the eleventh cranial nerve; (3) Schmidt's syndrome, with paralysis of the soft palate, pharynx, larynx, and the sternomastoid and trapezius muscles due to involvement of the tenth and eleventh cranial nerves at a higher level; (4) Vernet's syndrome, incorporating the clinical features of Schmidt's syndrome plus diminution of taste over the posterior third of the tongue and loss of pharyngeal sensation due to affection of the ninth, tenth and eleventh cranial nerves; (5) Hughlings Jackson's syndrome, with homo-lateral paralysis of the tongue, soft palate, neck muscles and larynx, due to a a lesion affecting the twelfth, eleventh and tenth cranial nerves; and (6) the Collet–Sicard syndrome in which paralysis of all the above regions is associated with diminished sensation and a reduced sense of taste, due to the simultaneous involvement of the last four cranial nerves in the region of the jugular foramen. Such an extensive lesion is usually caused by neoplastic extension.

The more common causes of these syndromes include the following.

(1) Lesions within the brain stem including lower motor neurone lesions in the medulla (bulb), such as (a) destructive lesions e.g. tumours in or outside the brain stem), (b) ischaemic lesions which are more likely to be bilateral, (c) degenera-tive lesions e.g. motor neurone disease in the form of a progressive bulbar palsy, or (d) demyelinating lesions. Upper motor neurone lesions must be bilateral to be effective by reason of the bilateral corticobulbar representation of the cranial nerve nuclei; progressive bulbar palsy (syn. motor neurone disease); pseudo-bulbar palsy; arterial obstruction, as in thrombosis of the posterior inferior cerebellar artery; tumours, either primary (glioma) or secondary; and acute anterior poliomyelitis of the bulbar type.

(2) Lesions within, or at the exit from, the skull, such as posterior fossa tumours, including acoustic "neuroma"; basal meningitis, either acute or chronic, the latter type including syphilitic or tuberculous meningitis; basal fractures; and new growths involving the jugular foramen.

The most common cause in this region is a neoplasm, including those which arise from the post-nasal space.

(3) Lesions high in the neck, where any combination of the last four cranial nerves may be involved in traumatic, inflammatory or neoplastic conditions, particularly by carcinoma in nearby tissues or by the reticuloses.

Combined paralysis of these nerves is not of serious consequence *per se* when it is unilateral, but it is of the utmost gravity when it is bilateral.

Their treatment is that of the causal condition, whenever that is possible. Some degree of recovery is to be expected when the cause is an inflammatory condition in the neck, or a toxic peripheral neuritis. In syphilitic pachymeningitis recovery is unlikely. Traumatic lesions of the nerves are usually irreparable. In lesions of the central nervous system the condition may remain stationary for a long time.

PSYCHOGENIC DISORDERS OF THE LARYNX

Anaesthesia, hyperaesthesia and paraesthesia

These may all be psychogenic in origin. The clinical features of these conditions have been described above.

Nervous laryngeal cough

This is not uncommon at the time of puberty, and it consists of repeated dry, irritating non-productive bouts of adductor spasm. It ceases during sleep or when the attention is otherwise diverted. The voice is unaffected.

It is important to eliminate any causal irritation in the nose or throat.

Hysterical spasm of the larynx

This is a form of inspiratory spasm of the glottis usually occurring in adults. It is often associated with sensations of choking and strangulation.

Functional aphonia

The larynx is one of the most vulnerable parts of the body to hysterical reaction, because it is so fundamental to such acts as swallowing, breathing, and speaking. Although aphonia is one of the most dramatic and least disabling "paralyses" for an hysteric to portray, and it is by far the commonest of the psychogenic conditions affecting the larynx, it is nevertheless relatively rare (cf. myasthenia laryngis, p. 552).

Typically it occurs in young women, not uncommonly after acute emotional stress. The onset and recovery are usually sudden and, although the patient can whisper audibly, she is unable to produce a normal voice.

The patient can laugh and cry normally, and she can also cough normally.

Examination with the laryngeal mirror is often surprisingly easy, with little or no tendency to gag or retch. On attempted phonation, the vocal cords come towards the midline, but they do not quite meet and they tend to have a bowed appearance. On the other hand, the glottis closes normally and explosively when the patient is asked to cough.

It is important to remember that adductor weakness of the vocal cords may be seen in phthisical subjects and a chest x-ray is always advisable with a first attack.

Treatment must be directed to psychological adjustment to the emotional cause, and if simple explanation and persuasion do not succeed in preventing recurrence, early psychiatric treatment is advisable before the condition becomes firmly established.

REFERENCES AND BIBLIOGRAPHY

Blackburn, G., and Salmon, L. F. (1961). "Cord Movements after Thyroidectomy". *Brit. J. Surg.*, **48**, 371.

Ellis, Maxwell (1954). *Modern Trends in Diseases of the Ear, Nose and Throat.* London; Butterworths.

Hawe, P., and Lothian, K. R. (1960). "R. C. N. Injury during Thyroidectomy". *Surg. Obstet. Gynec.*, **110**, 488.

Hoover, W. (1932). *Arch. Otolaryng.*, **15**, 339.

Kelly, J. D. (1941). *Arch. Otolaryng.*, **33**, 293.

King, B. T. (1939), *J. Amer. med. Ass.*, **112**, 814.

Lawson, H. P. (1955), *J. Laryng.*, **69**, 374.

Sharpey-Schafer, E. P. (1953). *Brit. med. J.*, **2**, 860.

Williams, A. F. (1958). "Recurrent Laryngeal Nerve Lesions during Thyroidectomy". *Surgery*, **43**, 435.

Williams, R. G. (1959). *J. Laryng.*, **73**, 161.

Wilson, T. G. (1962). *Diseases of the Ear, Nose and Throat* (2nd ed.). London; Heinemann.

Woodman, de Graaf (1946). *Arch. Otolaryng.*, **43**, 63.

21

OCCUPATIONAL DISORDERS OF THE LARYNX

John Ballantyne

LARYNGOCOELE

This rare dilatation of the ventricular saccule of the larynx is usually found in adult males, particularly in glass blowers and players of wind instruments. Although the laryngeal saccule is vestigial in man, it is dilated to form an air sac in many of the higher apes and other mammals; these air sacs are expansile and it is believed that they are used for re-breathing of air at times of physical stress (Negus, 1949).

Laryngocoeles may project internally into the larynx as a swelling beneath the ventricular band and aryepiglottic fold resembling a cyst; or alternatively, they present as external subcutaneous swellings in the subhyoid region, having expanded through the thyrohyoid membrane (Fig. 241). They are often bilateral and can be

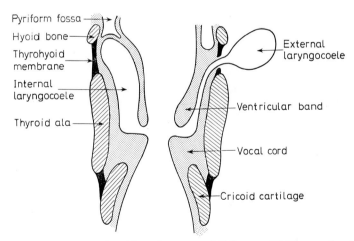

Fig. 241.—Laryngocoeles. (*From Simpson and Colleagues* (1960), *reproduced by courtesy of* John Wright.)

seen and felt to bulge on coughing or performing the Valsalva manoeuvre (Fig. 242), but completely disappear on pressure. They can be demonstrated radiologically by taking an x-ray during forcible Valsalva expiration. Differential diagnosis of the internal variety from ventricular cysts must be considered.

Symptoms. Internal laryngocoele if large may cause voice changes or attacks of dyspnoea. The external type may present as a large acutely inflamed cyst in the neck, if its narrow communication through the thyrohyoid membrane becomes obliterated by infection. Perhaps the majority of both types are asymptomatic and are only discovered accidentally in the course of routine laryngological or x-ray examination.

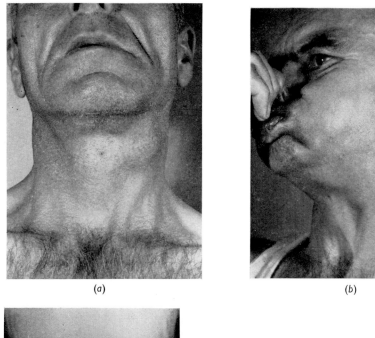

(a) (b)

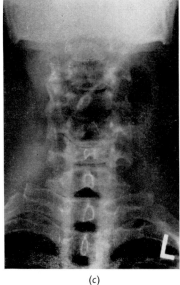

(c)

Fig. 242.—(a) and (b) Patient demonstrating large external laryngocoele; (c) postero-anterior x-ray of the same case.

Treatment, which is only indicated if symptoms are troublesome, consists of excision by an external approach to the thyrohyoid membrane. It may be necessary to divide the thyroid cartilage vertically to obtain access to the intralaryngeal

THE VOICE AND ITS DISABILITIES IN SINGERS AND OTHER VOICE-USERS

portion of the sac. The laryngocoele is dissected free, excised, and its stump closed and invaginated. The thyrohyoid membrane is meticulously repaired with sutures.

THE VOICE AND ITS DISABILITIES IN SINGERS AND OTHER VOICE-USERS

The subject of vocal disabilities in singers and other professional (and amateur) voice-users has for too long been shrouded in a sort of *mystique*, whose persistence has been due mainly to a false belief on the part of many laryngologists that these conditions are unique among vocalists and that their treatment requires special training. But the correct treatment of these vocal affections in singers differs in no way from the treatment which we advise for the same conditions in those whose living is not dependent upon the use of voice; and it is fair to say that all the conditions which affect singers can occur also in those who do not use their voices excessively but that, by virtue of the much greater insults to which these people subject their larynges, there are some affections which tend to occur with much greater frequency in professional voice-users than in the general population. It is advisable, therefore, to have some knowledge of their temperament and personality.

Most singers and actors are friendly, sociable people who tend to indulge freely in the pleasures of the table and the bottle; and they are great talkers, who give their voices far too little of the rest which they need and deserve. Extrovert yet sensitive, they are usually conscientious to a fault, having been brought up in the traditional belief that "the show must go on"; and they are loath to cancel any performance unless it is absolutely necessary. However, it is precisely this attitude of compulsion which may lead them sometimes into vocal trouble, coming on as it often does when they undertake an unfamiliar work whose excessive demands are artistic rather than purely vocal. The laryngologist may be at an advantage, therefore, if he has some knowledge of music and the stage, for only in this way can he assess fully the length and difficulty of a particular part.

Similarly, the daily background of these artists should be understood, and some of the most successful of them spend many of their waking, working hours in the dry, dusty, overheated atmospheres of old theatres, concert halls, opera houses, studios and night clubs, or in the air-conditioned dryness of aeroplanes flying them from one engagement and climate to another. Nothing, of course, could be worse for their throats; or, as Punt puts it: "When one considers the nature of vocal cord vibrations during singing or dramatic speaking, it seems clear that the cords can only be expected to withstand such exercise if they are lubricated with an adequate amount of their mucus, especially from the glands in the laryngeal ventricles." Smoking too, should be generally discouraged, particularly in singers, but it is impossible to lay down any firm "laws" about this and two of the greatest living singers of the German *lied* are quite heavy smokers.

The problem of the dry throat is well known to even the most occasional of public speakers, and it is one which may also affect the most experienced professional, especially during an attack of "stage-fright". Nor should one forget that many of the sore throats and husky voices seen and heard by a laryngologist may be but local manifestations of a failure to succeed in a chosen career of singing or acting.

THE HUMAN VOICE

Although it may be conceded that voice production is of secondary importance, both developmentally and functionally, compared with the protective role of the larynx, it is nevertheless true that it has acquired a unique position in man, as the main motor organ of communication through speech.

The muscles of the larynx, and the movements produced by them, are described in Volume 1, as also is the normal mechanism of speech; and the physiological mechanism of voice production. But we are concerned here solely with the voice as such, and in particular with the voice of singers.

The instrument of the voice

The human voice is a wind instrument which has three essential parts: the bellows; the reeds; and the resonators.

The bellows

"The bellows" of the vocal instrument are provided by the lungs, which supply the motive power to the vocal mechanism. In order to produce voice a prolonged and *controlled* act of respiration is necessary and in sustained singing the lungs must be capable of filling rapidly and of emptying in a steady, *controlled* manner. So important is this control of respiration to the singer that the late Elisabeth Schumann taught that "singing is breathing", and indeed she believed that, apart from articulation, breathing should be the only active part of singing. Ideally, singers' chests should be large, and Guthrie (1938), in his classical paper on the "Physiology of the Vocal Mechanism" suggested that an incorrect method of breathing was perhaps the chief cause of vocal failure.

In the so-called "old Italian method", probably the one most widely used by singers, the upward expiratory movement of the diaphragm is sustained and re-inforced by the controlled contraction of the muscles of the abdominal wall, known to teachers of singing as the "abdominal press".

The reeds

The "reeds", of course, are the vocal cords. But the "reeds" of the human vocal mechanism differ from mechanical reeds in that they are mobile and their tension can be varied; and being contractile they can be altered in consistency, shape and dimensions. Consequently a wide range of notes can be produced, with rapid changes in pitch, intensity and quality.

The air stream supplied by the lungs is forced through the narrow glottis and this causes the edges of the vocal cords to vibrate, thus cutting up the air stream into a very rapid series of puffs, and consequently producing a tone (Punt, 1952). The fundamental pitch of the note produced is determined by the frequency of these vibrations, but the vocal cords do not vibrate merely as a whole; they vibrate also in segments, it is thought, and the segmental vibrations add harmonics to the fundamental tone.

Recent work by von Leden (1960), in Chicago, supports this "aerodynamic theory" of phonation. Using ultra slow-motion cinephotography by indirect laryngoscopy, he demonstrated that the passage of air under pressure was a necessary prerequisite for normal laryngeal vibrations and voice production. In one patient with a tracheostomy, vibrations of the vocal cords ceased as soon as his breath bypassed the larynx, thus disproving the "neuro-chronaxie theory" of a French laryngologist (Husson, 1950) who purported that vibrations of the vocal cords were initiated and maintained entirely by nerve stimuli and not by the physical passage of air through the "reeds" from the "bellows". Some of the evidence for and against each of these theories is discussed in detail in Volume 1.

The resonators

The "resonators" of the voice are supplied by the cavities of the throat and mouth, and to some extent perhaps by the chest.

The vibrations of the vocal cords are communicated to the surrounding air, forcing it into waves and these waves pass into and through the pharynx and mouth. Without the resonators, the laryngeal tone is weak and indefinite, but by passing through these cavities the fundamental tones and the various overtones of the larynx are amplified selectively to varying degrees and the primary vocal sound is endowed with various qualities of resonance, such as volume, carrying power, timbre and "richness". In short, the resonators contribute to the beauty of the voice.

By virtue of the muscular elements within their walls, the cavities of the throat and mouth can be varied in shape, consistency and dimensions, and a large throat and mouth are desirable for powerful resonance; the chest cavity may also add volume and "richness". The exact rôle of the nose and sinuses is uncertain, but it cannot be doubted that vocal resonance is affected by disease of these structures, possibly by interfering with the subjective sensations experienced by the singer.

Some physiological aspects of singing

Pitch

There is nowadays more or less universal agreement that the pitch of the human voice is determined by the frequency of vibration of the vocal cords, but there is still much confusion about the way in which these variations in frequency are brought about. It has already been said that there is little support for the "neuro-chronaxie theory" of a certain French school which maintains that the vibrations of the vocal cords are initiated entirely by nervous stimuli, and the very great majority of investigators support the "aerodynamic theory" which postulates that the passage of air through the glottis under pressure is essential for normal vibrations of the cords. What is less certain is the role played by variations in the subglottic air pressure in the control of pitch.

Negus (1962), contributing to the *Encyclopaedia Britannica*, expresses the view that vocal pitch appears to depend on the relationship between the elasticity of the glottal margins and the pressure of air expelled from the trachea; and he believes that pitch can be increased by an increase in air pressure alone, the elasticity of the cords remaining almost unchanged. He even goes so far as to say that in the higher notes, a rise in pitch may be produced principally by a rise in air pressure.

Indeed it is one of the time-honoured axioms of laryngeal physiology that the pitch of the voice rises when the subglottic air pressure and air flow are increased, all other factors being constant. But this concept has recently been challenged by

545

Rubin (1963). In his investigations on dogs, he found that variations in air flow within physiological limits did *not* alter the resultant pitch, as determined by the intensity of contraction of the cricothyroid (external tensor) and thyro-arytenoid (internal tensor) muscles, although they did alter the volume (q.v., infra).

However, there is virtually unanimous agreement that the vocal cords elongate progressively as the pitch rises, and that this lengthening of the cords is a function of the cricothyroid muscle. During phonation, the cricoid cartilage rocks forward under the pull of the cricothyroid muscle. This in its turn increases the distance from the anterior to the posterior commissure and hence the glottis is elongated and the slack taken up. This powerful stretch tension of the external tensor provides a framework within which the internal tensor (the thyro-arytenoid muscle) can effect certain restricted variations in pitch.

Slow motion cinephotographic studies have demonstrated other changes in the vocal cords with variation in pitch and although there is no unanimity in the interpretation of these changes, there is much support for the following ideas. In the production of lower notes, for example, the whole length of the vocal cords (including the arytenoids) vibrates; the opposing surfaces of the cords present a "thick" edge (Fig. 243); and the period of approximation is prolonged. By contrast,

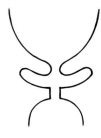

Fig. 243.—"Thick" cordal margins in low notes.

in the production of higher notes, the membranous cords alone are permitted to vibrate whilst the arytenoids are held firmly together; the opposing edges of the vocal cords are definitely thinned and come into contact with one another only with a sharp-edged "thin" margin (Fig. 244); and this contact is only momentary.

Fig. 244.—"Thin" cordal margins in high notes.

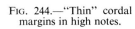
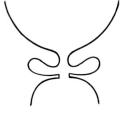

In the "falsetto" voice, heard mainly in tenors, the vibrations are much faster and there is even less contact between the sharpened edges of the vocal cords; and in some voices only the anterior segments of the cords appear to move at very high pitches (Fig. 245).

In inexperienced singers, the whole larynx will often be seen to rise as the pitch of the voice rises, but most experienced singers and teachers of singing believe that this is undesirable and indeed, in some celebrated singers, the larynx is known to descend as the pitch is raised. It is probable that the disadvantage of allowing the larynx to ascend as pitch rises is due in part to an elongation of the subglottic air column, and in part to the fact that it entails activity on the part of the accessory muscles, with consequent reduction in the resonating properties of the supraglottic structures of the throat and mouth.

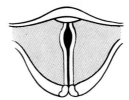

FIG. 245.—The "falsetto" voice

Although the breath pressure is under the conscious control of the singer, the action of the vocal cords is, or should be, entirely passive and is under the "automatic" control of the mind. As Madame Puritz (1956) expressed it "The mind determines pitch of the voice. The vocal cords must respond passively to the combined agents, mind and breath."

Loudness

The loudness (or volume or intensity) of the voice is determined largely by the air pressure from the "bellows" of the lungs, and a progressive increase in the air flow at any given pitch is accompanied by progressively greater vocal loudness. But vocal intensity is not influenced by air flow alone. A trained singer, for example, can sustain a singing tone *forte* about as long as he can sustain it *pianissimo*; furthermore, as Rubin has said, "he may be able to accomplish a maximal vocal effort without so much as causing the flame of a candle held before his open mouth to flicker".

There must therefore be some other factor which also contributes to the determination of vocal loudness, and this is thought to be the intensity of contraction of the tensor muscles, that is to say, sound pressure levels are greatly affected by the degree of glottic resistance above.

Hence vocal loudness is determined by the balance between the air flow from the lungs and the tension of the cricothyroid and thyro-arytenoid muscles.

Rubin's studies have emphasized the importance of correct breathing in speaking and singing. Since greater sound volume may be achieved by heightened tension of the vocal muscles alone, inadequate breath support and associated disturbances of the optimal relationships between air flow and glottal resistance will subject the vocal apparatus to undue and harmful stress (Rubin, 1963).

Timbre

The tonal quality of the voice is determined mainly by the relative amplitude of the harmonic partials, or overtones, generated in the resonating cavities.

The fundamental laryngeal frequency and the overtones caused by the segmental vibrations of the vocal cords are radiated from the larynx into the throat and mouth, and the harmonic structure of the voice sounds can thus be modified, by the singer or speaker, partly by the natural frequency and the resonance characteristics of the cavities themselves and partly by changes in the shape, dimensions and consistency of the "resonators".

It is possible that the "richness" of the voice may also be determined, to some extent, by minimal changes in the "thickness" of the cordal margins and by minor variations above and below the fundamental tone, similar to the vibrato effect produced by the violinist.

In recent experiments upon himself Donovan (1967), with many years of personal experience both as a singer and as a laryngologist, has also produced evidence that some at least of the total variations in singing have their origin in the larynx itself. By "fixing" his own oropharynx with an acrylic mould (thus preventing any alterations in its resonating properties) and recording his own voice on a "sonagraph", he has found that an increase of laryngeal intensity associated with a rise of subglottic pressure will lead to a progressive increase in the relative amount of energy in the higher harmonics, especially when singing low notes.

The range of the human voice

Nadoleczny, as long ago as 1926, wrote that the newborn infant cries on a note of approximately 435 Hz and, as growth proceeds, the vocal range is extended until, at the end of the first year, it encompasses six half-tones; at the end of the fourth year it covers about an octave, and just before puberty an octave and a half.

At puberty the male larynx grows very rapidly and the vocal cords increase appreciably in length. This process of "breaking" may take as little as six months or as long as two years to become complete; and the change may occur as early as the eighth year or be delayed as late as the eighteenth. The vocal pitch falls by one sixth at its upper limit, and by an octave at its lower limit.

In girls the change is much less marked. It is more rapidly completed and results merely in a slight extension of the upper and lower limits.

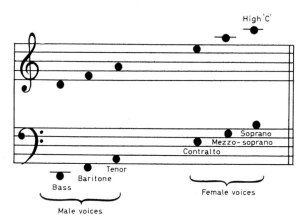

FIG. 246.—The range of adult singing voices.

In normal speech, the fundamental frequency of the adult larynx may range from as low as 80 Hz in men's voices to as high as 400 Hz in women's, with an average of 128 Hz in men and 256 Hz in women. The normal conversational range is rather less than one octave.

The vocal range in singing, however, is considerably wider, with an *overall range* (from bass to soprano) of about four octaves. But exceptional cases have been reported in which singers have been able to produce frequencies as low as 44 Hz and as high as 2048 Hz.

The average range of each individual is about two octaves (Fig. 246) but with training this may be extended to two (or even three) whole tones above and below this range.

"Registers"

If we listen carefully to a singer singing up or down a scale, we may often detect one or two changes—or "breaks"—in the quality of the sound he produces. These "breaks" occur as the singer passes from one "register" to another. Although there is much confusion about these registers, there is no doubt at all in the mind of any singer that these do exist, and some of the confusion about them is due to the fact that the singer (and the teacher of singing) uses one terminology which is based on his (or her) own sensations, while the physiologist and laryngologist tend to use a different terminology which is based on their observations of changes which occur within the larynx itself. Perhaps this is not a bad thing, for as the speech therapist Margaret Greene has said: "Success in singing is based upon natural physical endowment and artistic gifts; and no amount of insight into the mechanism of voice production will compensate for lack of these." Too carping an attention to detail can destroy the equilibrium of the whole, and the great singer doubtless achieves a perfect mastery of his art far better through unscientific and illogical verbal instruction than by a scientific approach which may destroy the really artistic interpretation necessary.

The singer talks of a *chest register* and a *head register* (with sometimes a middle register between them), whilst the physiologist and the laryngologist refer to a "thick" register and a "thin" register. The physiological basis of these latter terms has already been discussed (*see* Pitch *above*) and they describe fairly accurately one of the changes which occur in the opposed edges of the vocal cords, which are "thick" in approximately the lower octave of the singer's range, and "thin" in singing the upper octave. Indeed some highly-trained singers are even able to distinguish a "thick" or a "thin" sensation within the larynx itself as they sing in their lower or higher ranges respectively.

Much more evident to most singers, however, are the sensations of vibrations which they experience in the chest (in the lower range) and in the head (in the higher range). This becomes even more baffling when they refer to chest "resonance" and head "resonance". But surely this confusion is due, at least in part, to the fact that the singer and the scientist are talking at cross-purposes: that is to say, that the singer is referring to the sensation of vibrations (or "resonance") which he himself experiences in the "resonators" of the chest or the head while the scientist is more concerned with the sensations formed in the listener by the "resonators" of the larynx, throat and mouth.

It is perfectly true that the sinuses form no part of the wind-instrument of the voice: that, in this restricted sense, there can therefore be no justification for the use (by teachers of singing) of the expression "sinus tone production"; and that there can be no question of a singer "directing" the voice to a definite part of the face or head. But this negative attitude is not at all helpful in explaining why it is—and no singer has any doubt about this—that in the higher "register" every trained and experienced singer feels a sensation of *maximal* vibration somewhere in the head or face; and that many excellent teachers of singing will aver that few pupils are able to produce the best quality of sound in their higher registers unless and until they have experienced these sensations.

The voice is, after all, the only musical instrument which is actually a part of the instrumentalist. May it not be, therefore, that the large air-containing cavity of the chest "resounds" within the singer himself—in the true physical sense—when he sings his lower notes, whilst the smaller air-containing cavities of the sinuses "resound" when he sings in his higher register?

It would appear, in fact, that the main confusion about this subject arises from our failure to distinguish between the sensation produced in the listener by the "resonators" in the singer's throat and mouth from those produced in the singer himself by the "resonators" of his chest and head, and we must not dismiss "registers" simply because we cannot explain them.

As Guthrie said, over 30 years ago, "it is not easy to describe an art in terms of science".

VOCAL DISABILITIES

Although the conditions now to be described may occur to some extent in any person, they do, by the very nature of their origin, tend to be seen to a much greater extent in singers and in others who use their voices excessively, such as teachers and clergymen.

Non-infective laryngitis

This is a relatively common condition which usually results from screaming or shouting or other vocal excesses, either in duration or loudness. It may also be due to over-indulgence in coughing, smoking or the drinking of alcoholic drinks, especially spirits.

The condition may be acute or chronic. The main symptom is hoarseness, but even simple conversational speech may produce soreness in the throat, with a lowering of the pitch of the voice.

The vocal cords are dull, rough-looking and pink in colour, and the rest of the laryngeal mucosa is often diffusely reddened (Plate Xa). However, it must be emphasized that many professional singers, especially basses and baritones, have normally some slight pinkness of the cords, even when their voices are at their very best.

Treatment is mainly by vocal rest, and singers and actors so affected should be advised to avoid all such social engagements as cocktail parties, and others which involve much talking in an atmosphere of smoke and noise.

Punt (1968) has devised a very effective solution for local application to the pharynx and larynx in such cases, It is a 0·5 per cent solution of di-phen-hydramine hydrochloride (Benadryl), preferably made up in a vehicle of liquor *pro guttae*, to discourage contaminants. If there is much sticky mucus in the throat a tablet of Ascoxal (ascorbic acid 100 mg.; sodium percarbonate 70 mg.; copper sulphate 0·2 mg.; and menthol 2 mg.) may be added, with advantage, as a mucolytic agent. This is an excellent vasoconstrictor and a mild and comforting analgesic. Alternatively solvellae borac co., BPC, may be helpful.

One or other of these solutions may be applied, first to the pharynx with a de Vilbiss spray and then to the larynx with curved laryngeal spray. However, they should be reserved for use before an actual performance and in any event not more than once a day—until such time as the artist has an opportunity of resting his voice.

A distinct danger of such applications is that they may improve the voice so much that "the performer may throw caution to the winds and do more laryngeal damage by further vocal excesses". The laryngologist should warn him of this risk and his assessment of the situation, especially in terms of further vocal use, should be tempered with great restraint.

Submucosal haemorrhages of the vocal cords

This rather rare condition (*see* also p. 371) is due to a submucosal extravasation of blood following a sudden severe vocal strain.

The patient notices a sudden onset of hoarseness and local pain following immediately upon an intense vocal strain, and he (or perhaps more commonly she) may notice vocal fatigue on speaking.

Examination of the larynx discloses submucosal haemorrhages on one or both vocal cords, usually on or near the edge of the cord (Plate X*b*).

If treated properly, the haemorrhages will usually disappear entirely within a few weeks, leaving no scar nor other visible trace of their presence.

Vocal rest until they subside is absolutely essential, and if this is not adhered to very strictly, the haemorrhages rarely may become organized into vocal nodules.

In discussing the laryngeal problems of singers, Baker (1962) lays special emphasis on *recurrent* submucosal haemorrhages, and cites three cases in which a prominent vessel was seen on the upper surfaces of one or both cords. Meticulously careful removal of these vessels by forceps prevented any further recurrences in all these cases.

Singers' nodules (*see also* p. 363)

This is almost exclusively a disease of professional voice-users and, although occurring not uncommonly in singers (especially of the "pop" variety) it may also occur in teachers and actors. The present writer has seen vocal nodules in an actor who had "done a season" roaring the part of the lion in the play *Androcles and the Lion*. It is always due to faulty or excessive use of the voice, and among singers it is seen particularly in those who sing above their normal range (or tessitura), and especially in sopranos and tenors. It has been seen in one tenor whose reputation is based (at least in part) on the fact that he is the first tenor in a hundred years to have sung F above top C! It is said, furthermore, to be more likely to occur in singers who practise the so-called *coup de glotte* (or glottic shock technique), a forceful attack on the vocal cords somewhat akin to a cough but distinguished from it by the fact that the arytenoids remain together to prepare the vocal cords for phonation.

It has already been said that these nodules may result from the organization of submucosal haemorrhages, but nodules are usually symmetrical, haemorrhages are not. It would therefore seem more likely that, in most cases, the nodules are due to a hyperkeratosis, that is to say, that the vocal cords respond to the excessive strain by producing "corns" in the same way as the skin of the feet produces corns in response to the constant pressure of tight shoes.

At first the patient with vocal nodules may notice only a slight roughness of the voice, usually in his higher notes, especially when these are sung softly; indeed, it has been said that, ideally, a singer who cannot produce high notes softly should not sing them at all. As the nodules grow they affect the middle and, later, all the tones; and finally he is left with permanent huskiness.

Singers' nodules are usually bilateral and symmetrical (Plate X*c*). They are white or greyish-white and occur characteristically at the junction of the anterior and middle thirds of the cords.

Although an experienced singer may often be able to carry through with a particular performance, treatment is primarily by silence, and in advanced chronic cases vocal rest may be necessary for several months; in mild acute cases, however, the period need rarely exceed three weeks. Any septic focus, as in the teeth, tonsils or sinuses, should be treated before resort is made to local surgery. If these measures are not successful, the nodules may have to be removed by direct laryngoscopy with cupped forceps, one at a time, using the microsurgical technique recently introduced by Kleinsasser. Only the nodule must be removed and it is vitally important not to damage the underlying tissues of the cords. However carefully it may be performed, surgery should only be undertaken in these cases with the very greatest reluctance and, in any event, not without a generous period of vocal rest.

Vocal re-education by a singing teacher or speech therapist is an essential part of the treatment, for a return to early bad habits will almost certainly result in recurrence.

Contact ulcer

Contact ulcer (*see also* pp. 361, 362) is an uncommon condition which occurs almost exclusively in male adults.

It is largely a mechanical problem due to the hammering of one vocal process of the arytenoid against the other, and vocal abuse is an important contributory factor. *Coup de glotte* increases the risk, and coughing and constant clearing of the throat are always detrimental.

The symptoms range from mild discomfort and slight hoarseness to persistent pain, sometimes with referred otalgia, and severe persistent huskiness with vocal fatigue.

Ulceration is seen over one or both vocal processes, and in many cases the ulcer crater (usually on one side) is occupied by a granuloma which may become very large (Plate X*d*). When this is so, the prominence of the granuloma on one side may fit into the "cup" of the ulcer on the opposite side.

Von Leden and Moore (1960) recommend complete vocal abstinence, ideally for two or three weeks, followed by a period of vocal rehabilitation. The majority of ulcers will heal in three months with conservative treatment, but a granuloma must be removed by direct laryngoscopy if it persists.

Peacher (1961) has reported that most contact ulcers heal quicker with vocal therapy than with surgery, but she agrees that surgery is necessary when a large granuloma is present, advising its removal before therapy is started. She also found, however, that the healing process took longer as the number of surgical interventions increased. It is most important to treat any cough by appropriate drugs (*see* "General Management").

Myasthenia of the larynx (syn. phonasthenia)

This is the name given to a disorder of the phonatory muscles of the larynx.

Misuse of the vocal organ is common to all cases and the condition is due to indirect trauma in the form of overwork of the muscles, which become tired. This

PLATE X

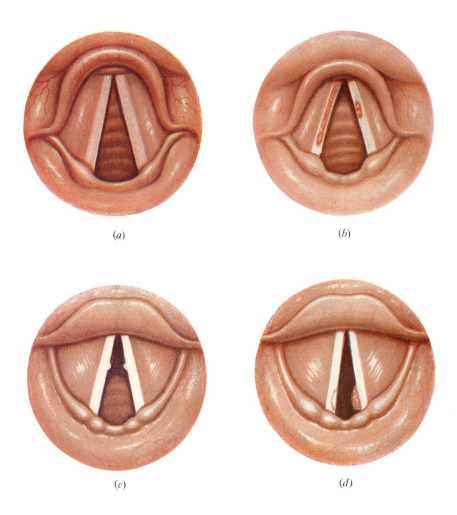

(a) Non-infective laryngitis. (b) Submucosal haemorrhages of the vocal cords. (c) Singers' nodules. (d) Contact ulcer.

may be caused by the strain of prolonged as well as violent overwork without proper intervals of rest, and is often seen in patients suffering from laryngitis due to upper respiratory infections.

The thyro-arytenoid muscles (the internal tensors) are the hardest worked muscles of the larynx in those who use their voices professionally, and it is these muscles which are most commonly affected; but the interarytenoid muscles may also be weakened.

Myasthenia of the larynx may also accompany other laryngeal diseases; and it should always be suspected if the voice *sounds* worse than the vocal cords *look* (Punt, 1968), especially inflammations of the larynx which are accompanied by myositis or associated with infections of the upper respiratory tract.

The voice is easily tired, intonation is impaired and the range is reduced. Further strain leads to hoarseness and even to complete aphonia. The throat becomes sore and dry, and may even be painful.

The acute form of phonasthenia results from a short period of excessive vocal abuse, but subacute and chronic forms also occur which are due to improper use over weeks, months or years.

When the internal tensors alone are involved, the vocal cords come together on phonation but they leave an elliptical space between them (Fig. 247a); when the interarytenoid muscles alone are affected, the cords approximate on phonation, but a triangular space is seen in the posterior commissure (Fig. 247b); and when both groups of muscles are weakened, a characteristic keyhole-shaped glottis appears on phonation (Fig. 247c).

FIG. 247.—Myasthenia of the larynx: (*a*) weakness of internal tensors; (*b*) weakness of inter-arytenoid muscles; (*c*) weakness of internal tensors and inter-arytenoid muscles.

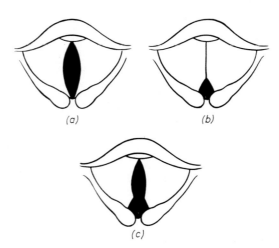

Myasthenia may be accompanied by a so-called *corditis marginatus*, which is characterized by hyperaemia of the vocal cords, especially along their free edges.

The proper treatment of the condition may demand prolonged vocal rest, which must include at least 24 hours absolute silence in acute cases; in those of longer standing the use of the voice must be stringently restricted for several weeks.

The life of a professional singer is precariously uncertain and it is not surprising, therefore, that if and when the opportunity presents itself, far too many singers are prepared to undertake far too heavy a programme of professional engagements, especially in the form of concert tours or "one night stands"; and if, as the result of these vocal excesses, a myasthenia develops, the singer is not unnaturally loath to cancel what may be his one and only engagement in a particular city, or with a particular orchestra; and so it happens that he may insist, unwisely, on fulfilling his contract, despite his laryngologist's advice to the contrary.

Although we must always recognize that it is wrong for a singer to sing with a phonasthenia—and it is our duty to advise him accordingly—we may sometimes be confronted with the singer who insists on rejecting advice which he knows to be right. But having discharged our main duty to him by proffering that advice, we cannot escape our further duty to "see him through" if he insists on singing.

The laryngologist who finds himself in such a predicament may often help his patient by referring him for a short exposure of the larynx to ultra short-wave diathermy (but never less than five or six hours before a performance), or by applying the Benadryl spray used in non-infective laryngitis (q.v.). Alternatively, he may use the well-known spray which was devised by the late Milsom Rees and named traditionally after the celebrated Australian soprano, Dame Nellie Melba. It is prescribed as follows:

Menthol	.. ..	0·3 g.
Spiritus Vini Rectificatus	.. ..	12 ml.
Amylocaine	.. ..	0·3 g.
Tinct. Ferri Perchlor. ..	.. ..	2 ml.
Glycerine	.. ..	12 ml.
Aqua. Dest.	.. ..	ad 30 ml.

This should never be used more than twice a day, and it should rarely be applied unless the singer is able to rest his voice at least until the following day.

Ventricular band voice (syn. dysphonia plicae ventricularis; psychogenic ventricular dysphonia)

Ventricular band voice is produced by the opposition of the false vocal cords in phonatory efforts. The ventricular bands normally form a closing sphincter, as in straining with breath held, and they may be used to some extent in phonation, in an attempt to compensate for myasthenia of the larynx or other vocal disabilities due to local laryngeal causes; most commonly, however, this condition is purely psychogenic in origin.

The voice is unpleasant and distorted, producing a low, gruff sound. Treatment is by vocal rest and speech therapy, but the outlook is always poor (*see also* p. 353).

Mogiphonia

Mogiphonia is the name given to a psychoneurotic form of phonic spasm which occurs in those who use their voices professionally, especially in singers, teachers and clergymen.

The vocal cords become firmly pressed together after uttering a few words, and no further sound can be emitted.

It occurs only in attempting to sing or speak in public, and disappears entirely in ordinary conversation.

The only treatment of any avail is by further training in the correct methods of voice production, but this is rarely successful and the condition has put an end to the professional careers of more than one aspiring singer.

All voices wear with age, and it is said that very few female singers are able to continue after the menopause. There are, of course, a few notable exceptions. During the course of an active professional career, however, most of the vocal failures are due to inadequacy of training (or even over-training); to excessive use and other forms of abuse, such as singing with an acute upper respiratory infection; to inadequate periods of professional abstinence, so great a problem in the present-day fashion of intensive concert tours and recording sessions; and to the singer's failure to recognize his or her own natural range, or tessitura. And in this latter respect, the singer's decision is too often based on financial, rather than purely artistic, considerations.

GENERAL MANAGEMENT

There are few *absolute* contra-indications to singing or dramatic performance, but they do exist and the chief amongst them are: uncontrolled asthma; severe acute laryngitis; and the presence of "singers' nodules", other than the very smallest of them, especially those of the acute type.

One of the most famous sopranos of all time was herself a severe asthmatic, but so effectively were her symptoms controlled that she continued to give public lieder recitals until her death at the age of 63. Occasionally, however, the condition may be so intractable that the sufferer may be better advised to give up all ideas of a singing career.

Any artist who insists on undertaking a performance in the presence of an acute infective laryngitis runs the very real risk of developing a permanent chronic laryngitis, or even nodules.

More than one famous theatrical reputation has been built on the foundations of a "gravelly" voice produced by chronic laryngitis, but none was ever enhanced by the presence of nodules. In the experience of the present author, nodules occur more commonly in untrained than in trained singers, and are due to incorrect use rather than over-use of the voice; whereas myasthenia of the laryngeal muscles (which may accompany either of the above conditions) tends to occur more commonly in classical singers, and is due usually to excessive vocal strain.

Any local laryngeal condition may call for vocal rest, but not infrequently the laryngologist is invited to proffer advice about the less serious problems of the professional voice-user.

Lubrication of the larynx

Reference has been made already to the adverse effects upon the respiratory tracts of actors and singers of those over-dry, over-heated atmospheres so often encountered in the daily round; and mention has been made also of their influence upon the lubrication of the larynx.

Some of our older theatres and concert-halls have a notorious reputation in this respect, but it would be counsel of perfection to expect managements to provide better working conditions for their artists; and it is in just these situations that the laryngologist is so often called in for help.

Simple lozenges, e.g. blackcurrant and glycerine, may be soothing when the throat is dry; and in more resistant cases tablets of 2, 3- (2- and 3-iodo-propyl-idenedoxy) propanol, usually prescribed under their proprietary name of Organidin, may be very useful, two (30 mg.) tablets being taken by mouth four times a day, for about one week.

Generally speaking, it is wise to discourage the use of "cold cures" in the treatment of simple upper respiratory infections, as most of them contain a mucus-drying agent which may increase the sense of discomfort in the nose and throat of such patients.

Treatment and prevention of upper respiratory infections

It is rarely necessary to forbid an artist to perform if he has only a mild, uncomplicated infection of the upper respiratory tract, provided that his general condition is good and his technique secure; but under such circumstances it may be helpful to spray an obstructed nose with a simple vasoconstrictor, and the pharynx and larynx with the Benadryl solution used in non-infective laryngitis or a dilute (5 per cent) solution of Argyrol, an hour or so before performing. Gargles should be discouraged, as the physical act of gargling may itself put further strain upon the already inflamed throat, and in any event they never penetrate beyond the level of the anterior faucial pillars.

Vitamin C, in the form of effervescent Redoxon tablets, one three or four times a day appears to shorten a cold in some instances; and although they are useless in pure viral infections, antibiotics may shorten the course of an acute upper respiratory illness when secondary bacterial infection has supervened.

To the average citizen, frequent colds are a nuisance; to an actor or singer they may lead to repeated cancellations of engagements, to the ultimate detriment of his career. Sometimes, but not by any means invariably, their incidence can be reduced by the use of a vaccine, preferably an autogenous one. When they do work, they can be extremely effective.

A useless cough is always positively harmful to the larynx, and it can often be suppressed by the use of physeptone methadone hydrochloride (Physeptone), one (5 mg.) tablet by mouth, not more than three times a day, for three or four days.

General supportive measures

Sometimes an artist, usually one who has been treated at one time or another in America or the mainland of Europe, will ask the laryngologist for "fortifying injections". Most commonly he has received some injections of vitamin B_{12}, apparently with some success: but strychnine is more rational as a muscle stimulant, and a dosage of 0·5 to 1 mg. may be given subcutaneously with advantage, about half an hour before a performance.

Although "pep-pills" generally are to be deprecated, one 10 mg. tablet of methyliphenidate hydrochloride (Ritalin) taken by mouth at a similar time may be helpful to someone who has been exhausted by a long tour or sleepless nights.

Anabolic steroids should be avoided, particularly in women, as they have been known to produce permanent virilizing changes in the voice; and so also should contraceptive pills. Zilstorff has reported voice changes in two sopranos, with temporary loss of their two highest tones, after only one week of taking "the pill". Fortunately, both of them recovered within one week of withdrawal.

Finally, a singer or actor who has lost confidence in his ability to see a performance through may be greatly comforted, on occasion, by the presence in the house of his laryngological adviser. This is a service which is rarely required or asked for, and treatment is hardly ever requested once the first interval has been reached.

REFERENCES AND BIBLIOGRAPHY

Baker, D. C. Jnr. (1962). "Laryngeal Problems in Singers." *Laryngoscope*, **72**, 902.

Ballantyne, J. C. (1968). "Vocal Disabilities of Singers." *Proc. R. Soc. Med.*, **61**, 1156.

Donovan, R. (1967). Personal communication.

Greene, M. C. L. (1968). "Vocal Disabilities of Singers." *Proc. R. Soc. Med.*, **61**, 1150.

Guthrie, D. (1938). "Physiology of the Vocal Mechanism." *Brit. med. J.*, **2**, 1189.

Husson, R. (1950). "Etude des phénomènes physiologiques et acoustiques fondamentaux de la vox chantée." Thesis, Faculty of Science, Paris.

von Leden, H. (1960). "Laryngeal Physiology." *J. Laryng.*, **74**, 705.

— and Moore, P. (1960). "Contact Ulcer of the Larynx—Experimental Observations." *Arch. Otolaryng.*, **72**, 746.

Nadoleczny, M. (1926). *Lehrbuch der Sprach- und Stimmheilkunde*. Leipzig; Vogel.

Negus, Sir Victor (1949). *Comparative Anatomy and Physiology of the Larynx*. London; Heinemann.

— (1962). Article on "Voice". *Encyclopaedia Britannica*.

Peacher, Georgiana M. (1961). "Vocal Therapy for Contact Ulcer of the Larynx." *Laryngoscope*, **71**, 37.

Pressman, J. J. (1938). *Proc. R. Soc. Med.*, **31**, 1179.

Punt, N. A. (1952). *The Singer's and Actor's Throat*. London: Heinemann.

— (1968). "Applied Laryngology—Singers and Actors." *Proc. R. Soc. Med.*, **61**, 1152.

Puritz, Elizabeth (1956). *The Teaching of Elisabeth Schumann*. London; Methuen.

Rubin, H. J. (1963). "Experimental Studies on Vocal Pitch and Intensity in Phonation." *Laryngoscope*, **73**, 973.

Simpson, J. F., Robin, I. G., Ballantyne, J., and Groves, J. (1960). *Synopsis of Otolaryngology*. Bristol; John Wright.

Stein, L. (1942). *Speech and Voice*. London; Methuen.

Zilstorff, K. (1965). *Nord. Med.*, **74**, 724.

22

DISORDERS OF SPEECH

C. H. EDWARDS

INTRODUCTION

Spoken speech is the commonest and nearly the most primitive part of a larger whole of communication that started with, and still includes, mime and gesture and later added picture-drawing, writing, singing, music and, lately, the extensions derived from telephone, radio and television. Speech, in the narrower sense, is perhaps the skill that most clearly separates us from the rest of the animal kingdom though the extent to which other animals can pass information in certain ways exceeds our own. We are more ignorant of the origins and derivations of speech than of mankind itself. There is no philological equivalent of Darwin's theory. We quickly realize that the subject has many facets and that each is scored with narrow crannies so that one expert may know nothing of the beliefs of another and may even be using a different set of words for his ideas. There are the philosophies such as the origins, growths and comparisons of languages. Linguistics, semantics, philology, grammar, and literary style reflect somewhat differing interests and none includes the anatomy, physiology or psychology of speech, much less elocution or speech therapy. In discussion of speech we are constrained by the difficulties of language. We find ourselves at variance as to what is the smallest unit of speech or how to define a sentence. It is therefore imperative that we confine ourselves here to one small part of a great subject, that we state which part and that we start by admitting much ignorance about it. The part is a brief discussion of the essentials of speech disorders as they are seen by the clinician and particularly by the ear, nose and throat surgeon. Those who wish to read further than this programme will find a modest bibliography at the end of the chapter.

Speech demands that we carry in our mind, that is our brain, a store of remembered symbols in which to clothe our thoughts for communication to others. This store consists of symbols used in the comprehension of the heard word, the spoken word, the read word and the written one; accumulated slowly in that order in the first few years of life. Later they may be added to, or adapted for, skills such as typewriting, shorthand and the varied aspects of music. Their form and style and number we can only surmise. It is likely that we use them to think as well as to speak, to commune with ourselves as well as with others and herein lies one of the many dilemmas. Can speech be disturbed without affecting intellect if the latter is itself dependent on internal speech? Or, in what form do we think and how much of it could we do if we were removed at birth from our fellows? Would we be the equal or not of an untrained deaf mute? The items in this store have been given many names by those conjuring them for an exploration of speech mechanisms. Brain (1965), for instance, used the word "schema". Speech disorder can happen by preventing the learning of it. This can be the result of closing a peripheral channel, such as hearing or seeing, or interfering with the complex physiology of laying down the store. It can be disrupted by disease affecting these same receptive channels, or by interfering with the mechanism of recall from the store or by destroying the contents (the schemas) of the store itself. Similarly, the expressive (executive) channels of output from the central store can be involved, that for speaking or for writing. We know some of the anatomy of this complex. There are several places in the complex where disease may fall and harm its workings. On the receptive side congenital deafness or blindness will prevent proper speech being learnt, the first more fundamentally than the other. Acquired total deafness in later life brings relatively trivial changes and disability, blindness much more. Disturbance at the point in the complex of laying down or recall, into or from the schema store, brings faults of reception. But the store, itself unharmed, is still available for internal speech (thinking) and spontaneous utterance and writing. Obviously both may happen together. Expressive speech may fail from damage to the schemas or to the ability to select them and propagate them onward. All this so far described is at a high physiological level, confined to man, and its faults are named *dysphasia*. It is a different category of disorder from *dysarthria* and *dysphonia*, both at a lower level.

It is as well to bear in mind that pure discrete forms of speech disturbance, as described below, partly for convenience of explanation of the whole complex, are not the rule whilst mixed forms are. A little thought makes this obvious. The anatomy of reception is fairly close and discrete, that of comprehension and laying down and recall of schemas is even more so. The physiological manoeuvres are even more intertwined. The evocation of schemas by heard speech and by written words is so intimate that damage to one is likely to affect the other. Expression, distal in the complex, in talking and writing also uses physiological paths in common and these are often disabled together. We monitor our own words and writing by our own intact auditory and visual skill of comprehension, so that purely receptive lesions are likely to involve execution. The speech complex of reception, mulling, thinking, preparation, expression and monitoring is carried out in swift holistic unison so that the results of damage tend to be functionally "all or none".

Anatomy and physiology

Cerebral dominance

Perhaps the most reliable knowledge of anatomy concerning the higher realms of speech is that the two sides of the brain do not usually have equal importance in this respect. Evidence about this has slowly emerged from clinicopathological correlation and the use of sodium amytal injected into the human carotid artery of one side at a time, so as to cause temporary unilateral selective paralysis. The old-fashioned simple clinical tests of a person's cerebral dominance are as reliable as any of the more complicated ones. This is determined by questions of the family history, personal preferences for early and later writing, games playing and other more or less self-taught activities such as punching, polishing and throwing; these being less subject to prejudice from parent and teacher and therefore more natural. Footedness tends to confirm handedness. The finding that the major or dominant eye, of two with roughly equal acuity, is on the same side of the body adds its considerable weight to the evidence. Thus it is possible to divide people into four groups; right handers, left handers, clear ambidextrals and uncertain. The alternatives are put into the order of their frequency. The last three together are no more than 10 per cent of the population of this country. Left handedness is twice as common in boys as in girls.

The great majority of dextrals have their speech centres in the opposite, left, hemisphere. More than one half of "truly" left handers also have their left as the dominant half-brain. More left handers and more "truly" ambidextrals have brains which seem to store the speech skills between the two sides and these people suffer dysphasia from unilateral lesions less often and less severely and recover from it better. In other words, cerebral dominance for language skill is even more prevalent to the left than is handedness to the right. It has been suggested that right handedness is determined as a Mendelian dominant and left handedness as a recessive. One can only feel certain of individual hemisphere speech dominance in full dextrals of similar stock, without the positive evidence that brain disease sometimes gives.

There are other functions of the brain which are also not equally allotted to both sides; recognition of objects and sounds, manipulative skills, topographical ability and memory, awareness of outside space and the body image and the ability for construction in building or drawing are some of them. None of them is of the same importance to the otologist as speech. These varied functions need not be accepted by the same hemisphere in the one person, some of them are indeed more often provided in the side opposite to speech, the minor or non-dominant half. The evidence suggests that the decision, so to say, as to which side should be dominant for speech is not made at birth or for some years afterwards. Both halves play an equal role in the first few experimental years perhaps and then usually one side "majors" and continues whilst the other fails to develop further in this skill. The practical outcome is that unilateral brain damage in the youngster tends to cause less immediate dysphasia and that the subsequent recovery and subsequent ability to learn further speech skill is better than in the adult, often indeed unimpaired.

Speech learning and speech centres

The anatomy of speech is perhaps best described as we trace the development of this skill in the child. We need not discuss the peripheral elements except to emphasize that they are, to a varied extent, fundamental to learning of speech and that the receivers (ears and eyes) from each side serve both halves of the brain and that the effectors of spoken speech (muscles of mouth, tongue and larynx at least) although moved on both sides of the body by either cerebral hemisphere are only made to speak by the dominant one. Thus the learning and the prosecution of the spoken and the written word is dependent upon one (or other) ear and eye and upon one (a particular one) side of the brain.

The normal infant at birth is endowed with immediate means of communication. It can cry and yell to indicate various discomforts and soon can make vague noises of contentment. With less accuracy its face may convey primitive emotion and other body movements may suggest pain. From these the psychologist can begin to evaluate crudely its capacity to react and therefore its brain potential and therefore the likelihood of it achieving intellectual normality. This simple state of affairs remains seemingly unchanged for some months until the next step in communication is taken. This is a gradually improving appreciation of what it

561

hears and sees, expressed as eye following and later a facial response to seeing its mother and a similar response to voice. These are initially and largely exercises in reception. Later, vocal mimicry by babbling and the utterance of simple sounds and words proclaims the growing accuracy of reception and the beginnings of enunciation. It is in these early months that clues may be noted of a deficiency of one or more of the needs of speech. Bilateral complete deafness is an absolute bar to the normal acquisition of spoken speech. Even skilled teaching brings a poor image of human spoken words to the congenitally deaf child. Bilateral brain damage to those parts subserving receptive speech has the same result. Blindness has a later effect on other aspects of speech. To underline that we are not dealing with the programming of a machine there are formidable delays and disorders of speech in children who have been deprived of the innumerable exogenous stimuli that come from loving care and the turmoil of an appropriate environment. Although the aetiology of autism is under dispute it occurs in physically normal children and may well be due solely to a psychological fault. The methods used to teach the deaf mute to utter words that he has never heard and to monitor them remind us that other sensations than hearing and seeing play a part in producing the finished product of spoken speech; proprioceptive impulses from the vibrating skull and movements of the muscles, tendons, joints and other peripheral tissues used in speaking. In addition, for speech to proceed to greater things than this, the child needs a sufficiency of what we term intelligence. The anatomy and physiology of intelligence is not understood beyond our knowing that it has phylogenetically to do with brain size and that too little tissue, whether by disordered growth or damage, is inconsistent with its fulfilment. However, this is not to say that a normal-looking brain is necessarily the seat of a normal intellect. The fine distinction that may be drawn between a supposed absence of particulate areas of brain on the one hand, to cause developmental speech fault with normal intelligence, and a more diffuse fault to cause amentia (carrying with it speech disturbance) is one of the reasons for disagreement between authorities.

Gradually the growing infant with normal endowments learns by repetition to attach meaning to sounds and to words and by association comes to connect these with objects seen. In this way he assembles a growing storehouse of meanings attached to words, other sounds and objects. These are available to him also in his own spoken speech. The complexity quickly grows as he finds that he has to place the same meaning to words uttered in different tones and accents and later that he must recognize different meanings in small differences of pronunciation. Later still he finds that a single word with a single pronunciation may have different meanings, e.g. hair/hare, air/heir, bear/bare. It is the means by which this storehouse is laid down and used that forms the basis for most of the theorizing, argument and quarrelling that has surrounded the subject for so long. A few simple anatomical facts such as cerebral dominance are broadly agreed but the physiology and the psychology as well as finer anatomy is disputed. This has led to the narrowest unitarianism on the one hand and the most permissive, vague holism on the other, with every compromise between. However, we may find some firm ground for belief if we proceed briefly to describe speech development in the normal.

Having achieved some proficiency in the understanding of the spoken word and its utterance, in the formation of sentences to receive others' thoughts, and in collecting words together to clothe his own, the child progresses to identify pictures. A few years later he learns the meaning attached to symbols of the written word, numbers and perhaps, as a rule later still, music. In the English language he then tussles with and overcomes the vagaries of spelling, pronouncing and meaning. Having for some time scribbled pictures he now has to learn to copy the alphabet and numbers and thus the skill of writing and arithmetic. Depending upon his natural habit and the variable press of teaching opinion he has to store further memory-meanings of letters, syllables, whole words and figures or their dotted equivalents. Later he has to recognize the same meanings to the same word, however it is written or printed, and he has to acknowledge the laws of arithmetic and music. As the years go by, depending upon his inherent gifts (about which we know no anatomy, physiology or psychology), environment, and education his vocabulary will grow and he will understand rapid and complex speech, read as quickly, transfer his ideas (perhaps even with enough elegance to profess) to others by talk or hand or typescript, memorize word-perfectly parts in many different plays, memorize tracts of music, execute music, do mental arithmetic, master foreign tonques and if necessary learn braille. All this and more is within the realm of speech All of it is peculiar to man and peculiar to the brain of man and indeed usually to one side of that brain. Our difficulty is to divine quite where and how this happens in the brain. If we now turn to what we observe in disease we shall be able to assemble what we do know, what we do not know and a vast field between. Obviously it may be easier to recognize, in oneself or another, the loss of a part or a function than its congenital absence. For example, people spend a lifetime unaware that they have a congenital homonomous hemianopia or abnormal balance or that their child has always been clumsy in movement. However, the appearance, particularly if sudden, of the same fault is immediately appreciated. For similar reasons acquired speech disorders of adult life are apt to be more amenable to analysis than children's inborn or early acquired failures. However, it would be wrong to assume that a congenital defect in one facet of speech must be equal or comparable with an acquired one in the same part of the speech mechanism or even the same part of the brain. To prevent the brain in some way from learning a skill may be a different affair from destroying the faculty already learnt.

RECEPTIVE SPEECH DISORDERS

Auditory

Congenital deafness (deaf mutism)

It will have been obvious from the foregoing brief account of the child's learning to speak that one essential key is hearing and a growing understanding of what is heard. In the normal child the back of the learning of his native tongue is broken by the time he is five or six years old. This phenomenal achievement is dependent upon a more or less constant bombardment with meaningful noises of many kinds. This is what his parents and family give him, particularly his mother. Deprivation of this stimulus can be as damaging to speech learning as deafness and this gives the clue to the management of the deaf child. He needs his hearing not only to hear and to put meaning to spoken words but to monitor and to mould his own speech into increasingly exact replica-words of his parents and teachers so that they emerge from him with the same packaging of vowels, consonants and syllables, enunciated with the same accents, and with the same content of meaning as theirs. Later he may learn to alter both sound and meaning to comply with a wider horizon than his home but at first he is as exact a copying machine as the size and shape of his tissues of speech allow. This auditory monitoring is assisted by kinaesthetic sensations from the periphery; of touch, tension in muscles and ligaments and skin and vibrations set up in the caverns of the nose, mouth, larynx and chest. When hearing is lost or never present these assume greater importance. But the flat, improperly pitched voice of the severely deaf adult shows how poor an aid to speaking they are as compared with hearing.

It used to be thought that the infant at birth was endowed with a pre-set level of intelligence, measured perhaps by the number of neurones in his brain. This share was looked upon as genetically determined and subject only to an absence of damage. Now it is shown that the measure of intelligence can fluctuate according to the amount and quality of the stimulus applied to it. The same is shown to be true of the sense of hearing in its broadest concept, that the ability to learn the meaning of words and other sounds is dependent upon the practice that the appropriate part of the brain is given and that much depends, as in other skilled learnings, on how early in life the practice is begun. Delay cannot be brooked if a good quality is to be reached.

It is the congenital or very early acquired deafness, preventing the learning of speech, that is the main concern of the otologist so far as speech is concerned. To overlook this as the cause of mutism or as the mimic of amentia or of psychologically determined backwardness or withdrawing is to make an irreparable error far more costly than to misjudge a later dysphasia or dysarthria. It is now widely accepted that absolute congenital deafness is rare and that some hearing is nearly always present. The manipulation of that remnant, by any means, so as to use this normal physiological channel into the mind gains far better results than the only alternative methods, the manual or the oral. The first uses hand signs and the other lip reading. Both condemn the child to spend his communication mostly with those equally deprived.

The identification of the deaf child and its management is dealt with in Volume 2. The separation of the deaf child from the imbecile and the psychologically distressed and the one with auditory agnosia is not always easy. The precise assessment of the degree and quality of his deafness and the best means of surmounting it whilst at the same time guiding the parents and husbanding their essential aid is demanding and specialized work with rich spiritual rewards.

Auditory agnosia

Here there is no deafness that matters and intelligence is not impaired greatly if at all. But the person, having previously done so, fails to understand the meanings of any sounds. The fault may be complete or partial in two senses. It may cover all kinds of sounds or not, and it may be total or partial in depth for any particular kind of noise. For instance, the patient may fail to comprehend the means or the meaning or the message of a ringing bell (though hearing it perfectly) or of any other noise. He may be unable to separate speech sounds from any other. If there is a partial fault in depth, so to speak, the sounds of more complex meanings suffer the most. Thus speech and music, for instance, are not spared if agnosia exists for grosser sounds. One might describe the new-born baby, without experience and with brain of virgin soil, as being near completely sound agnostic. Not quite so however, for it will show some primitive, feeble defence responses to certain noises indicating that the stimulus has some inherent "meaning". The adult sufferer from acquired disease may not even show that.

Clearly this state of affairs is not easy to diagnose but one is helped by the fact that the patient's spontaneous speech and writing are usually normal and that he can read accurately and therefore communication with him is possible on a high level. It is rare. The evidence from morbid anatomy is that the cause is a lesion of the dominant hemisphere close to, perhaps sometimes involving, the posterior part of the first temporal convolution and the adjoining part of the parietal lobe.

Word or speech deafness

This is a less gross and more particulate example of auditory agnosia. The patient hears normally and understands the meaning of other sounds but fails to a greater or lesser degree to comprehend the spoken word. Indeed, the patient hears his own tongue as though it was a foreign language. As for many of us, in a language in which we are unskilled, the patient may understand a word or two and a simple linkage of them. Other facets of speech may be normal so that reading, spontaneous speaking, reading aloud and writing or copying are all unimpaired. This situation too is rare and as a pure entity has been denied by some. In other cases the same word deafness exists in combination with a profound loss of the ability to read and this double fault always seems to be associated with expressive difficulty. The fact that word deafness may exist in two forms or stages (as a pure entity or combined with dyslexia and then with expressive dysphasia) suggests that there is a central pool lying physiologically between the receptive speech stations and the executive or expressive ones. The pure form could then be imagined as a fault confined to the function of giving meaning to heard symbols, the mixed form being a disturbance of a physiological complex subserving more than that.

This brings us to the central core of the problem in more than one sense. Upon receipt of the information from without by ways of ears and eyes, how and where is it manipulated into food for thought, the production of ideas, the stimulation of emotion or the pronunciation of utterance? Many different authors through the decades have imagined these processes and given different names to the pieces, so to speak, in the puzzle. These theories have come from widely differing disciplines and have carried the imprint of their authors' persuasion. Brain and Critchley in this country particularly have written widely on this aspect. Some of their contributions are listed at the end of this chapter. Brain, very briefly, considers that we build up in our mind a growing collection of images or schemas, as he calls them, that are evoked by letters, words and sentences, both heard and read. This process is regarded as physiological rather than psychological. The word-schemas are the keys to meaning and are the product of repeated evocation by ear and eye with cross reference between both. These schemas are either available to executive speech mechanisms or "copies" of them are. They are moulded more finely or etched more deeply by the repeated action of ear and eye and by the smoothing action of manipulating them by using them in speech and writing, and the proprioceptive impulses from the moving parts of tongue and mouth and throat that are essential to this skilled juggling. We have already seen that their very presence depends upon a sufficiency of hearing and seeing, though schemas of less general use can be made by one of those senses alone and are then not transferable to the use of the other. If these schemas are spared by the damage causing a receptive dysphasia then they are available to internal speech, and therefore thinking, to speaking thoughts aloud or to writing them. In these circumstances the fault is only that heard speech cannot evoke the proper schemas. If the schemas share in the damage then the comprehension of the written word, internal speech (thinking) and expressive speech are all involved and the disability is greater. This state is what Wernicke described as central aphasia. Such a dysphasia can be more or less severe. One variety of it concerns chiefly or only the names of objects and is called *nominal dysphasia*.

Visual

Comparison and analogies between hearing and seeing in speech communication are not exact or even close. Reading is a later learnt and more highly evolved and rarer skill than the understanding of the spoken word. Indeed, a proportion of our population of normal intelligences have not been pressed, or impelled by curiosity, to learn to read more than the simplest and most clearly printed words. They can follow the pictures in comic papers and read the title but not the text. Such a person can inevitably write no better, usually a scrawled signature only. This sorry state in someone of normal intellect shows us how much more there is to speech than anatomy and physiology. High degree mental defective persons can understand much of what is said simply, so indeed can some animals. The fundamentally basic nature of spoken speech, receptive and expressive, is emphasized by a consideration of how much more disabled and deprived the congenitally deaf person is as compared with the blind. The former is imprisoned by silence, in a state of ignorance comparable with a domestic animal, a prison whose walls have to be breached by patience and ingenuity from without. His experience is gained without the softening and easing of spoken explanation until he learns to comprehend the moving signals of hands, lips and face. His exquisite gift of discriminative touch is of no avail in communication. Only by most arduous means can an understanding of the symbols of written speech be achieved, unless electrical amplification makes him hear. How different are the problems of the congenitally blind person. He learns to understand the spoken word and to speak himself with no added difficulty. All that he fails to receive by sight is amenable to description and explanation so that his fingertips (or lips if he lacks them) can be educated to perform the equal in communication of reading. The same fingers can probe the outside world and clothe his imagination, already well provided for by his friends, with facts of size and shape and texture. However, all these differences in privilege between the congenitally deaf and the blind in their formative years are lost or levelled by time so that the adult is much less disabled by the acquisition of complete deafness than by the onset of blindness unless his calling particularly demands the ear. Many of us would unhesitatingly choose to be afflicted by deafness rather than blindness and yet all would surely elect for the opposite in an infant.

Congenital blindness

This can happen at any anatomical level of the visual system, from eye to visual cortex, and for a number of different reasons. If the intelligence be good, however, we have already seen how other channels into it may be used to provide a normal educational diet. The ears and the finger tips can successfully by-pass the blocked visual channel to the mind.

Visual agnosia

Analogous with auditory agnosia is the situation when, with a normal ability to see, the person fails to understand the meaning of what he sees—visual agnosia. This may apply to all objects or, at a higher physiological level, may only concern written symbols of speech; dyslexia or alexia, depending upon severity. As in the case of hearing a gross agnosia, for common objects for instance, does not allow a sparing of a higher function such as recognition of written words. Thus dyslexia can be alone without general visual agnosia but not vice versa.

Dyslexia

Acquired dyslexia is not of prime importance to the otologist. He is far less likely to be confronted by an undiagnosed example of it than his ophthalmologist colleague and will more often be asked to identify a fault of receptive speech in the auditory range. However, it is of interest for analogy. Acquired brain disease, most often ischaemia, may rob a person of his ability to read yet leave untouched his acuity of sight. He ceases to comprehend the meaning of written or printed symbols of speech yet seeing them clearly. The fault may be of variable degree. It may be so pure that no other department of communication is touched, so that writing from dictation and copying and the spontaneous writing of thoughts are unimpaired or only minimally affected. However, it is rare for handwriting not to be changed at all and copying is usually slower than normal. This pure form has been called agnosic alexia, pure word blindness or simply alexia. Not surprisingly the disturbance may extend so as to affect the skill of writing and this too may be totally or partly abolished. Since we monitor our writing by our ability to read it is clear how a disorder of the last might involve the quality of the other. The mixed variety, when both skills are severely damaged, is named visual asymbolia or better alexia with agraphia. In both examples the responsible lesion is found to have damaged an area of the posterior part of the dominant cerebral hemisphere known as the angular gyrus, lying at the meeting point of three lobes, the occipital, parietal and temporal. Here the fibres from both occipital lobes converge, those from the minor half-brain having travelled through the corpus callosum. Always there is an accompanying opposite (usually right, of course, in dextrals) homonymous hemianopia. Such a visual fault alone, from damage to the major hemisphere, may exist without any reading disability other than a slight clumsiness of line finding. We know therefore that alexia is not merely an ingredient of such an hemianopia.

Acquired disorder of the comprehension of numbers and the ability for arithmetic, in the realm of writing and reading, may be side by side with alexia or a separate fault on its own, dyscalculia.

The analogies between the various forms of dyslexia and auditory agnosia are obvious. Of particular theoretical interest is the fact that, as in the realm of heard and spoken speech, the written word may merely fail to arouse the mental imagery of meaning from the storehouse of word schemas and cause pure dyslexia without dysgraphia or "go deeper" and disturb the schemas themselves and therefore bring dysgraphia as well.

Developmental dyslexia (*congenital dyslexia or word blindness*)

The acquired disorders of speech at a dysphasic level are morbid tragedies to the patient and his family, perhaps making a stroke more difficult to bear for both, or happening as a pure discrete entity. But they are fortuitous accidents in the natural history of living and disease. In another category is developmental dyslexia; as far apart in respect of speech as congenital deafness is from that acquired in adult life. However difficult to isolate and to manage, congenital deafness at least has the merit of being recognized by everyone as an entity and one of importance. Not so word blindness as an inborn error. The reasons are easy to see. The sufferer is normal in build and body, he hears and sees and moves normally. He usually achieves his early mental milestones normally. He usually learns to speak normally and understands what is said. All is well until he approaches the later, and intellectually higher, hurdles of reading and writing. He then falls back in the same way and at the same time as the dullard at the lower levels of intelligence or as one just outside that boundary. His disability slows back to a trickle the flow of formal educational information which at his age begins to be so largely through the printed and written word. He does not understand his difficulty and no one does around him. Almost inevitably he reacts to this dilemma by withdrawing from it in one of a number of ways. He may choose merely to stop trying when he will be called lazy: he may become aggressive and undisciplined; he may retire into a silent shell of apparent psychological disturbance; he may play the part to increasing perfection of the stupid dullard he has been called or even taken for. If we believe, as we have said, that the ultimate intelligence depends not only upon an inborn endowment of nerve cells and their interactions but upon their constant usage by their owner and his teachers, then this boy actually does become what at first he only appeared to be, dull and backward.

Prejudice has played a large part in misunderstanding or denying this disability. Different people and disciplines have seen these children through different eyes; parents, neurologists, psychologists, psychiatrists and school teachers have formed rigid opposing views and sometimes proclaimed them with more vigour than logic. The greatest mistake, and injustice to the child, has been the assumption that pure inborn dyslexia does not exist and that it is always an euphemism for low intelligence or, not much better, that it is one part of a spectrum that contains imbecility and gross brain damage.

As information about these children was slowly gathered over the decades some of it argued for the neurological concept of a specific inborn speech disability unconnected with visual defect or a lack of potential intelligence or psychological inadequacy. For instance, it became known that a statistically significant proportion of the subjects had strong family history of difficulty in learning to read. The sufferers in previous generations were usually seen to have achieved positions consistent only with normal intelligence, having successfully breached or circumvented the barrier to learning, to being tested and to communication in general. It became known that boys were significantly more often affected and that, amongst them, there was a high incidence of departure from the rule of cerebral dominance. Thus delayed achievement of handedness, left handedness, ambidexterity and dissociated dominances were common. The last refers to preference for hand or foot or eyedness not being, as is usual, ipsilateral. Further, that the common childhood fault of transposing letters, alone or in words, such as "d" for "b" and "dog" for "god", was perpetuated far beyond the normal span. Mirror writing, usually denied the strongly dominant hander, is commoner amongst this group than any other; a bizarre extra skill in the midst of a lack. The growing skill of manipulating in the mind one's body image and the projection of laterality to outside objects, i.e. knowing one's own and another's right and left and so on, may be delayed or lastingly imperfect in these people. The application of this ability to practical things such as dressing, buttoning, shoe-lacing, time-telling and riding a bicycle may be noticeably late or imperfect. All these pieces of evidence point to an inherited defect of some of the duties of a dominant hemisphere, perhaps one of slowness of maturation or delay in dominance decision and not a missing piece of structure. The fact that on occasion the dyslexic child has previously been late in other milestones such as talking, or that his relatives may have been, seems not to detract from this thesis. Nor does the fact that some children seem to fall a little outside the pure concept of dyslexia necessarily condemn the proposition of its existence.

Congenital dyslexia is an uncommon cause of illiteracy. The incidence given for Denmark is much the same as for Edinburgh, 10 per cent of the total population of school children of appropriate age. To the neurologist this figure from psychologists seems high.

Most neurologists, and many others too, including psychologists and school teachers, have come to agree that there is such an entity as specific developmental dyslexia existing in pure form, set within a larger heterogeneous group of children who have one thing in common—difficulty in learning to read. Immediately on either side of this pure form, within the group, there is a child or two who has this defect as the more important one amongst others that have been mentioned above; minor neurological faults that of themselves would be no hindrance to learning and finding a place in the world. The detection of specific dyslexia in the individual case depends upon a number of more or less fortuitous circumstances. However, if it runs in the family this is not by chance and it alerts a parent or other relation to take some action. If the defect is sporadic much depends upon the shrewdness of the parents in noticing, as they often do, that there is a discrepancy between the child's intelligence in general and its specific performance with written symbols. Then the attitude of the teacher or the family doctor is crucial for the reference will be to one or both of them. If one of them is not prejudiced against the concept the chances are that neurological or psychological opinion will be sought and it is in these two fields that the definitive diagnosis is likely to be made. Then comes the most important decision of all. Have the teachers, or one teacher, at the child's school an acceptable or at least open mind to this problem and have they the dedication to do two main things for the child. These are to provide for him individually an education based largely or wholly on the auditory channel into his mind, and extra teaching to overcome the defect or to "flatten it out" to some extent? If not, is there a special school available? So often unfortunately this special school has a population and a bias towards the mentally handicapped or the psychologically abnormal and if this goes with a lack of the specific training required the situation is worse than before for the child is confirmed in his belief that he is thought to be, or even is, lacking intelligence or balance of mind. If all this fails the parents are the only hope but, however helpful, they are likely to be battling against prejudice or disinterest from the school. At the best they will be shouldering a formidable task. Much depends upon the character of the child. One who is easily disheartened or unduly sensitive to separation or to ridicule clearly fares worse. Some strong ones take a grip of their own problem and succeed by themselves in mastering it to an extent to allow them later a normal place in the world without becoming soured. The demands on such a person are formidable. He must be tough enough to be proof against ridicule, calm to tolerate misunderstanding, imaginative to understand his own disability, determined to overcome or circumvent and wise enough to find a niche where his failing can be hidden. Two such particularly come to the author's mind. A successful self-made market gardener who cannot even read unfamiliar road signs or maps or do his own arithmetic, whose wife guides him on holiday and whose assistants do all the book-work. Another, a highly placed sports coach, who can shrewdly circumvent and hide his difficulty with reading and simple arithmetic.

CENTRAL SPEECH DISORDERS

It will be recalled that on p. 560 we spoke of the concept of a store of word and sentence meaning schemas accumulated by the receptive apparatus. An incoming spoken or written sentence is recognized and given meaning by recall from the store. The store is available for making received messages meaningful, for internal speech or thinking and for giving our ideas to others by the spoken or written word. A disturbance of the schema complex then is apt to cause confusion to all three elements; receptive, internal and expressive. This is of moderate practical importance to the otolaryngologist for occasionally a sufferer may be thought merely to be deaf or to be unable properly to pronounce.

The appropriate lesion is about the posterior part of the superior temporal convolution of the dominant hemisphere with a tendency in some examples to spread to the adjacent part of the parietal lobe.

The symptoms may vary somewhat from case to case in degree and quality and, like most dysphasias, from time to time and from one to another circumstance. The fault is always mixed, receptive and expressive, though either may suffer the most. The miscomprehension may vary from absolute to trivial with occasional difficulty in understanding a word or phrase. The more difficult the meaning the worse the comprehension, the closer it is to the patient's life the better he understands. The quicker he is spoken to and the more tense he is the more he misses. All these variabilities apply to the heard and the read word about equally, sometimes with a preference for one.

Difficulties with expression commonly involve speaking and writing equally. There may even be hesitation and confusion with simple mime such as waving goodbye, or this means of expression may be enthusiastically taken up by a patient in a way quite foreign to his culture. The patient may be virtually speechless with a few, often repetitive, words to use on all and every occasion. For instance, a woman with an appropriately placed embolus from a rheumatic heart said only "South Africa" but with such a variety of emphasis as to be surprisingly eloquent. Months of speech therapy merely improved the elocution of the same two words. The speech contains many kinds of mistake. Utterly wrong but existent words jostle with neologisms, proper ones and those that are recognizably near-right. The latter may be so according to sound, spelling or meaning, e.g. "case" for "face", "broad" for "bread", "cutting" for "knife". Words are mispronounced and grammar has gravely deteriorated from the patient's norm. These faults apply both to spontaneous speech and in reply. A contemporary utterance is adulterated with perseverations from minutes previously. Sometimes the monitoring by auto-reception momentarily improves to bring embarrassment to the patient. But most of what he says he finds satisfactory. The extreme extension of this into a voluble flow of totally meaningless sentences is called jargon aphasia. As in a child the ability to repeat another's words is sometimes preserved, for the edification of the speech therapist. As befits a higher skill, writing is usually more damaged with perhaps some preservation of copying.

Nominal dysphasia

This is a special example of a central dysphasia. The description above shows that such a global fault must involve the more particulate nominal one. Except in the mildest examples the disorder is deeper than a mere inability to name objects and people. As Brain puts it "Nominal aphasia is in a peculiar sense a disturbance of the symbolic element in speech for it is the use of words in their capacity of symbols . . . that is primarily the fault". There is a fault in the reproduction of what a word or group of words stand for. The disorder lies right in the midst of the schema storehouse complex, in the linkage between word schemas and meaning-schemas. To the student of speech disorder the differences between nominal and central aphasia are discernible and important, but here it is sufficient to recognize that the former as a rule causes less devastation in communication and more emphasis on the misnaming of objects with a peculiar reiterative, seemingly stupid, inability to carry forward a correction. The patient seems satisfied, despite insight into his errors, in mis-naming single objects.

The lesion lies about the dominant temporoparietal area close to the one for central aphasia and therefore symptomatically merging with it. Nominal dysphasia in its mildest forms is the most likely speech disorder to present as part of the clinical picture of a dominant-side otogenic temporal lobe abscess.

EXPRESSIVE DISORDERS OF SPEECH

There are two expressive, or executive, disorders of speech; disorder of speaking, dysphasia, and of writing, dysgraphia. We have already seen that expressive dysphasia may be part of a receptive or central fault and also that writing may suffer too in such a case. However, there are more or less pure examples of discrete expressive dysphasia and dysgraphia. The first is, for obvious reasons, more likely to attend the ear, nose and throat surgeon.

Expressive dysphasia

There has been at least as much confusion amongst authors about this department of speech disturbance as any other. The synonyms betoken that; Broca's, cortical motor, verbal and expressive have all been employed as prefixes. Word dumbness has been used by some as meaning the same, by others as a separate entity.

Again the degree of disorder varies greatly from one patient to another, the worst making the patient unable to speak. Especially in the less severe forms the patient, by gesture, is able to show that his powers of receiving and comprehending talk and writing are normal and that his ability to use internal speech is at least partly spared. He also shows that he is aware of his mistakes. All this suggests that the lesion is "distal" in the speech complex, at the stage when the correctly chosen word and sentence schemas are about to be propelled into spoken utterance. The more words left to him the better the chance of portraying some of the mistakes already described for other dysphasias. Perseveration, repetition, mispronunciation, errors of syntax, neologisms and jargon utterance are some of them. In this form, more than any other, dysarthria may accompany the dysphasia, indeed be a symptom of it. Hence the aphorism that dysarthria may be a symptom of dysphasia but never vice versa. There may be strange dissociations of speech when, for instance, words may be used normally in a commonplace automatic utterance and yet next moment be lost when commanded. Similarly emotional oaths are often preserved when propositional speech is entirely lost or may be only present at the behest of anger or surprise. Speech performance varies much from moment to moment, a mistake or an attempt to hurry or tension may precipitate a gush of errors tumbling over one another whilst at another time the few available words will be hesitatingly dispensed one at a time.

The anatomy has been disputed but the region of the posterior part of the third frontal lobe convolution and the immediate surrounds form the centre of the lesions described.

Word dumbness and dyspraxia

Soon we shall be discussing dysarthria and dysphonia, symptoms of damage to the peripheral moving tissues of speech or their innervation. One of the lesions is at the neuromuscular junction, myasthenia gravis. In the same way that this gap has to be bridged and that we have to take account of happenings in it we have to accept a point of physiology that lies between speech determination and speech articulation, belonging perhaps to neither. Examples, not concerned with speech, may aid description and understanding. Neurologists well recognize a somewhat rare state in which a patient with full understanding, a normal mind, intact power, sensation and co-ordination is quite unable to perform a previously simple task, with, for instance, his hand. The hand, or more exactly the brain working the hand, has lost its skills but not its strength. This can affect execution, by any part of the body but clearly only parts endowed with the ability and the practice for expertness, such as the mouth and limbs, can lose them. The fault is called dyspraxia. Physiologically identical faults happen to the receiving mechanisms, apart from speech. These are called agnosias. Examples are the ability to see but failure to comprehend the meaning; to feel with the finger tips but, blindfold, to be unaware of the meaning of the object; to have normal common sensation but to have lost the body image. Visual agnosia, astereognosis and somatognosis are names given to these three examples. There are other apraxias and agnosias. Dysgraphia might be called a special example of hand dyspraxia. Dysgraphia can occur alone as the only deficiency of a hand but dyspraxia of the major hand always includes dysgraphia.

Word dumbness is a situation in which the patient becomes unable to speak voluntarily, repeat words or read aloud yet remains able to comprehend heard and written speech, to think clearly with internal speech and to write normally. Some authors classify this disorder as apraxic and not dysphasic. The fault may be of any severity. Causative lesions have been too widespread to allow of discrete isolation but one thing common to most has been a subcortical situation between the insula and the putamen of the basal ganglia.

Gesture, mime and foreign tongue dysphasia

Perhaps these topics are remote from everyday otology but they have interest. Critchley has suggested that gesture is a part of ordinary speech and dependent upon national culture, changing fashion and personal inclination. It tends to suffer with ordinary speech from disease, but less so. It therefore tends to be partially or wholly preserved. This can be well shown to a group by telling them to block their ears to the voluble jargon of a severe dysphasic and watch the normal accompanying face and mouth movement enriched by accompanying gesture. The appearance is of someone talking volubly and sensibly; which he may be to himself. Pantomine on the other hand is a relatively cold, unemotional alternative to speech used by a subject who has lost the powers of his tongue. Deaf and dumb manual communication is pantomime. It can suffer from damage to the dominant hemisphere like normal speech but the place of damage might have to be somewhat different from the normal anatomy of speech. The blind, limbless boy who reads braille with hisnose-tip might be rendered dyslexic by unusually placed morbid anatomy.

Usually the mother tongue suffers less from dysphasia than one learnt later, but there are inexplicable exceptions to this general rule.

Aetiology, pathology, prognosis and treatment of the dysphasias

Because of the complications and the dangers inherent in the delayed diagnosis or poor management of congenital or early acquired deafness and of developmental dyslexia these two stand out from the rest as being of paramount importance. The cause and morbid anatomy of dysphasia is manifold. The cases can be put into two groups, the transient and the installed. *Transient dysphasia* lasting minutes or an hour or so is commonplace as one ingredient, in some episodes the chief one, of an attack of migraine. Because it tends, in the lay and professional mind, to be equated with a stroke it may cause concern to both. It can be as fleeting, though commonly somewhat longer lasting, as part of a transient ischaemic attack of structural arterial disease. These are identical effects caused by identical physiological fault, ischaemia, but with different morbid anatomy; arteriolar constriction or blockage or haemorrhage. The differentiation is made partly by the time factor.

Obviously the separation and detailed classification described above for the dysphasias cannot be realized in such short-lived happenings nor is such dysphasia of any importance except to signal one or other of these two diseases with such different prognosis. The differential diagnosis of transient ischaemic attack of the brain is discussed in Volume 2. The morbid anatomy of *installed dysphasia* is as wide as the whole of intracranial disease. Head injury, arterial blockage, intracranial haemorrhage and primary and secondary tumours form the bulk of causes. To the otologist, however, the relatively rare brain abscess is perhaps the chief reason for attention to acquired dysphasia and because nearby purulent infection spreads or jumps inevitably to the nearest piece of brain it is the otogenic one that causes speech disturbance of this variety (*see* Volume 2).

The prognosis concerns life, morbidity of body generally and of speech in particular. Clearly for the first all depends upon the cause and any complications. Dysphasia never makes a good recovery when once installed. This is for two reasons. The anatomy of speech is well defined and there are no alternative channels in the adult brain to take over from a damaged one. The physiological mechanism is delicate and less brutish than, for example, the relatively simple act of walking. The prognosis for installed dysphasia then is always poor, the natural recovery is small at the best. A good deal of emotional heat is generated about the treatment of dysphasia, most of which concerns whether or not it is of any use rather than the relative merits of various devices. Neurologists on the whole take an agnostic view, speech therapists naturally have some degree of belief in their powers in this particular field, whilst most other disciplines tend to take a calm, uncritical view. The therapist points to the difference between the patient a week after the installed stroke and three months or so later, claiming the livelier mind and a few additional words, better strung and more clearly pronounced as her due. As with many of her medical colleagues she is ignorant of, or rejects, the natural history of events. Her critics see comparable results without treatment. They claim that it is the fortuitous preservation of some of the anatomophysiological necessity and its stimulation by the environment, and the repetitive practice that comes from it, that produces the difference. At the best, they say, speech therapy is an occupation for the patient; at the worst an expensive indulgence for the relatives and a source of irritation to the patient. Certainly a number of patients, whose thinking and emotion are relatively preserved, are angered by the indignity of being pressed to say their pitiful few words in a way to please their teacher.

DYSARTHRIA AND DYSPHONIA

Speech is the total function of communication between people, the comprehension and expression of ideas in words. Articulation is a part of this process; the expression into sounds by lips, tongue, palate, larynx and respiratory muscles, of ideas formulated in the mind and clothed with words chosen from the central schemas. Dysarthria is the disorder of articulation. Dysphonia is the special example of dysarthria, from faulty working of the vocal cords. The dysarthric patient may have full command of speech comprehension and the formulation of words and sentences so that what he says is fully meaningful yet, perhaps, made incomprehensible by distorted articulation. Writing and typing are of course normal unless there is an accompanying paralysis of limbs. The essentially peripheral nature of dysarthria is shown by causing it with a pebble in the mouth or a dental local anaesthetic, of dysphonia by inflammation of the larynx. Therefore we have to take account of the physiology of movement of all the parts mentioned above.

Upper motor neurone

We have already said that slight dysarthria may be a part of dysphasia. This is an integral part of the disorderly speech function of dysphasia and not just due to clumsy facial movements on the hemiparetic side. The fibres of the upper neurone used for speech are the same, or lie close to, those used to move the same muscles and parts for other reasons. For instance, the tongue movements of eating are innervated by the same neurones as for talking. The place of initial command and formulation is different and the complexity of the physiology is vastly greater too. Dysphasia is dependent upon damage to one, and one only, side of the brain. Bilateral upper neurone damage makes no difference to dysphasia unless it be to disturb the mind and thereby lessen the quality of ideas. However, except for the slight dysarthria caused by dysphasia, disordered articulation from upper neurone lesions is dependent upon bilaterality. So richly bilateral are the cranial nuclei of speech muscles supplied from the hemispheres that a one-sided lesion causes no more than a transient dysarthria, commonly the result of temporary facial weakness. The seventh cranial nerve, though sharing the advantage of bilateral innervation, does so to a sufficiently less extent to allow of temporary partial paralysis from a one-sided stroke or tumour or other lesion. Bilateral corticospinal tract damage, to cause dysarthria, must of course be high enough; in fact above the pons and medulla.

It may be from chronic progressive disease affecting both sides at the same time, it may be acute on both sides simultaneously, or it may be that a second stroke contralateral to an earlier one completes the total anatomical needs for dysarthria. The majority of cases are found to have disease where the brunt falls particularly at an upper brain stem level rather than higher in the hemispheres. There are a number of causes and pathologies. Agenesis and birth trauma account for most of the children so affected. Degenerative arterial ischaemia, acute or chronic in effect, motor neurone disease and disseminated sclerosis form the majority in later life, tumours being a rare cause of this particulate, bilateral, high brain stem situation. There is semantic confusion here. Congenital diplegia is the name given to the causes of bilateral corticospinal tract disease of a number of kinds that happen before, at or soon after birth. Dysarthria is the rule in them. Other parts of the nervous system and the body may be affected, particularly the intelligence and the cerebellum, so that there is often more than one reason for speech disorder. Amyotrophic lateral sclerosis is the title for that form of motor neurone disease where the upper motor neurone is involved with the lower neurones, so that a mixture of muscle wasting and fasciculation with evidence of pyramidal tract damage occurs. Pseudobulbar palsy is the overall name for the clinical picture that is the result of high bilateral upper motor neurone damage. Therefore amyotrophic lateral sclerosis is one of the causes of pseudobulbar palsy, the others being chronic atherosclerotic ischaemia, degeneration of uncertain aetiology, head injury, disseminated sclerosis and very rarely primary and secondary tumours. The results so far as speech is concerned are the same.

Originally, as now, "bulbar palsy" referred to the clinical picture of lower motor neurone paralysis of the muscles supplied by the medulla oblongata, for instance by acute poliomyelitis. Later it was realized that a similar symptomatic result, so far as these muscles were concerned, was achieved by damage to the corticospinal tract (upper motor neurone) fibres of the bulb. The clumsy title "pseudobulbar" palsy was used for this.

Upper motor neurone weakness of all the primary muscles of speech, facial, lingual, palatal and laryngeal, contrive together to produce a characteristic effect. We have to remember that the facial muscles are used, not only in speech, but to express our emotions. Speech is slow, laboured and indistinct. The effort to force it out can be seen from the puckered and grimacing face and lips. It sounds strangled, nasal and the voice high pitched. The muscles are not wasted but tautly spastic and the tongue of small, slow-moving bulk. Choking, spluttering and explosiveness are common. Little involuntary grunts or giggles or gasps show how difficult it is for the patient to do his will with the unruly neurones. The effort to speak, often with exasperating failures, may provoke a similar uncontrollability of emotional facial play to bring an excessive or even inappropriate laughter or tears. This does not necessarily register the quality or the amount of emotion happening within the mind. There is indeed a dyspraxia of emotional facial play. The outward facial play of emotional response may be altered in a characteristic way so that it is inverted or precipitate or slowed or prolonged or too great or all of these. Joy, humour or surprise may cause weeping when the face may behave in the delayed slow-motion fashion often seen in the child. Sadness may bring similarly uncontrolled laughter. To some extent many of these changes are parts of growing older; senility mimics many diseases throughout the body or, perhaps more accurately, old age brings disease of many parts. An interesting social convention is uncovered; to cry with joy is commonplace and wholly acceptable, to laugh in sorrow is horrific and embarrassing.

Lower motor neurone

Here we are concerned with the same muscles but now with disease of the cranial nuclei or their axons, the lower motor neurone or, as Sherrington regarded it, the final common path along which all the many supranuclear forces and effects are brought to bear on the muscles. There is no other route for the corticobulbar, rubrobulbar, cerebellar, tectal and basal ganglia effects to pass. Hence unilateral and even mononeuritic damage can be disabling to speech. If they occur abruptly and completely they tend to upset speech more and, even though there may be no neural recovery, time allows for compensatory adjustments.

A complete unilateral facial palsy brings buccal dysphasia. Palatopharyngeal palsy on one side usually brings a temporary nasal and choking quality to words. The dysphonia of unilateral cord palsy of acute onset is unmistakably husky and vibratory until the healthy cord learns to oppose itself more vigorously to the other. The amount to which speech is affected by a twelfth nerve lesion is an even better example of how much is dependent on speed of onset, degree and the functional improvement from practice. The kind is much the same as for facial palsy but without the flapping quality given by the inert cheek. It is exactly reproduced by a suitably-sized pebble in the mouth.

As would be expected bilateral paralysis of the above muscles brings added dysarthria of the same qualities. This is less so with facial weakness than the others, the speech like the appearance being reminiscent of some normal subjects. However, the dysarthria, which may become anarthria, tends later to be less disabling than the accompanying damage to vital functions such as getting air and food down and secretions up. Apart from the cranial nerve damage the intercostal, diaphragmatic and abdominal muscles of respiration are often weakened.

Because there is a wider field of anatomy involving central nuclei and lengthy peripheral axons, and because one-sided lesions are symptomatic in all cases the aetiology and morbid anatomy of lower motor neurone dysarthria is a wider subject than in the previous section. However, there is no merit in doing more here than to make mention, especially since much of it is discussed in the chapter on laryngeal paralysis (p. 525) and in another part of this chapter. The cause may be within the brain stem (intramedullary), immediately outside it (intracranial), intra-osseous or intraforaminal or extracranial, even as far from the skull as the neck or chest in some instances. Intramedullary lesions usually involve more than one nucleus or nerve and the long tracts. Expanding intracranial causes may bring the symptoms and signs of increased pressure. Extracranial lesions are more likely to show themselves to inspection, plain radiology and biopsy. Bilateral intracranial palsy has two features which contrive to puzzle the ear, nose and throat surgeon, symmetry of inspected form and movement and the absence of a responsible lesion that he can see or feel. Bilateral deformity is often less obvious than unilateral, for instance bilateral facial palsy may be more acceptable to a patient's vanity than one-sided. Many cases of motor neurone disease have been unrecognized by a laryngologist before appearing to a neurologist. Difficulty in swallowing, chewing or talking, caused by symmetrical paralysis may elude the surgeon's eye. Ironically the speech therapist is more likely to make the anatomical diagnosis by ear alone, not being prejudiced by eye.

The basal ganglia

Disease here is likely to cause dysarthria when it is advanced. Usually, however, the speech disorder is too late in the natural history to be useful to diagnosis and later it is one of the least distressing symptoms. All cases eventually come to have slow monotonous speech. Many speak in low volume, often inaudibly. Failure to get rid of saliva may give a wet sound whilst later the drying effects of many of the drugs used may bring a tacky quality, such as may be heard in the normal subject under nervous tension. The voice may become tremulo either because the speech muscles are affected or because the whole person may be shaken by transmission from larger muscles. Rarely, speech muscles may be included in the spasmodic crises that more often involve eye movements in the encephalitic variety of parkinsonism, caused by the virus of Von Economo.

The cerebellum

So far as speech is concerned, damage to the cerebellum is eloquent. The cerebellum might be called the organ of co-ordination of movement for which purpose it needs to receive information on which to act, carried by the fibre tracts afferent to it. In speaking with normal speed and fluency we need to pronounce collections of letters, i.e., syllables and words and sentences, so that each of these parts are joined together with a nicety to avoid jumbling or too much separation. This seems to be one of the tasks of the cerebellum, sustained constantly by information coming from the muscles, joints and tendons of speech. Impairment of its contribution to the final common path leads to a number of ingredient faults, together called inco-ordination. They may concern the use of the mouth and throat or the larynx. The primary fault seems to be repeated collision between adjacent syllables and words so that they run into one another, slurring. A secondary phenomenon is the pulling apart of contiguous syllables and words, scanning, so as to make the sentences slow, stilted and staccato. This part of the fault is an outcome of the slurring tendency; a more or less voluntary effort to prevent the bumping together of the items of speaking. Both faults can be heard in the unpracticed young child as he learns to juggle to achieve the rapid, smooth flow of his elders. The intoxicated adult also breaks down to similar faults, his words being as ataxic, or as carefully dispensed, as his steps. The fine collaboration between the laryngeal muscles to set the cords and the respiratory ones to blow them into vibrations is lost. Noises are prepared but not executed, meaningless gasps of air carrying no voice. The pitch or tone may vary in an unwonted and discordant fashion. The effort for clarity may bring facial grimacing. Accompanying ataxia of eyes (nystagmus), swallowing, breathing, standing, walking and the arms may be seen. In severe cases the resultant speech may be largely incomprehensible. Bilateral cerebellar hemisphere disease or that confined to the unpaired midline structures causes more disturbance to speech than unilateral damage.

The aetiology, pathology and prognosis differs in no essential from what has been said for disease of the rest of the brain. Cerebellar ataxy of any part is a frequent accompaniment of hind-brain arterial block or rupture in which dysphagia may direct the patient to the surgeon.

577

Muscle disease

Faults in the physiology at the neuromuscular junction are rare but, relatively, speech disorder is common in the presenting symptomatology. Palatal, pharyngeal, and facial dysarthria and dysphonia may happen alone or in combination as transient, intangible symptoms, puzzling until the true diagnosis is considered. Myasthenia gravis is the disease proper to the junctional tissues whether or not in association with overt disease of the thymus gland. The myasthenic syndrome is the euphemism proposed for the examples of myasthenia associated with, and seemingly caused by, carcinoma other than of the thymus gland. The myopathies are all rare and unlikely in any case to present to the E.N.T. surgeon. Particularly they are unlikely to cause dysarthria as a major symptom though this is always present when the facial muscles are involved as they are in the facioscapulo-humeral variety of muscular dystrophy. Macroglossia causing progressive and finally severe dysarthria is common in amyloid disease. Dysphagia is much commoner than dysarthria in polymyositis and could well be presenting.

Dysphonia

Paralysis of the lower motor neurones concerned with vocal cord movement is discussed in another chapter (p. 525). We have already made it clear that dysphonia may be caused by cerebellar divorce, by myasthenia gravis or the myasthenic syndrome or by one of the myopathies. Intrinsic disease of the cords may of course closely mimic neurological disorder. Dysphonia is one of the common symptoms of hysteria or of malingering for nothing is easier to pretend, and few things are more dramatic, than loss of voice. In addition it is painless and demands some withdrawal from active life, a status much desired by the hysterical subject.

STUTTERING

Stuttering and stammering are taken to be synonymous words. Andrews and Harris (1964) define it as "an interruption in the normal rhythm of speech of such frequency and abnormality as to attract attention, interfere with communication or cause distress to a stutterer or his audience". No description is necessary. Everyone has met it. No two cases are quite the same in their exact symptomatology. It is taken for granted that the sufferer has no anatomical barrier to normal speech such as congenital or acquired distortion of the parts used in speaking. The E.N.T. surgeon will have patients referred to him because such a fault is wrongly thought to be the cause, in part or whole, or because he is thought to be closer to speech therapy than most clinicians. It is thought to be world wide but the frequency is difficult to know. The published figures for this and other countries vary. One possible reason for this is the uncertainty of measure of what does, and does not, constitute a stammer. Another source of difference is whether or not the early transient stutter of the child learner is to be included. Many children have a stutter sometime between the age of three and eight out of which they grow naturally and which is about equally distributed between boys and girls. All are agreed that males suffer an installed stutter more commonly than females but the figures diverge by as much as 2 and 10 to 1. Most doctors would not agree to the lower figures and feel that the highest is an understatement for severe adult stutter. It is indeed rare to see a woman with a disabling stutter. There is a significantly higher incidence of stutter amongst the children of stutterers but whether this is genetic or environmental is not known. Because the cause is not known and there is no morbid anatomy aetiological imagination has run riot especially in the psychological field. There is hardly a psychological perversion that has not been blamed, followers of Freudian principles having perhaps the richest vein for fancy. Andrews and Harris (1964) have arrayed the present knowledge and ignorance about stuttering.

Intelligence.—The evidence suggests that the average I.Q. of all stutterers is slightly lower than normal and that the opposite belief is founded on a natural selection along at least two ways; those that achieve academic success have had to surmount the additional barrier of their stammer and may therefore be some-what superior to the average of their normally spoken colleagues, and those who seek treatment may be of relatively higher I.Q.

Cerebral dominance.—Perhaps the biggest surprise in this context has been the recent unequivocal denial that left-handedness, ambidexterity and natural changeover are all unconnected with stuttering. A number of studies underlie this denial. However, one still wonders whether these experiments, conducted since 1940, might have given different results had they been done at a time when sinistrals were regarded and made to feel as their descriptive adjective implied. There is now no psychological stress laid on the left-hander and no attempt is made to convert him.

Structural disease.—Many attempts have been made to salvage stutter, and indeed the stutterer, from theory so far as cause and therefore treatment are concerned by proposing and finding a morbid anatomy. All have failed. Known structural disease of the brain does not include the symptoms of installed stutter although hesitancy and trivial inco-ordination of speech may accompany expressive dysphasia.

Emotion and environment.—All the surveys show that a disturbed family back-ground procures more stutterers of the installed variety. Although there are no figures to confirm it the feeling is that stutterers tend to be neurotic and lack confidence but this may be provocative or perpetuating rather than truly causative; indeed it may be effect.

Since no convincing evidence is forthcoming to incriminate structural brain fault and the theories of such faults fail to last it is tempting to regard a physiological or psychological "weakness" as, at least in part, the cause. If the latter then any-thing that provoked it, such as domestic unhappiness, would also tend to worsen stutter as one of its symptoms. Speech, a highly organized and therefore vulnerable piece of physiology, a skill hesitantly learned from relatives at a time of potential insecurity and inferiority, and a function designed to communicate the child's present state of mind and achievement is perhaps the most likely to break down. One of the ways it might do so would be to become hesitant or inco-ordinate. We have already said that such a state is common as a transient fault in the natural history of speaking. Certainly the factors that tend to inflame an incompletely cured stammer seem to be psychological. No matter whether or not a disturbed mind may distort speech the opposite is overtly true. It seems possible then that the birth and natural history of stutter may depend upon an inherited tendency balanced between emotional factors in the environment and the moral fibre of the individual; flourishing, being stifled at onset, rising, falling and capable of being held down or even made to disappear by effort combined with ingenuity. However it is distinctly rare for an installed stutter to be cured to the point of being forgotten by the patient.

Treatment and other observations

There are some disorders of the mind or the body which seem to attract therapists of remarkable strength in several ways; obsessional rigidity of belief, dedication and forceful personality amongst them. The diseases, though disparate, tend to have a number of common factors. They are long lasting, lacking agreed cause, benign so far as life and limb go, distressing to patient and those around him, causing or arising from a particular disposition which seeks for placebo attachments and tending toward spontaneous improvement or remission. Such disorders include some examples of pain in the head, face or back, blushing, adolescent obesity, juvenile delinquency, academic laziness and stutter. It is difficult to be sure in the individual case of stutter whether an improvement comes from the treatment or not. But it is clear that many successes are achieved by, or alongside, considerably different methods.

The theories and means of treatment may be divided as follows:

Psychological.—The pure psychological approach is to believe that the mind, and what is working on it from within and without, is all important. More or less the physical and mechanical aspects are ignored.

Physical.—Attention is directed to the distorted mechanics of speech in one or more of a number of ways although, inevitably, the psyche of the giver and the receiver are intimately concerned and reflected.

Mixed.—When both aspects are believed to be interdependent and both receive attention.

This is not the place to describe the details or to discuss the results. Andrews and Harris (1964) either do this fully or give appropriate references. However, it might be useful to make some further observations and comments. Most sufferers from all but the transient physiological or the most trivial installed stammer soon find that their symptoms are amenable to a variety of influences. To speak with immoderate slowness so as to separate the syllables or better still to drawl them loses the stutter. A change of pitch of voice as in singing or shouting immediately banishes it. The slowness may be self-imposed or by metronome. An associated act such as walking, running, hand clapping, sighing or innumerable others including grimaces and contortions, that often stamp the patient with exact individuality, may smooth away the stammer at the expense perhaps of congruity. Posture alone may make all the difference so that to lie down or rise or stand on the head may help. Masking the whole face or the eyes alone by dark glasses or being behind a curtain can reduce or abolish the fault. There is no limit to the variety or the bizarre nature of these catalysts. The sufferer becomes adept at scanning prospectively his ideas and the possible words to clothe them and thereby avoid awkward items or combinations, particularly first syllables and prefixes. This is why the inevitability contained in reading aloud is so disastrous to many stutterers. Mechanical preventatives such as a pebble in the mouth or a half a matchstick propping it open may transform the speaker. The spoken words of an acted script may make possible a flow that was denied without the movement and pretence. Parental disapproval or pedagogic ridicule freeze most sufferers into contorted silence or splutter. It needs no imagination to dissect out of these commonplace examples the appropriate psychology and physiology of stutter. They are the basis of much of the methodology of professional treatment. It is the author's belief that a successful outcome depends upon some or all of the following. The most important single item, as indeed in many cures, is the personality and strength of purpose of the patient—whether he has the drive to find the tricks for himself, or to transfer them from his teacher, and apply them with growing ingenuity. At first they will be as clumsy as children's stitching, later as skilfully woven into the cloth of speech as the best invisible patch. As he gets older his experience will make him bolder and less vulnerable to ridicule. The best end result is almost perfect in all situations but tending to crack a little on occasion and nearly always apparent to the expert eye and ear of a fellow sufferer who can detect the inter-polations, reversals and other invisible "stitches". The modern imprecision of speaking and cluttering with meaningless repeats such as "I mean" and "you know" have been most helpful to the recovering stutterer who no longer has to face the syntactic criteria that daunted his stammering forbears. The teacher may be of great help as a guide and moral support in his understanding. Syllable-timed speech, the metronome, breathing exercises, delayed feedback and the many means of instilling a confidence not naturally present are no more than ways round a disorder of uncertain cause. Stammer, like mutism or dysphonia or paralysis of any other part, may be a symptom of hysteria or malingering. It may also be a mannerism in children or adults, used in much the same way as a tem-porary change of accent.

BIBLIOGRAPHY

Andrews, G., and Harris, M. (1964). *The Syndrome of Stuttering*. London; The Spastics Society and Heinemann.
Brain, W. R. (1965). *Speech Disorders* (2nd ed.). London; Butterworths.
Critchley, M. (1964). *Developmental Dyslexia*. London; Heinemann.
Head, H. (1926). *Aphasia and Kindred Disorders of Speech*. London; Cambridge University Press.
Whetnall, E., and Fry, D. B. (1964). *The Deaf Child*. London; Heinemann.

23

LOWER RESPIRATORY CONDITIONS IN THE PRACTICE OF EAR, NOSE AND THROAT SURGERY

E. H. Miles Foxen

INTRODUCTION

During the last two decades the management of numerous lower respiratory conditions has passed from the province of the ear, nose and throat surgeon to that of the thoracic surgeon, and it is sometimes forgotten that much pioneer work in such conditions as carcinoma of the bronchus and bronchiectasis was carried out by laryngologists.

In spite of the rapid growth of thoracic surgery, however, there are certain conditions of the lower respiratory tract which are of particular importance to the ear, nose and throat surgeon and in which his advice may be sought. The object of this chapter therefore is to dwell for a time on these conditions but not to deal exhaustively with all the diseases of the lungs and thorax, for this would fill many books and would be outside the scope of the present volume.

BRONCHIAL FOREIGN BODIES

The ear, nose and throat surgeon may be called upon at any time to deal with bronchial foreign bodies, which are sometimes classified as endogenous and exogenous. Exogenous foreign bodies are, of course, much more common than endogenous, and are further subdivided into vegetable and non-vegetable varieties which cause very different problems.

Endogenous foreign bodies

Saliva and *mucopurulent* material may be inhaled by patients who are in deep coma, or by patients in whom there is serious disturbance of the neuromuscular mechanism of deglutition, for example bulbar palsy. The causes are numerous, and great advances in the management of these cases took place following the Copenhagen poliomyelitis epidemic of 1952 (Lassen, 1953). In a single hospital, in less than five months, special measures, such as tracheostomy and artificial respiration, had to be applied to 316 cases, the main problem in such cases, apart from respiratory failure, being inhalation of upper respiratory secretions. It became apparent that where this risk exists frequent aspiration of the bronchial tree is essential, and that the most suitable method of implementing such treatment is by way of a cuffed rubber tracheostomy tube, which not only allows the passage of an aspirator tube but prevents the entry of upper respiratory tract secretions into the lower respiratory tract.

Blood may be inhaled by the comatose patient with injuries of the jaws or mouth, in cases of cut-throat, and during or after an upper respiratory tract operation. In the latter connection it is of supreme importance to ear, nose and throat surgeons. Fortunately, thanks to the development of modern endotracheal anaesthesia, the hazard of blood inhalation during operation has been reduced to a minimum, but it can occur and, if suspected, bronchoscopy, with aspiration, should be carried out in order to avert post-operative pulmonary collapse.

Asphyxial deaths due to the inhalation of blood after adenotonsillectomy and other upper respiratory operations still occur from time to time, and medical and nursing staff must always be aware of the possibility of this disastrous complication. It is completely fallacious to suppose that such deaths are the result of blood loss; they are caused by the occlusion of the main bronchi by blood clots which have not, in every case, resulted from excessive haemorrhage.

Gastric contents are liable to inhalation under certain circumstances. The dangers attending this occurrence have been recognized since the dawn of general anaesthesia, but the particularly injurious effect of inhaled gastric juice has received attention only in more recent times. The patients likely to be at risk are ill-prepared dental or out-patient cases, obstetric cases (Mendelson, 1946), and cases of intestinal obstruction, and the ideal management when gastric juice inhalation is suspected is a matter of some dispute. Scurr (1960) advocates tracheobronchial lavage with normal saline or water, 20 ml. at a time being instilled by syringe or catheter down the endotracheal tube or bronchoscope and followed by suction; experimental work by Simenstad, Galway and MacLean (1963) supports the validity of this advice. On the other hand, Bannister, Sattilaro and Otis (1961), in a series of animal experiments, found that attempts to prevent pneumonitis by introducing diluent or neutralizing solutions following the introduction of hydrochloric acid were not beneficial in effect. Recently bronchial lavage has been found to be of considerable value in obstructive lung disease, for example in cases of asthma with bronchitis in which bronchi are plugged with inspissated mucus (Thompson and Pryor, 1964).

The management of the pulmonary oedema consequent upon the inhalation of gastric juice may include the employment of oxygen under pressure, antibiotics, anti-foam agents and intravenous hydrocortisone (Hausmann and Lunt, 1955).

Adenoid or *tonsil fragments* must occasionally be inhaled and no doubt account for a number of cases of post-operative pulmonary collapse. As a rule, however, this type of foreign body causes little mucosal reaction.

Dental foreign bodies when aspirated into a bronchus may give rise to an acute mucosal reaction, which may be almost as severe as that caused by a vegetable substance. Their removal is an urgent necessity.

Exogenous foreign bodies

Non-vegetable foreign bodies include such objects as pins, tacks, screws, buttons, beads, portions of dental plates, toys, tracheostomy tubes, etc. Perhaps the most common foreign body to be aspirated is *water*, and in recent years the difference in the sequence of events following the inhalation of salt water and fresh water has been stressed. When salt water is inhaled fluid passes from blood stream to alveoli, and may cause pulmonary oedema and increasing anoxia. On the other hand, when fresh water is inhaled it is absorbed rapidly into the blood, and if excessive may cause haemodilution, haemolysis, a rise in the K–Na ratio and death from ventricular fibrillation (Birch, 1963).

Solid foreign bodies are of particular importance to the ear, nose and throat surgeon, for their management constitutes an onerous, if relatively infrequent, part of his work.

Aspiration of foreign bodies occurs more often in children than in adults, and Jackson (1936) has stated that in America 66 per cent of tracheobronchial and oesophageal foreign body accidents happen to patients under five years of age. Carelessness in holding articles such as pins and tacks in the lips or mouth frequently leads to the entrance of foreign bodies into the tracheobronchial tree. Hasty eating may lead to the aspiration of portions of food, and edentulous patients with artificial dentures are more prone to this accident, as the absence of palatal sensation lessens the chance of detection of hard objects in the bolus.

In conscious patients aspirated foreign bodies enter the right main bronchus more frequently than the left one owing to the following anatomical and physiological facts: (1) the right main bronchus has a greater diameter than the left main bronchus; (2) the right main bronchus has a lesser degree of deviation from the tracheal axis than has the left main bronchus; (3) the carina is situated to the left of the midline of the trachea; and (4) the volume of air which enters the right main bronchus is greater than that which enters the left one. As a rule a foreign body is arrested in the main, lower or one of the basal bronchi of the right lung; less frequently in the main, lower or one of the basal bronchi of the left lung. The upper and middle lobe bronchi in conscious patients are invaded in less than 4 per cent of cases. On the other hand an unconscious patient (*see* anatomy of larynx, Volume 1) in the recumbent position is more likely to aspirate a foreign body into the apical segment of a lower lobe if supine, or the upper lobe if lying in one or the other lateral positions (Brock, 1956).

Foreign bodies tend to move distally in the bronchi, and very occasionally may traverse the lung, pleural space and chest wall (Seydell, 1937).

The changes which take place when a foreign body remains for any considerable time in the tracheobronchial tree vary with the character of the aspirated object (Jackson, 1936) and, as one would expect, inert objects, such as glass beads, set up only minimal reaction.

Clinical picture

Aspiration of a foreign body in a conscious patient is usually followed by immediate choking and gagging, and this is followed by a symptomless interval varying in duration from a few hours to several months depending on the nature of the foreign body and upon the degree of bronchial obstruction which it causes.

In the case of an inert non-vegetable foreign body mucosal reaction occurs perhaps after a fairly prolonged symptomless period, when the cough may return, heralding the onset of pulmonary collapse. If the cause is not then removed, suppuration—and ultimately bronchiectasis or lung abcess—may ensue.

When a vegetable foreign body has been aspirated an acute or so-called "vegetal" bronchitis rapidly supervenes, and the foreign body may cause a valvular obstruction in the bronchus with emphysema distally, or alternatively a large object, such as a bean, may cause complete occlusion of the bronchial lumen and collapse.

Aspirated peanuts cause a particularly acute reaction owing, it is thought, to the presence of highly irritative free fatty acids.

The bronchitis resulting from the inhalation of vegetable matter is characterized by its rapid onset and by the intensity and diffuseness of the pathological changes which take place. There is at first a profuse serous exudate, which rapidly becomes purulent, and pathogenic organisms appear in the sputum.

Diagnosis

A history suggesting the possible inhalation of a foreign body places the medical attendant under immediate obligation to prove either the presence or the absence of the foreign body in the patient's respiratory tract.

Interpretation of the physical signs may be made difficult by change of position of the foreign body, but broadly speaking the physical signs of a bronchial foreign body are as follows:

(1) Limited expansion of the affected side of the chest.
(2) Impaired percussion note of the pulmonary area distal to the foreign body.
(3) Decreased vocal fremitus.
(4) Diminished or absent air entry into the affected area.
(5) Decreased vocal resonance.
(6) Adventitious sounds in the affected area.

X-ray examination is essential and, as a rule, dense and metallic objects can readily be recognized. If, however, the foreign body is not radio-opaque the radiological diagnosis has to be made on the evidence of the bronchial obstruction which it has produced.

Removal of foreign bodies from the tracheobronchial tree

It is unwise to delay bronchoscopy in the hope that a foreign body will be coughed up. Jackson (1934) has recorded that only 2–4 per cent of foreign bodies are expelled spontaneously in this manner, whereas about 99 per cent of bronchial foreign bodies can be removed with the bronchoscope.

Delay also renders removal more difficult, as most bronchial foreign bodies tend to move distally towards the periphery of the lung, and the bronchial mucosa becomes oedematous, partially obscuring the foreign body or even completely occluding the lumen of a small bronchus.

The bronchoscope is introduced under general anaesthesia. Advantage should be taken of the assistance that can be gained from the lip of the bronchoscope, which may be used to afford counter-pressure to form a protector to slip over sharp points and to assist in the conversion of an unfavourable presentation into a favourable one.

In some cases the removal of bronchial foreign bodies requires the utmost skill. It is often essential to aspirate secretions from above the foreign body, and in order to obtain a clear view of the latter it may be necessary to swab the area with an adrenaline–cocaine solution.

Numerous instruments have been designed for the removal of bronchial foreign bodies (see Figs. 248, 249), and it is mandatory that the bronchoscopist should acquaint himself with these instruments before attempting to use them. For example, he must learn to close the forceps without causing their tips to recede from the target.

In some cases it is not possible to remove a foreign body by means of the broncho-scope. This may be because it is situated at the periphery of the lung and beyond the field of bronchoscopic vision. In the days before the development of modern thoracic surgical techniques biplane radioscopy was used with success in such cases and the foreign body removed under radiological guidance only, but this method is not without hazard, and today thoracotomy is preferred.

Pins and needles usually present point uppermost, and it may be necessary to disimpact the point, which is then worked gently into the bronchoscopic lumen.

An open safety-pin with the point uppermost should be dealt with by using the Clerf–Arrowsmith safety-pin closer (Fig. 248).

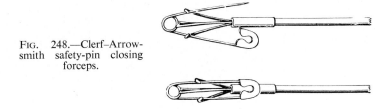

Fig. 248.—Clerf–Arrow-smith safety-pin closing forceps.

Staples may require version, but if this is not possible both points should be engaged in the lumen of the bronchoscope or grasped by special forceps before removal (Fig. 249).

Small ferrous foreign bodies have on occasion been removed by magnets. An alloy named alnico, which has remarkable powers of attraction, has been mounted on both rigid and vertebrated introducers which can be introduced through the bronchus.

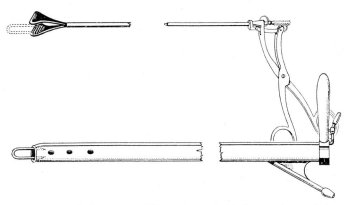

Fig. 249.—Staple forceps, used in cases unsuitable for version, and the staple bronchoscope. (*Reproduced by courtesy of W. B. Saunders, Philadelphia.*)

Vegetable foreign bodies have been referred to in connection with the marked local pathological changes which so rapidly follow their aspiration. Extreme gentleness of manipulation and lightness of touch must be exercised in the extraction of friable vegetable foreign bodies, for fragmentation may readily occur and minute particles may be aspirated into smaller bronchi.

POST-OPERATIVE PULMONARY COLLAPSE

Post-operative pulmonary collapse occurs most commonly following upper abdominal operations but may follow a nose or throat operation such as tonsillectomy.

Basically the collapse is the immediate result of bronchial obstruction caused by blood, mucus or other secretion which cannot be coughed up but stagnates, affecting a greater or lesser area of lung tissue. Unless treatment is rapidly instituted infection becomes established, and if this is allowed to progress unhindered lung abscess and bronchiectatic change may ensue.

Prophylaxis

Operations should be postponed if there is any possibility that respiratory tract infection—for example, a common cold—might be present. Few ear, nose and throat operations can be regarded as emergencies, and it is unwise medical practice to carry out a routine operation merely to avoid inconvenience, when such doubt exists. It has indeed been advocated that pre-operative chest radiography should be carried out in all non-emergency cases (Loder, 1955). Such advice may be justified, but in any case, the house surgeon's pre-operative history-taking and clinical examination are of supreme importance. In patients whose respiratory function may be impaired pre-operatively the opinion of a physician should be sought, and such measures as breathing exercises, curtailment of smoking and postural percussion-drainage may be advised.

The routine adoption of the "head-low" position in unconscious patients after upper respiratory operations is of importance in preventing the aspiration of secretions, and if, at the conclusion of the operation, there is any suspicion that blood or mucus has been aspirated bronchial suction with a catheter should be carried out. If doubt still exists a bronchoscope should be passed in order to permit more thorough suction.

Needless to say, deep-breathing, encouragement to cough and early mobility are important prophylactic measures in the case of the convalescent patient.

Clinical picture

The earliest manifestations of post-operative pulmonary collapse occurring as a rule within 48 hours of operation are pyrexia and cough. The latter is at first dry but later may become productive of mucopurulent sputum which is not blood-stained. If blood is present in the sputum the diagnosis should be re-considered. There may also be dyspnoea, cyanosis and chest pain, but these are inconstant.

The pulse and respiratory rates are found to be raised, chest movement is limited, and there may be displacement of the heart and mediastinum. Dullness is present on percussion over the affected area and breath sounds are diminished or absent; later there are moist sounds and bronchial breathing.

The radiological appearances are characteristic. The shadow is dense and homogeneous, and there may be elevation of the diaphragm and narrowing of the intercostal spaces. Displacement of the heart, trachea and mediastinum to the affected side are confirmed.

Treatment

As soon as the diagnosis of post-operative pulmonary collapse has been made vigorous measures should be instituted to clear the blocked air passages. Cough is encouraged, and postural drainage with percussion is commenced. Post-operative pain is the great inhibitor of cough, and such inhibition must be removed, if necessary, by the administration of morphine or similarly acting drugs. Skilled physiotherapy circumvents any ill-effects which might result from the depressive properties of such drugs. The relief of pain is essential.

Pulmonary collapse marches hand-in-hand with pulmonary infection. The longer the collapse is allowed to persist, the greater is the likelihood of severe infection. Antibiotic treatment is therefore commenced at the outset. In the first place penicillin is the antibiotic of choice, but if the sputum is found to contain resistant organisms the appropriate antibiotic is substituted.

If the measures described above (that is, postural drainage with percussion, etc.), are not rapidly successful in removing the obstruction and aerating the collapsed lobe, no time should be lost in resorting to bronchoscopy with suction. In some patients this procedure may need to be repeated, and in a few patients tracheostomy may be necessary in order that bronchial suction may be carried out frequently (Pitman and Wilson, 1955).

Once collapse has become established the resulting lesion will depend upon the type and virulence of the infecting organisms. In some cases the collapsed lung tissue may fail to re-expand, with the ultimate development of fibrosis and bronchiectasis, and in other cases infection of the tissue may lead to the formation of a pulmonary abscess.

BRONCHIECTASIS

Bronchiectasis was first described by Laennec in 1819, and its incidence has undergone a dramatic decline since the introduction of antibiotics. To quote Hinshaw and Garland (1963) "Physicians who practised in the days prior to definitive surgical and antimicrobial therapy of bronchiectasis may recall the patient with this truly loathsome disease as it then manifested itself. Such patients produced large quantities of foul-smelling sputum hourly; some were offensive at considerable distances, making it impossible for them to occupy a room with other people or even to eat a meal with a person having normal olfactory sense. These patients frequently were in the adolescent age group or their early twenties; few lived beyond the third or fourth decade. The psychological problems related to such a condition were often overwhelming, and suicide was not uncommon. Severe bronchiectasis in young persons carried about the same prognostic import as severe rheumatic heart disease, with the expectation that death would occur between the ages of 30 and 45 years. Death commonly was due to a severe respiratory tract infection which led to pneumonia or to bronchial obstruction with pulmonary abscess and death from sepsis, metastatic brain abscess or generalised blood stream infection. Since 1950, disease of such severity and with lethal complications has become a rarity because of improvement in medical and surgical treatment."

For a full description of bronchiectasis the student is advised to consult one of the many excellent textbooks on diseases of the chest, for it is the intention in this chapter merely to stress certain aspects of the condition which are of immediate interest to the otolaryngologist.

Bronchial foreign body and post-operative pulmonary collapse have already been mentioned as possible aetiological factors in the production of bronchiectasis, but it is the association of bronchiectasis and chronic infection of the paranasal sinuses which more frequently comes to the notice of the ear, nose and throat surgeon.

The syndrome of bronchiectasis, chronic sinusitis and dextrocardia described by Kartagener (1933) is well known, but relatively uncommon. On the other hand, the association of the first two participants in this alliance, i.e. bronchiectasis and chronic sinusitis, is common. Ormerod (1914), investigating a group of 40 cases of bronchiectasis, found that 42·5 per cent were suffering from sinusitis, and Hogg (1950), in a survey of 110 cases of bronchiectasis, found evidence of sinusitis in 60·9 per cent. In 49 of these cases lobectomy or pneumonectomy was carried out, and of these 57·1 per cent had operative treatment for sinusitis.

Why should this common association between bronchiectasis and sinusitis exist ?

Hitherto it was often stated that chronic sinusitis was an aetiological factor in the production of bronchiectasis, but it is more likely that the sinuses are infected by droplet infection from the lungs, as evidenced: (1) by the scientific work of Proetz (1932), demonstrating that expired air currents are in close communication with the ostia of the sinuses; and (2) by clinical observations such as those of Ormerod and Hogg. Nevertheless, it must not be supposed that the traffic is all one-way. Infected sinuses are a constant source of re-infection of the bronchial tree, and this brings us to the important consideration of the rôle of sinus treatment in bronchiectasis.

Treatment of infected sinuses in bronchiectasis

The principles underlying the treatment of infected sinuses in cases of bronchiectasis scarcely differ in any way from those principles which should be applied to cases in which bronchiectasis is absent. Sinuses which are the seat of constant or recurrent infection must be adequately drained, but surgery should not be more radical than necessary, and every effort is made to spare healthy ciliated mucosa.

Each case should be treated on its own merits, and Hogg (1950), dealing with the problem in some detail, considers that in cases where there is a chance of curing the pulmonary suppuration by thoracic surgery preliminary nasal surgery should be as complete as possible. On the other hand he advises a more conservative policy in the patient with extensive bronchiectasis in whom there is no hope of eradicating the pulmonary disease by surgical means.

Lavage through indwelling polythene tubes or Walford's cannulae is of value in children, and bilateral intranasal antrostomy bestows on patients the enormous benefit of enabling them to wash out their own antra, if necessary, at frequent intervals after leaving hospital.

More advanced cases of sinus suppuration, however, with diseased and polypoidal mucosa, will probably require Caldwell–Luc operations and possibly frontal, ethmoidal or sphenoidal drainage.

BRONCHITIS

In the British Isles bronchitis in its various forms is associated with enormous morbidity, loss of wage-earning capacity and physician's time and attention. It is of course undoubtedly influenced by such factors as overcrowding and air-pollution, and the magnitude of the social and medical problem which it presents, for example, in the "Industrial North" is not always appreciated by those who practise in more healthy and less heavily populated areas.

The laryngologist may be consulted at any stage. In childhood, adenoidal hypertrophy, tonsillar sepsis and maxillary sinusitis are not infrequently associated with bronchitis and may require appropriate attention. A case of acute bronchitis which is slow to resolve should always have a careful clinical and radiological examination of the sinuses as antral lavage may be necessary as an adjunct to medical treatment. Finally, in chronic bronchitis continued patience and skill may be required, for sinus lavage or more permanent drainage, septal resection and polypectomy are likely to be called for in certain cases with a view to reducing upper respiratory infection and improving the upper airways. The unfortunate patient may have permanent damage due to fibrosis and emphysema affecting the lower respiratory tract and the least we can do is to attempt to ease his burden by improving the health of the upper air passages.

BRONCHIAL ASTHMA

Bronchial asthma is characterized by paroxysmal attacks of expiratory dyspnoea due to muscular constriction of the bronchi and bronchioles, mucosal oedema and the accumulation of viscid secretion.

Its onset may occur at any time of life, and the severity of the attacks varies enormously. A mild attack may cause scarcely any disturbance yet a severe one is surely one of the most terrifying experiences known to man.

Few medical conditions have excited more interest or research than asthma and as the otolaryngologist is likely to encounter numerous patients suffering from this condition it is essential that he should be conversant with the current thought regarding its aetiology, pathogenesis, and the means by which he may influence its course.

Aetiology and precipitating factors

Heredity is undoubtedly an important predisposing factor particularly in cases of early onset, and few asthmatic patients can claim a complete absence of asthma, hay fever or other allied conditions amongst their close relatives.

Allergy to dusts, pollens and occasionally ingestants is present in about 50 per cent of cases which are sometimes referred to as *extrinsic asthma*. Whereas in other cases—*intrinsic asthma*—no hypersensitivity can be demonstrated.

Reflex nasal factors are undoubtedly present in many cases of asthma and it is well known that there exists in the nose a reception area for the nasopulmonary reflex. It is situated in the olfactory region of the nose, spreading down to the lower margin of the middle turbinal, and the corresponding area of the septum, and over the anterior surface of the sphenoid. The nasopulmonary reflex pathway connects the nose with the bronchial muscles and mucous membranes. It consists of an afferent path from the nasal mucous membrane through branches of the fifth cranial nerve, and an efferent path through the vagus.

Experimentally, Brodie and Dixon (1903) were able to cause reflex bronchoconstriction in dogs by electrical stimulation of the asthmagenic zone. Stimulation of the area by a variety of different factors may initiate an attack of bronchospastic asthma in the susceptible, but not in the normal, human subject.

In the human subject, these reflexes may be excited by any inflammatory, allergic, hypertrophic or neoplastic swelling of the nasal mucous membrane, or by deformities of the septum or turbinates, causing the mucous membrane of the septum and lateral nasal walls to come into close contact.

Infections of the nose or nasal sinuses play an important part in causing asthma in those patients in whom a bacterial allergen is a causative factor.

Emotional stress is clearly a precipitating factor of attacks in many cases of asthma. The rôle it plays varies enormously from case to case; in some patients it appears to have an overwhelming effect whilst in others it plays a negligible part.

Pathogenesis

It is probable that an antigen–antibody reaction is present in most cases of asthma, certainly in the *extrinsic cases,* and even in the *intrinsic* cases where no hypersensitivity can be demonstrated. The reaction releases histamine and the so-called "slow-reacting substance" (SRS–A) in the bronchial muscles which con-tract, causing constriction of the lumina of the bronchioles. The latter are moreover usually plugged by the excessive secretion of tenacious mucus. It is interesting to note that SRS–A is not inhibited by antihistamine drugs.

Laryngology in the treatment of asthma

The treatment of bronchial asthma in its entirety is beyond the scope of this work but attention must be drawn to the special rôle of the otolaryngologist. He is often consulted by the parents of asthmatic children who, grasping at straws, feel convinced that if only the tonsils and adenoids are removed all will be well. Considerable reserve must be shown in such circumstances and collaboration with paediatric colleagues is advisable. No hope of "cure" can be tendered; on the other hand infected tonsils and sinuses and adenoidal hypertrophy should certainly receive appropriate treatment which, though unlikely to cure, may certainly have a beneficial effect.

In other cases treatment for nasal allergy, sinus operations, submucous resection of the septum or nasal polypectomy may be required but these conditions should be treated "on their own account" and the patient should be warned that though the treatment is indicated for the well-being of his respiratory tract he must not expect the asthma to undergo miraculous improvement. It is sometimes necessary to cover operations on asthmatic patients with antihistamines or corticosteroids.

LUNG ABSCESS

It is customary to classify lung abscesses on an aetiological basis, and they may fall into the following categories: bronchogenic; suppurative pneumonic; haematogenous; and subdiaphragmatic.

Abscesses which arise by blood stream spread or by spread from an amoebic hepatic or subdiaphragmatic abscess are rare. The suppurative pneumonic variety are those resulting from the necrosis of lung tissue in some forms of pneumonia particularly where the organism concerned is very virulent or perhaps insensitive to antibiotics, for example in cases of infection with Friedländer's bacillus or *Staphylococcus aureus.* But the most common variety of lung abscess and that which concerns the ear, nose and throat surgeon most closely falls into the bronchogenic group.

Aetiology of bronchogenic lung abscess

Operations on the upper respiratory tract have in the past been considered likely causes of lung abscesses, and writers have asserted that almost 25 per cent of solitary lung abscesses occurred after operations for the removal of tonsils and adenoids. Happily, this is by no means the picture today. Bosher (1951) in describing 130 cases of lung abscess asserted that 21 followed tonsillectomy, but Pickar and Ruoff (1959), writing eight years later, found that in a series of 70 cases of lung abscess only one case followed tonsillectomy.

Tartar and fragments from septic teeth are suspect. Brock (1946), in a series of 316 lung abscesses, showed that 7 per cent followed dental extractions, and there is no doubt that inhaled foreign bodies, both endogenous and exogenous, may be responsible for the ultimate development of a lung abscess

For the most likely distribution of pulmonary suppuration consequent upon the inhalation of blood or debris the reader is again referred to Brock's important work *Anatomy of the Bronchial Tree* (1946). *See also* "Bronchial foreign bodies" (p. 583).

Bronchial obstruction caused by bronchogenic carcinoma frequently leads to abscess formation, and it is estimated that at least 25 per cent of cases of bronchogenic abscess are caused in this way.

Diagnosis and treatment

It is not the intention in a work of this scope to give the detailed clinical picture of lung abscess, to enumerate the methods of investigation, or to deal in full with the question of treatment. Mention must, however, be made of the important rôle of bronchoscopy.

The bronchoscope is an instrument of enormous importance in the prophylaxis, diagnosis and treatment of lung abscess. In the first connection bronchoscopy, with the removal of foreign bodies or the relief of pulmonary collapse, is undoubtedly responsible for averting the development of a large number of lung abscesses. In the case of an established abscess the bronchoscopic technique is used to exclude or remove any foreign body, to examine and biopsy an underlying tumour or to remove by aspiration secretions which may be subjected to cytological and bacteriological examination.

Bronchoscopy with aspiration may be curative in the case of the early acute abscess and, if necessary, can be repeated to maintain drainage. In chronic abscesses, however, it is unlikely to be curative, and recourse has to be made to lobectomy or, in the case of abscess with carcinoma, pneumonectomy.

CONGENITAL STENOSIS OF TRACHEA

Fortunately this anomaly is of considerable rarity but it is important that the surgeon should be aware that it may occur for if ignored it is likely to be fatal, though if recognized it may be corrected.

Most commonly there is an hour-glass narrowing at some point in the trachea causing inspiratory and expiratory stridor from, or soon after, birth. Radiography may be of some value in diagnosis and bronchography using water-soluble media may be employed. Bronchoscopy, though confirmatory is intensely hazardous as any instrumentation may cause sufficient oedema to obstruct the airway completely.

Cantrell and Guild (1964) believe that correction of the anomaly must be achieved as early as possible and describe in detail their surgical approach and excision of the stenotic area.

BENIGN TUMOURS OF THE TRACHEA AND BRONCHI

Although benign tumours of the trachea and bronchi are relatively rare the occurrence of many different types has been recorded from time to time. These are as follows: adenoma; papilloma; endothelioma; chondroma; osteoma; fibroma; myoma; lipoma; angioma; neurofibroma; and neurilemmoma. Cylindroma may also occur and may have malignant tendencies. Adenoma of the bronchus deserves special mention.

Adenoma of the bronchus

These are the most frequently encountered of all benign tracheobronchial tumours and occur more commonly in the main or secondary bronchi. They are extremely vascular and give rise to spontaneous haemoptyses. There is no marked difference between the incidence in men and in women, and the patients are often between 30 and 50 years of age.

Microscopically, well-differentiated cells are found in glandular pattern, and in some tumours the vascular stroma is extremely abundant. The diagnosis is based on a history of haemoptysis, with perhaps wheezing and the signs of bronchial obstruction. Confirmation is obtained by radiography and bronchoscopic examination with biopsy.

Bronchoscopy must be carried out with care, for even slight contact with the end of the bronchoscope or suction tube may cause profuse haemorrhage. The tumour is smooth and non-ulcerated and varies in colour from pale to bright pink; on close inspection blood vessels may be seen coursing beneath its epithelial covering.

With regard to treatment, it is not now considered advisable to attempt the bronchoscopic removal of these tumours, or to employ radiotherapy. Segmental resection is occasionally satisfactory, but lobectomy is more often the method of choice.

MALIGNANT TUMOURS OF THE TRACHEA

Malignant disease of the trachea occurs either as a primary or as a secondary lesion. Primary malignant tumours are usually adenocarcinomata or squamous-celled growths. Secondary malignant disease of the trachea arises by direct spread from the larynx, the thyroid gland, the hypopharynx, the oesophagus or from adjacent neoplastic lymph nodes.

Clinical picture

The predominant symptom is dyspnoea, and its onset may be abrupt or insidious. A characteristic low-pitched expiratory and inspiratory stridor is often present. The degree of dyspnoea is often influenced by the patient's position, and frequently made worse when he is supine. The growth gradually encroaches further into the tracheal lumen, causing constant dyspnoea, which may be accompanied by cough and haemoptysis. Later, the recurrent laryngeal nerves are likely to become involved, and extension to the oesophagus may take place with the development of a tracheo-oesophageal fistula and all its attendant misery. Extension to the thyroid gland and the paratracheal lymph nodes is usually early.

Diagnosis

Sometimes a glimpse of the growth is obtained in the laryngeal mirror, but tracheoscopy with biopsy is necessary as a confirmatory measure. Tomography is of value in delineating the growth and giving information about its local spread.

Treatment

Various attempts to cure carcinoma of the trachea have been made by means of diathermy destruction, radon seeds, teleradiotherapy or radical surgical removal, but it must be admitted that these attempts have been, as a general rule, unsuccessful.

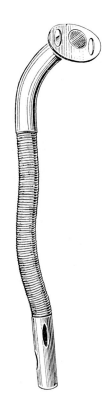

FIG. 250.—Koenig's long tracheal tube.

Diagnosis is not usually established until the growth has spread into adjacent structures, by which time surgical ablation is no longer feasible, and the chief task left to the medical adviser is that of palliation. In this connection the Koenig tracheostomy tube (Fig. 250) may be of value.

In those cases where surgical removal can be accomplished, reconstruction of the trachea has, in the past, presented a great problem, but more recently successful reconstruction has been achieved by the use of fascia lata braced with tantalum gauze, or a spiral of stainless steel wire (Belsey, 1946 and 1950). Rob and Bateman (1949) reported a case of tracheal replacement with tantalum gauze covered on both sides with fascia lata in which the defect in the trachea was 9 cm. long. The same patient was referred to later (Rob and Bromley, 1953) and was alive and well five years after the reconstruction which had followed excision of a recurrence of thyroid carcinoma. Greenberg (1960), in a review of the subject of tracheal reconstruction quoting from an extensive bibliography and basing his conclusions on animal work, found that freeze-dried tracheal homografts were unsatisfactory, but Marlex plastic mesh, Merilene cloth and tantalum gave more hopeful results.

CARCINOMA OF THE BRONCHUS

The incidence of carcinoma of the bronchus continues to increase, and the disease is of enormous interest to clinicians not only on account of its relative frequency but by virtue of the varied nature of the symptoms with which it may present. For detailed descriptions of its aetiology, pathology, clinical features and treatment the reader is advised to consult the current textbooks on thoracic medicine and surgery, but certain facets of the diagnosis which are of particular interest to the ear, nose and throat surgeon are now given.

Clinical picture

Cough is the most common and, as a general rule, the earliest presenting symptom of carcinoma of the bronchus. The complaint of cough by a patient attending the E.N.T. clinic, perhaps for some entirely separate condition, calls for an exclusory chest x-ray. Examine the patient's fingers for *clubbing*. Pulmonary osteo-arthropathy is not uncommon in patients suffering from a malignant new growth of the bronchus, and the rapid development of clubbing in middle-aged patients should always arouse suspicion of such a neoplasm. This sign may appear before any other clinical manifestations of the disease. *Haemoptysis, chest pain, dyspnoea* and *wheezing* are frequently among the first symptoms; they are seldom neglected by the patient, who usually seeks medical advice as soon as they develop. *Hoarseness* or *weakness of voice*, however, may have been present for some considerable time before the patient consults his doctor, who will then direct him to the E.N.T. clinic. The hoarseness is due to left recurrent nerve paralysis resulting from involvement of the nerve by malignant mediastinal lymph nodes under the aortic arch. Asherson (1952) describes a laryngeal and pharyngeal syndrome as a presenting symptom in some cases of lung cancer. Disordered deglutition occurs as the nerve supply which the cricopharyngeal sphincter receives from the recurrent laryngeal nerve is interrupted. In cases where only one recurrent nerve is paralysed the disorder is confined to the swallowing of fluids.

Occasionally, a *mass in the neck* brings the patient to the ear, nose and throat surgeon. Clinical and radiological examination is unrevealing, and biopsy is performed, the result suggesting a malignant deposit in a lymph node. If bronchoscopy has not been performed in such a case it should certainly be the next step, for a small primary tumour may be found in the bronchus. In some cases even the bronchoscopic findings are normal and time alone confirms the diagnosis.

Bronchoscopy in the diagnosis of bronchial carcinoma

Bronchoscopy is of great importance to the surgeon as an aid not only in the diagnosis of bronchial carcinoma but in the establishment of operability. As the situation of 75–80 per cent of all bronchial carcinomas is in the main bronchus or at the commencement of a secondary bronchus, all of which are visible through the bronchoscope, it is unnecessary to emphasize the need for this examination.

The carina must be inspected carefully. Widening of this normally sharp structure suggests involvement of the subcarinal (inferior tracheobronchial) lymph nodes and is a sign of inoperability, as is any involvement of the trachea. The mobility of the carina and the walls of the main bronchi should be determined.

The tumour itself may occur as a thickening of the submucosa with or without surface ulceration; sometimes sessile or pedunculated nodular growths are present. The most frequently observed lesion, however, is a mass of fungations filling one of the bronchi and possibly covered by purulent and necrotic material. A biopsy is taken.

In other cases no tumour may be seen, but the presence of bloodstained secretion exuding from a subsidiary bronchus is highly suspicious, and the aspirated fluid should be submitted for cytological examination.

Other methods of investigation

Apart from radiology and bronchoscopy with cytological examination of biopsy, other methods sometimes employed in establishing the diagnosis of bronchogenic carcinoma are needle biopsy of the pleura or lung, pre-scalene biopsy, mediastinoscopy and, of course, in some cases, exploratory thoractomy.

Whilst needle biopsy of the pleura is of value in certain circumstances, lung biopsy should be avoided in any case which might be operable, as it may cause dissemination of disease. Pre-scalene biopsy, from the patient's point of view a relatively minor operation, may obviate the necessity of the more major operation —thoracotomy.

Treatment and prognosis

Briefly, operable cases treated by lobectomy or pneumonectomy have a five year survival rate in the region of 20 per cent but, unfortunately, for every case which is operable at least five cases presenting for treatment bear the criteria of inoperability.

For these there remain radiotherapy and cytotoxic drugs. Although occasionally fairly good palliation is achieved with both these methods, it must be admitted that the chief duty of the medical attendant to the patient with inoperable bronchogenic carcinoma is to ease his suffering.

REFERENCES

Asherson, N. (1952). *Brit. J. Tuberc.*, **46**, 95.
Bannister, W. K., Sattilaro, A. J., and Otis, R. D. (1961). *Anaesthesiology*, **22**, 440.
Belsey, R. (1946). *Thorax*, **1**, 647.
— (1950). *Brit. J. Surg.*, **38**, 200.
Birch, C. A. (1963). *Emergencies in Medical Practice* (7th ed.). Edinburgh and London; Livingstone.
Bosher, L. H., Jr. (1951). *J. thoracic Surg.*, **21**, 370
Brock, R. C. (1964a). *Guy's Hosp. Rep.*, **95**, 40.
— (1946b). *Anatomy of the Bronchial Tree*. London; Oxford University Press.
Brodie, T. G., and Dixon, W. E. (1903). *J. Physiol.*, **29**, 97.
Cantrell, J. R., and Guild, H. G. (1964). *Amer. J. Surg.*, **108**, 297.

Greenberg, S. D. (1960). *Arch. Otolaryng.*, **72**, 565.
Hausmann, W., and Lunt, R. L. (1955). *J. Obstet. Gynaec. Brit. Emp.*, **62**, 509.
Hinshaw, H. C., and Garland, L. H. (1963). *Diseases of the Chest* (2nd ed.). Philadelphia and London; Saunders.
Hogg, J. C. (1950). *Proc. R. Soc. Med.*, **43**, 1087.
Jackson, Chevalier (1934). *Bronchoscopy, Oesophagoscopy and Gastroscopy* (3rd ed.). Philadelphia; Saunders.
— (1936). *Diseases of the Air and Food Passages of Foreign Body Origin.* Philadelphia; Saunders.
Kartagener, M. (1933). *Beitr. klin. Tuberk.*, **83**, 489.
Lassen, H. A. C. (1933). *Lancet*, **1**, 37.
Loder, R. E. (1955). *Lancet*, **1**, 1150.
Mendelson, C. L. (1946). *Amer. J. Obstet. Gynec.*, **52**, 191.
Ormerod, F. C. (1941). *J. Laryng.*, **56**, 227.
Pickar, D. N., and Ruoff, W. F. (1959). *J. thoracic. Surg.*, **37**, 452.
Pitman, R. G., and Wilson, F. (1955). *Lancet*, **2**, 523.
Rob, C. G., and Bateman, G. H. (1949). *Brit. J. Surg.*, **37**, 202.
— and Bromley, L. L. (1953). *Thorax*, **8**, 269.
Scurr, C. F. (1960). *Med. Press*, **243**, 5.
Seydell, E. M. (1937). *Arch Otolaryng.*, **26**, 189.
Simenstad, J. O., Galway, C. F., and Maclean, L. D. (1963). *Anaesth. Analg.*, **42**, 616.
Thompson, H. T., and Pryor, W. J. (1964). *Lancet*, **2**, 8.

INDEX TO VOLUME 4

Abbé's skin flap, 477–479
Abscess,
  acute cervical, 70
  intratonsillar, 116
  larynx, of 323–325
  lung, of, 592–593
  parapharyngeal, 70, 109, 116
  peri-oesophageal, 228
  peritonsillar, 109, 113–116
    incision of, 115
    tonsillectomy in, 115
Abscess tonsillectomy, 115
Accelerator, linear, 490, 493
Achalasia of cardia, 231–234
Actinomycosis,
  larynx, of, 343
  mouth, of, 24
  salivary glands, of, 49
Adamantinoma, 34
Addison's disease, 5
Adenitis (see "Lymphadenitis")
Adenocarcinoma,
  larynx, of, 395
  pharynx, of, 148
  trachea, of, 594–596
Adenoidectomy, 136–140
  anaesthesia for, 136
  complications of, 140
  haemorrhage from,
    primary, 137
    reactionary, 138
    secondary, 139
  indications for, 136
  post-operative care in, 139
  technique of, 137
Adenoiditis,
  acute, 111
  chronic, 133–136
    complications of, 135
    symptoms and signs of, 134
    treatment of, 136
Adenoids,
  enlargement of, 104–105
  retention cyst of, 135
Adenolymphoma, 54
Adenoma,
  bronchus, of, 594
  laryngopharynx, of, 173
  larynx, of, 387–388
  mouth, of, 31

oropharynx, of, 163
palate, of, 31
pleomorphic, salivary gland, of, 51–53,
    56, 57, 63
trachea, of, 594
Adenovirus, 83
Agnosia,
  auditory, 564–565
  visual, 567, 572
Agranulocytosis, 88–89, 107
  pharyngitis in, 143
  stomatitis in, 22
Ameloblastoma, 34
Amyloidosis of larynx, 386–387
Anaemia,
  hypochromic, 87
  microcytic, 87
  normocytic, 87
  pernicious, 87
  stomatitis in, 22
  tonsillectomy in, 121
Anaesthesia of pharynx, 94
Anastomosis, portacaval, 239
Angina, 140–143
  agranulocytic, 88–89, 107, 143
  aphthous, 142
  leukaemic, 143
  Ludwig's, 68
  monocytic, 141–142
  Vincent's, 141
Angiofibroma, juvenile, 161–162
Angioma,
  bronchus, of, 594
  larynx, of, 384–385
  trachea, of, 594
Ankyloglossia, 18
Anti-metabolites, 498–499
Aorta, aneurysm of, 212, 213
Aphonia, functional, 540
Apple-jelly nodules, 81
Artery,
  aberrant subclavian, 212
  internal carotid, injury of, adenoidec-
    tomy, in, 140
  posterior inferior cerebellar, thrombosis
    of, 539
Arthritis,
  crico-arytenoid, 313, 325
  laryngeal, 372–373
Aryepiglottic folds, carcinoma of, 401

Astereognosis, 572
Asthma, bronchial, 591–592
  laryngology in treatment of, 592
Atresia,
  larynx, of, 292–293
  oesophagus, of, 217
Avellis' syndrome, 538

Behçet's disease, 26, 92
Betatron, 490
Blastomycosis,
  larynx, of, 343–344
  mouth, of, 24
Blindness, congenital, 566
Block dissection of neck, 459–471
  carcinoma of larynx, in, 416, 467
Bornholm disease, 83
Brain stem, tumours of, 539
Broder's classification of carcinoma of
  larynx, 395
Bronchi,
  diseases of, 583–597
  foreign body in, 583–589
    removal of, 586–587
Bronchiectasis, 589–590
  sinusitis in, 590
Bronchitis, 590–591
  sinusitis in, 591
Bronchoscopy, 268–279
  anaesthesia for, 274
  carcinoma of bronchus, in, 597
  foreign body, for, 586–587
  lung abscess, in, 593
  normal appearances at, 277–279
  pulmonary collapse, in, 588–589
  technique of, 274–279
Bronchus, tumours of,
  benign, 594
  malignant, 596–597

Caesium-137, half-life of, 491
Calculus, salivary, 44–45, 47
Cancrum oris, 26, 73
Carcinoma,
  bronchus, of, 596–597
    bronchoscopy in, 596, 597
    mediastinoscopy in, 597
    treatment of, 597
  glottic region, of, 399
  laryngopharynx, of, 173–195
  larynx, of, 389–455 (see also "Larynx,
    carcinoma of")
    in situ, 399
  lip, of, 36
  mouth, of, 35
  nasopharynx, of, 152–160

oesophagus, of, 239–244
  achalasia, in, 233
oropharynx, of, 164–172
pharyngeal pouch, of, 199
pharynx, of, 148
salivary glands, of, 54
  adenoid cystic, 53
subglottic region, of, 400
supraglottic region, of, 400
tongue, of, 7, 35
trachea, of, 594–596
  treatment of, 595–596
Cardia, achalasia of, 231–234
Cardiomyotomy, 234
Cardiospasm, 231
Carditis, neonatal, 83
Celestin's tube, 242
Cerebellum, diseases of, 577
Cervical node dissection, 459–471
  incisions in, 460–464, 471
  laryngectomy, with, 467–469
Chancre,
  extragenital, 78
  mouth, of, 23
Chemotherapy, malignant disease, in,
  principles of, 489, 494–502 (see also
  "Drugs, cytotoxic")
Chest, injuries of, 509
Chicken-pox, 73
Chondroma,
  bronchus, of, 594
  larynx, of, 385–386
    congenital, 297
  oropharynx, of, 163
  pharynx, of, 147
  trachea, of, 594
Chondrosarcoma,
  larynx, of, 395
  pharynx, of, 148
Chorditis nodosa, 363–364
  children, in, 367
Chorditis tuberosa, 360
Chordoma,
  nasopharynx, of, 160
  pharynx, of, 149
Chorea in tonsillitis, 110
Christmas disease, tonsillectomy in, 121
Clergyman's throat, 76
Cobalt bomb, 493
Cobalt-60, half-life of, 491
Cold, common, 84
Collapse, post-operative, pulmonary, 588–
  589
Collet–Sicard syndrome, 539
Coma, 509
Commando operation, 170
Contact ulcer, 361, 362
  larynx, of, 552
Cord, vocal,
  excision of, bilateral recurrent laryngeal
    nerve paralysis, in, 533

Cord (*continued*)
  hyperkeratosis of, 394
  nodule of, 363–364, 551
  pachydermia of, 359
  paralysis of, 313 (*see also* "Nerve, recurrent laryngeal")
  submucosal haemorrhage of, 551
Cordopexy, 534–536
Corona veneris, 5 79
Coryza, 67
Costen's syndrome, 6, 28
Cough, laryngeal, 827
Coup de glotte, 363, 551, 552
Coxsackie virus, 83
Crossling's Bougies, 242
Croup, 282, 326
Cyclophosphamide, 498
Cylindroma,
  bronchus, of, 594
  trachea, of, 594
Cyst,
  branchial, larynx, of, 296
  branchiogenic, 149, 151
  dental, 30
  dentigerous, 30
  dermoid, larynx, of, 296
  epiglottis, of, 173
  eruption, of, 30
  larynx, of, 382–384
    congenital, 296–297
  mouth, of, 29
  nasopalatine, 29
  oesophagus, of, 239
  primordial, 29
  retention, 31
    adenoids, of, 135
  salivary gland, of, 43, 55
  thyroglossal, 19
  tonsil, of, 117
Cytology, exfoliative, carcinoma of oeso-phagus, in, 209

Deafness, congenital, 563–564
Decannulation after tracheostomy, 288
Degeneration, subacute combined, 87
Dehiscence, Killian's, 197
Diathermy, endoscopic, pharyngeal pouch, of, 203, 204
Dieffenbach's skin flap, 479
Diphtheria,
  laryngeal, 327–331
    diagnosis of, 329
    pathology of, 328
    symptoms of, 329
    treatment of, 330
  oesophagus, of, 228
  pharyngeal, 70, 107
Diverticulo-oesophagostomy, 205

Diverticulum,
  hypopharyngeal, 197–206
  oesophagus, of, 234–236
D.N.A. virus, 83
Dohlman's operation in pharyngeal pouch, 204
Drugs, cytotoxic, 494–502
  administration of, 499–502
  choice of, 496–499
Duct, parotid,
  injury of, 44
  ligation of, 48
  stricture of, 47
Dysarthria, 574–581
  disease, in,
    basal ganglia, of, 577
    cerebellum, of, 577
    muscle, of, 578
  lower motor neurone disease, in, 576
  upper motor neurone disease, in, 574–576
Dysgraphia, 572
Dyslexia, 567
  congenital, 567–570
Dysphagia lusoria, 212
Dysphasia, 560
  aetiology of, 573
  expressive, 571–572
  foreign tongue, 572
  gesture, 572
  mime, 572
  nominal, 566, 571
  pathology of, 573
  prognosis of, 573
  treatment of, 573
Dysphonia, 574–581
  disease, in,
    basal ganglia, of, 577
    cerebellum, of, 577
    muscle, of, 578
  lower motor neurone disease, in, 576
  upper motor neurone disease, in, 574–576
Dysphonia plicae ventricularis, 353, 554
Dyspraxia, 572

E.C.H.O. virus, 83
Electrogustometry, 9
Emphysema, surgical,
  neck, of, 221
  tracheostomy, after, 517, 521
Endocarditis, subacute bacterial, 110
Endothelioma,
  bronchus, of, 594
  trachea, of, 594
Enterocytopathogenic human orphan virus, 83
Enterovirus, 83
Epiglottis,
  bifid, 292
  carcinoma of, 400

Epiglottitis,
    acute, 316–317
    lingual tonsillitis, in, 111
Epulis
    fibrous, 32
    giant-celled, 32
Erythema migrans linguae, 19
Erythema multiforme, 5
Estlander's skin flap, 477–479

Fauces, examination of, 10
Fever,
    glandular, 91–92, 107, 141–142
    pharyngoconjunctival, 84
    rheumatic, 110, 117
    scarlet, 72, 107
Fibroma,
    bronchus, of, 594
    laryngopharynx, of, 173
    larynx, of, 382
        congenital, 297
    mouth, of, 32
    oesophagus, of, 239
    oropharynx, of, 163
    salivary glands, of, 55
    trachea, of, 594
Fibrosarcoma,
    larynx, of, 395
    oesophagus, of, 239
    pharynx, of, 148
Finzi–Harmer operation, 421
Fistula,
    salivary, 44, 58
    tracheo-oesophageal, 595
        congenital, 217–219
Foramen, jugular, tumours of, 539
Fordyce spots, 18
Foreign body,
    bronchial, 583–589
        endogenous, 583–584
        exogenous, 584–585
        removal of, 586–587
    larynx, in, 304–306
    oesophagus, in, 223–228
    pharynx, in, 225
    tonsil, in, 144
    tracheobronchial tree, in, 583–589
        removal of, 586–587

Gamma-rays, 490
Ganglia, basal, diseases of, 577
Gastrostomy in carcinoma of oesophagus, 243
Gillies' fan-flap, 479–481
Gingivitis, 6

Gland,
    parotid,
        oncocytoma of, 54
        surgical anatomy of, 37–39
        tumours of, 55–58
    salivary,
        acinic cell tumours of, 53
        actinomycosis of, 49
        adenoid cystic carcinoma of, 53
        calculus of, 44–45
        carcinoma of, 54
        connective tissue tumours of, 55
        cysts of, 43
        diseases of, 37–66
        enlargement of, 49
        infections of, 45–49
        management of tumours of, 55–65
        minor,
            surgical anatomy of, 37–41
            tumours of, 59–63
        muco-epidermoid tumours of, 53
        mucoviscidosis, in, 49
        neoplasms of, 50–65
        pleomorphic adenoma of, 51–53, 56, 57
        sarcoidosis of, 48–49
        secondary tumours of, 54
        syphilis of, 49
        tuberculosis of, 48
    submandibular,
        excision of, 59
        surgical anatomy of, 39–40
        tumours of, 58–59
Glandular fever, 91–92, 107, 141–142
    stomatitis in, 22
Globus hystericus, 93
Glomerulonephritis, acute, tonsillitis, in, 110, 117
Glossectomy, 170, 172
Glossitis,
    anaemia, in, 88
    median rhomboid, 19
Glottis, carcinoma of, 399
Gougerot's syndrome, 49
Granuloma, benign reparative giant-celled, 34
Gumma,
    larynx, of, 341
    mouth, of, 23
    pharynx, of, 79

Haemangioma,
    congenital, larynx, of, 297–299
    mouth, of, 33
    oesophagus, of, 239
    salivary glands, of, 55
Haematoma of larynx, 372
Haemophilia, tonsillectomy in, 121

Haemorrhage after tracheostomy, 517, 520
Hamartoma of pharynx, 149, 151
Hare lip, 4
Heerfordt's syndrome, 49
* Heller's operation, 234
Hernia,
    para-oesophageal, 229, 230, 231
    sliding, oesophageal hiatus, of, 230, 231
Herpangina, 9, 83, 84
Herpes,
    labialis, 4
        recurrent, 24
    larynx, of, 325–326
    simplex, mouth, of, 24
    zoster, mouth, of, 24
Hiatus hernia, 229–231
Histoplasmosis of mouth, 24
Hughlings Jackson syndrome, 539
Hurst's mercury bougie, 234, 237
Hutchinson's teeth, 6, 79
Hygiene, oral, 17
Hygroma, cystic, larynx, of, 296
Hypernasality after adenoidectomy, 140

Immunization in poliomyelitis, 99
Infectious mononucleosis, 91–92, 107, 141–142
    stomatitis in, 22
Infusion, regional arterial, 496, 501–502
Intubation, laryngeal, infants, in, 287–290
Iodine-131, half-life of, 491

Jackson's gum-elastic bougie, 237
Jaws (see also "Mouth")
    benign reparative giant-celled granuloma of, 34
    osteoma of, 33
    sarcoma of, 36
    tumours of, 31

Kartagener's syndrome, 590
Kelly's operation, 534
Keratoconjunctivitis, epidemic, 84
Keratosis pharyngis, 82, 143
Killian, dehiscence of, 197
King's operation, 534
Koplik's spots, 5, 73

Laryngectomy, 172, 183–194
    abscess of larynx, in, 325

block dissection, with, 467–469
    partial, 415, 417, 418, 425–437
        supraglottic, 432–437
    total, 415, 416, 417, 418, 423, 437–453
        complications of, 450–451
        post-operative care of, 447–449
        rehabilitation after, 451–453
        technique of, 438–446
Laryngismus stridulus, 527
Laryngitis,
    acute, 301–331
        children, in, 315–320
        measles, in, 73
    acute catarrhal, 311–315
    atrophic, 369–371
    chronic, 333–373
        childhood, in, 367–368
        diffuse hyperplastic, 348–353
            aetiology of, 348
            diagnosis of, 340
            pathology of, 348
            prognosis of, 352
            signs of, 350
            symptoms of, 349
            treatment of, 351
        localized hyperplastic, 353–359
        non-specific, 345–371
            aetiology of, 345–347
            classification of, 347–348
            pathology of, 347
        systemic disease, in, 368
    granular, 360–361
    haemorrhagic, 371
    lingual tonsillitis, in, 111
    membranous, 326–327
    non-infective, 550
    ozaenatous, 369
Laryngitis sicca, 369
Laryngocoele, 541–543
Laryngofissure, 415, 424, 425–432
    amyloidosis of larynx, in, 387
    chondroma of larynx, in, 386
    complications of, 430–432
    laryngeal injuries, in, 303
    leucoplakia, in, 366
    scleroma, in, 345
    stenosis of larynx, in, 308
Laryngogram, 267, 268
Laryngomalacia, 291–292
Laryngopharynx,
    examination of, 14
    malignant neoplasms of, 173–195
    tumours of, 172–195
        benign, 173
Laryngoscopy,
    direct, 253–265, 376–379
        anaesthesia for, 255–259
    indirect, 15, 249–253
    infants, in, 284–287
Laryngotomy, 505, 522–523
Laryngotracheobronchitis, acute, 317–320

Larynx,
  abscess of, 323–325
    syphilis, in, 342
  actinomycosis of, 343
  acute perichondritis of, 322–323
  adenocarcinoma of, 395
  adenoma of, 387–388
  amyloidosis of, 386–387
  anaesthesia of, 525–526
  angioma of, 384–385
  angioneurotic oedema of, 320
  atresia of, 292–293
  blastomycosis of, 343–344
  burns and scalds of, 304
  carcinoma of, 389–455
    chemotherapy in, 418
      symptomatic relief of, 419, 420
    radiotherapy in, 416, 417, 419, 420–423
    treatment of, 415–455
      results of, 453–455
      surgical, 415, 416, 417, 418, 423–455
  chondroma of, 385–386
    congenital, 297
  chondrosarcoma of, 395
  closed injuries of, 302–304
  congenital diseases of, 281–299
  contact ulcer of, 552
  cyst of, 382
    branchial, 296
    congenital, 296–297, 383
    dermoid, 296
    retention, 383
  cystic hygroma of, 296
  diphtheria of, 327–331
    diagnosis of, 329
    pathology of, 328
    symptoms of, 329
    treatment, of, 330
  examination of, 249–268
  fibroma of, 382
    congenital, 297
  fibrosarcoma of, 395
  foreign body of, 304–306
  haemangioma of, congenital, 297
  haematoma of, 372
  herpes of, 325–326
  hyperaesthesia of, 526
  infantile, 281–282
  intubation of, 505–523
    complications of, 519–520
    diphtheria in, 331
    indications for, 505–510
    infants in, 287–290
    laryngotracheobronchitis, 319
    oedema of larynx, in, 322
  leiomyoma of, congenital, 297
  leptothricosis of, 343
  leucoplakia of, 364–366
    diagnosis of carcinoma, from, 414
  lipoma of, 389
    congenital, 297

  lupus vulgaris of, 340–341
  lymphangioma of, 296
  lymphoma of, malignant, 395
  melanoma of, malignant, 395
  motor disorders of, 526–539
  myasthenia of, 552
  mycoses of, 343–344
  myoblastoma of, 388–389
  neurofibroma of, 389
  neurological affections of, 525–540
  obstruction of, infants, in, 282–299
  occupational disorders of, 541–557
  oedema of, 314, 320–322
    intubation, after, 517, 519
    radiotherapy, after, 422
  palpation of, 266
  papilloma of, 379–382
  paraesthesia of, 526
  paralytic disorders of, 529–539
  perichondritis of, syphilis, in, 342
  plasmacytoma of, 389, 395
  pseudocyst of, 384
  psychogenic disorders of, 539–540
  radiography of, 267–268
  rhabdomyoma of, 389
  scleroma of, 344–345
  sensory disorders of, 525–526
  spasmodic disorders of, 526–529
  stenosis of, 306–309
  stroboscopy of, 266
  submucous haemorrhage of, 371–372
  syphilis of, 341–343
  telangiectasia of, congenital, 384
  tomography of, 268
  trauma of, 301–309
  tuberculosis of, 333–340
    diagnosis of, 336
    pathology of, 334–335
    prognosis of, 339
    symptoms of, 336
    treatment of, 337–339
  tumours of, 375–455
    benign, 375–389
    congenital, 297–299
    malignant, 389–455
      causation of, 393
      classification of, 389–393
      diagnosis of, 403–415
      histopathology of, 395–399
      incidence of, 393–395
      spread of, 401–402
      symptoms of, 402–403
  ulceration of, intubation, after, 517, 520
  vascular polyp of, 384
  wounds of, 301–302
  web of, 292–293
  xanthoma of, 389
Leiomyoma,
  laryngopharynx, of, 173
  larynx, of, congenital, 297
  oesophagus, of, 239

Leiomyosarcoma of oesophagus, 239
Leptothricosis of larynx, 343
Leucoplakia,
   larynx, of, 364–366
   mouth, of, 5, 27
   oesophagus, of, 229
Leukaemia, 90–91, 107
   stomatitis in, 22
Lichen planus of mouth, 27
Lip,
   carcinoma of, 36
   congenital haemangioma of, 4
   salivary tumours of, 60
Lipoma,
   bronchus, of, 594
   laryngopharynx, of, 173
   larynx, of, congenital, 297
   mouth, of, 33
   salivary glands, of, 55
   trachea, of, 594
Lobectomy in carcinoma of bronchus, 597
Ludwig's angina, 8, 68
Lung abscess, 592–593
Lupus vulgaris,
   larynx, of, 340–341
   pharynx, of, 81
Lymphadenitis,
   acute cervical, 109
   acute, pharyngitis, in, 69
Lymphangioma,
   larynx, of, 296
   salivary glands, of, 55
Lympho-epithelioma of oropharynx, 164
Lymphoma,
   larynx, of, malignant, 395
   pharynx, of, 149
Lymphosarcoma,
   oesophagus, of, 239
   oropharynx, of, 164
   pharynx, of, 149

Macroglossia, 18
Marginal zone of larynx, carcinoma of, 400
Measles, 73–74
Mediastinoscopy in carcinoma of bronchus, 597
Mediastinotomy, 222
Megavoltage therapy, 493
Melanoma, malignant,
   larynx, of, 395
   mouth, of, 36
Melanosarcoma of oesophagus, 239
Melphalan, 498
Meningitis,
   aseptic, 83
   basal, 539
Methotrexate, 499
Microglossia, 18

Microlaryngoscopy, 263–265, 377–378
   chronic laryngitis, in, 348
Mikulicz' syndrome, 49
Mogiphonia, 554–555
Monilia,
   mouth, of, 23
   oesophagus, of, 228
Mononucleosis, infectious, 91–92, 107, 141–142
Motor neurone disease, 539
Mousseau–Barbin tube, 241, 242, 243
Mouth (see also "Glossitis", "Jaw", "Stomatitis", "Tongue")
   adenoma of, 31
   carcinoma of, 35
   chancre of, 23
   congenital anomalies of, 18–20
   cysts of, 29
   diseases of, 17–36
   examination of, 3
   fibroma of, 32
   floor of, examination of, 7
   fungal infections of, 23
   haemangioma of, 33
   hygiene of, 17
   leucoplakia of, 27
   lichen planus of, 27
   lipoma of, 33
   melanoma of, 36
   myoma of, 33
   myxoma of, 33
   papilloma of, 31
   pemphigoid of, 27
   pemphigus of, 26
   plasmacytoma of, 34
   salivary tumours of, 62
   sarcoma of, 36
   tumours of, 31
Mutism in congenital deafness, 563–564
Myasthenia gravis, 97
Myasthenia of larynx, 552–554
Mycoses of larynx, 343–344
Myoblastoma of larynx, 388–389
Myoma,
   bronchus, of, 594
   mouth, of, 33
   trachea, of, 594
Myotomy in pharyngeal pouch, 201, 202
Myxoma,
   mouth, of, 33
   pharynx, of, 148]
Myxoviruses, 83

Nasopharyngoscope, 14
Nasopharynx,
   carcinoma of, 152–160
   chordoma of, 160
   examination of, 12
   juvenile angiofibroma of, 161–162

Nasopharynx (*continued*)
  neoplasms of,
    benign, 152
    malignant, 152–162
  tumours of, 150–162
Negus' hydrostatic bag, 234
Neoplasms (*see under* anatomical region affected)
Nephritis, acute, tonsillitis, in, 110, 117
Nerve,
  accessory, paralysis of, 538
  glossopharyngeal, paralysis of, 538
  hypoglossal, paralysis of, 538
  recurrent laryngeal,
    injury of, 302
    paralysis of, 207, 313, 529–536
      bilateral, 531–536
      carcinoma, in,
        bronchus, of, 596
        trachea, of, 595
      pharyngeal pouch, in, 199, 200
      therapeutic, 339
  superior laryngeal,
    injection of, 338
    paralysis of, 536–537
    resection of, 338
  vagus, paralysis of, 538
Neuralgia, glossopharyngeal, 94
Neurectomy, tympanic, 48
Neurilemmoma,
  bronchus, of, 594
  trachea, of, 594
Neurofibroma,
  bronchus, of, 594
  salivary glands, of, 55
  trachea, of, 594
Neuroma, acoustic, 539
Neurone,
  lower motor, diseases of, 576
  upper motor, diseases of, 574–576
Neurotomy, glossopharyngeal, 94
Nitrogen mustard, 495, 496
Nodules,
  apple-jelly, 81
  singers', 551
  vocal cord, of, 363–364
    children, in, 367
Noma vulvae, 73
Nystagmus of palate, 100

Odontome, 31
Oedema, angioneurotic, larynx, of, 320
Oesophagectomy,
  carcinoma of oesophagus, in, 244
  non-malignant stricture, in, 238
Oesophagitis, 228, 229
Oesophagogastrectomy in oesophageal varices, 239

Oesophagoscopy, 211–215
  achalasia of cardia, in, 233
  anaesthesia for, 214
  carcinoma of oesophagus, in, 241
  contra-indications to, 213
  foreign body, for, 226–228
  hazards of, 215
  stricture of oesophagus, in, 237, 238
  technique of, 214, 215
Oesophagostomy, cervical, 218, 223
Oesophagotomy, 216
  foreign body, for, 228
Oesophagus,
  abnormalities, congenital, 216–220
  atresia of, 217–219
  carcinoma of, 239–244
    achalasia in, 233
  diseases of, 207–245
    symptoms and signs, 207–211
  diverticula of, 234–236
  foreign bodies in, 223–228
  injuries of, 220–223
    corrosive, 222, 223, 236–238
  neoplasms of, 239–244
  perforation of, accidental, 221, 222
  radiography of, 210, 211
  rupture of, spontaneous, 220
  stenosis of, congenital, 220
  stricture of, 207
    non-malignant, 236–238
  surgical exposure of, 215–216
  varices of, 235, 238–239
Oncocytoma of parotid gland, 54
Oropharynx,
  examination of, 9
  neoplasms of,
    benign, 163
    malignant, 163–172
  tumours of, 162–172
Osler–Rendu disease, 384
Osteoma,
  bronchus, of, 594
  jaws, of, 33
  oropharynx, of, 163
  pharynx, of, 148
  trachea, of, 594
Osteosarcoma of pharynx, 148
Otitis media, acute
  adenoiditis, in, 135
  tonsillitis, in, 110

Pachydermia laryngis, 359–366
  interarytenoid, 362–363
  posterior hypertrophic, 361
  red, 359–363
  white, 363–366
Pachydermia verrucosa, 360
Palate (*see also* "Mouth")
  adenoma of, 31
  cleft, 9

Palate (*see also* "Mouth") (*continued*)
 deformity of, adenoids, and, 135
 examination of, 9
 nystagmus of, 100
 paralysis of, 9, 94–100
 salivary tumours of, 59–62
Palsy,
 progressive bulbar, 539
 pseudobulbar, 539
Papilloma,
 bronchus, of, 594
 laryngopharynx, of, 173
 larynx, of, 379–382
 trachea, of, 594
 mouth, of, 31
 oesophagus, of, 239
 oropharynx, of, 163
Paralysis,
 diphtheritic,
  palate, of, 96
  pharynx, of, 96
 facial,
  parotidectomy, after, 48, 58
  sarcoidosis, in, 48
Parotidectomy, 48, 57–58, 64–65
Parotitis, 46–49
Paterson–Brown Kelly syndrome, 4, 7, 88, 176, 208, 209, 236
Pemphigoid of mouth, 27
Pemphigus, 5
 mouth, of, 26
Perfusion, extracorporeal, 495, 500
Perichondritis, acute, larynx, of, 322–323
Pierre–Robin syndrome, 284
Pharyngitis,
 acute, 67–73
  coryza, in, 67
  lymphadenitis in, 69
  measles, in, 73–74
 acute diphtheritic, 70–72, 107
 acute lymphonodular, 84
 agranulocytosis, in, 88–89, 107, 143
 aphthous, 142
 Behçet's disease, in, 92
 chronic, 73–82
  aetiology of, 73–75
  signs of, 76
  symptoms of, 75–76
  treatment of, 77
 chronic atrophic, 77–78
 chronic catarrhal, 76
 chronic hypertrophic, 76
 glandular fever, in, 91
 leukaemia, in, 90–91, 107
 virus infections, and, 83–85
Pharyngitis sicca, 78
Pharyngoconjunctival fever, 84
Pharyngolaryngectomy, 183–194
 plastic reconstruction after, 487
Pharyngotomy,
 lateral trans-thyroid, 170, 173

 median, 170
 median translingual, 170
 supraglottic carcinoma, in, 424, 425
Pharynx,
 adenocarcinoma of, 148
 anaemia in, 87, 88
 anaesthesia of, 94
 carcinoma of, 148
 chondrosarcoma of, 148
 chordoma of, 149
 fibrosarcoma of, 148
 foreign body in, 225
 functional disorders of, 93
 hamartoma of, 149, 151
 herpes of, 93
 keratosis pharyngis, 82
 lupus vulgaris of, 81
 lymphoma, 149
 lymphosarcoma, 149
 myasthenia gravis, in, 97
 neoplasms of, benign, 147
 nervous diseases of, 93–100
 neuralgia of, 94
 osteosarcoma of, 148
 paralysis of, 94–100
 plasmacytoma of, 149
 pleomorphic tumours of, 147
 poliomyelitis, in, 97–100
 reticulum cell sarcoma, of, 149
 rhabdomyosarcoma of, 148
 spasm of, 100
 stenosis of, 82
 syphilis of, 78–80
 tuberculosis of, 80–82
 tumours of, classification of, 150
Phonasthenia, 552–554
Phosphorus-32, half-life of, 491
Plasmacytoma,
 larynx, of, 395
 mouth, of, 34
 oropharynx, of, 163
 pharynx, of, 149
Plummer Vinson syndrome, 4, 88
Pneumonectomy in carcinoma of bronchus, 597
Pneumothorax after tracheostomy, 517, 521
Poliomyelitis, 83, 97–100, 509
 tonsillectomy, and, 122
Polyneuritis, 509
Polyp, vascular, larynx, of, 384
Polypus, mucous, larynx of, 356–357
Pouch, pharyngeal, 197–206
 diathermy of, 203, 204
 excision of, 201–203
Pregnancy tumour, 33
Process, elongated, styloid, 144
Prolapse of ventricle of larynx, 354

Quinsy, 109, 113–116
 incision of, 115

Quinsy (*continued*)
  lingual, 110
  tonsillectomy in, 115

Radiation, ionizing, 489–492
  biological effect of, 491–492
  production of, 489
  sources of, 490–491
  wavelengths of, 490
Radiography of oesophagus, 210–211
Radiotherapy,
  carcinoma of larynx, in, 416, 417, 419, 420–423
    complications of, 422
  malignant disease, in,
    methods of, 492–494
    principles of, 489–502
Radium bomb, 493
Radium, half-life of, 491
Radon, half-life of, 491
Ramsay Hunt syndrome, 9
Ranula, 31
Reiter's syndrome, 26
Rhabdomyoma of pharynx, 148
Rhabdomyosarcoma,
  oesophagus, of, 239
  pharynx, of, 148
Rheumatic fever, 110, 117
Rhinolalia aperta, 95
  adenoidectomy, after, 140
Rhinolalia clausa in adenoiditis, 135
Rhinoscopy, posterior, 11
Rhinovirus, 84
Rotation skin flap, 477

Saliva, secretion of, 42–43
Sarcoidosis of salivary glands, 48–49
Sarcoma,
  jaw, of, 36
  mouth, of, 36
  pharynx, of, 149
  reticulum cell, oropharynx, of, 164
  tongue, of, 36
Scarlet fever, 72, 107
Schick test, 328
Schmidt's syndrome, 538
Schmiegelow's operation, 309
Scleroma of larynx, 344–345
Scurvy, 6
Semon's law, 531
Sengstaken's tube, 239
Sialectasis, 47
Sialography, 46–47
Sickle-cell disease, tonsillectomy in, 121
Sinusitis,
  adenoiditis, in, 135

  bronchiectasis in, 590
  bronchitis, in, 591
Sjögren's syndrome, 49
Skin graft,
  Abbé flap, 477–479
  abdominal flap, 480–481
  Dieffenbach flap, 479
  Estlander flap, 477, 479
  fan-flap of Gillies, 479–481
  free eyebrow, 475
  Imre flap, 486
  rotation flap, 477
  thin split, 473–474
  three-quarter thickness, 474
  transposition flap, 476–477
  Tripier flap, 486
  tubed pedicle, 481–483
  types of, 473–483
  whole thickness, 474–475
  Wolfe, 474–475
  Z-plasty, 476
Skin grafting, principles of, 483–487
Somatognosis, 572
Souttar's tube, 241, 242
Spasm,
  glottic, 528
  laryngeal, 527–529
Speech,
  anatomy and physiology of, 560–561
  cerebral dominance and, 560–561
  development of, 561–563
  disorders of, 559–581
    central, 570–571
    expressive, 571–574
    receptive, 563–570
      auditory, 563–566
      visual, 566–570
Speech centres, 561–563
Speech deafness, 565–566
Speech learning, 561–563
Spots, Koplik's, 73
Staging of cancer of larynx, 390–393
Starck's dilator, 234
Status epilepticus, 509
Stenosis,
  congenital,
    oesophagus, of, 220
    subglottic, 293–294
    trachea, of, 593
  larynx, of, 306–309·
  pharynx, of, 82
  subglottic,
    intubation, after, 517, 520
    tracheostomy, after, 521
  tracheal, 517, 519
Stomatitis, 21–28
  acute ulcerative, 23
  allergic, 25
  angular, 4
  aphthous, 25
  avitaminosis and, 21–22

Stomatitis (*continued*)
Behçet's syndrome, in, 26
blood diseases and, 22
catarrhal, 24
coccal, 23
Coxsackie virus infections, in, 25
drugs and, 25
fungal, 23
gangrenous, 26
herpes simplex, in, 24
herpetic, recurrent, 24
injury and, 21
metals and, 25
recurrent ulcerative, 25
Reiter's syndrome, in, 26
syphilis, in, 23
tuberculosis, 23
Vincent's infection, in, 23
virus diseases, in, 24
Stricture, oesophagus, of, 207, 236–238
congenital, 220
Stridor,
congenital laryngeal, 291–292
infants, in, 282
Stroboscopy of larynx, 266
Stuttering, 578–581
cerebral dominance in, 579
treatment of, 580–581
Sweating, gustatory, parotidectomy, after, 58
Synchrotron, 490
Syndrome,
Avellis', 538
Behçet's, 26
Collet–Sicard, 539
Costen's 6, 28
Gougerot's 49
Heerfordt's, 49
Hughlings Jackson's, 539
Kartagener's, 590
Mikulicz', 49
Paterson–Brown Kelly, 4, 7, 88, 176, 208, 209, 236
Pierre–Robin, 284
Plummer Vinson, 4, 88
Ramsay Hunt's, 9, 93
Reiter's, 26
Schmidt's, 538
Sjögren's, 49
Tapia's, 538
Vernet's, 538
Syphilis,
larynx, of, 341–343
mouth, of, 23
oesophagus, of, 228
pharynx, of, 78–80
salivary glands, of, 49

Tapia's syndrome, 538
Taste, 8

Teeth,
examination of, 5
Hutchinson's, 79
Telangiectasia, congenital, larynx, of, 384
Temporomandibular joint, disorders of, 28
Tetanus, 509
Thrush, 5, 23
Thyroid gland in block dissection, 467
Thyroid, lingual, 19
T.N.M. staging of laryngeal cancer, 392–393
Tongue,
anaemia, in, 88
bifid, 18
black hairy, 7, 20
carcinoma of, 7, 35
examination of, 7
furrowed, 19
geographical, 19, 20
lymphangioma of, 18, 19
malformations of, 18
"raspberry", 7
salivary tumours of, 62
sarcoma of, 36
"strawberry and cream", 7
syphilis of, 23
Tongue-tie, 8, 18
Tonsil (palatine, faucial),
cyst of, 117
enlargement of, 104–105
examination of, 10
foreign body of, 144
functions of, 103–104
lingual, 103
nasopharyngeal (*see* "Adenoids")
Tonsillectomy, 118–133
abscess, 115
anaesthesia for, 123
local, 124
risks of, 121–122
case selection for, 119–123
complications of, 132–133
dissection method of, 124
guillotine method of, 124
haemorrhage in,
reactionary, 131–132
risks of, 120–121
secondary, 132
indications for, 113
infection in, risks of, 122
instruments for, 125
menstruation, in, 122
morbidity of, 119
mortality of, 119
poliomyelitis in, risks of, 122
post-operative care in, 130–132
pregnancy, in, 122
premedication for, 123
preparation for, 123
technique of, 124–130
voice changes after, 122

Tonsillitis,
  acute, 105–110
    aetiology, 105
    complications of, 109
    diagnosis of, 107
    symptoms and signs of, 106
    treatment of, 108
  acute lingual, 110
  agranulocytosis, in, 143
  chronic, 109, 111
    aetiology of, 111
    complications of, 113
    diagnosis of, 112
    symptoms and signs of, 111
    treatment of, 113
  chronic lingual, 133
  glandular fever, in, 141
  leukaemia, in, 143
  Vincent's angina, in, 141
Tonsillolith, 117
Torus mandibularis, 33
Torus palatinus, 33
Trachea,
  congenital stenosis of, 593
  excision and reconstruction of, 596
  stenosis of, tracheostomy, after, 517, 519
  tumours of,
    benign, 594
    malignant, 594–596
  ulceration of, tracheostomy after, 517, 518
Tracheitis after tracheostomy, 517, 518
Tracheobronchial tree, diseases of, 583–597
Tracheoscopy, 278, 279
Tracheostomy, 505–522
  abscess of larynx, in, 325
  bilateral recurrent laryngeal nerve paralysis, in, 532, 535
  carcinoma of trachea, in, 595
  complications of, 290, 516–519, 520–522
  decannulation after, 516, 522
  diphtheria, in, 331
  indications for, 505, 510
  infants, in, 287–290
  laryngeal injuries, in, 303
  laryngotracheobronchitis, in, 319, 320
  oedema of larynx, in, 322
  papillomatosis of larynx, in, 382
  poliomyelitis, in, 99
  post-operative management of, 513–516
  stenosis of larynx, in, 308
  technique of, 510–513
Transposition skin flap, 476–477
Tripier's skin flap, 486
Trismus, 11
Tuberculosis,
  larynx of, 333–340
    diagnosis of, 336
    pathology of, 334–335
    prognosis of, 339
    symptoms of, 336
    treatment of, 337–339

miliary, pharynx, of, 80
  mouth, of, 23
  oesophagus, of, 228
  pharynx, of, 80–82
  salivary glands, of, 48
Tumours (see also under anatomical region affected)
  acinic cell, salivary glands, of, 53
  connective tissue, salivary glands, of, 55
  muco-epidermoid, salivary glands, of, 53
  secondary, salivary glands, of, 54

Ulcer,
  aphthous, pharynx, of, 142
  snail track, 79

Ventricle,
  larynx, of,
    carcinoma of, 400
    cystic protrusion from, 355
    prolapse of, 354
Ventricular bands, carcinoma of, 400
Vernet's syndrome, 538
Vertigo, laryngeal, 349, 528–529
Vincent's angina, 141
Vincent's stomatitis, 23
Vinson's bougie, 237
Virus infections of pharynx, 83–85
Vocal cord, congenital paralysis of, 294–296
Voice,
  disabilities of, 550–557
    treatment of, 555–557
  falsetto, 545
  loudness of, 547
  mechanisms of, 544–545
  pitch of, 545–547
  range of, 548
  singing, 545–550
  timbre of, 547
  registers, 549
Voice-users, professional, 543–544
von Willebrand's disease, tonsillectomy in, 121

Web of larynx, 292–293
Wegener's granuloma of larynx, 368
Wolfe's skin graft, 474–475
Woodman's operation, 535
Word blindness, 567–570
Word deafness, 565–566
Word dumbness, 572

Xerostomia, 50

Yttrium-90, half-life of, 491

Z-plasty, 476